Practical Anatomic Pathology

Series Editors

Fan Lin
Geisinger Health System
Danville, PA, USA

Ximing J. Yang
Feinberg School of Medicine
Northwestern University
Chicago, IL, USA

This Book Series is designed to provide a comprehensive, practical and state-of-the-art review and update of the major issues and challenges specific to each subspecialty field of surgical pathology in a question and answer (Q&A) format. Making an accurate diagnosis especially from a limited sample can be quite challenging, yet crucial to patient care. This Book Series, using the most current and evidence-based resources 1) focuses on frequently asked questions in surgical pathology in day-to-day practice; 2) provides quick, accurate, terse, and useful answers to many practical questions encountered in daily practice; 3) emphasizes the importance of a triple test (clinical, radiologic, and histologic correlation); 4) delineates how to appropriately utilize immunohistochemistry, in situ hybridization and molecular tests; and 5) minimizes any potential diagnostic pitfalls in surgical pathology. These books also include highly practical presentations of typical case scenarios seen in an anatomic pathology laboratory. These are in the form of case presentations with step-by-step expert analysis. Sample cases include common but challenging situations, such as evaluation of well-differentiated malignant tumors vs. benign/reactive lesions; distinction of two benign entities; sub-classification of a malignant tumor; identification of newly described tumor and non-tumor entities; workup of a tumor of unknown origin; and implementation of best practice in immunohistochemistry and molecular testing in a difficult case. The Q&A format is well accepted, especially by junior pathologists, for several reasons: 1) this is the most practical and effective way to deliver information to a new generation of pathologists accustomed to using the Internet as a resource and, therefore, comfortable and familiar with a Q&A learning environment; 2) it's impossible to memorialize and digest massive amounts of new information about new entities, new and revised classifications, molecular pathology, diagnostic IHC, and the therapeutic implications of each entity by reading large textbooks; 3) sub-specialization is a very popular practice model highly demanded by many clinicians; and 4) time is very precious for a practicing pathologist because of increasing workloads in recent years following U.S. health care reforms. This Book Series meets all of the above expectations. These books are written by established and recognized experts in their specialty fields and provide a unique and valuable resource in the field of surgical pathology, both for those currently in training and for those already in clinical practice at various skill levels. It does not seek to duplicate or completely replace other large standard textbooks; rather, it is a new, comprehensive yet concise and practical resource on these timely and critical topics.

More information about this series at http://www.springer.com/series/13808

Ximing J. Yang • Ming Zhou
Editors

Practical Genitourinary Pathology

Frequently Asked Questions

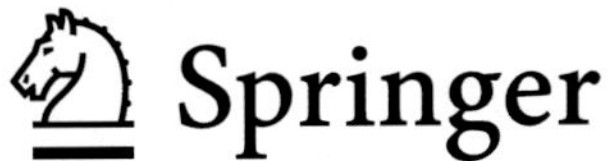

Springer

Editors
Ximing J. Yang
Department of Pathology
Northwestern Memorial Hospital, Northwestern
University Feinberg School of Medicine
Chicago, IL
USA

Ming Zhou
Department of Pathology and Laboratory
Medicine
Tufts Medical Center, Tufts School of Medicine
Boston, MA
USA

Practical Anatomic Pathology
ISBN 978-3-030-57143-6   ISBN 978-3-030-57141-2   (eBook)
https://doi.org/10.1007/978-3-030-57141-2

This Springer imprint is published by the registered company Springer Nature Switzerland AG
The registered company address is: Gewerbestrasse 11, 6330 Cham, Switzerland

Preface

Today's pathologists are inundated with a huge amount of information generated from constantly evolving disease classification, grading and staging criteria, and novel and emerging diagnostic methods and tools. They need easy access to an organized collection of information that will facilitate their daily work and sign out. Using the format of "Questions and Answers," this book aims to address frequently encountered diagnostic challenges in the genitourinary system, including the prostate, kidney, bladder, testis, urethra, ureter, penis, and adrenal gland. The emphasis is placed on formulating differential diagnosis and rendering correct diagnosis based on integrating morphology, clinical findings, and immunohistochemical and molecular ancillary tests. The book will also review current topics, controversies, and diagnostic dilemmas in diagnostic genitourinary pathology. The answers to the questions are supplemented by ample illustrations, tables, and updated references. It can serve as a quick reference for busy practicing pathologists, pathologists in training, urologists, medical students, and other physicians with questions regarding genitourinary conditions.

We are enormously grateful to the contributors of this book. They spent countless hours out of their very busy schedules to make this book possible. Special thanks is given to Barbara Lopez-Lucio (Developmental Editor) and Sarah Simeziane (Assistant Developmental Editor) for their patience and persistence in keeping this book on track.

Chicago, IL, USA

Boston, MA, USA

Ximing J. Yang

Ming Zhou

Contents

Editors

Ximing J. Yang, MD, PhD Department of Pathology, Northwestern Memorial Hospital, Northwestern University Feinberg School of Medicine, Chicago, IL, USA

Ming Zhou, MD, PhD Department of Pathology and Laboratory Medicine, Tufts Medical Center, Tufts School of Medicine, Boston, MA, USA

Contributors

Fang-Ming Deng, MD, PhD Department of Pathology, New York University Langone Health, New York, NY, USA

Charles C. Guo, MD Department of Pathology, The University of Texas MD Anderson Cancer Center, Houston, TX, USA

Liwei Jia, MD, PhD Department of Pathology, University of Texas Southwestern Medical Center, Dallas, TX, USA

Xunda Luo, MD, PhD Pathology and Laboratory Medicine, Pennsylvania Presbyterian Hospital, Philadelphia, PA, USA

Gregory T. MacLennan, MD Department of Pathology, University Hospitals Cleveland Medical Center, Cleveland, OH, USA

Qinghu Ren, MD, PhD Department of Pathology, New York University Langone Health, New York, NY, USA

Jenny Ross, MD Department of Pathology, Northwestern Memorial Hospital, Northwestern University Feinberg School of Medicine, Chicago, IL, USA

Steven Shen, MD, PhD Department of Pathology and Genomic Medicine, Houston Methodist Hospital, Houston, TX, USA

Ngoentra Tantranont, MD Department of Pathology, Siriraj Hospital, Faculty of Medicine, Mahidol University, Bangkok, Thailand

Maria Tretiakova, MD, PhD Department of Pathology, University of Washington, Seattle, WA, USA

Sean R. Williamson, MD Department of Pathology, Cleveland Clinic, Cleveland, OH, USA

Debra L. Zynger, MS, MD Department of Pathology, The Ohio State University Medical Center, Columbus, OH, USA

Maria Tretiakova and Sean R. Williamson

Evaluating a Renal Epithelial Tumor in a Biopsy Specimen

In many institutions, renal mass biopsy is used conservatively, since most renal neoplasms will be treated with partial or radical nephrectomy. However, renal mass biopsy is often undertaken when the results may influence clinical management. Some goals of renal mass biopsy include distinguishing primary renal cell neoplasms from other tumors that would necessitate different treatment, particularly metastases, lymphoma, urothelial carcinoma, or rare variants (medullary, collecting duct, or sarcomatoid carcinomas). Secondly, subclassification and grading of primary renal epithelial neoplasms may lead to differences in management. For example, elderly patients with multiple comorbidities may be candidates for surveillance or ablation of nonaggressive tumor subtypes.

- Benign tumor types that can be recognized by biopsy include oncocytoma and angiomyolipoma, among other rarer entities (metanephric adenoma, mixed epithelial and stromal tumor).
- Lower-risk primary renal epithelial tumors include oncocytic neoplasms (possible or definite oncocytomas) and chromophobe renal cell carcinoma (RCC; particularly eosinophilic variant).
- Of note, some pathologists are unwilling to diagnose oncocytoma in a biopsy sample, instead giving a diagnosis of "oncocytic neoplasm" or "oncocytic tumor" with a comment that the features would be compatible with oncocytoma if representative of the entire tumor (since distinguishing eosinophilic chromophobe from oncocytoma remains challenging).

Table 1.1 shows clues to well-differentiated "clear cell tumors" in renal mass biopsy, and Table 1.2 shows high-grade carcinomas in renal mass biopsy (see also Fig. 1.1).
References: [1–9].

Effectively Sampling a Renal Mass in a Resection Specimen

Sampling a renal mass and determining the pathologic stage are among the most critical steps to determine patient prognosis. RCCs often invade structures (renal sinus or veins) with subtle, finger-like outpouchings that are relatively easy to miss if the individual performing gross examination is not familiar with the usual growth patterns of tumors, especially clear cell RCC.

- The renal sinus is the central fat compartment that surrounds the hilar structures (renal pelvis, arteries, and veins).
- With increasing tumor size, the likelihood of clear cell RCC invading the renal sinus increases dramatically, to the point that >90% of tumors over 7 cm invade the renal sinus (Fig. 1.2a), making pT2 clear cell RCC rare.
- For tumors larger than 4–5 cm, the likelihood of renal sinus invasion increases to over 50%. Histologic assessment of the entire tumor-sinus interface should be strongly considered.
- Any deviation from a well-circumscribed, spherical tumor shape should be viewed with great suspicion for extension into a vein branch or tributary (Fig. 1.2b).
- Changes to the 2016 American Joint Commission on Cancer (AJCC) staging system include removal of the requirements that vein invasion be recognized grossly and that the vein wall contain muscle microscopically.

M. Tretiakova (✉)
Department of Pathology, University of Washington, Seattle, WA, USA
e-mail: mariast@uw.edu

S. R. Williamson
Department of Pathology, Cleveland Clinic, Cleveland, OH, USA

© Springer Nature Switzerland AG 2021
X. J. Yang, M. Zhou (eds.), *Practical Genitourinary Pathology*, Practical Anatomic Pathology,
https://doi.org/10.1007/978-3-030-57141-2_1

Table 1.1 Clues to well-differentiated "clear cell tumors" in renal mass biopsy

	Frequency in adult renal tumors	Clues	Helpful immunohistochemistry
Clear cell RCC	>50–60%	Solid, nested, alveolar growth patterns; often purely clear cytoplasm (less often vacuolated; Fig. 1.1a–d)	PAX8 positive, carbonic anhydrase IX diffuse membrane positive, cytokeratin 7 and high molecular weight cytokeratin usually focal/limited, alpha-methylacyl-CoA racemase (AMACR) variable
Papillary RCC with clear cell change	15% (overall incidence, of which up to 39% may have clear cell change)	Vacuolated cytoplasm, foamy macrophages, hemosiderin	AMACR diffuse/strong, cytokeratin 7 positive in type 1 tumors, carbonic anhydrase IX negative or minimal (except with necrosis/ischemia)
Clear cell papillary RCC	3–4%	Branched glandular configuration, nuclear alignment	PAX8 positive, carbonic anhydrase IX "cup-shaped" pattern, cytokeratin 7 diffuse, high molecular weight cytokeratin frequently positive, GATA3 frequently positive, CD10 negative, AMACR negative/minimal
Adrenal rest/adrenal-renal fusion	Rare	Vacuolated cytoplasm	PAX8 negative, inhibin positive, Melan-A positive
Hemangioblastoma	Rare	Solid, foamy cytoplasm, lack of glandular structures	Inhibin positive, neuron-specific enolase (NSE) positive, S100 positive, keratin negative (note: PAX8 may be unexpectedly positive in primary renal hemangioblastoma)
Hemangioma	Rare, increased incidence in end-stage renal disease	No epithelial component, often requiring immunohistochemical verification; anastomosing subtype often contains hematopoiesis and hyaline globules	CD31/CD34/ERG positive; keratin, carbonic anhydrase IX, PAX8 negative

Table 1.2 High-grade carcinomas in renal mass biopsy

	Helpful immunohistochemistry	Notes
High-grade clear cell RCC (Fig. 1.1e)	PAX8 positive, carbonic anhydrase IX positive (usually maintained in high-grade tumors), cytokeratin 7 usually minimal/negative	PAX8 and GATA3 are not always perfect for distinguishing RCC from urothelial carcinoma in the upper urinary tract
Urothelial carcinoma	GATA3 positive, p63 positive, high molecular weight cytokeratin positive	PAX8 and GATA3 are not always perfect for distinguishing RCC from urothelial carcinoma in the upper urinary tract
Metastatic carcinoma of another origin	Organ-specific markers (TTF1, etc.)	Lung cancer is among the more common metastases to the kidney and may mimic a primary tumor
Medullary carcinoma	OCT3/4 often positive, INI-1 loss	Sickle cell trait essentially a requirement (without sickle trait = "RCC unclassified with medullary phenotype")
Fumarate hydratase (FH)-deficient RCC	Abnormal negative FH immunohistochemistry, positive 2-succino-cysteine	If germline, hereditary leiomyomatosis and RCC (HLRCC) syndrome; or FH-deficient if unknown germline status
Collecting duct carcinoma	PAX8 positive	Diagnosis of exclusion if medullary and FH-deficient carcinoma excluded

- Invasion of the renal pelvis has been added as a route to pT3a for RCC in the AJCC system.
- Invasion of the perinephric fat is less common than renal sinus or vein branch invasion in RCC, but qualifies for pT3a.
- In modern practice, surgeons usually attempt to spare the adrenal gland; however, pathologic assessment of adrenal involvement, when present, should aim to discern direct invasion (pT4) from metastatic involvement (pM1).
- Gerota fascia involvement (pT4) is quite rare but usually occurs in the context of RCC extending to the soft tissue surface of a radical nephrectomy, in conjunction with clinical/intraoperative impression of Gerota fascia involvement.
- RCC tumors can extend into the main renal vein and rarely follow the inferior vena cava (pT3b–pT3c) to the level of the heart.
- RCC tumor may be protruding from the vein margin; however, consensus among urologic pathologists is

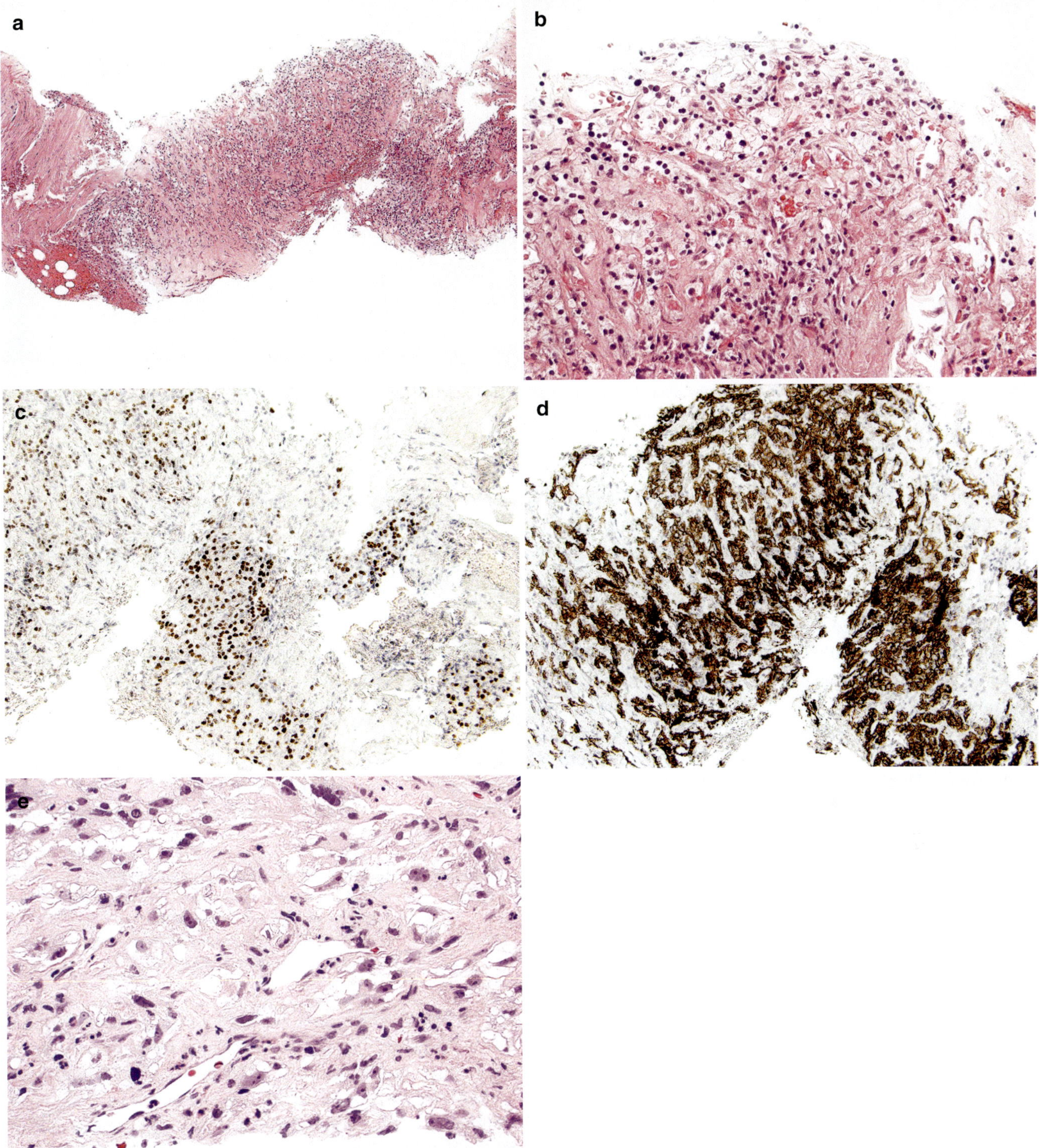

Fig. 1.1 (**a**) Clear cell renal cell carcinoma in renal mass biopsy is composed of fibrosis and bland epithelial cells. (**b**) Higher magnification demonstrates cells with clear cytoplasm. (**c**) Positive PAX8 immunohistochemistry supports a primary renal cell neoplasm and argues against an adrenal rest or non-renal lesion. (**d**) Diffuse membrane staining for carbonic anhydrase IX supports clear cell subtype. (**e**) A different case of high-grade clear cell renal cell carcinoma in renal mass biopsy shows clusters of cells with clear cytoplasm in fibrous stroma with marked nuclear atypia

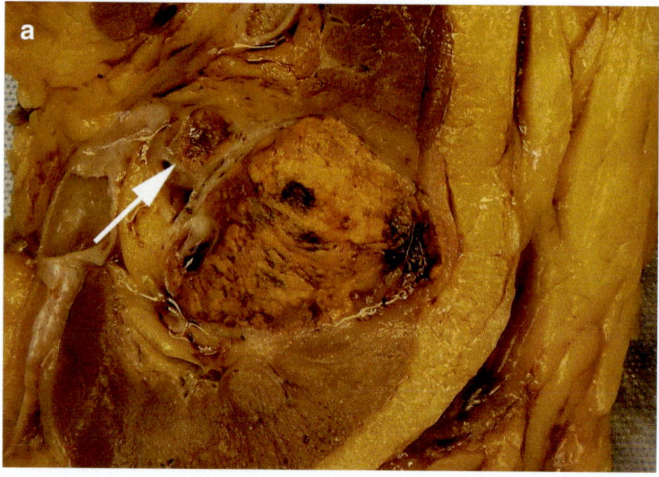

Fig. 1.2 (**a**) This clear cell renal cell carcinoma abuts the renal sinus (the fatty compartment containing the renal pelvis and vasculature) with an outpouching (arrow), concerning for renal sinus invasion. (**b**) This clear cell renal cell carcinoma has multiple outpouchings (arrows) that likely represent extension of the tumor into renal vein branches, which would qualify for pT3a

that this only constitutes a positive margin if the tumor is confirmed histologically to be adherent to or invading the vein wall at the margin (as the surgeon would not have necessarily transected tumor when freely mobile).

- Separately submitted vena cava "thrombus" should be examined histologically (at least 2–3 sections) to evaluate for adherent/invaded vein wall, which defines pT3c.
- In some cases (5–8%), RCC extending into the main renal vein subsequently spreads backwards into tributary veins, creating multiple nodules in the kidney (retrograde venous invasion). This can be misinterpreted as multiple tumors or a multinodular tumor by those unfamiliar with the phenomenon.

Table 1.3 shows recommended sampling of renal epithelial tumor specimens.

References: [10–16].

Table 1.3 Recommended sampling of renal epithelial tumor specimens

Normal kidney	1–2 sections away from the tumor, if possible
Hilar margins	1 or more cassettes containing: Artery, vein*, and ureter margins (there may be more than one artery or vein) *Vein with tumor can be sampled by trimming the vein wall circumferentially (if freely mobile from the tumor) or cutting a complete cross section of vein containing tumor (to assess for microscopic adherence)
Tumor to renal sinus	2–3 sections routinely; consider entire interface if tumor is larger than 4–5 cm
Tumor to perinephric fat	1–2 sections routinely; more if gross impression of invasion
Secondary tumors	International Society of Urological Pathology (ISUP) guidelines recommend measuring and sampling at least the 5 largest tumors
Other	Any finger-like outpouching of the tumor, to assess for possible vein branch invasion

What Are the Typical Gross Features of Renal Tumors?

Gross examination is an important part of the pathology of renal tumors for two major reasons: (1) Staging of RCC, as discussed in question 1.2, and (2) differential diagnosis of renal neoplasms. In general, RCC tumors and other renal neoplasms are predominantly spherical, and deviation from this round shape should be viewed with caution for invasion of structures, as discussed previously. Tumors can bulge well beyond the contour of the normal kidney, markedly distorting its shape, which does not necessarily indicate invasion. Gross "necrosis" should be confirmed histologically to be coagulative tumor necrosis, as large zones of hemorrhage and fibrosis are relatively common and do not have the same prognostic implications as true necrosis. The significance of necrosis in papillary RCC is less clear, perhaps due to an increased tendency of the fragile papillary structures to undergo necrosis.

Table 1.4 shows gross features of renal neoplasms (see also Fig. 1.3).

References: [10, 14, 17–24].

Table 1.4 Gross features of renal neoplasms

	Classic gross appearance	Variations	Notes
Clear cell RCC	Golden-yellow to orange, heterogeneous (Fig. 1.3a)	White or tan (fibrotic areas or sarcomatoid dedifferentiation), red-brown (hemorrhage), cystic	Sampling of any golden-yellow areas may be helpful to verify a low-grade clear cell component for poorly differentiated tumors
Papillary RCC	Variable, tan, yellow, or red-brown	Yellow (with abundant foamy cells), red-brown (with abundant hemosiderin)	A granular cut surface can sometimes be appreciated as a clue to the papillary architecture; necrosis is common
Chromophobe RCC	Pale tan	Red-brown resembling oncocytoma for eosinophilic variant	Can have central scar resembling oncocytoma
Clear cell papillary RCC	Tan-white, fibrous, solid and cystic		Usually does not have golden-yellow/orange cut surface of clear cell RCC, despite histologic similarity
Oncocytoma	Red-brown ("mahogany"; Fig. 1.3b)	Rarely microcystic with hemorrhage ("telangiectatic" oncocytoma)	Often unencapsulated or poorly encapsulated; can involve veins or fat, which has not been reported to alter its benign behavior
Angiomyolipoma	Tan-white/fibrous (if myoid predominant), resembling a smooth muscle neoplasm	Resembles normal fat or lipomatous tumor (if fat predominant)	Surgical specimens tend to be myoid predominant, since those containing fat can be recognized by imaging and removed only if there is concern for large size or rupture
Tubulocystic RCC	"Bubble wrap" appearance with uniform cystic cut surface		
Multilocular cystic renal neoplasm of low malignant potential	Entirely cystic architecture with fluid-filled cysts (no grossly visible solid areas)		Formerly known as multilocular cystic RCC; tumors with a visible solid component should be classified as extensively cystic clear cell RCC

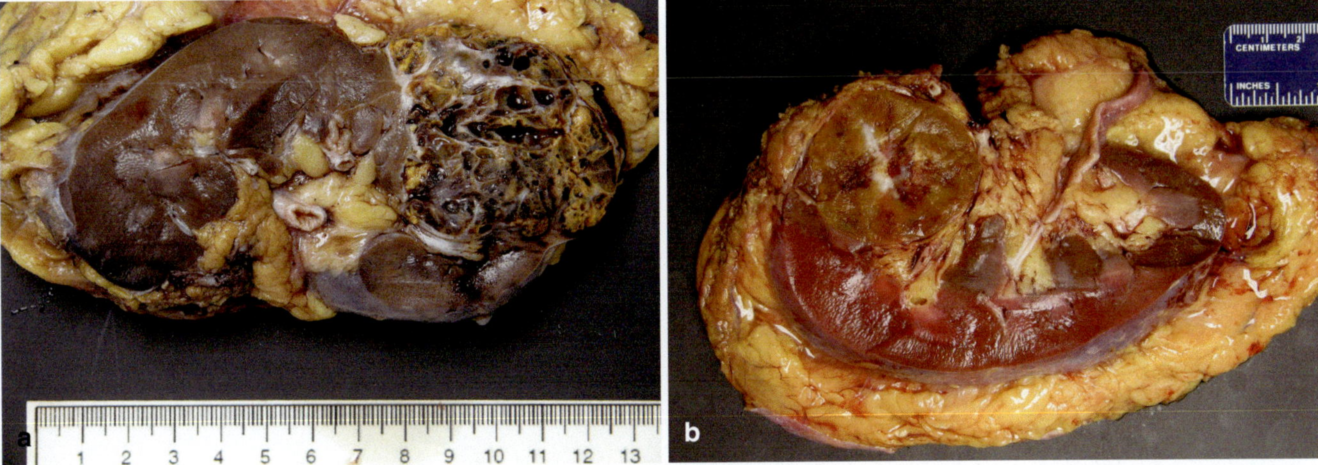

Fig. 1.3 (**a**) This clear cell renal cell carcinoma is solid and cystic with a heterogeneous red-brown to golden-yellow cut surface. (**b**) This oncocytoma is a uniform tan-brown color with a central scar, which is classic but not specific for oncocytoma

What Are the Key Histologic Features for Common Renal Epithelial Tumors?

Most renal tumors can either be diagnosed based on histologic features alone, or a narrow differential diagnosis can be readily discerned based on the tumor histology.

Table 1.5 shows key histologic features of common renal epithelial tumors (see also Fig. 1.4).

References: [17, 21].

What Are the Key Features of Cystic Renal Tumors?

Most renal tumors have the potential to be at least partly cystic; however, tumors that are most commonly cystic include clear cell RCC, multilocular cystic renal neoplasm of low malignant potential (formerly multilocular cystic RCC), clear cell papillary RCC, and tubulocystic RCC. In general, a cystic component is thought to be favorable for

Table 1.5 Key histologic features of common renal epithelial tumors

	Histology	Pitfalls	Notes
Clear cell RCC	Cells with clear cytoplasm arranged in nests, tubules, or alveolar structures	Eosinophilic cytoplasm (Fig. 1.4a) and/or marked pleomorphism are not unusual in high-grade tumors	Thorough sampling for straightforward low-grade component is helpful for high-grade or eosinophilic cases
Papillary RCC, type 1	Basophilic cuboidal cells lining papillary, tubular, or solid structures	Cytoplasmic clearing is not uncommon (at least focally; Fig. 1.4b), but is usually highly vacuolated rather than entirely clear	Foamy macrophages, psammoma bodies are helpful ancillary clues in cases with less evident papillary architecture
Papillary RCC, type 2	Eosinophilic cells with elongated, pseudostratified nuclei (Fig. 1.4c)	Eosinophilic cells alone are not sufficient for classification as type 2	In modern practice, it has become a relative diagnosis of exclusion after FH-deficient RCC/HLRCC syndrome and other RCC types are excluded
Chromophobe RCC	Cells with pale cytoplasm, prominent cell borders, variable nuclear size, wrinkled nuclear contours; some cells appear to have no nuclei (due to sectioning artifact; Fig. 1.4d)	Eosinophilic variant can closely resemble oncocytoma (Fig. 1.4e); clues include perinuclear clearing, trabecular architecture	Immunohistochemistry may be needed to distinguish difficult cases of eosinophilic variant
Oncocytoma	Granular eosinophilic cytoplasm, round/uniform nuclei, occasional nuclei with smudged degenerative chromatin, nested/solid/tubular architecture (Fig. 1.4f), central scar	Succinate dehydrogenase (SDH)-deficient RCC can have monotonous eosinophilic cell morphology that mimics oncocytoma	
Clear cell papillary RCC	Tubular, cystic, papillary architecture with branched glandular structures, small papillae into cystic spaces, alignment of nuclei at the same height within the cytoplasm (Fig. 1.4g)	Some areas closely resemble clear cell RCC (immunohistochemistry often required); papillary component is not always prominent	Immunohistochemistry often needed for confirmation

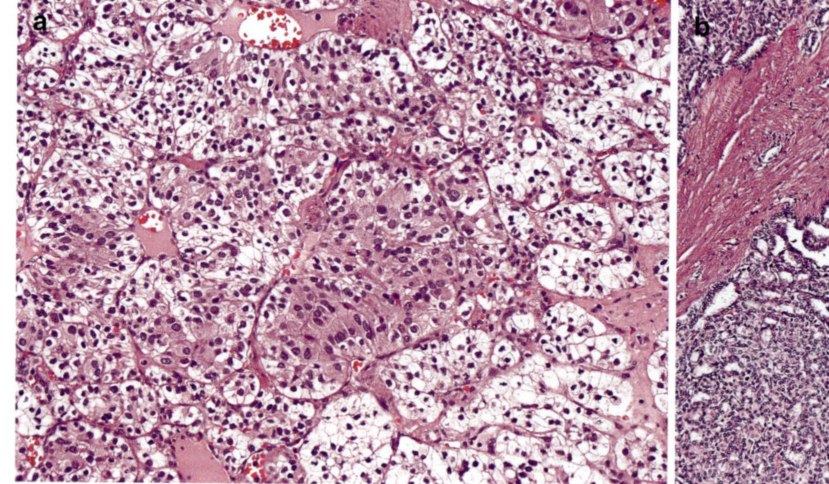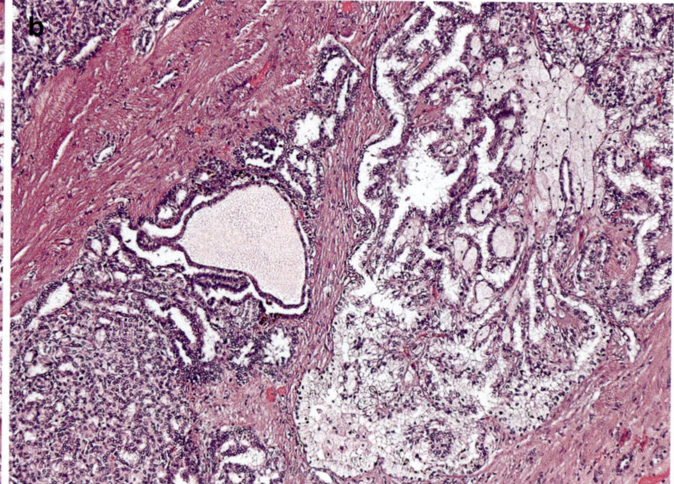

Fig. 1.4 (**a**) Clear cell renal cell carcinoma can have substantial areas with eosinophilic cells, shown in this case with abrupt transition from clear cells to eosinophilic cells. (**b**) Papillary renal cell carcinoma, type 1, is characteristically composed of papillary structures lined by basophilic cells (left) but can also have substantial clear cell changes, often caused by vacuolated cytoplasm (right). (**c**) Papillary renal cell carcinoma, type 2, exhibits elongated nuclei with pseudostratification and eosinophilic cytoplasm. (**d**) Classic chromophobe renal cell carcinoma exhibits prominent cell borders and low nuclear-cytoplasmic ratio with some cells appearing to have no nucleus (due to sectioning artifact). (**e**) Eosinophilic chromophobe renal cell carcinoma remains difficult to distinguish from oncocytoma. However, clues can include prominent trabecular architecture and perinuclear clearing. This case also contains cystic spaces with pigment. (**f**) Oncocytoma is characteristically composed of uniform eosinophilic cells with round, regular nuclei. Although large areas may appear solid, often discrete round nests are present in areas of edematous stroma. (**g**) Clear cell papillary renal cell carcinoma exhibits branched glandular structures with variable amounts of clear cytoplasm. Often, the nuclei appear to be aligned at the same height within the cytoplasm

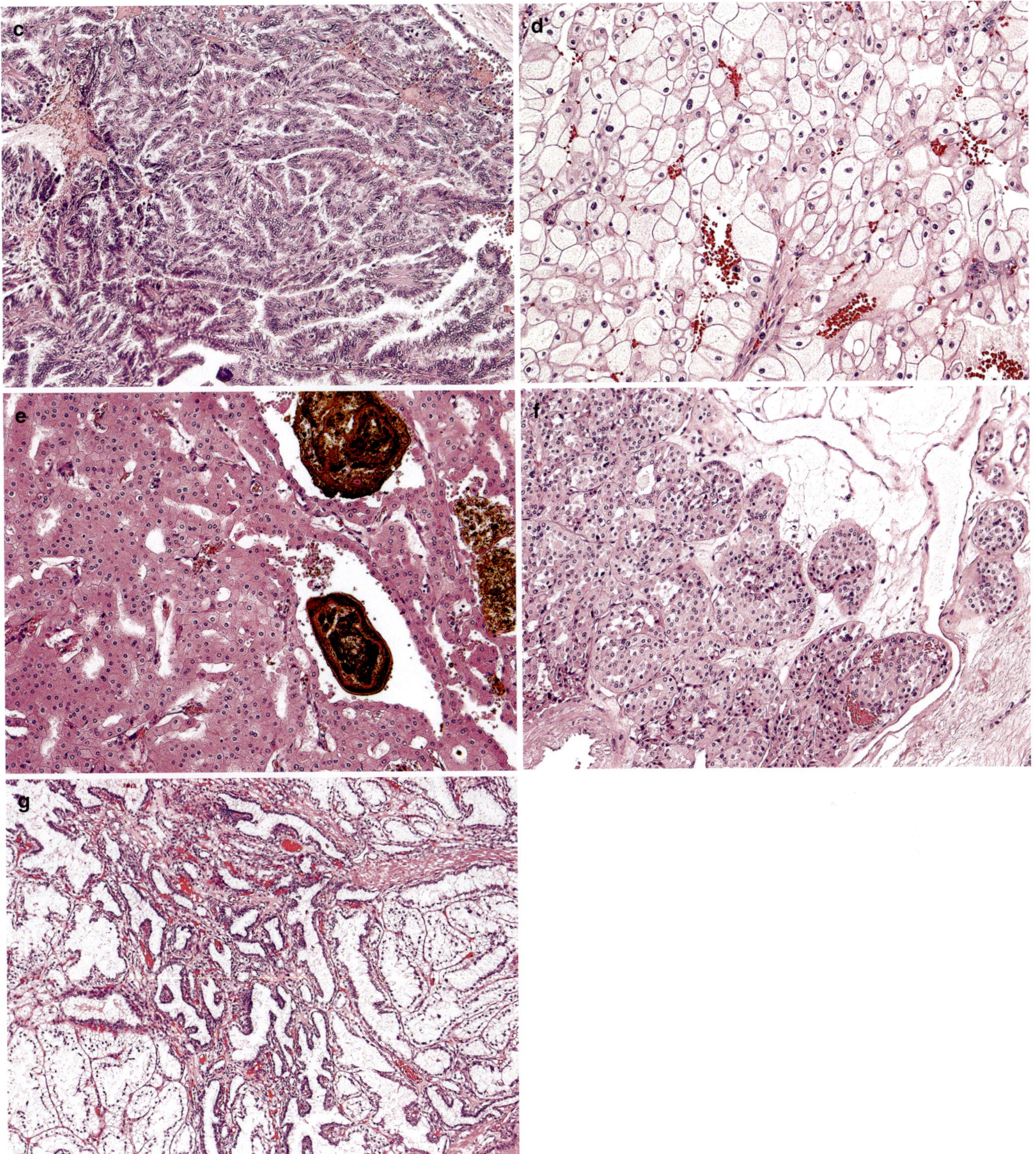

Fig. 1.4 (continued)

clear cell RCC, even if the tumor does not meet the strict definition for a multilocular cystic tumor. Most tumors have a mixture of cystic and tubular architecture throughout the neoplasm; however, rarer variations that have been described include predominant central cystic necrosis or degeneration, leaving only a rim of viable neoplasm around a central cavity, and a single solid tumor growing in the wall of a cyst.

Table 1.6 shows key features of cystic renal tumors (see also Fig. 1.5).

References: [4, 25–31].

Table 1.6 Key features of cystic renal tumors

	Histology	Components	Immunohistochemistry	Genetics
Clear cell RCC	Cells with clear cytoplasm	Solid, tubular, cystic (no true papillary structures except non-cohesive areas)	Carbonic anhydrase IX positive, cytokeratin 7 focal/limited	*VHL* mutation, 3p25 deletion
Multilocular cystic renal neoplasm	Cells with clear cytoplasm, small clusters of cells within septa	Exclusively cystic (no solid component; Fig. 1.5a); papillary structures favor clear cell papillary RCC	Carbonic anhydrase IX positive, cytokeratin 7 often substantial, CD10 positive	*VHL* mutation, 3p25 deletion, possibly lower rates than conventional clear cell
Clear cell papillary RCC	Cells with clear cytoplasm, nuclei aligned above the basement membrane, branched glandular structures, small or complex papillae in cystic spaces	Tubular/glandular, cystic, solid, papillary (Fig. 1.5b)	Carbonic anhydrase IX positive (cup shaped), cytokeratin 7 diffuse, CD10 negative (except cysts), high molecular weight cytokeratin often positive, GATA3 often positive, AMACR negative/minimal	Negative for *VHL* mutation or 3p25 loss, no consistent copy number abnormalities
Mixed epithelial and stromal tumor	Variable epithelium, most commonly cuboidal cells, spindle cell stroma	Cystic and solid (variable percentages)	Common estrogen and progesterone receptor positivity, positivity for CD34, WT1, smooth muscle actin, or desmin; minimal or negative carbonic anhydrase IX	
Tubulocystic RCC	Eosinophilic cells with prominent nucleoli lining tubular and cystic spaces with fibrous stroma (Fig. 1.5c)	Tubular and cystic	AMACR positive, cytokeratin 7 negative or focal, carbonic anhydrase IX negative or focal	Usually lacking trisomy 7/17 (contrast to papillary RCC), if pure

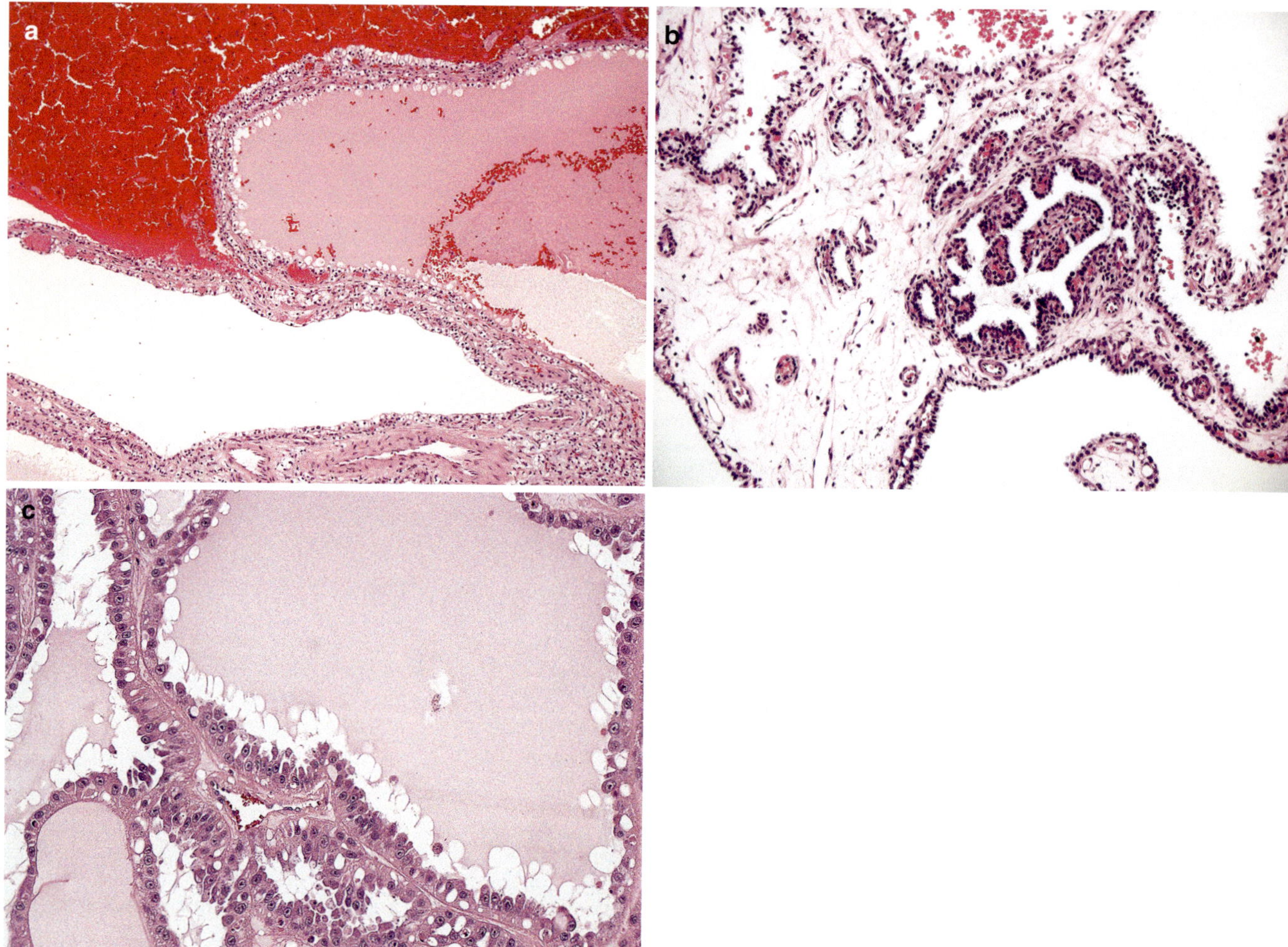

Fig. 1.5 (**a**) Multilocular cystic renal neoplasm of low malignant potential is composed entirely of cysts lined by cells with clear cytoplasm. The septa can contain small clusters of tumor cells, but there should be no mass-forming solid component. (**b**) Clear cell papillary renal cell carcinoma can have an extensive cystic component, resembling multilocular cystic neoplasms; however, the presence of papillary structures or branched glands within the stroma favors clear cell papillary renal cell carcinoma. (**c**) Tubulocystic renal cell carcinoma is composed of eosinophilic, hobnail-shaped cells with prominent nucleoli lining cystic and tubular spaces. The nuclear grade is usually equivalent to ISUP/WHO grade 3

What Are the Commonly Used Immunohistochemical Markers in Differentiating Renal Tumors?

Immunohistochemistry can be helpful in resolving differential diagnoses of renal tumors; however, it is important to take immunohistochemical (IHC) markers in the context of the histologic appearance and to know their limitations, as very few are highly specific in isolation. Predominant results are described in Table 1.7, with some notable exceptions or caveats as follows:

- Carbonic anhydrase IX is a robust marker of clear cell RCC, showing diffuse membranous staining in most cases (Fig. 1.6a). However, since carbonic anhydrase IX is part of the hypoxia pathway, many tumors and tissues can have some positivity in areas of ischemia or necrosis. In large tissue sections with abundant viable tumor cells, this typically does not account for more than focal positivity (Fig. 1.6b), but interpretation should be approached with caution for small biopsies with limited viable cells.
- Specificity of carbonic anhydrase IX is also lower in the context of unknown primary cancer, as many non-renal cancers can have positivity.
- Diffuse strong intensity for AMACR is characteristic of papillary RCC (Fig. 1.6c); however, many other tumors can have some degree of positivity. A very strong positive reaction (similar to normal proximal renal tubules) is supportive of papillary RCC but should be taken in the context of the other findings.
- In chromophobe RCC vs. oncocytoma, the classic expectation is that chromophobe will exhibit diffuse membranous cytokeratin 7 reactivity. However, this is most reliable only in tumors with classic (pale cell) features.

- In oncocytoma, a pattern of only scattered rare cells positive for cytokeratin 7 is expected (Fig. 1.6d).
- A cutoff for an amount of cytokeratin 7 positivity that warrants a diagnosis of eosinophilic chromophobe is not well agreed upon, but the amount of positivity can be much more limited than that of classic chromophobe.
- Positivity for cytokeratin 7 is most consistent in type 1 papillary RCC. In type 2 papillary RCC or tumors with eosinophilic features, reactivity for cytokeratin 7 is often focal or absent.
- TFE3 and TFEB protein immunohistochemistry may be helpful for raising suspicion for translocation-associated RCC (if strong); however, weak reactivity is less specific for gene rearrangement and often is better confirmed with molecular studies.

References: [4, 21, 29, 32–36].

What Are the Useful Molecular Tests in Diagnosis of Renal Epithelial Tumors?

Classification of renal cell neoplasms has evolved over the years based on integration of tumor histology with immunohistochemistry and genetics; however, fortunately in current practice, classification can still be achieved without using routine genetic assays, rather by relying on immunohistochemical and histologic surrogates of existing genetic knowledge. Still, several molecular techniques can be helpful in select instances, ranging from mutation analysis to copy number studies to fluorescence in situ hybridization (FISH).

Table 1.8 shows helpful molecular markers for renal tumor diagnosis (see also Fig. 1.7).

References: [17, 21, 37–49].

Table 1.7 Most widely used immunohistochemical markers for differential diagnosis of renal tumors

	Carbonic anhydrase IX	AMACR	Cytokeratin 7	KIT (CD117)	High molecular weight cytokeratin	GATA3	Vimentin	Melanocytic	Cathepsin-K
Clear cell RCC	+++	+/−	−/+	−	−/+	−	+/−	−	−
Papillary RCC, type 1	−/+	+++	+++	−	+/−		+/−	−	−
Papillary RCC, eosinophilic or type 2	−/+	+++	−/+	−			+/−	−	−
Chromophobe RCC, classic	−/+	+/−	+++	+		+/−	−	−	−
Chromophobe RCC, eosinophilic	−/+	+/−	+/−	+			−	−	−
Oncocytoma	−/+	+/−	−/+*	+		−/+	−	−	−
Clear cell papillary RCC	+++	−	+++		+	+/−	+	−	−
Translocation RCC (*TFE3* or *TFEB*)	−/+	+/−	−/+	−		−	−/+	+/−	+/−

Note: +++ = consistent diffuse strong positive, + = positive, +/− = may be positive but not consistent, −/+ = usually negative but can be rarely or focally positive, − = negative, * = only rare scattered cells positive

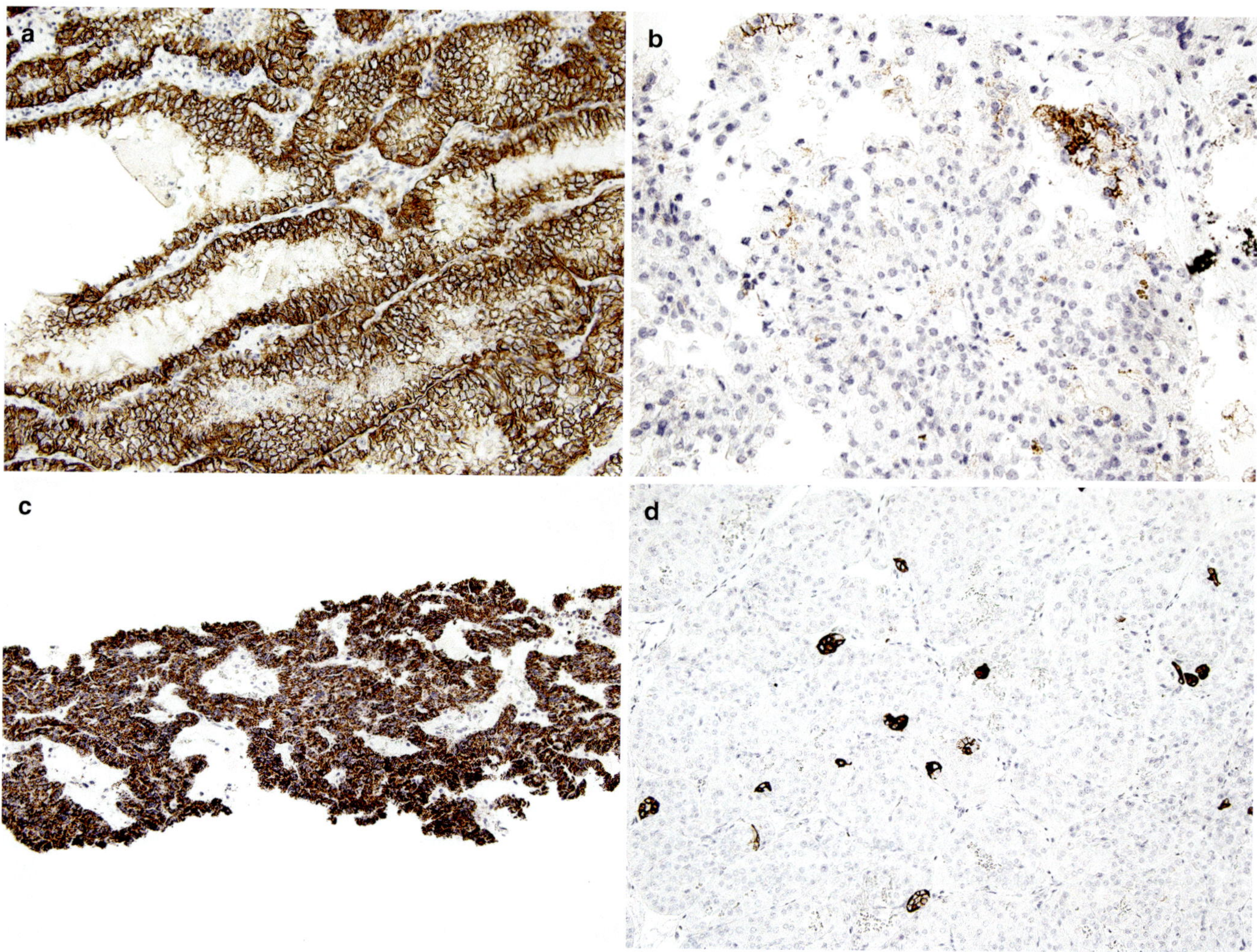

Fig. 1.6 (**a**) Clear cell renal cell carcinoma characteristically exhibits diffuse membrane positivity for carbonic anhydrase IX. (**b**) In contrast to clear cell cancer, other subtypes of renal cell carcinoma may exhibit focal nonspecific staining for carbonic anhydrase IX, which should not be interpreted as favoring clear cell subtype. (**c**) Diffuse strong staining for alpha-methylacyl-CoA racemase (AMACR) similar to that of the proximal renal tubules is supportive of papillary renal cell carcinoma in the appropriate context, although other renal cell neoplasms may exhibit some degree of positivity. (**d**) Oncocytoma characteristically exhibits a pattern of scattered cells positive for cytokeratin 7, usually not accounting for more than a few percent of tumor cells

Table 1.8 Helpful molecular markers for renal tumor diagnosis

	Tumor type	Comments
VHL mutation	Clear cell RCC	Over 50% of clear cell RCCs have mutation; however, other mechanisms of inactivation occur, including promoter hypermethylation and chromosome arm loss. Therefore, absence of mutation does not exclude a clear cell RCC
3p25 FISH	Clear cell RCC	Many clear cell RCCs have a copy loss of the chromosome 3p arm, which contains *VHL* and several other genes now known to be frequently altered in clear cell RCC (*PBRM1, SETD2, BAP1*). The specificity is less clear, however, as other reports have occasionally described 3p loss in non-clear-cell tumors. When combined with other mechanisms of *VHL* inactivation, over 90% of tumors have an alteration of *VHL*/3p25
Trisomy 7/17; loss of Y	Papillary RCC	Trisomy of chromosomes 7 and/or 17 is common in type 1 papillary RCC; however, the specificity of these alterations is less clear, as they have been reported in other neoplasms
TFE3/TFEB studies	Translocation RCC	Molecular studies to evaluate the *TFE3* and/or *TFEB* genes are helpful in confirming a diagnosis of translocation-associated RCC. The most common assay is break-apart FISH, which often can detect rearrangement (Fig. 1.7). However, a few recent fusions have been noted to result in a chromosomal inversion with a subtle, potentially false-negative FISH result (notably *NONO-TFE3* and *RBM10-TFE3* fusions). Next-generation sequencing studies or real-time polymerase chain reaction (RT-PCR) may be alternate methods to detect these gene fusions; however, these are less widely available. Recently, a subset of aggressive RCCs has been found to have amplification of 6p21 including *TFEB*, which can be detected by FISH or other copy number analyses

Table 1.8 (continued)

	Tumor type	Comments
FH studies	FH-deficient RCC/HLRCC syndrome	The simplest way to detect alterations of *FH* is immunohistochemistry for the FH protein. An abnormal result is loss (negative staining of the tumor cells with positive internal control of normal tissues). However, a subset of neoplasms exhibits a normal staining pattern even in the presence of confirmed mutation. Therefore, routine histopathology with immunohistochemistry and recommendation for genetic counseling may be necessary to capture all patients with the HLRCC syndrome. FH-deficient is used for tumors that are abnormal for FH in the absence of known germline mutation
Copy number analysis	Other RCC types	Other RCC types sometimes have recurrent copy number changes that can be detected by copy number analyses, such as FISH, comparative genomic hybridization (CGH), or single nucleotide polymorphism (SNP) array. For example, mucinous tubular and spindle cell carcinoma has some overlapping features with papillary RCC; however, it has been shown to have multiple chromosomal losses involving chromosomes 1, 4, 6, 8, 9, 13, 14, 15, and 22 rather than 7/17 gain. For oncocytoma vs. chromophobe RCC, the latter tends to have multiple losses involving chromosomes 1, 2, 6, 10, 13, 17, and 21, in contrast to loss of chromosome 1 only or 11q rearrangement in oncocytoma
CCND1 rearrangement	Oncocytoma	Recent data have shown that a subset of oncocytomas has rearrangement of *CCND1* (cyclin D1). The precise role for using this knowledge for diagnosis remains incompletely understood; however, it appears that tumors with immunohistochemical positivity tend to be those with rearrangement (although incompletely specific), whereas those with negative immunohistochemistry are usually not rearranged

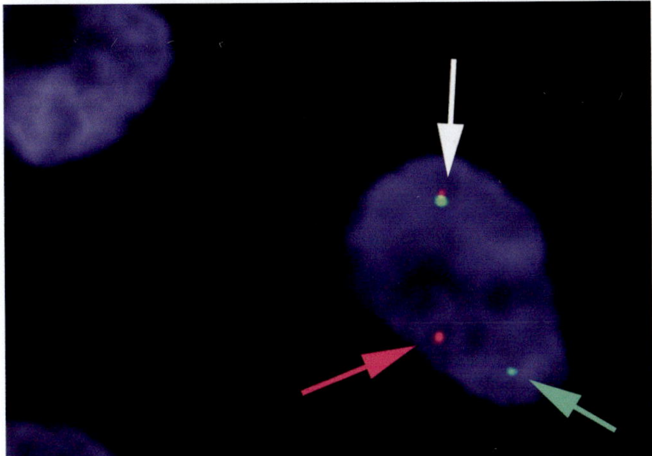

Fig. 1.7 Break-apart fluorescence in situ hybridization (FISH) for the *TFEB* gene in this case of *TFEB* rearranged renal cell carcinoma shows one normal signal result (white arrow). The other copy of the 6p21 region shows a split signal pattern (red and green signals and arrows)

Accurate Grading of Renal Cell Carcinoma in Small Tissue Biopsy and Nephrectomy Specimens

- The original Fuhrman grading system for renal cell carcinoma relied on several parameters to assign grade, including nuclear size, nuclear irregularity, and nucleolar prominence.
- Based on the difficulty of assessing multiple nuclear parameters at once, combined with data supporting nucleolar prominence as the key parameter, the 2013 ISUP Vancouver Consensus and 2016 WHO Classification recommend a modified grading system that relies primarily on the nucleolar prominence (Table 1.9, Fig. 1.8).

Table 1.9 ISUP/WHO grading of RCC

ISUP/WHO RCC grading	Features
1	Nucleoli inconspicuous or absent at 400x magnification (40x objective)
2	Nucleoli conspicuous/eosinophilic at 400x magnification (40x objective) but not at 100x magnification (10x objective)
3	Nucleoli conspicuous/eosinophilic at 100x magnification (10x objective; Fig. 1.8)
4	Extreme nuclear pleomorphism, tumor giant cells, or sarcomatoid/rhabdoid features

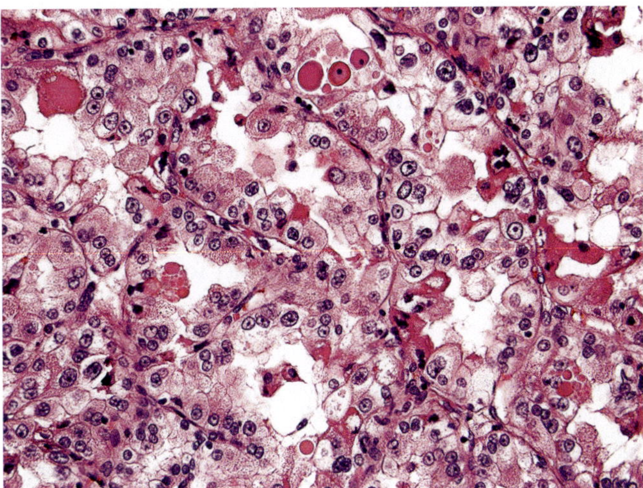

Fig. 1.8 The main defining criterion for nuclear grade in the modified grading system is prominent nucleoli recognizable at 100x magnification (10x objective), which warrants grade 3. Prominent nucleoli recognizable only at higher magnification warrant grade 2, whereas inconspicuous nucleoli even at high magnification warrant grade 1

- The minimum number of cells showing a higher grade required to assign the higher grade overall is debatable; however, the most established method is to identify at least an entire high-power field composed of the higher grade.
- An alternate system incorporating tumor necrosis has also been proposed; however, in most practices, the nucleolar method endorsed by ISUP/WHO is now used, with presence or absence of necrosis also noted in synoptic reports.
- The nucleolar grading system is recommended for use in clear cell and papillary RCC. For other RCC subtypes, it can be used descriptively, but has not been validated as a prognostic factor.
- Chromophobe RCC has a favorable prognosis, yet often has inherent nuclear atypia. It is recommended that grading not be applied to chromophobe RCC, as it has not been shown to have definite prognostic value.
- An alternate grading system has been proposed for chromophobe RCC based predominantly on nuclear crowding (chromophobe tumor grade), although reporting this is currently not required (Table 1.10).
- Grading is approached in a similar way for core biopsy samples. Recent attention has been drawn to risk stratifying tumors in the biopsy setting based on histologic subtype of tumor and grade, such that grade 1–2 tumors of specific histologies may be more amenable to surveillance or less aggressive therapy.

References: [1, 50–55].

What Are the Histologic Growth Patterns and Variants for Clear Cell RCC?

- Clear cell RCC can have a variety of patterns, especially when tumors are high-grade.
- A common pattern is that of eosinophilic cells (which likely often fell into the now defunct former category of "granular cell" RCC) (Fig. 1.9a).

Table 1.10 Proposed "chromophobe tumor grade" as an alternate grading scheme for chromophobe RCC

Chromophobe tumor grade (Paner et al. [53])	Features
1	Lack of nuclear crowding or anaplasia, as defined for grades 2 and 3
2	Nuclear crowding detectable at 100× magnification (10× objective), some nuclei in direct contact with each other at 400× magnification (40× objective), and threefold nuclear size variation (non-degenerative)
3	Frank anaplasia, including multilobated nuclei, tumor giant cells, or sarcomatoid change

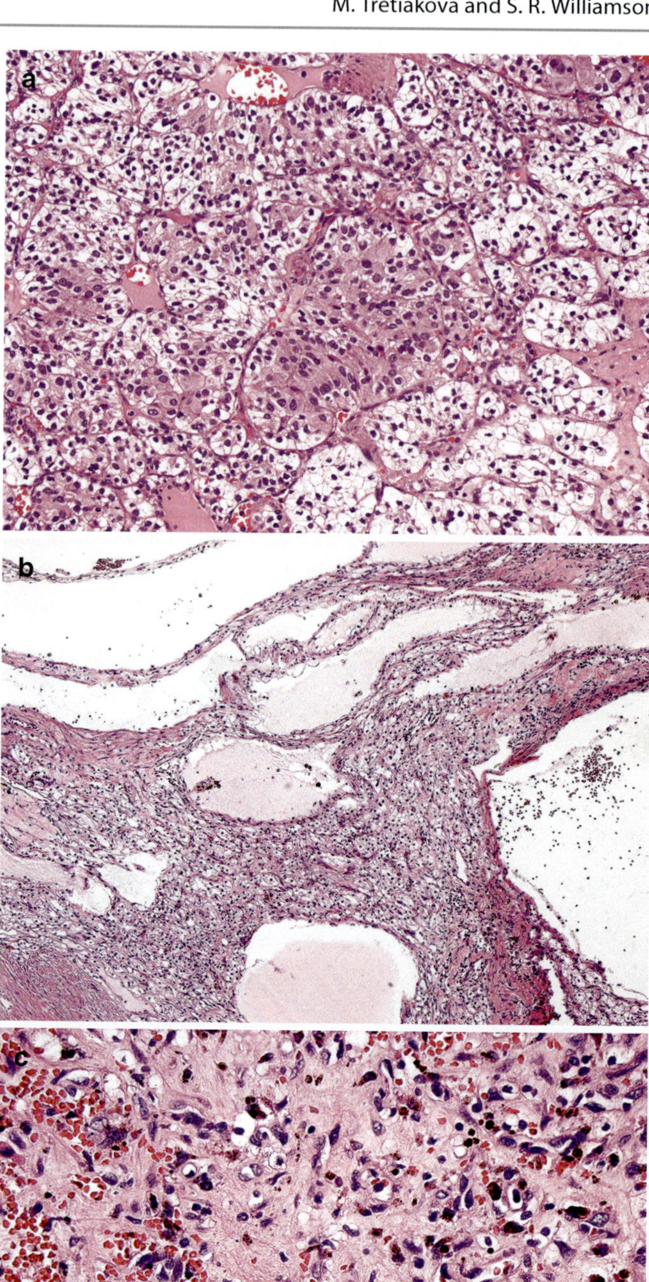

Fig. 1.9 (**a**) Clear cell renal cell carcinoma can have a transition to granular eosinophilic cytoplasm (formerly known as granular cell renal cell carcinoma); however, identification of a classic low-grade clear cell component supports interpretation as clear cell renal cell carcinoma. (**b**) Some clear cell renal cell carcinomas are extensively cystic such that they mimic multilocular cystic low malignant potential tumors; however, a solid mass-forming component, as shown here, precludes a diagnosis of multilocular cystic neoplasm. Still, the behavior may be favorable, and a comment regarding extensive cystic change can be included. (**c**) In some cases, the epithelial component of a clear cell renal cell carcinoma is subtle or obliterated by scarring, which can mimic a hemangioma. Identification of classic clear cell areas or confirmation of epithelial tumors cells with immunohistochemistry can resolve this distinction

- Clear cell RCC can often have cystic change (often accompanied by fibrosis and hemorrhage), with some areas mimicking multilocular cystic neoplasm of low malignant potential. Any solid component (defined as an expansile nodule that would be grossly visible, Fig. 1.9b) precludes a diagnosis of multilocular cystic neoplasm and favors clear cell RCC.
- Some clear cell RCCs have extensive degeneration and sclerosis, so that the vascular component predominates, mimicking hemangioma (Fig. 1.9c).
- Keys to recognizing an unusual RCC as clear cell RCC include: identification of classic golden-yellow/orange areas grossly (even if focal), identification of classic low-grade clear cell areas histologically (may require additional sampling), and diffuse membrane positivity for carbonic anhydrase IX.
- A list of select variants is discussed in Table 1.11.

References: [8, 56–62].

What Are the Differential Diagnoses for Renal Epithelial Tumors with both Clear Cell and Papillary Features?

- Renal epithelial tumors with both clear cell and papillary features can include several different diagnostic entities, ranging from clear cell RCC to translocation RCC to the entity clear cell papillary (tubulopapillary) RCC.
- Key features helpful in distinguishing these entities are shown in Table 1.12 (see also Fig. 1.10).

References: [4, 9, 17, 47–49, 60–63].

Clear Cell RCC vs. Chromophobe RCC

Usually, distinction of clear cell RCC and chromophobe RCC is straightforward, based on their characteristic histologic features; however, some tumors may exhibit overlapping features that necessitate immunohistochemistry or other studies to resolve the differential diagnosis (Fig. 1.11). The behavior of chromophobe RCC is considered favorable, with few demonstrating progression or metastasis, compared to clear cell RCC, which can be less predictable, especially with larger tumor sizes.

Table 1.13 shows how to distinguish clear cell from chromophobe RCC.

References: [17, 32, 57, 64].

Table 1.11 Deceptive variants of clear cell RCC

Variant pattern	Notes
Cystic clear cell RCC	Solid nodule (grossly appreciable) precludes diagnosis of multilocular cystic neoplasm of low malignant potential. immunohistochemistry may help identify tumor cells in areas of bland cyst lining or lymphocyte-like tumor cells within the stroma (PAX8, carbonic anhydrase IX)
Clear cell RCC with eosinophilic cells	Additional sampling may help in identifying classic low-grade areas (may focus on areas of golden-yellow/orange grossly). Diffuse positivity for carbonic anhydrase IX (not limited to necrosis or ischemic areas) supports clear cell subtype
Clear cell RCC with syncytial-type giant cells	Bizarre giant tumor cells with numerous nuclei and marked pleomorphism, often associated with necrosis and sometimes containing emperipolesis. Frequently has an abrupt transition to clear cell RCC with classic features. Even areas of severe atypia usually have similar immunohistochemical features to low-grade clear cell RCC (carbonic anhydrase IX and epithelial markers)
Hemangioma-like clear cell RCC	Epithelial component is subtle/inconspicuous, with associated capillary vascular network mimicking hemangioma. Additional sampling or careful search for epithelial areas may be helpful. immunohistochemistry for epithelial markers (keratin, epithelial membrane antigen [EMA], PAX8) or carbonic anhydrase IX can highlight a subtle epithelial component that resembles capillaries or inflammatory cells
Sarcomatoid clear cell RCC	The most helpful clue to recognizing a sarcomatoid neoplasm as clear cell RCC is additional sampling in search of conventional clear cell areas. Positivity for PAX8 would support a sarcomatoid carcinoma over sarcoma and generally favors RCC over urothelial carcinoma; however, some overlap in the patterns of GATA3 and PAX8 in upper urinary tract sarcomatoid neoplasms has been reported. almost any type of RCC can undergo sarcomatoid dedifferentiation; however, clear cell RCC accounts for the most cases due to its higher incidence. Some studies have suggested that chromophobe RCC has a paradoxically high incidence of sarcomatoid change
Clear cell papillary RCC-like pattern	Although clear cell papillary (or tubulopapillary) RCC is now recognized as a distinct entity with favorable prognosis, there occur cases of clear cell RCC with overlapping morphology. If the immunohistochemical features are not perfect for the entity clear cell papillary RCC (such as incomplete cytokeratin 7 positivity or positivity for CD10 and/or AMACR), it appears that these are better classified as clear cell RCC. These sometimes have higher-stage parameters, larger tumor size, necrosis, etc., which are unexpected in the indolent clear cell papillary RCC. The same also holds true of patients with von Hippel-Lindau (VHL) disease (tumors that resemble clear cell papillary RCC occur, but their immunohistochemical profile is usually not a perfect fit)

Table 1.12 Differential diagnosis of renal epithelial tumors with clear cell and papillary features

	Features	Immunohistochemistry	Genetics
Clear cell RCC with pseudopapillary structures (Fig. 1.10a)	Usually some areas with conventional clear cell features, usually high-grade (ISUP/WHO grade 3). Debatable whether clear cell can have true papillae or this represents loss of cohesion and exclusively pseudopapillary structures	Carbonic anhydrase IX diffuse membrane positive, cytokeratin 7 and high molecular weight cytokeratin negative or partial, AMACR variable, CD10 often positive, melanocytic markers negative	*VHL* mutation and/or 3p25 loss
Papillary RCC with clear cytoplasm (Fig. 1.10b)	Cytoplasm usually vacuolated, with or without hemosiderin, rather than totally clear. Foamy macrophages with similar cytoplasm or psammoma bodies often present	AMACR diffuse strong positive, carbonic anhydrase IX focal or negative, cytokeratin 7 usually diffuse (for type 1 tumors)	Trisomy 7 or 17, loss of Y
Clear cell papillary (tubulopapillary) RCC (Fig. 1.10c)	Branched glandular structures with nuclei aligned above the basement membrane, stubby to complex papillae into cystic spaces, usually small tumors (pT1a)	Carbonic anhydrase IX diffuse positive with "cup-shape" (spares cell apex), cytokeratin 7 diffuse positive, high molecular weight cytokeratin frequently positive, GATA3 frequently positive, AMACR extremely weak or negative, CD10 positive in cysts only or negative	Few/no recurrent genetic alterations
Translocation RCC (Fig. 1.10d)	Variable nested, papillary, clear cell, and eosinophilic cell features. May have voluminous cytoplasm, hyalinized stroma, pigment, or psammoma bodies	Carbonic anhydrase IX minimal or negative, sometimes negative for keratins or vimentin, often melanocytic markers or cathepsin-K positive, AMACR variable, TFE3 or TFEB immunohistochemistry positive	*TFE3* or *TFEB* gene fusion (or rarely *MITF*); occasional false-negative FISH (*RBM10-TFE3* and *NONO-TFE3*)
Clear cell RCC with overlap resembling clear cell papillary RCC (Fig. 1.10e, f)	Branched glands or nuclear alignment mimicking clear cell papillary RCC	Cytokeratin 7 ranges from focal to diffuse, but other markers not supportive of clear cell papillary (CD10 and/or AMACR positive), high molecular weight cytokeratin minimal or negative	At least two-thirds with 3p25 deletion like clear cell RCC

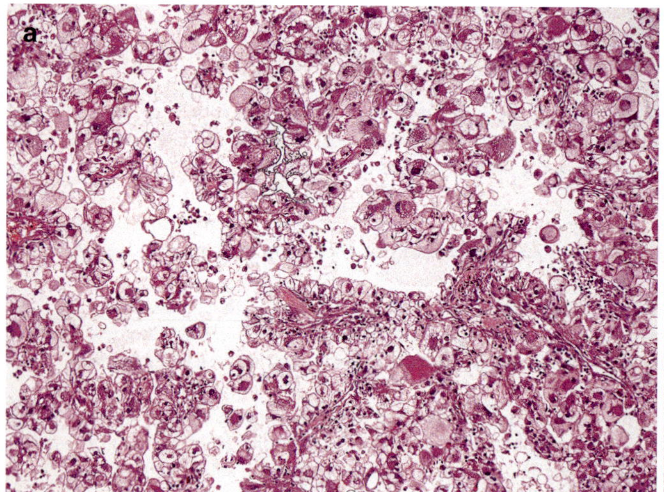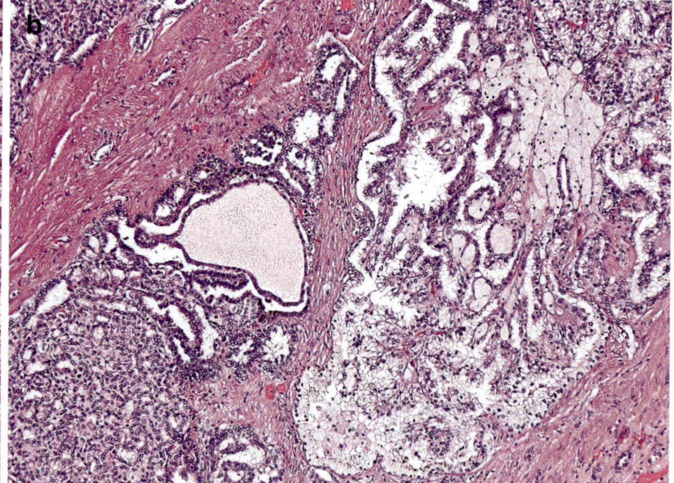

Fig. 1.10 (**a**) Rarely clear cell renal cell carcinoma can exhibit papillary structures, often likely resulting from lack of cohesion in higher-grade tumors. (**b**) Clear cytoplasmic change can be observed in a subset of papillary renal cell carcinomas, often manifesting as numerous cytoplasmic vacuoles. (**c**) The entity clear cell papillary (tubulopapillary) renal cell carcinoma is composed of branched glandular structures with alignment of the nuclei at a similar height within the cytoplasm. (**d**) Translocation renal cell carcinomas often have mixed clear cell and eosinophilic patterns, as well as mixed nested and papillary patterns. The presence of psammoma bodies, as in this case, favors a translocation renal cell carcinoma over clear cell renal cell carcinoma. (**e**) Some clear cell renal cell carcinomas can have overlapping features of clear cell papillary (tubulopapillary) renal cell carcinoma. However, if the immunohistochemical phenotype is not perfect, a diagnosis of clear cell renal cell carcinoma should be used. (**f**) The same case as shown in 10E demonstrates areas more suggestive of typical clear cell renal cell carcinoma

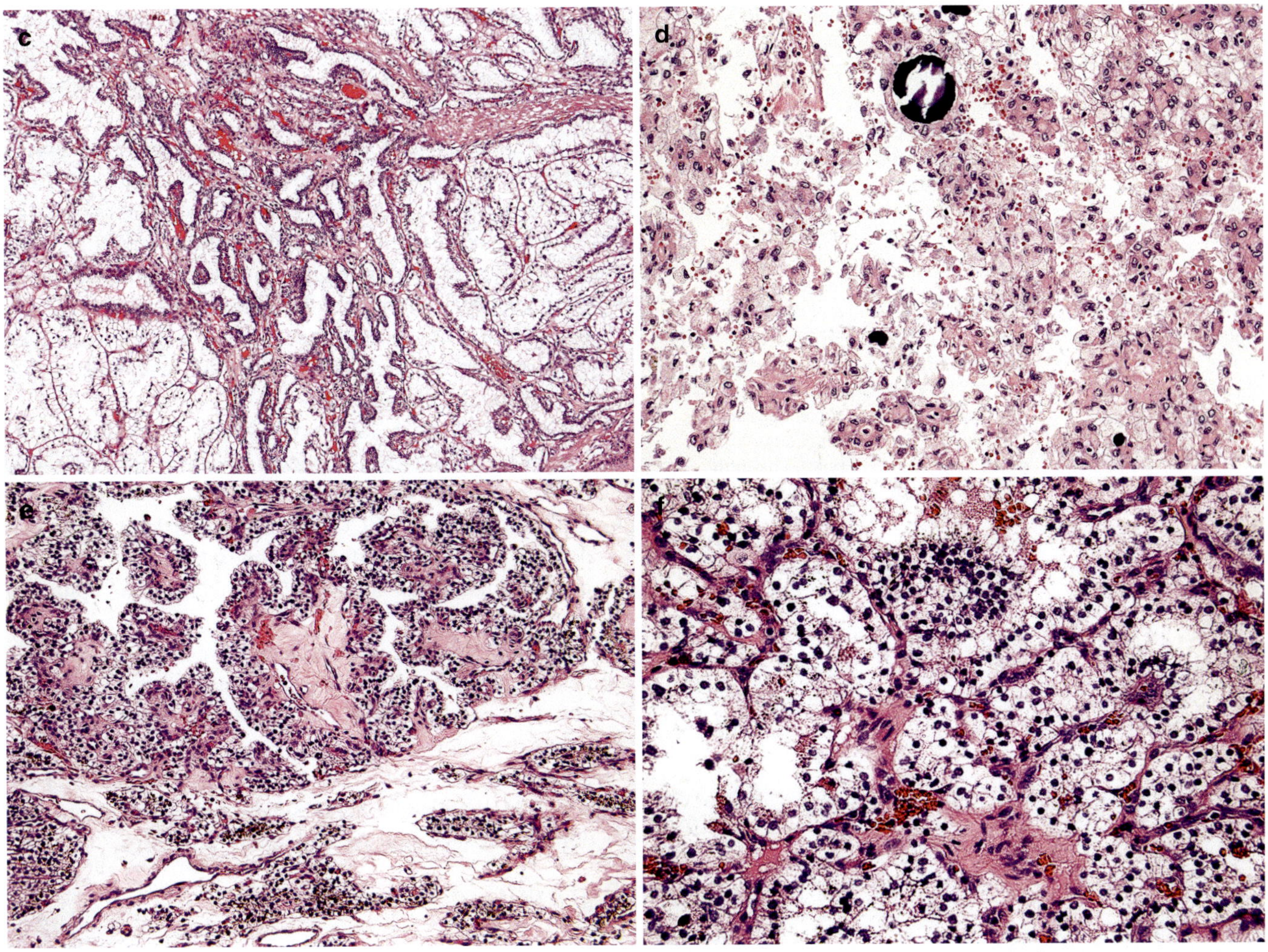

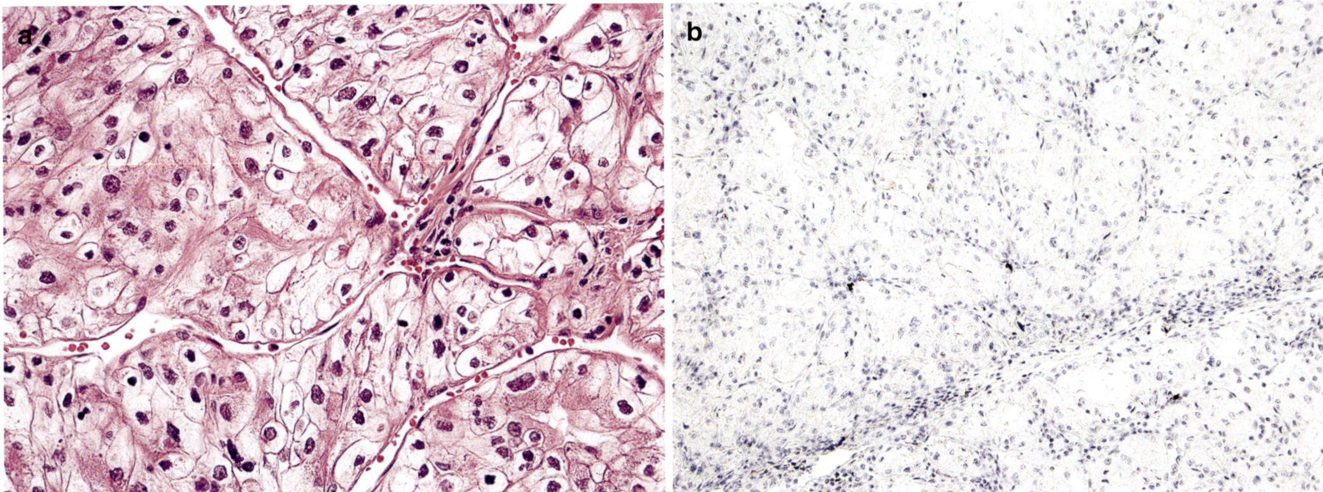

Fig. 1.10 (continued)

Fig. 1.11 (**a**) This clear cell renal cell carcinoma demonstrates some nuclear wrinkling and prominent cell borders, raising consideration of chromophobe renal cell carcinoma. (**b**) The same case shows negative immunohistochemistry for KIT (CD117), arguing against chromophobe renal cell carcinoma. Other results included positive carbonic anhydrase IX and negative cytokeratin 7, further supporting this classification (not pictured)

Table 1.13 Distinguishing clear cell from chromophobe RCC

	Clear cell RCC	Chromophobe RCC
Gross	Golden-yellow, orange	Pale, tan
Histology	Nests of cells with complex vascular network, clear cytoplasm	Solid or trabecular architecture with voluminous cytoplasm, prominent cell borders, wrinkled nuclei
Immunohistochemistry and other staining	Carbonic anhydrase IX diffuse positive, KIT (CD117) negative, vimentin frequently positive (especially with higher grade), cytokeratin 7 negative or focal. colloidal iron may have reticular positive pattern	KIT (CD117) positive, cytokeratin 7 usually diffuse positive (for classic chromophobe, less for eosinophilic type), vimentin negative (consistently). Diffuse colloidal iron positive
Genetics	*VHL* mutation, loss of 3p25	Loss of chromosomes 1, 2, 6, 10, 13, 17, and 21

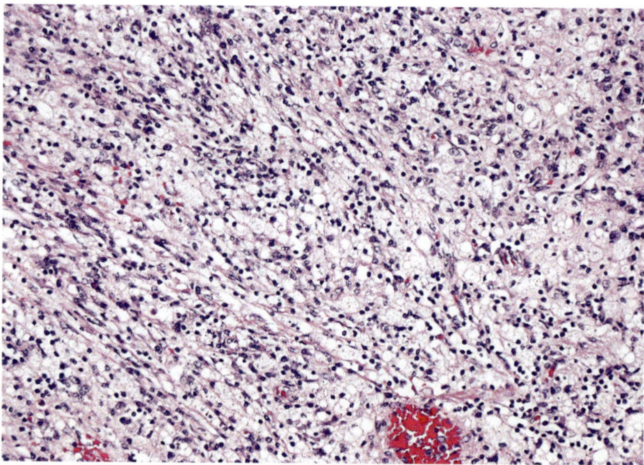

Fig. 1.12 The foamy histiocytes of xanthogranulomatous pyelonephritis can mimic a renal cell carcinoma microscopically

RCC vs. Xanthogranulomatous Pyelonephritis

Xanthogranulomatous pyelonephritis is an unusual granulomatous process that may involve the kidney entirely or partially. This can variably mimic a renal neoplasm clinically, grossly, or microscopically (Fig. 1.12).

- Xanthogranulomatous pyelonephritis is associated with urinary tract infection, particularly with organisms like *Escherichia coli* or *Proteus mirabilis*, and obstruction.

- "Staghorn" calculus of the renal pelvis is also common.
- Extension of xanthogranulomatous pyelonephritis locally can mimic high-stage renal cancer, such as with involvement of the psoas muscle.
- Gross appearance of xanthogranulomatous pyelonephritis includes yellow nodules reminiscent of clear cell RCC, although often arrangement around the calyces is a clue to the infectious/inflammatory nature of this entity.
- Histologic differential diagnosis of xanthogranulomatous pyelonephritis could include sarcomatoid or poorly differentiated RCC, due to sheets of lipid-laden histiocytic cells (mimicking clear cell RCC cells), with lack of distinct glandular architecture.
- Cells of interest in xanthogranulomatous pyelonephritis are predominantly histiocytic and positive for histiocytic markers, such as CD68 or CD163.
- Cells of interest in RCC should have at least some evidence of epithelial differentiation, which with immunohistochemistry can include PAX8, keratin, or epithelial membrane antigen (EMA) positivity.
- Vimentin, although frequently positive in clear cell RCC, is also positive in xanthogranulomatous pyelonephritis and does not distinguish these entities.
- Other differential diagnostic considerations for xanthogranulomatous pyelonephritis include malakoplakia (in which Michaelis-Gutmann bodies can be found) or other nonspecific infectious/inflammatory processes.

Ref: [65].

Papillary RCC vs. Papillary Adenoma

- Papillary RCC and papillary adenoma are analogous lesions, with distinction based predominantly on a few key parameters.
- In the prior WHO Classification (2004), the definition of papillary adenoma required size 5 mm or less to distinguish papillary adenoma from RCC.
- The current WHO Classification (2016) has increased the size threshold for papillary adenoma to 15 mm.
- Other requirements include lack of a fibrous pseudocapsule and low nucleolar grade (ISUP/WHO grades 1 and 2) (Fig. 1.13a, b).
- This change is based on data showing a lack of aggressive behavior from RCC tumors in general under 2.0 cm.
- Otherwise, the features of papillary adenoma are essentially identical to those of type 1 papillary RCC, including basophilic cuboidal cells, papillary or tubular architecture, and psammoma bodies or foamy macrophages.
- In view of this size threshold, it is now conceivable that papillary adenomas could be intentionally subjected to renal mass biopsy, in which case a diagnosis for a tumor up to 1.5 cm could be "papillary renal cell neoplasm"

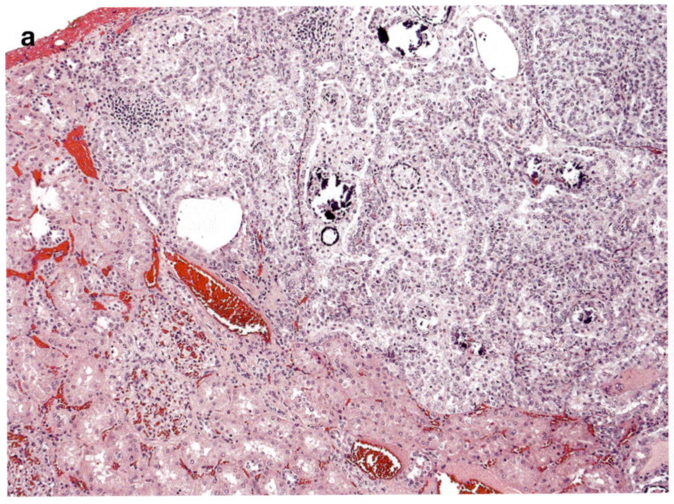

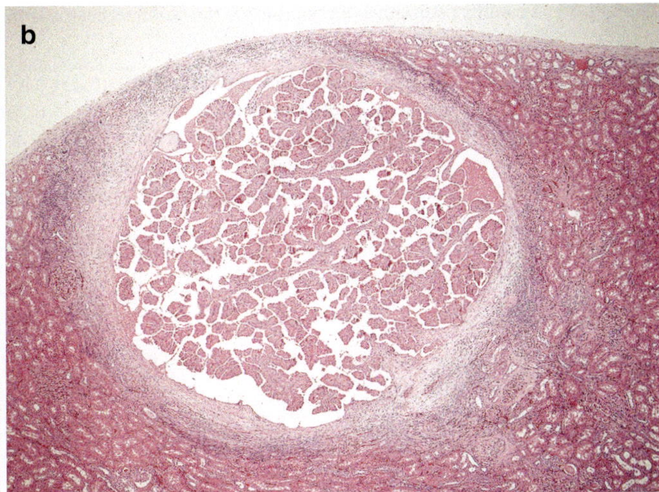

Fig. 1.13 (**a**) Papillary adenomas generally resemble a grade 1–2 papillary renal cell carcinoma, but they are less than 15 mm (in the 2016 World Health Organization Classification) and lack a fibrous pseudo-capsule. (**b**) This papillary lesion meets the size criteria for adenoma, but would in the current classification warrant designation as a small renal cell carcinoma due to fibrous pseudocapsule

with a comment that distinction between adenoma and RCC is based on size, encapsulation, and grade, which cannot be entirely assessed in a biopsy.

References: [66, 67].

Papillary Adenoma and RCC vs. Metanephric Adenoma and Wilms Tumor

- Differential diagnostic considerations for unusual patterns of papillary renal cell neoplasms include metanephric adenoma and Wilms tumor (nephroblastoma).
- In contrast to papillary neoplasms, metanephric adenomas typically have highly monotonous cells with very small, bland nuclei (Fig. 1.14).
- Conversely, Wilms tumor (nephroblastoma) exhibits prominent atypia and mitotic activity, especially in the blastemal component, and often will have more than one of the characteristic patterns of blastema, tubules, and stroma.
- Studies for chromosomes 7, 17, and Y can be used, as trisomy 7/17 and loss of Y appear largely specific to papillary RCC in this context and typically lacking in metanephric adenoma and Wilms tumor.
- Metanephric adenomas are often *BRAF* mutant and many label for mutant BRAF protein with immunohistochemistry.

Table 1.14 shows features distinguishing papillary renal cell neoplasms from metanephric adenoma and nephroblastoma.

References: [68–70].

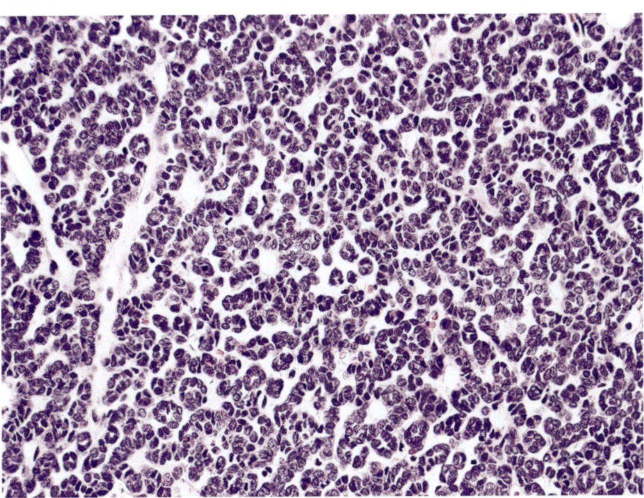

Fig. 1.14 Metanephric adenomas may closely resemble papillary renal cell carcinomas in several ways; however, they are notable for their highly monotonous small, bland nuclei forming tight tubular structures or papillae (not pictured)

Type 1 Papillary RCC vs. Type 2 Papillary RCC

Type 1 and type 2 papillary RCC have been distinguished for many years, based on more aggressive behavior in the latter; however, some recent increased understanding of these two morphological types has challenged the thinking about some cases, particularly the subset of type 2 tumors that are now considered a distinct entity, fumarate hydratase (FH)-deficient RCC/HLRCC syndrome.

Table 1.15 shows a comparison of type 1 vs. type 2 papillary RCC and HLRCC syndrome/FH-deficient RCC (see also Fig. 1.15).

References: [6, 17, 71–73].

Table 1.14 Features distinguishing papillary renal cell neoplasms from metanephric adenoma and nephroblastoma

	Morphology	Immunohistochemistry
Papillary RCC/ adenoma	Nuclei variable, ranging from ISUP grades 1 to 3, sometimes prominent nucleoli. Papillary structures, foamy macrophages, psammoma bodies	AMACR diffuse strong positive, cytokeratin 7 typically positive (type 1 tumors), WT1, CD57 negative
Metanephric adenoma	Highly monotonous small bland nuclei. Can have papillary structures and psammoma bodies, mimicking papillary RCC	AMACR and cytokeratin 7 negative (or focal), WT1 and CD57 positive, epithelial membrane antigen usually negative
Wilms tumor/ nephroblastoma	Often more than one pattern of: Blastema, tubules, stroma. Atypical with brisk mitotic activity	WT1 positive, lesser CD57 than metanephric adenoma, AMACR and cytokeratin 7 typically negative

Table 1.15 Comparison of type 1 vs. type 2 papillary RCC and HLRCC syndrome/FH-deficient RCC

	Type 1 papillary	Type 2 papillary	HLRCC/FH-deficient
Morphology	Basophilic, cuboidal cells (Fig. 1.15a)	Elongated eosinophilic cells with pseudostratified nuclei (Fig. 1.15b)	Cells with very prominent nucleoli (Fig. 1.15c) and perinucleolar clearing; heterogeneous architectural patterns including tubulocystic, papillary, sarcomatoid, or collecting duct carcinoma-like
Immunohistochemistry	Cytokeratin 7 typically positive, AMACR positive	Cytokeratin 7 typically negative or minimal, AMACR positive	Largely nonspecific, but with abnormal negative staining for FH protein and positive 2-succino-cysteine (2SC). Note: Normal FH staining in the presence of mutation is still possible and requires genetic testing
Genetics	Trisomy 7/17, *MET* alterations (especially in the hereditary papillary RCC syndrome)	*CDKN2A* silencing, *SETD2* mutations. Note: Must exclude FH-deficient RCC/HLRCC syndrome	Alterations of *FH* gene, predominantly germline, but likely rare sporadic
Behavior	Nonaggressive	More aggressive	Highly aggressive
Notes	Most common	Diagnosis of exclusion if FH-deficient/HLRCC excluded	Now a distinct entity from papillary RCC

Papillary RCC vs. Mucinous Tubular and Spindle Cell Carcinoma

Mucinous tubular and spindle cell carcinoma is an unusual renal cell neoplasm composed of tubular structures resembling those of papillary RCC, mixed with areas of spindle-shaped cells (likely representing unusual compressed epithelial structures), and extracellular mucinous material. Papillary RCC and mucinous tubular and spindle cell carcinoma share several overlapping features, such that it has been speculated whether the latter is a variant of the same entity. Nonetheless, enough differences, including a distinct copy number profile, have been recognized such that mucinous tubular and spindle cell carcinoma is recognized as a distinct entity in the WHO Classification. Distinct features are summarized in Table 1.16 (see also Fig. 1.16).

References: [74–80].

Papillary RCC vs. Papillary Urothelial Carcinoma

Papillary RCC and urothelial carcinoma are usually readily distinguished, due to their different clinical presentations (involvement of the renal pelvis with or without extension into the kidney vs. renal parenchymal spherical tumor with rare extension into renal pelvis) and different histologic features. However, rare cases can be challenging, such as for papillary RCCs that extend into the calyceal system (Fig. 1.17) or high-grade sarcomatoid tumors that overgrow the kidney. Features that may be helpful in such cases are summarized in Table 1.17.

References: [8, 34, 81].

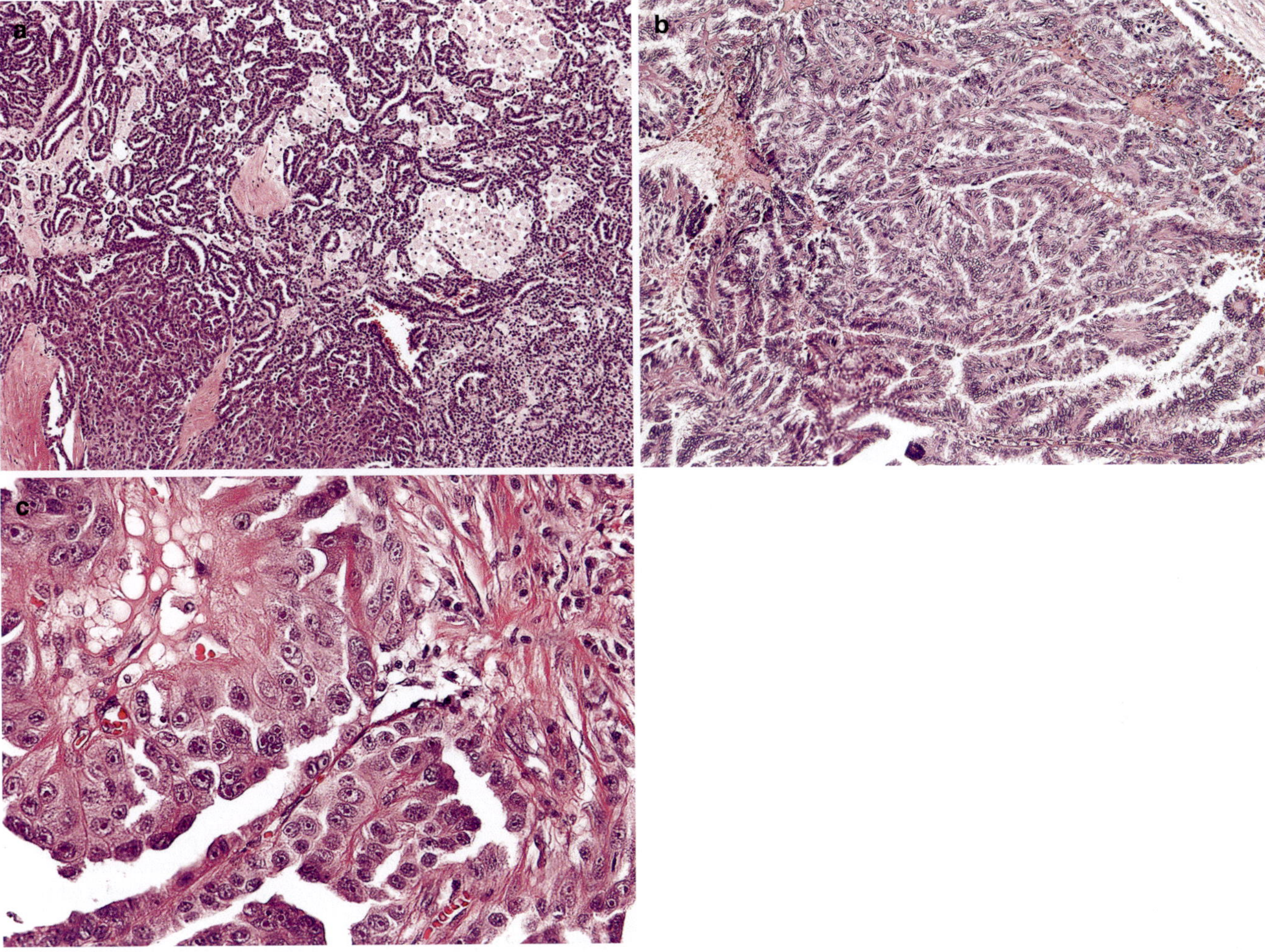

Fig. 1.15 (**a**) Type 1 papillary renal cell carcinomas are characteristically composed of cuboidal basophilic cells, often associated with foamy macrophages or psammoma bodies. (**b**) Type 2 papillary renal cell carcinomas contain eosinophilic cells with elongated pseudostratified nuclei. (**c**) A renal cell neoplasm with mixed histologic patterns (papillary, tubulocystic, collecting duct-like) and prominent nucleoli should raise concern for the possibility of hereditary leiomyomatosis and renal cell carcinoma syndrome/FH-deficient renal cell carcinoma

Table 1.16 Comparison of papillary RCC and mucinous tubular and spindle cell carcinoma

	Papillary RCC	Mucinous tubular spindle cell carcinoma
Morphology	Papillary structures, tubules, solid, psammoma bodies, foamy macrophages	Tubular structures (similar to those of papillary RCC; Fig. 1.16a), elongated spindle-shaped cells (likely compressed glandular structures; Fig. 1.16b), mucinous stromal material
Immunohistochemistry	Strongly positive AMACR, cytokeratin 7 (type 1 tumors)	Similar positivity for AMACR and cytokeratin 7, mixed results for markers of distal nephron. Overall, limited significant differences. Recent study found VSTM2A overexpression by in situ hybridization, different from papillary RCC
Genetics	Trisomy 7/17, loss of Y	Loss of chromosomes 1, 4, 6, 8, 9, 13, 14, 15, and 22 in typical cases. Those with overlapping features of papillary RCC have been reported to have 7/17 gains. Recent discovery of alterations in hippo pathway, including *NF2* and *PTPN14* genes
Behavior	Generally nonaggressive with small, organ-confined tumors	Generally nonaggressive but local recurrence, metastasis, and sarcomatoid cases have been described

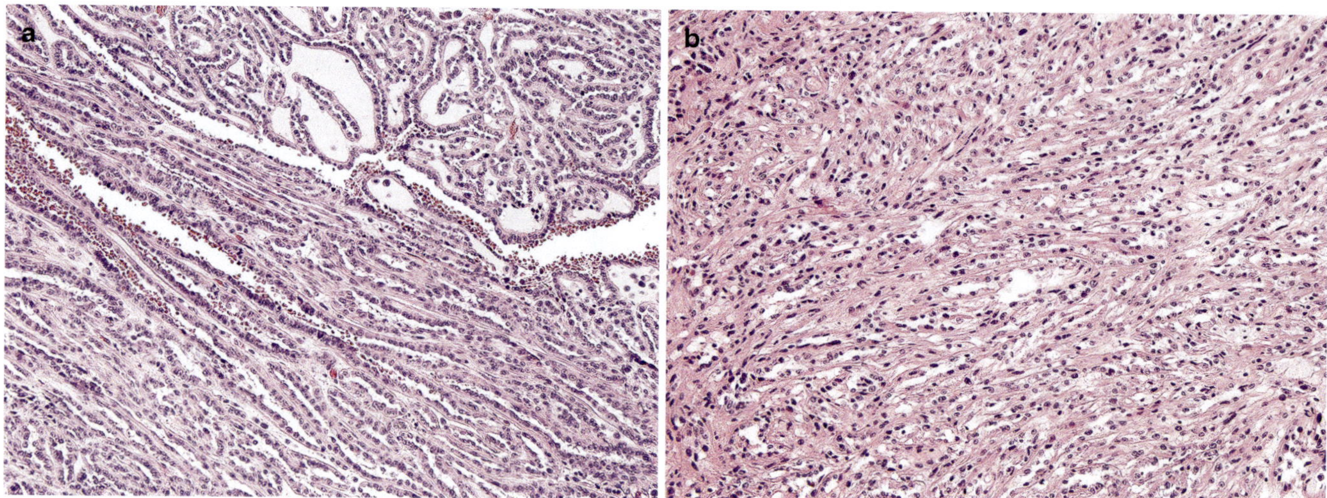

Fig. 1.16 (**a**) Mucinous tubular and spindle cell carcinoma is composed of cuboidal glandular cells, similar to those of papillary renal cell carcinoma, with associated basophilic mucinous material. (**b**) Mucinous tubular and spindle cell carcinoma also contains areas of compact spindle-shaped cells, which despite their mesenchymal appearance are likely of epithelial origin (same case)

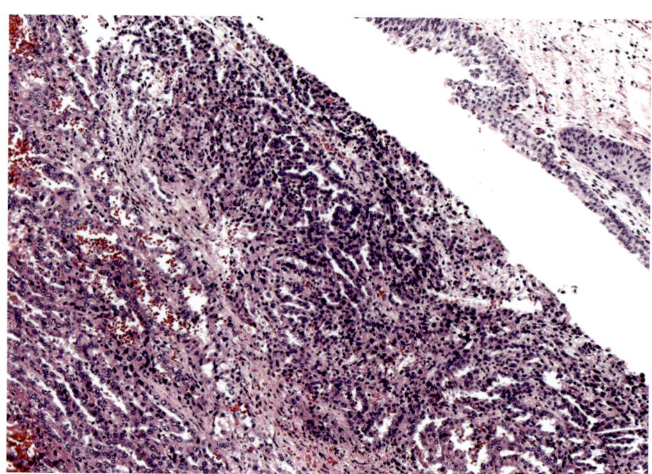

Fig. 1.17 This papillary renal cell carcinoma extended into the renal pelvis and was originally diagnosed by a ureteroscopic biopsy, clinically mimicking urothelial carcinoma. Renal pelvis mucosa is evident at far right

Chromophobe RCC vs. Oncocytoma

Despite being recognized as distinct tumors for decades, chromophobe RCC vs. oncocytoma continues to be a challenge for urologic pathologists, even today, owing to a lack of robust discriminatory markers. It remains incompletely understood whether these are two entirely unrelated entities that sometimes mimic each other, or if they exist as parts of a spectrum. Numerous histochemical and immunohistochemical markers have been explored over the years; however, only a few are widely used, with the most prevalent being cytokeratin 7. Helpful features are summarized in Table 1.18 (see also Fig. 1.18). Classic chromophobe RCC

Table 1.17 Features distinguishing papillary RCC from urothelial carcinoma

	Papillary RCC	Urothelial carcinoma
Gross growth pattern	Spherical/ovoid tumor, well circumscribed, with infrequent extension into renal pelvis	Renal pelvis or ureter-based but may infiltrate the kidney; usually poorly circumscribed if mimicking a renal mass
Histologic features	Cuboidal or columnar cells lining papillae, usually monolayered; psammoma bodies or foamy macrophages often present	Often multilayered cells lining papillae, but may be monolayered in areas of partial mucosal denudation; pleomorphism usually greater
Immunohistochemistry	PAX8 positive, AMACR strongly positive, cytokeratin 7 usually positive (type 1/non-eosinophilic tumors), p63 and GATA3 typically negative, cytokeratin 20 typically negative	GATA3 and p63 typically positive, AMACR variable, cytokeratin 20 often positive. Note: PAX8 would be ideally negative but has been reported in some urothelial carcinomas, including sarcomatoid urothelial carcinoma of the upper tract
In situ lesion of renal pelvis or ureter	None, except with rare coexistence of concurrent unrelated tumors	If present, favors urothelial carcinoma, but cannot always be found

Table 1.18 Features distinguishing oncocytoma from chromophobe RCC with eosinophilic features

	Oncocytoma	Chromophobe RCC (eosinophilic)
Gross appearance	Red-brown ("mahogany"), similar in color to normal kidney, sometimes central scar	Pale tan but can closely mimic oncocytoma, sometimes central scar
Histology	Discrete round nests or tubules composed of oncocytic cells with round regular nuclei	Solid growth or trabecular structures (Fig. 1.18c), perinuclear clearing
Atypical cells	Can have smudged cells with degenerative chromatin (Fig. 1.18a)	Nuclear wrinkling and irregularity (raisin-like), low nuclear-cytoplasmic ratio
Colloidal iron histochemistry	Negative or minimal apical positivity	Uniform cytoplasmic positivity
Cytokeratin 7	Rare scattered individual cells (Fig. 1.18b), can be increased in central scar areas	Ranges from oncocytoma-like pattern to small contiguous patches of positive cells (Fig. 1.18d) to diffuse
Vimentin	Negative, except in central scar	Negative
KIT (CD117)	Often positive, may be weak	Often positive
Chromosomal	No chromosomal alterations, or loss of 1, loss of Y, translocation of 11q (*CCND1* gene)	Multiple losses of 1, 2, 6, 10, 13, 17, and 21, possibly chromosomal gains, may have less abnormalities in more eosinophilic cases
Deceptive features	Can extend into fat or vein branches, which does not appear to alter the benign behavior; clear cytoplasmic change or basophilic features can occur in central scar areas	Very oncocytic cases may have minimal differences from oncocytoma, making distinction challenging

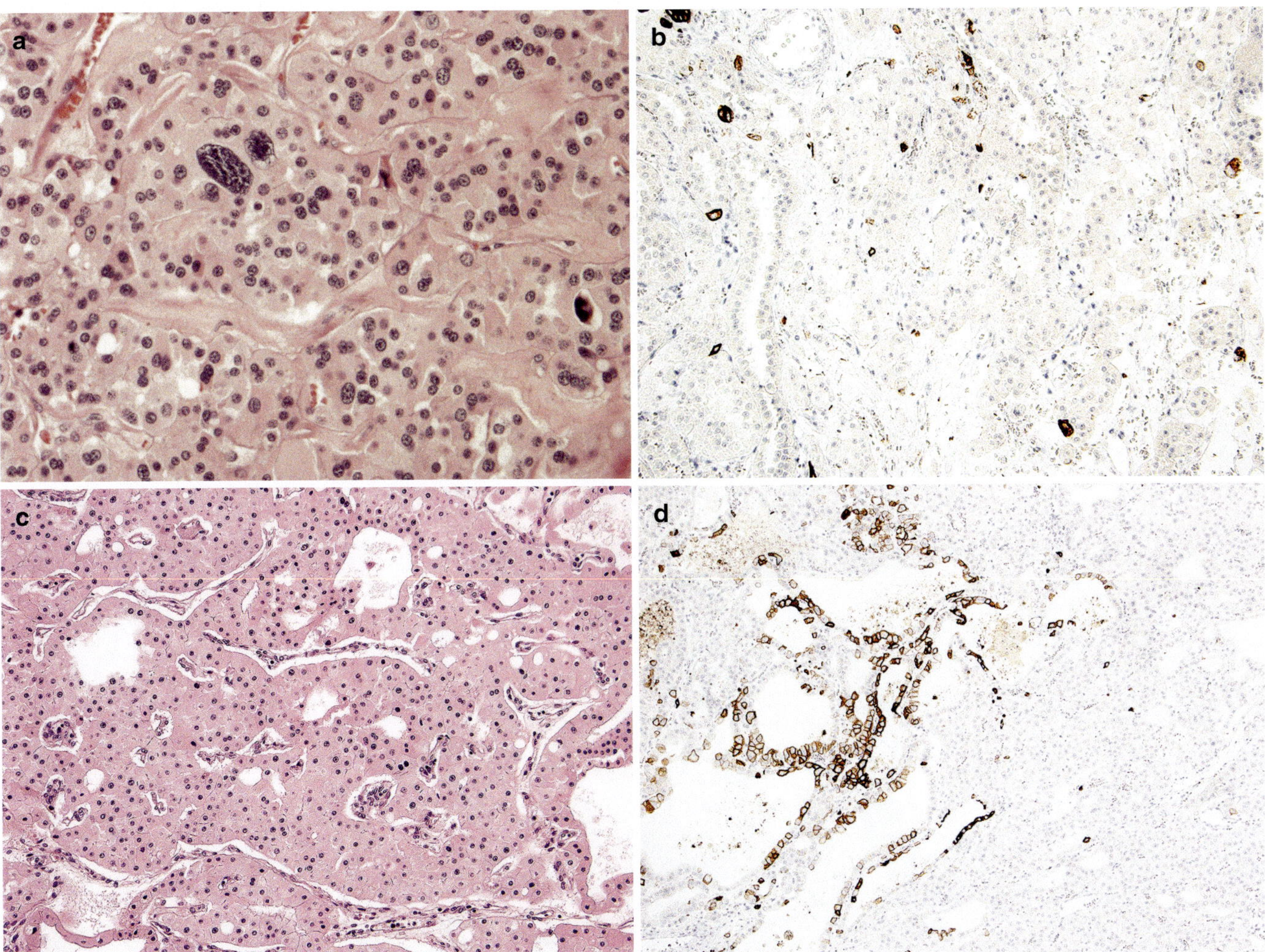

Fig. 1.18 (**a**) Oncocytoma can contain occasional atypical cells, generally considered to represent degenerative atypia. (**b**) The expected staining pattern of cytokeratin 7 in oncocytoma is labeling of scattered individual cells. (**c**) Eosinophilic chromophobe can mimic the cytology of oncocytoma, but extensive trabecular growth is a clue to the diagnosis. (**d**) Eosinophilic chromophobe may not necessarily exhibit diffuse cytokeratin 7, as expected of classic cases. However, patch-like contiguous areas of staining, as shown here, would be an argument against oncocytoma

with pale cells rarely presents a diagnostic challenge with oncocytoma, and so this discussion focuses on eosinophilic chromophobe.

References: [20, 21, 23, 32, 36, 57, 64, 82–85].

Collecting Duct Carcinoma vs. Mimics

With increased understanding of the pathology and genetics of renal cancer, collecting duct carcinoma has become essentially a diagnosis of exclusion, after several other entities are excluded. These tumors are highly aggressive renal malignancies, often necessitating aggressive therapy more akin to that of urothelial carcinoma than renal cell carcinoma. Features distinguishing this group of closely related entities are summarized in Table 1.19.

- All of the mimics of collecting duct carcinoma can have similar histologic features, including: infiltrating glands or cords/sheets/nests, papillary or tubular-papillary structures, or cribriform structures.
- Recently, disruption of INI-1 (*SMARCB1* product) has been recognized in renal medullary carcinoma (Fig. 1.19a). Although medullary carcinoma occurs essentially by definition in the setting of sickle cell trait, an emerging subgroup of tumors with INI-1 loss in the absence of sickle

Table 1.19 Collecting duct carcinoma vs. mimics

	Collecting duct carcinoma	Medullary carcinoma	Fumarate hydratase-deficient RCC	Urothelial carcinoma	Secondary metastatic carcinoma
Gross features	May be partly centered on medulla	May be partly centered on medulla	Less medullary centered	Renal pelvis or ureter involvement with careful search, may overrun the kidney	Often single mass (not necessarily multiple)
Clinical scenario	None of the others apply and metastasis from another organ argued against	Sickle cell trait (if not, then "RCC unclassified with medullary phenotype")	HLRCC syndrome (uterine and cutaneous leiomyomas); if no germline alteration, "FH-deficient RCC"	Association with in situ lesion(s) of renal pelvis or ureter	History of cancer of another organ, may be long duration (10–20 years)
Helpful immunohistochemistry	PAX8 positive, other phenotypes excluded	INI-1 (*SMARCB1* product) abnormal negative	Abnormal negative FH, positive 2-succino-cysteine	GATA3 or p63 positive	Positive markers of another primary cancer (e.g., TTF1 for lung cancer)
Genetics	Alterations of *NF2, SETD2, CDKN2A*; alteration of *SMARCB1* has been reported, but may represent "medullary phenotype"	*SMARCB1* (INI1) alterations/ translocations	*FH* mutations (usually germline, possible rare sporadic cases)	*TP53* alterations, *TERT* promoter mutations	As applicable to patient's primary cancer

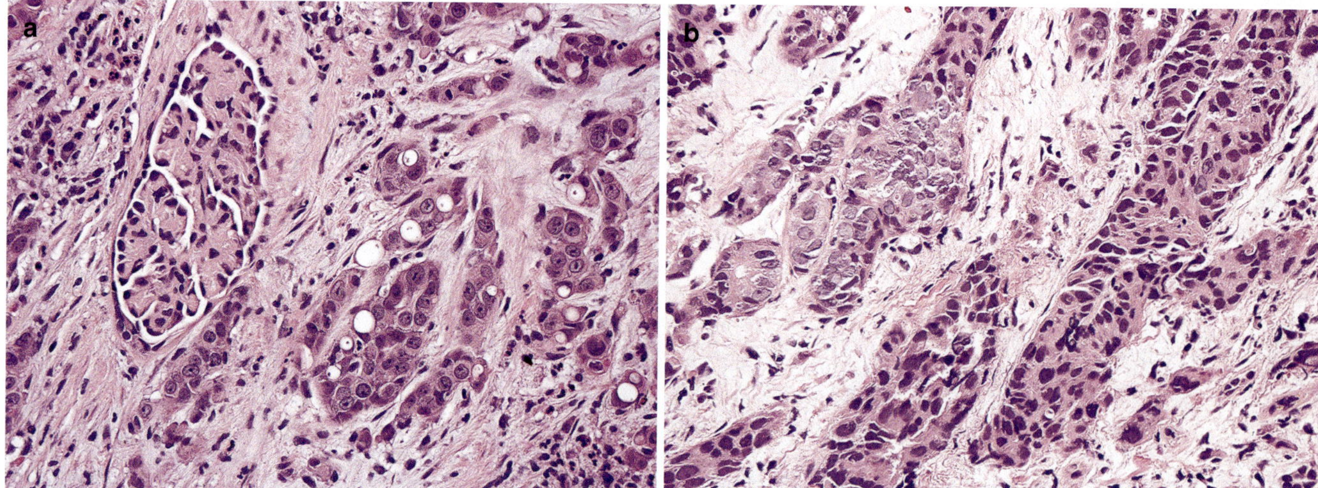

Fig. 1.19 (**a**) Histologic features of renal medullary carcinoma (pictured), collecting duct carcinoma, fumarate hydratase-deficient carcinoma, and urothelial carcinoma can overlap significantly, such that the clinical scenario and special studies are routinely needed. This example is a medullary carcinoma in a 16-year-old boy with sickle trait. (**b**) Metastases to the kidney can mimic primary neoplasms. This is a metastatic adenocarcinoma of lung origin involving the kidney in a renal mass biopsy

trait has been described, under the proposed name "RCC unclassified with medullary phenotype."

- Metastases to the kidney can mimic primary tumors, including solitary masses mimicking a primary tumor many years after original diagnosis.
- Most common metastases to the kidney include those of: lung (Fig. 1.19b), breast, gynecologic, colorectal, and head and neck primary origins.

References: [6, 7, 72, 73, 86–92].

Diagnostic Criteria for Sarcomatoid RCC and Clinical Significance

- The presence of sarcomatoid (sarcoma-like) histology is associated with a poor prognosis in cancers arising from various organs, and renal cell carcinoma with sarcomatoid differentiation represents the most aggressive, treatment-resistant group of renal tumors.
- RCC with sarcomatoid features is not currently recognized as a specific type of RCC mainly because sarcomatoid areas can be observed in all histologic subtypes of RCC. If no underlying RCC subtype is detected, then a tumor with pure sarcomatoid differentiation falls into the category of unclassified RCC and should be distinguished from sarcoma.
- The presence of sarcomatoid features is an independent predictor of poor survival and by many studies considered the most influential prognostic variable for patient outcome.
- Several studies have looked at the effect of the percentage of sarcomatoid differentiation on prognosis and demonstrated that greater amounts were associated with a worse outcome, however there is no agreed upon cut-point for risk stratification at this time. Therefore, any amount of sarcomatoid morphology and underlying RCC subtype should be reported.
- Recognition and reporting of sarcomatoid change in RCC is also required due to potential treatment implication (i.e., using more aggressive systemic therapy, targeted therapy after molecular profiling, including or excluding patients from experimental clinical trials).
- Sarcomatoid RCC is often considered and managed as a single clinical entity, regardless of the underlying parent RCC subtype with which it is associated. However, recent molecular studies have shown that sarcomatoid RCC is a heterogeneous disease requiring precise molecular classification to improve diagnosis, prognosis, and therapeutic management.
- Detailed characteristics of RCC with sarcomatoid features are listed in Table 1.20 (see also Fig. 1.20).

References: [50, 93–96].

Table 1.20 Detailed diagnostic criteria of sarcomatoid RCC

Criteria	Sarcomatoid RCC
Incidence	1–8% of RCCs, ~1/6 of advanced kidney cancers
Epidemiology	Mean age 60 years
Pathogenesis	Dedifferentiation of a lower-grade RCC (multiple mutational steps)
Presentation	90% patients are symptomatic with pain, hematuria, weight loss, fatigue, and other signs of primary mass or metastases
Associated tumors	Reported in all main RCC subtypes; >80% cases with clear cell RCC
Gross	Large (>10 cm) heterogeneous tumor with multiple solid white or gray areas with fleshy or firm cut surface, infiltrative margins (Fig. 1.20)
Histology: Biphasic—Sarcoma-like plus underlying RCC	Atypical spindle cells arranged into sheets and fascicles with storiform pattern (fibrosarcoma-like) or pleomorphic undifferentiated sarcoma pattern; occasional areas of heterologous elements (osteosarcoma, chondrosarcoma, or rhabdomyosarcoma)
Lower-grade RCC component	Present in the majority of cases with careful sampling (mean ~ 40%, median ~ 50% tumor volume); pure sarcomatoid extremely rare (4%)
Grade	ISUP/WHO grade 4 by definition
Stage	45–85% present at advanced tumor stage 3 or 4
Metastases	~40% patients with distant metastases to lung, bone, nodes, liver, and brain
Molecular findings	Complex set of chromosomal gains and losses, common −13q (75%) and −4q (50%) plus mutations of PTEN, TP53, and RELN
Median survival	4–9 months after diagnosis; 5-year cancer-specific survival 15–22%

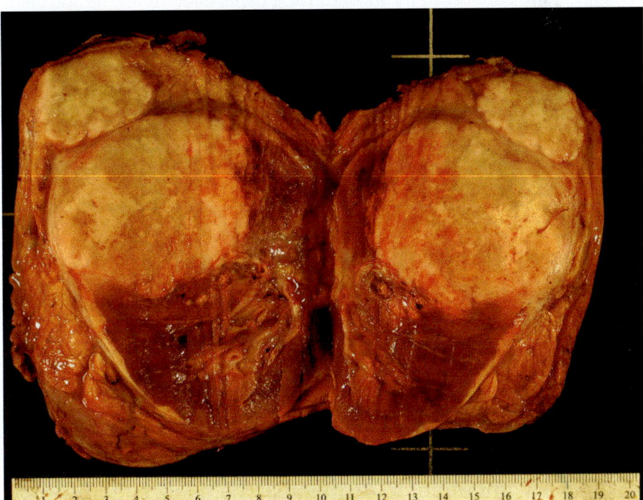

Fig. 1.20 Gross image of clear cell renal cell carcinoma with extensive sarcomatoid dedifferentiation showing heterogeneous fleshy grayish cut surface and areas of geographic necrosis

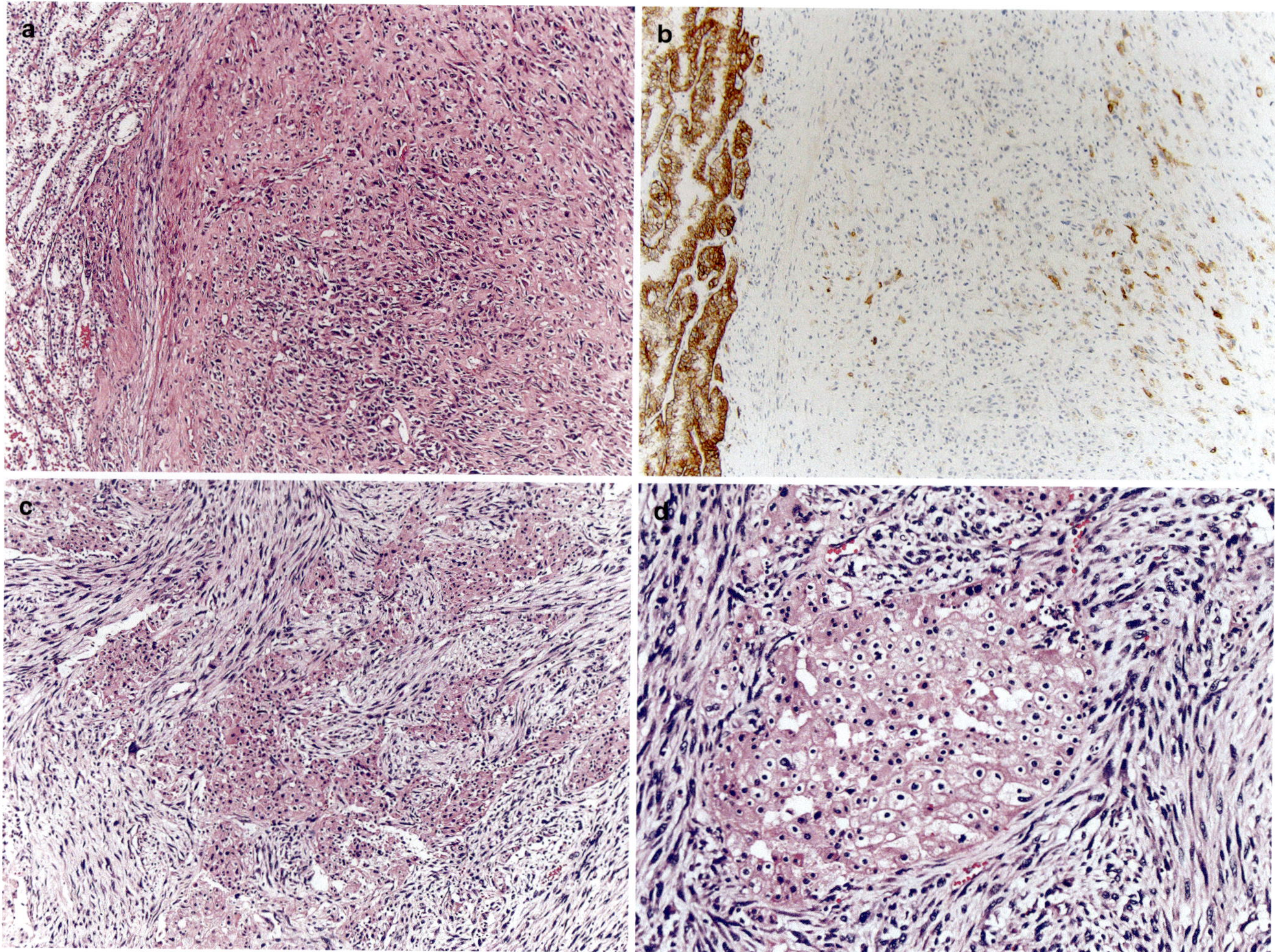

Fig. 1.21 (**a**) Clear cell renal cell carcinoma (left) with abrupt transition to area of sarcomatoid dedifferentiation (right). (**b**) Immunostaining with carbonic anhydrase IX shows strong expression in low-grade clear cell renal cell carcinoma area (left) and only focal scattered positivity within sarcomatoid area (right). (**c**) Microscopic image of sarcomatoid carcinoma arising in a background of chromophobe renal cell carcinoma (100×). (**d**) Higher magnification of sarcomatoid carcinoma surrounding area of low-grade classic chromophobe RCC with plant-like membranous accentuation, raisinoid nuclei, perinuclear halos, and cohesive solid growth pattern (200×)

How to Distinguish Sarcomatoid RCC from a Sarcoma?

Sarcomatoid dedifferentiation can be found in association with any of main subtypes of renal cell carcinoma (RCC). Sarcomatoid dedifferentiation is not very common (<5% of all RCC), but its prevalence is ten times higher than of primary kidney sarcoma.

- Although sarcomatoid RCCs resemble classic sarcomas, it is very important to distinguish them since the prognosis and treatment for both tumors are different.
- Grossly sarcomatoid RCC is centered in the kidney parenchyma, while a sarcoma is often developed from the renal capsule or soft tissue adjacent to the kidney.

- Sarcomatoid RCC can be derived from either low-grade (30%) or high-grade RCC (70%). Therefore, sarcomatoid RCC is typically composed of a low-grade or high-grade RCC component and a high-grade spindle cell sarcomatoid component (Fig. 1.21a–d).
- Sarcomatoid RCC is typically composed of multiple heterogeneous nodules in a large mass greater than 10 cm. Sufficient sampling from different tumor nodules is necessary to identify the lower-grade RCC component.
- Sarcomatoid RCC is usually positive for pan-cytokeratins and PAX8 (at least focally), whereas other markers of RCC subtypes may be negative.
- The comparison between sarcomatoid RCC and sarcoma is listed in Table 1.21.

References: [93–95, 97, 98].

Table 1.21 Sarcomatoid RCC vs. sarcoma

	Sarcomatoid RCC	Sarcoma
Pathogenesis	Dedifferentiation of a lower-grade RCC	Malignant transformation of mesenchymal cells
Tumor epicenter	Renal parenchyma	Renal capsule or perinephric tissue
Gross	Multiple areas of heterogeneous tumor	Large homogenous tumor with fleshy appearance
Presence of lower-grade RCC component	Yes (mean ~40%, median ~50% tumor volume); pure sarcomatoid extremely rare	No
Typical histology	Highly cellular areas of atypical haphazard spindle cells admixed with RCC components	Variable histological patterns: i.e., leiomyosarcoma (most common), liposarcoma, osteosarcoma, angiosarcoma, synovial sarcoma
Immunohistochemical (IHC) with epithelial markers	AE1/AE3, CAM5.2, and EMA are positive at least focally	Negative except for epithelioid angiosarcoma and leiomyosarcoma
Renal marker PAX8	Positive in ~100% lower-grade components and ~70% of sarcomatoid components	Negative
Other IHC markers	Desmin sometimes positive; lower-grade RCC components could be positive for CAIX, AMACR, CK7, CKIT, and TFE3	Expression of histogenesis-specific markers (i.e., SMA, desmin, MDM2, CD31, CD34, ERG, TLE1, and CD99)
Behavior	Always high grade (4); very aggressive malignancy	Low grade can be slow growing, high grade aggressive
Prognosis	Very poor (<30% survival)	Depending on the grade and location, but generally poor
Treatment	Surgery and chemotherapy	Surgery

Table 1.22 Sarcomatoid RCC vs. sarcomatoid urothelial carcinoma (UC)

Parameter	Sarcomatoid RCC	Sarcomatoid UC
Epidemiology	Mean age 60; slight male predominance	Mean age 71; male:Female ratio 3:1
Incidence	1–8% of all RCC	0.3–1.6% of all UC
Pathogenesis	Dedifferentiation of a lower-grade RCC through multistep mutational changes	Dedifferentiation toward mesenchymal lines from pluripotent stem cells of a carcinoma
Associated tumors	Lower-grade RCC (mean ~40%, median ~50% tumor volume)	In situ or invasive urothelial carcinoma
Pure sarcomatoid morphology	Extremely rare (0.2%), called unclassified RCC with sarcomatoid component	Pure sarcomatoid accounts to 0.6% of all urothelial carcinomas
Gross	Large (>10 cm) heterogeneous multinodular tumor with white-gray firm fleshy areas	Large polypoid and infiltrating mass with fleshy cut surface, hemorrhage, necrosis, and cavitation
Typical histology	Highly cellular areas of atypical haphazard spindle cells arranged in fascicles or sheets of pleomorphic cells admixed with RCC components	High-grade spindle and undifferentiated pleomorphic cells admixed with less prominent conventional urothelial, squamous, glandular, or small cells areas (Fig. 1.22a, b)
Heterologous elements	Very rare (case reports), most commonly osteosarcoma	More common (~10%), including osteo-, chondro-, rhabdomyo-, leiomyo-, angio-, and liposarcoma
IHC with epithelial markers	Low molecular weight cytokeratin, AE1/AE3, EMA	High molecular weight cytokeratin, AE1/AE3, EMA
Renal cell markers	PAX8 positive in ~100% lower-grade RCC and ~70% of sarcomatoid components; could also express CK7, AMACR, CD10, and CKIT	Negative, except for 18% cases from upper urinary tract
Urothelial markers	Negative	Positive GATA3 (70%), p63
Prognosis	Median survival 4–9 months	Median survival 14 months

Sarcomatoid RCC vs. Sarcomatoid Urothelial Carcinoma

- Sarcomatoid carcinomas are highly aggressive tumors that demonstrate biphasic epithelial carcinomatous and mesenchymal sarcoma-like differentiation. The mesenchymal or sarcomatoid component of these tumors consists of either undifferentiated spindle cells or elements showing heterologous differentiation.

- Sarcomatoid carcinomas arise from almost any organ system with an epithelial component, including the kidney and urinary tract, and often have overlapping morphology. Distinction between sarcomatoid RCC and sarcomatoid urothelial carcinoma is very important due to different prognosis and patient management (see Table 1.22 and Fig. 1.22).

References: [8, 50, 93, 99–101].

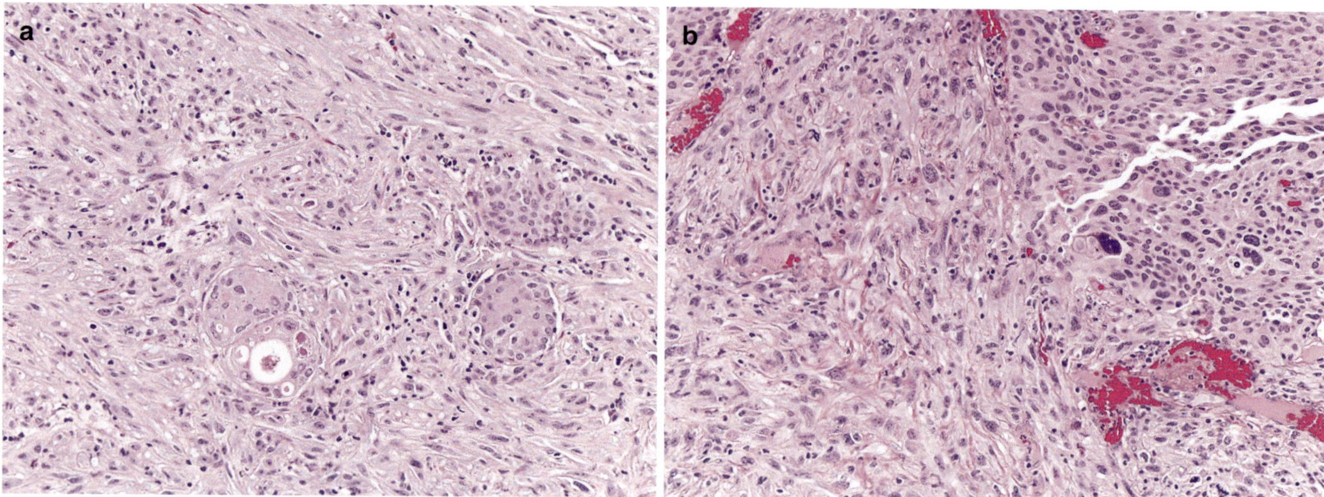

Fig. 1.22 (**a**) Small focus of low-grade urothelial carcinoma embedded into the sarcomatoid carcinoma. (**b**) High-grade urothelial carcinoma transitioning to sarcomatoid area

What Are the Histological Variants of Angiomyolipoma?

- Renal angiomyolipoma (AML) is a mesenchymal tumor composed of three main components in variable proportions: (1) angio—abnormal vasculature, (2) myo—smooth muscle cells, and (3) lipoma—mature adipocytes. Renal AML is believed to originate from pluripotent perivascular epithelioid cells (PEC) and also called PECOMA.
- The vast majority of renal AML are benign indolent tumors, although large tumors have tendency to massive retroperitoneal bleeding, and AML with epithelioid atypical features could show aggressive behavior. Multifocal and bilateral AMLs are often associated with tuberous sclerosis and genetic alterations in tuberous sclerosis genes *TSC1* (hamartin, 9q34) and *TSC2* (tuberin, 16p13.3). All renal AMLs are typically positive for smooth muscle markers actin and caldesmon, as well as melanocytic markers Melan-A (MART-1), HMB-45, MITF, tyrosinase, and cathepsin-K. Renal AMLs are negative for PAX8 and epithelial markers (EMA and cytokeratins) (Fig. 1.23a–f).
- Histological variants of renal AML in decreasing frequency are as follows: typical triphasic AML, predominantly leiomyomatous (fat-poor), lymphangiomyomatous AML, predominantly lipomatous (fat-rich), epithelioid AML, AML with epithelial cysts (AMLEC), oncocytoma-like AML, sclerosing AML, microscopic hamartomatous AML.

Table 1.23 provides description of all histologic variants of AML and differential diagnoses for each of them.

References: [102–106].

Renal Angiomyolipoma vs. Medullary Fibroma

- Both renal angiomyolipoma (AML) and medullary fibroma (also known as renomedullary interstitial cell tumor) represent relatively common mesenchymal neoplasia with overlapping morphology in some cases.
- Monophasic, sclerosing, and microhamartomatous variants of AML are more likely to have similar to medullary fibroma presentation (Fig. 1.24a, b).
- The overwhelming majority of renal AML and medullary fibroma with overlapping morphology are incidental small tumors with benign biological behavior.
- Distinction of renal AML from medullary fibroma is most important in case of multifocal and bilateral tumors due to association with tuberous sclerosis complex.
- The comparison between renal AML and medullary fibroma is listed in Table 1.24.

References: [103, 106–109].

Renal Angiomyolipoma vs. Mixed Epithelial and Stromal Tumor

- Mixed solid mesenchymal and cystic epithelial components could be seen in two unrelated renal tumors: angiomyolipoma with epithelial cysts (AMLEC) and mixed epithelial and stromal tumor (MEST). Despite striking radiologic, morphologic, and even some immunophenotypic overlap between these two neoplasms, their distinction could be made based on our understanding of etiology, pathogenesis, and molecular differences.

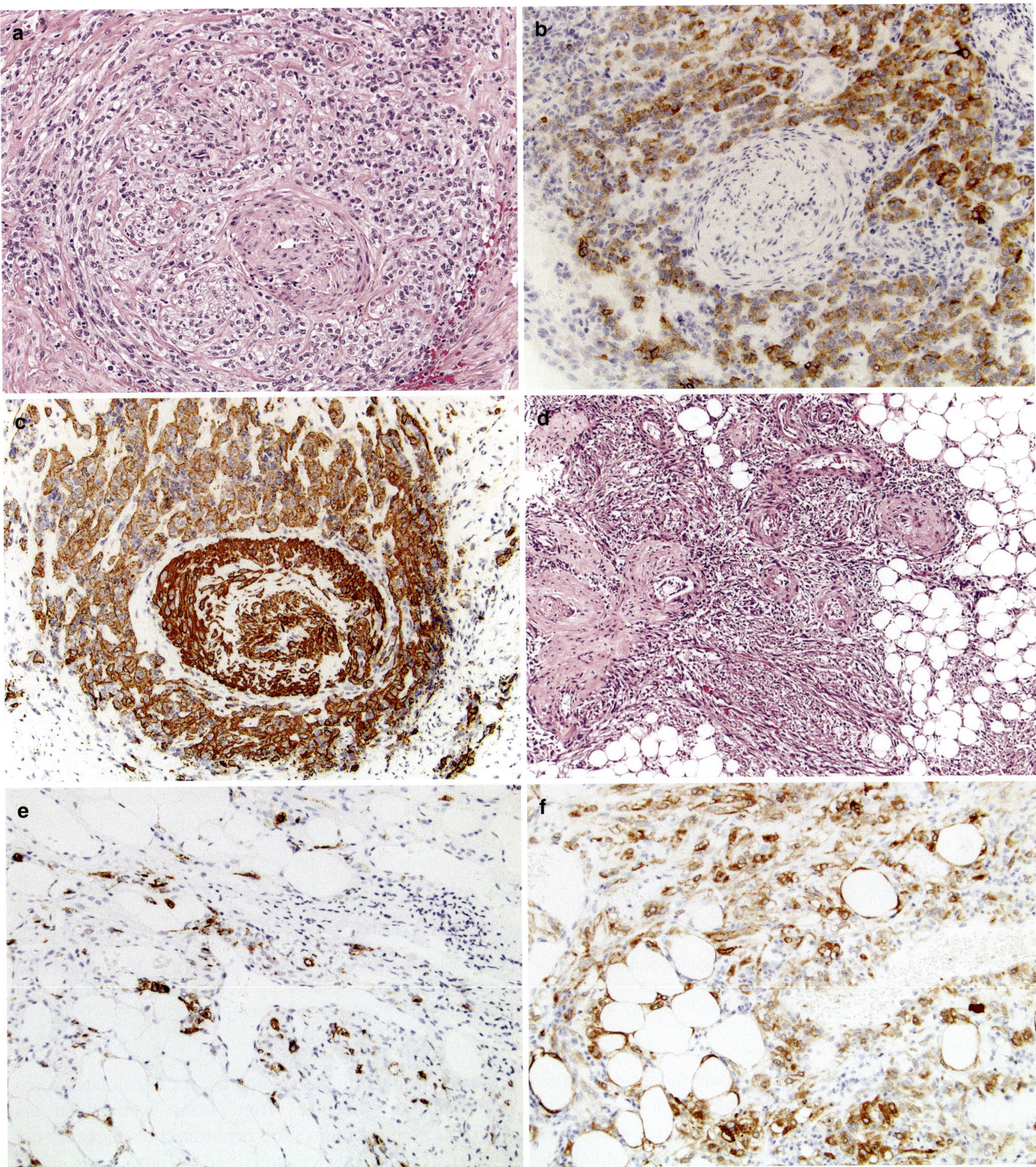

Fig. 1.23 (**a**) Perivascular epithelioid cells (PEC) surrounding abnormal vessel in PECOMA. (**b**) Strong reactivity with Melan-A in perivascular epithelioid cells. (**c**) Smooth muscle actin exhibiting bright labeling of abnormal vessel and spinning out perivascular epithelioid cells of PECOMA. (**d**) Classic morphology of triphasic angiomyolipoma (AML) with clusters of dysmorphic hyalinized vessels, spindled smooth muscle cells, and adipocytes. (**e**) Triphasic AML demonstrating scattered HMB45 positivity. (**f**) Triphasic AML exhibiting strong expression of Melan-A

Table 1.23 Variants of angiomyolipoma (AML)

AML variant	Components	Top differential Dx
Triphasic/classic (most common)	Dysmorphic thick-walled eccentric vessels, mature fat, epithelioid and spindle smooth muscle cells	Clear cell RCC with abundant stroma or sarcomatoid RCC
Predominantly leiomyomatous (fat-poor)	Usually subcapsular; fascicles of spindled or epithelioid smooth muscle cells often radiating of the vessel walls	Leiomyoma and leiomyosarcoma
Lymphangiomyomatous AML	Smooth-muscle proliferation growing in fascicles with clefts and associated thin-walled, branching vessels	Leiomyoma of renal pelvis
Predominantly lipomatous (fat-rich)	Mature adipose tissue with abnormal thick-walled vasculature and scattered small vessels with epithelioid cells	Normal fat, lipoma, and liposarcoma
Epithelioid AML	Sheets and compact nests of large eosinophilic polygonal or plump spindled epithelioid cells comprising >80% of tumor	RCC with oncocytic phenotype, metastatic melanoma
AML with epithelial cysts (AMLEC) or so-called cystic AML	Mixed solid and cystic architecture with epithelial cysts lined by cuboidal to hobnail cells	Mixed epithelial and stromal tumor (MEST) and cystic nephroma
Oncocytoma-like	Homogeneous population of eosinophilic polygonal cells with small nuclei	Oncocytoma
Sclerosing AML	Sheets and cords of spindled cells within abundant sclerotic stroma	Leiomyoma with sclerosis
Microscopic AML (microhamartomatous)	Small nodules of epithelioid perivascular smooth muscle cell proliferations	Medullary fibroma

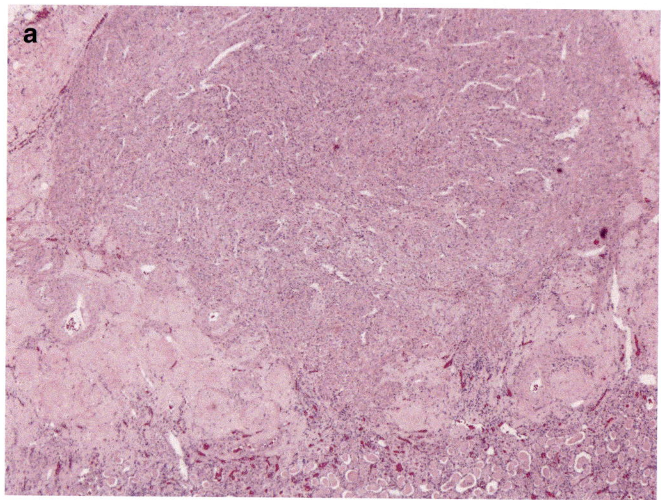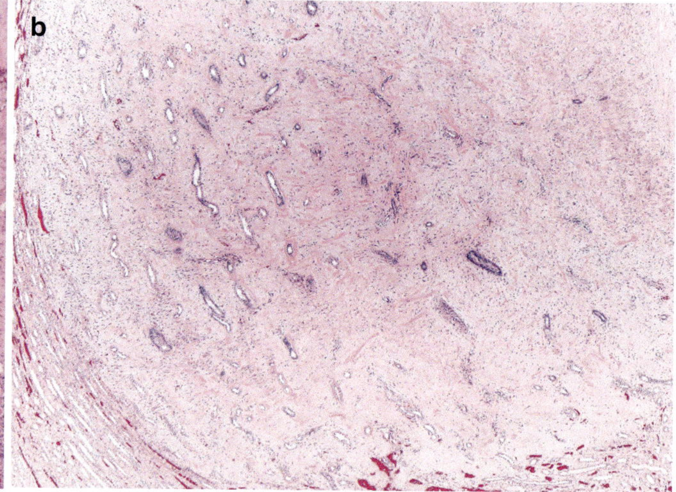

Fig. 1.24 (**a**) Monophasic AML composed of spindled leiomyomatous cells with vascular clefts, abnormal thickened vessels with hyalinization and fibrosis at the periphery. These tumors frequently arise in the kidney capsule (hence the name "capsuloma"). (**b**) Renomedullary fibroma composed of spindled and stellate cells embedded into the myxoid or sclerotic stroma with abundant but normal vessels

- AMLEC represents a very rare variant of fat-poor angiomyolipoma with characteristic combination of dysplastic vessels and plump epithelioid smooth muscle cells, plus cystically dilated epithelial tubules with cuboidal to hobnail lining and underlying compact "cambium-like" Mullerian-like stroma. Like any other angiomyolipoma, AMLEC shows prototypical co-expression of melanocytic and smooth muscle markers within the solid mesenchymal component (Fig. 1.25a, b).
- MEST is another rare biphasic tumor that typically occurs in perimenopausal women and consists of variably sized cysts and glands separated by more or less abundant stroma. Epithelial cells could be cuboidal, hobnailed, columnar, endometrioid, or intestinal type with eosinophilic, amphophilic, or vacuolated cytoplasm. Stroma ranges from scant hypocellular and fibrotic septa (adult cystic nephroma) to markedly cellular, condensed, edematous, and ovarian-like in classic MEST (Fig. 1.25c, d).
- Both AMLEC and MEST stromal component is positive for smooth muscle markers (actin, desmin, caldesmon), estrogen receptor (ER), progesterone receptor (PR), and CD10 highlighting condensed subepithelial Mullerian-like stroma underlying epithelial cysts.
- The detailed comparison focusing on differentiating features between AMLEC and MEST is listed in Table 1.25.

References: [104, 110–114].

Table 1.24 Renal angiomyolipoma (AML) vs. medullary fibroma

	Renal AML	Medullary fibroma
Epidemiology	Adults; peak age fifth decade; female predilection (4:1)	Adults; peak age sixth decade; very common; 10–40% on autopsy
Pathogenesis	Derived from perivascular epithelioid cells (PEC)	Renomedullary interstitial cells producing vasoactive agents
Etiology	Sporadic (>50%) or associated with tuberous sclerosis; mutations in genes *TSC1* or *TSC2*	Sporadic only; >40% multifocal (range 1–23 tumors per patient, mean = 3)
Presentation	Imaging surveillance; pain or hematuria if large	Incidental finding
Localization	Cortical or medullary; often subcapsular or renal pelvis	Renal medulla
Size	Mean size 4–6 cm	Very small; mean size 1.7 mm
Gross	Well circumscribed, unencapsulated with heterogeneous cut surface	Small solid nodules; white or pale-gray
Typical histology	Spindle and epithelioid smooth muscle cells admixed with adipocytes and hyalinized eccentric blood vessels; usually quite cellular although could be sclerotic	Spindle and stellate cells within pale myxoid stroma or densely collagenized low-cellularity tumors with amyloid-like material (typical for older patients)
IHC: Epithelial and renal cell markers	Negative (EMA, pan-cytokeratins, PAX8)	Positive only in occasionally trapped tubules (younger patients)
IHC: Smooth muscle markers	Positive (actin, caldesmon)	Positive (actin)
IHC: Melanocytic markers	Positive (HMB45, Melan-A, MITF, tyrosinase, cathepsin-K)	Negative
IHC: Other markers	ER/PR, CD34, S100 could be positive	ER/PR, CD34, S100 negative; COX2 and PGE2 positive
Behavior	Benign, but risk of retroperitoneal bleeding due to rupture when large and in pregnant patients	Benign, hardly any clinical significance; suspected association with hypertension is not proven
Prognosis	Very good	Excellent
Treatment	Surgery; mTOR inhibitors	None required

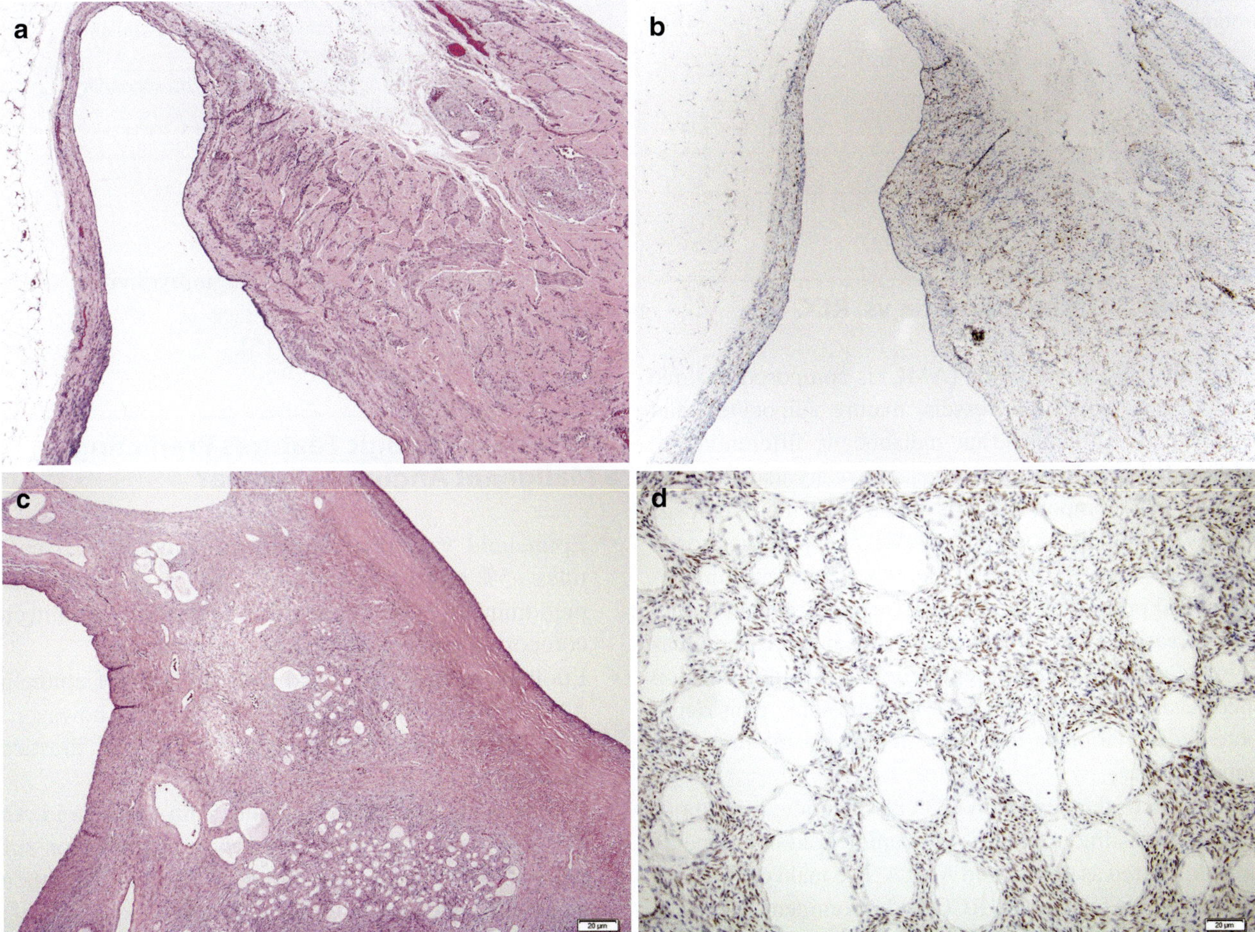

Fig. 1.25 (**a**) Angiomyolipoma with epithelial cysts (AMLEC) consists of solid areas with spindled smooth muscle cells and dysplastic vessels and cystically dilated epithelial cysts (40×). (**b**) Immunohistochemical expression of melanocytic marker HMB45 in AMLEC. (**c**) Mixed epithelial and stromal tumor (MEST) with variably sized cysts and solid component composed of tubules surrounded by spindle cells reminiscent of ovarian-type stroma (40×). (**d**) Mullerian-like stroma of MEST if highlighted by strong diffuse expression of estrogen receptor (ER)

Table 1.25 Renal AMLEC vs. MEST differentiating features

	AMLEC	MEST
Incidence	Very rare, ~20 cases reported; mean age 44; slight female predilection	Rare, mean age 52–53 years; almost exclusively in females
Pathogenesis	Derived from perivascular epithelioid cells (PEC)	Cell of origin is uncertain; hormonally dependent
Etiology	Majority are sporadic; few cases associated with history of tuberous sclerosis or multifocal	Sporadic
Hormonal imbalance	No association	Sex steroid exposure in men; diagnosed during pregnancy or perimenopause due to size increase
Presentation	Majority incidental	Majority symptomatic
Localization	Unilateral, subcapsular	Unilateral, medulla-centered
Size	Mean ~4 cm	Mean ~9 cm
Gross	Well-demarcated partially cystic mass	Multilocular complex cystic mass with firm solid areas
Epithelial component	Cuboidal or hobnailed; reported to express Melan-A and HMB45 in addition to keratins and PAX8	Highly variable: Glands, small and large cysts; cells could be flat, cuboidal, hobnailed, columnar, endometrioid, or urothelial-like
Stromal component	Muscle-predominant cellular stroma with compact subepithelial layer of "cambium-like" Mullerian stroma with chronic inflammation	Variable, ranging from hypocellular fibrotic to markedly cellular; ovarian type; myxoid; edematous or smooth muscle type
Abnormal vasculature	Always contains dysmorphic thick-walled eccentric vessels; muscle cells radiating from vessels	Absent, but have prominent normal vasculature
Stromal luteinization	Not reported	Reported with inhibin and calretinin expression
IHC: Melanocytic markers	Positive (HMB45, Melan-A, MITF, tyrosinase, cathepsin-K)	Negative
Malignant transformation	No reports	In large tumors: Stromal sarcoma, carcinosarcoma, chondrosarcoma, rhabdomyosarcoma, synovial and undifferentiated sarcoma
Behavior	Benign	Benign except for aggressive tumors with secondary malignant transformation
Prognosis	Very good	Good

Epithelioid Angiomyolipoma vs. RCC

- Typically, angiomyolipoma (AML) is composed of three components: abnormal vessels, mature adipocytes, and spindle cells with muscle and melanocytic differentiation. Although it may have focal degenerative atypia within the spindle cell component, it is not a difficult diagnosis. However, epithelioid variant of AML may post diagnostic challenges due to marked pleomorphism, multinucleation, and prominent carcinoma-like appearance reminiscent of various types of high-grade renal cell carcinomas (Fig. 1.26a–d). Moreover, epithelioid AML may develop metastasis or recurrence and is, therefore, considered potentially malignant neoplasm in contrast to other variants of AML.

- According to the current WHO classification, only those AMLs consisting of at least 80% epithelioid components are considered as epithelioid AMLs. The main differential diagnosis is a high-grade RCC with prominent oncocytic change and/or rhabdoid dedifferentiation.

Table 1.26 shows epithelioid angiomyolipoma (eAML) vs. high-grade RCC.

References: [17, 102, 115–118].

What Are Histologic Features Predicting a Malignant Angiomyolipoma?

- Epithelioid variant of angiomyolipoma (AML) constitutes ~5% of all resected AMLs and is characterized by predominantly carcinoma-like epithelioid architecture composing more than 80% of tumor volume.

- Etiology, pathogenesis, and epidemiology of epithelioid AML are similar to other AML variants; however, its morphology and biological behavior are drastically different.

- Five to sixty percent of patients with epithelioid AML develop distant metastases, have recurrence, or suffer death from disease, depending on the study. Although prognostic factors of malignant epithelioid AML are largely undetermined, several histological features have

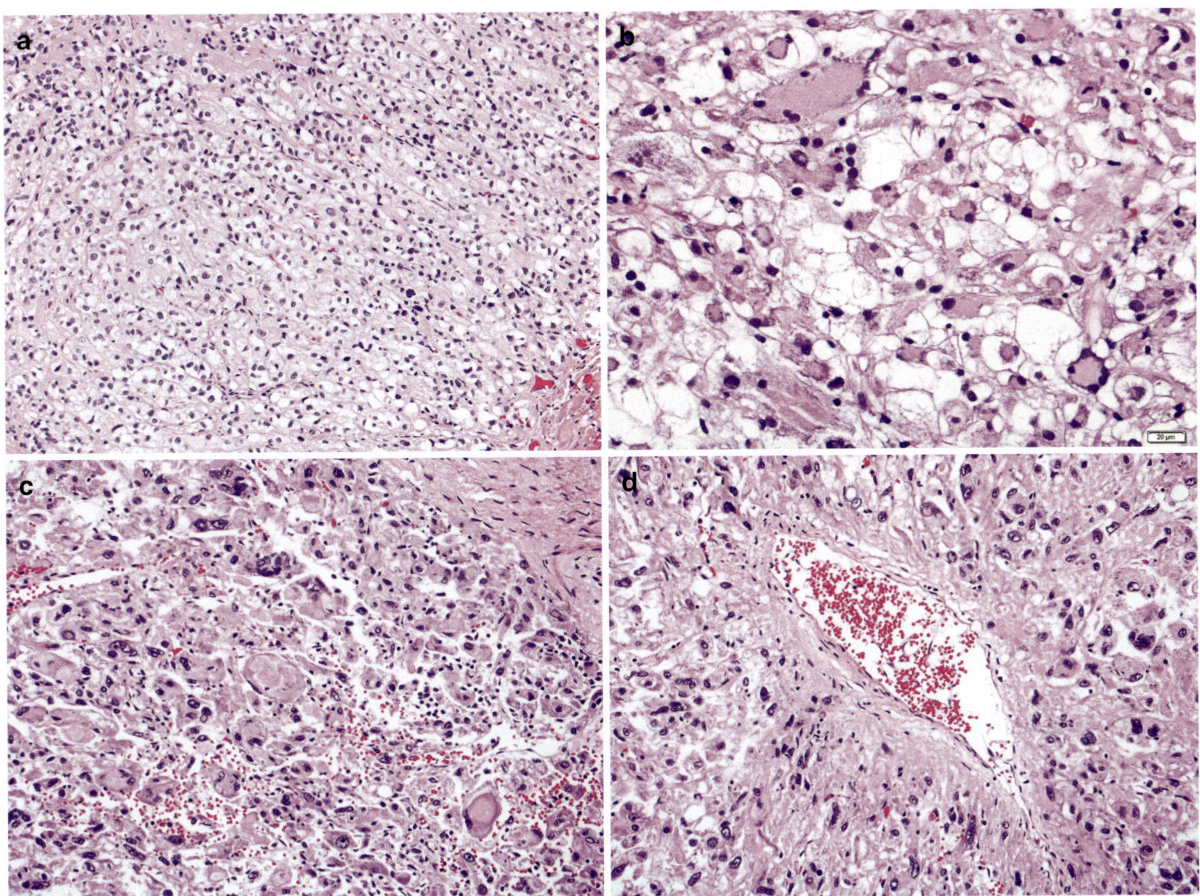

Fig. 1.26 (**a**) Epithelioid AML with "carcinoma-like" growth pattern imitating clear cell RCC. (**b**) Epithelioid AML mimicking clear cell RCC with pleomorphism and multinucleation. (**c**) Epithelioid AML with discohesive high-grade morphology and rhabdoid cells. (**d**) Epithelioid AML featuring perivascular growth pattern characteristic for PECOMAs

Table 1.26 Epithelioid angiomyolipoma (eAML) vs. high-grade RCC

Features	eAML	High-grade RCC
Incidence	Very rare; <5% of all AML	High; 30–50% of all RCC are high-grade tumors
Epidemiology	Peak age fourth decade; women > men	Peak age sixth decade; men > women
Etiology	Alterations in tuberous sclerosis genes *TSC1* (hamartin, 9q34) and *TSC2* (tuberin, 16p13.3)	Alterations of genes *VHL*, *cMET*, or *MiTF/TFE3* family; chromosomal gains and losses depending on RCC type
Pathogenesis	Derived from perivascular epithelioid cells (PEC)	Derived from tubular epithelial cells
Gross characteristics	Solid and circumscribed; gray-tan cut surface; size variable	Solid or cystic, multinodular; bright yellow or patchy cut surface; large size
Necrosis/hemorrhage	Could be present	Frequent
Architecture/morphology	>80% tumor with nests, alveoli, or sheets of plump epithelioid cells with large eosinophilic cytoplasm or smaller uniform cells with clear cytoplasm	Clear cell, papillary, or chromophobe growth patterns with clear and eosinophilic cytoplasm; ISUP/WHO grade 3/4
Atypia	Often markedly pleomorphic cells, multinucleation, giant cells, and ganglion-like cells	Scattered pleomorphic cells with rhabdoid or sarcomatoid features
Typical AML component	Absent or present (0–19%)	Usually absent, although has been reported
Mitoses	Common in pleomorphic tumors; some cases with brisk (>5/10 HPF) and atypical forms	Present, including atypical forms, but usually not brisk
Vasculature	Occasional thick-walled dysmorphic vessels	Usually well-formed, chicken-wire thin vessels
Vascular invasion	May have	Common
Melanocytic markers: HMB45, Melan-A, MITF, cathepsin-K	Positive, usually strong and diffuse, but can be focal	Negative, but TFE3 translocation RCC may be positive
SMA	Positive	Negative
PAX8	Negative	Positive
Pan-cytokeratins, EMA	Negative	Positive
Other markers: CAIX, AMACR, CKIT, TFE3	Negative	Positive depending on subtype
Prognosis	~5% aggressive; risk of malignancy increases if large size (>7 cm), high mitotic rate, atypical mitoses, necrosis, mostly atypical epithelioid morphology (>70%)	Mostly aggressive

been linked to increased risk of aggressive behavior of this tumor and are summarized in Table 1.27.

- The majority of published series agree that presence of three of more of such adverse parameters as large tumor size (>7 cm), necrosis, atypical mitoses, severe atypia, perinephric fat, or renal vein invasion significantly increases the risk of malignant behavior (Fig. 1.27a–c).

References: [115, 117, 119–125].

Renal Angiomyolipoma vs. Sarcoma

- Renal angiomyolipoma (AML) is a mesenchymal tumor that classically exhibits triphasic morphology including abnormal vasculature (angio), smooth muscle cells (myo), and adipose tissue (lipoma). All three components are derived from pluripotent perivascular epithelioid cells (PEC) expressing melanocytic markers, thus renal AML is also known as PECOMA.

Table 1.27 Histologic features of primary epithelioid AML differentiating patients with and without tumor progression

Histologic features	Progressors	Non-progressors
Tumor size	>7 cm or >9 cm	<7 cm
Necrosis and hemorrhage	Often present	Usually absent
Carcinoma-like	Always	Sometimes
Morphological pattern	Large polygonal cells with deeply eosinophilic cytoplasm and high N/C ratios growing in nests, alveoli, or discohesive sheets	Small monomorphic epithelioid cells with uniform nuclei, clear to granular cytoplasm, arranged in densely packed cohesive sheets
Adipocyte differentiation	Absent	Often present
Pleomorphism	Abundant multinucleated, giant, rhabdoid, and ganglion-like cells	Scattered clusters
Atypia/pleomorphism	>70% (severe)	<25%
Intranuclear inclusions	Common	Rare
Mitotic count	>2/10 high-power fields of view	<2/10 high-power fields of view
Atypical mitoses	Often present	Absent
Renal vein invasion; tumor thrombus	Common	Absent
Perirenal fat invasion	May be present	Absent
P53 overexpression	Present	Absent
Tuberous sclerosis complications	May be present	Not reported

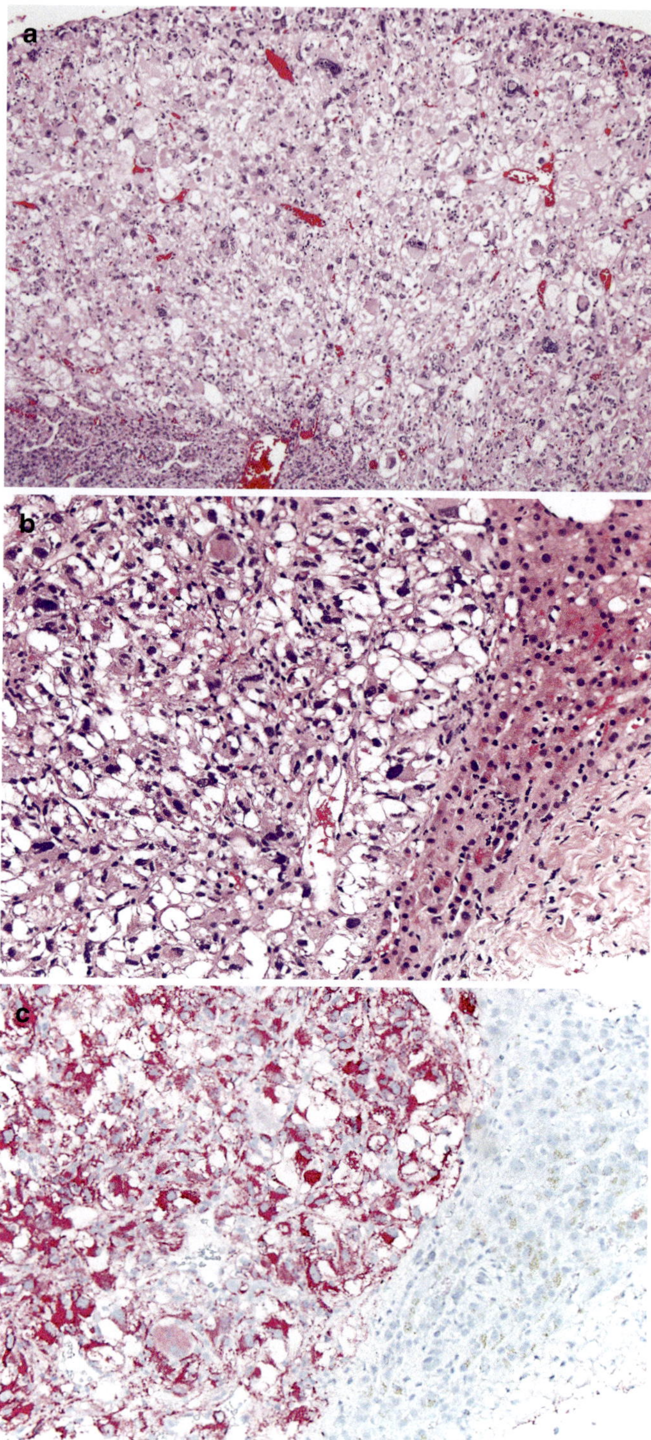

Fig. 1.27 (**a**) Epithelioid AML with severe atypia in >70% cells arising in the background of monophasic leiomyomatous AML. (**b**) Liver metastasis of high-grade neoplasm with marked pleomorphism and atypia mimicking clear cell renal cell carcinoma. (**c**) Diffuse strong expression of Melan-A supports the diagnosis of metastatic epithelioid AML

- Approximately 13% of renal AML have predominantly leiomyomatous (fat-poor) and 5% have predominantly lipomatous (fat-rich) morphology resembling well-differentiated leiomyosarcoma (Fig. 1.28) or liposarcoma, respectively. Their comparisons are presented in Tables 1.28a and 1.28b.

References: [97, 103, 126–128].

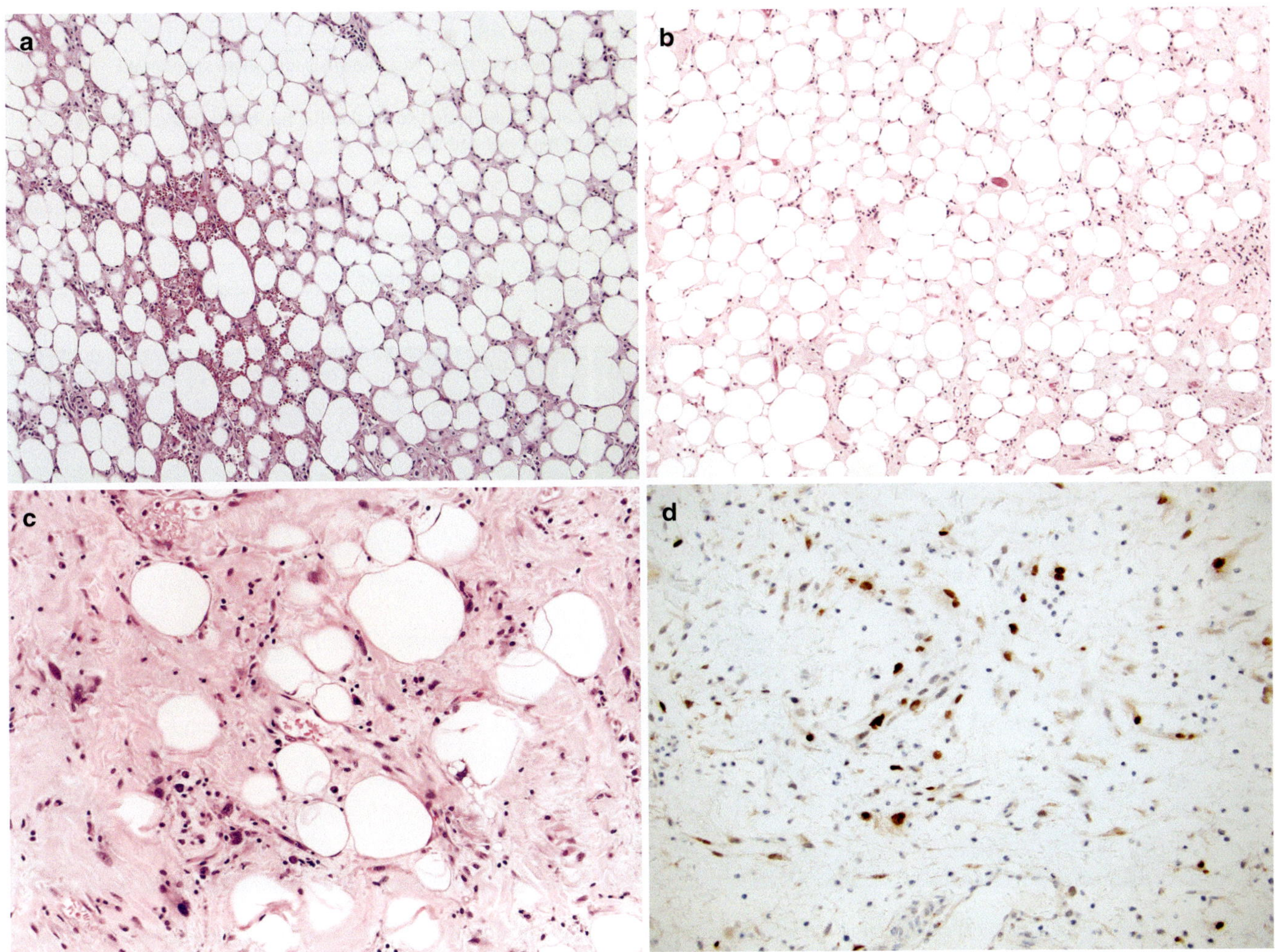

Fig. 1.28 (**a**) Lipomatous AML comprised of large sheets of variably sized fat cells closely resembling atypical lipomatous tumor/well-differentiated liposarcoma. (**b**) Well-differentiated liposarcoma composed of rather mature-looking fat cells with minimal atypia. (**c**) Examination of the same case at higher power allows identification of fibrotic areas with enlarged hyperchromatic cells and lipoblasts. (**d**) Immunohistochemical staining shows strong nuclear reactivity with MDM2 further supported by *MDM2* gene amplification by in situ hybridization in this case of well-differentiated liposarcoma

Table 1.28a Comparison of fat-poor AML and leiomyosarcoma

Feature	Leiomyomatous (fat-poor) AML	Leiomyosarcoma
Epidemiology	5th decade	6th decade
Prevalence	2nd most common AML variant	Most common sarcoma type
Location	Subcapsular cortical or medullary	Commonly involves entire kidney
Gross	Usually small solid rubbery mass; could be multiple and bilateral; extrarenal extension is not a sign of malignancy (common in tuberous sclerosis complex [TSC])	Large (mean 13 cm) encapsulated gray-white solid mass often involving perirenal or hilar fat
Histology	Fascicles of spindled or epithelioid smooth muscle cells often radiating of the vessel walls	Well-formed fascicles with occasional pleomorphic cells with haphazard growth
Mitotic activity	Low	On average 10/HPF
Necrosis	Absent	Common
Other features	Atypical vessels and rare fat cells	Marked atypia, plexiform growth
Melanocytic markers	Positive (HMB45, Melan-A, MiTF, tyrosinase, cathepsin-K)	Negative
Prognosis	Excellent	Poor

Table 1.28b Comparison of fat-rich AML and well-differentiated liposarcoma

Feature	Lipomatous (fat-rich) AML	Liposarcoma
Epidemiology	5th decade	6th decade
Prevalence	3rd most common AML type	2nd most common sarcoma type
Location	Subcapsular or hilar	Perinephric or hilar fat encasing renal parenchyma; true intrarenal tumors are very rare
Gross	Yellow, lobulated; smaller	Large yellow, lobulated
Histology	Mature adipose tissue with abnormal small and medium size thick-walled vessels	Sheets of adipocytes of variable sizes and shapes; enlarged hyperchromatic nuclei
Other features	Scattered epithelioid cells and radial smooth muscle collarets present with careful sampling	Atypical multinucleated stromal cells, lipoblasts, myxoid change; areas of necrosis and sclerosis
Melanocytic and smooth muscle markers	Positive focally	Negative
Prognosis	Excellent	Poor: Locally aggressive tumor

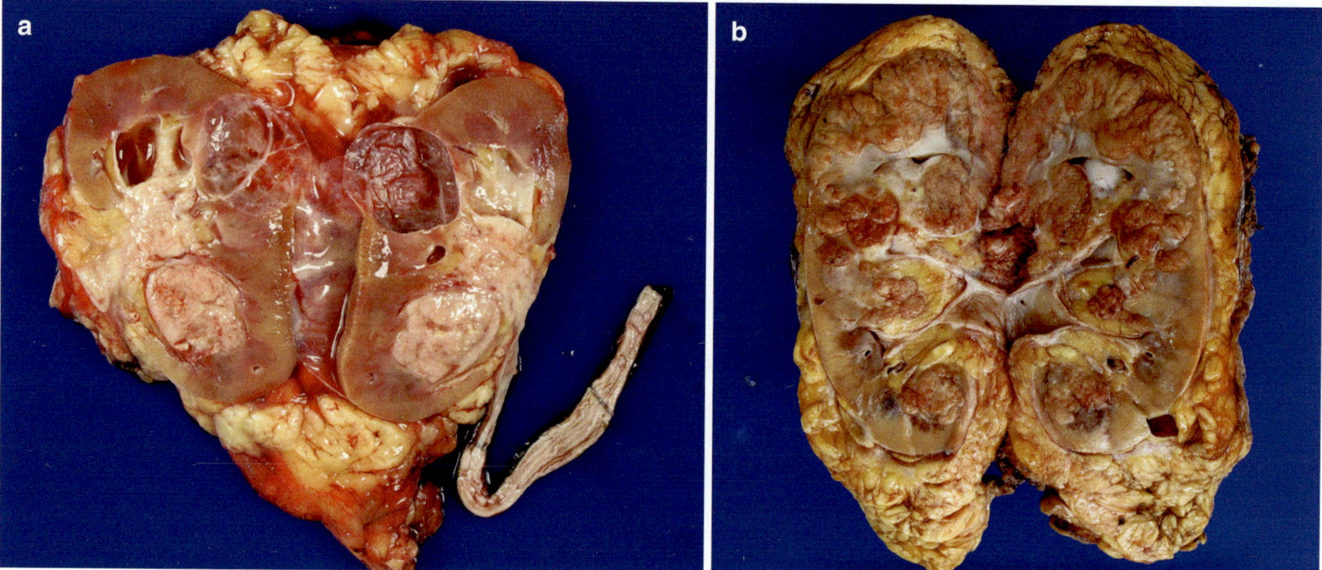

Fig. 1.29 (**a**) Gross photo of radical nephrectomy and ureterectomy performed for resection of urothelial carcinoma of the renal pelvis. (**b**) Gross photo of radical nephrectomy specimen performed for renal cell carcinoma, papillary type

Clinical Significance of Distinguishing Renal Cell Carcinoma from Urothelial Carcinoma of the Renal Pelvis

- Urothelial carcinoma of the renal pelvis (UCRP) develops from the renal pelvic urothelium. In general, UCRP is more aggressive than bladder urothelial carcinoma. In addition, there is a great risk of involving lower urinary tract because of tumor seeding. Therefore, UCRP will be treated more aggressively than either bladder urothelial carcinoma or RCC.
- Invasive and noninvasive UCRP are typically subject to more extensive surgical procedure, which includes radical nephrectomy, ureterectomy, and resection of portion of bladder (bladder cuff) (Fig. 1.29a). Since RCC is not a urothelial disease, it only requires a partial or radical nephrectomy without ureterectomy (Fig. 1.29b).

- If RCC is misdiagnosed as UCRP, the patient would undergo an unnecessary extensive resection including a ureter and portion of bladder. On the other hand, if UCRP is misdiagnosed as RCC, partial or radical nephrectomy alone is not sufficient for its treatment.
- Furthermore, the medical oncologists will use regimens such as gemcitabine or cisplatin-based neoadjuvant chemotherapy for UCRP patients, which are significantly different from treatment for RCC patients such as tyrosine kinase inhibitors (sorafenib, sunitinib), mTOR pathway inhibitors (i.e., everolimus), immune therapy with IL2, specific monoclonal antibodies (bevacizumab against VEGF), or PD1/PD-L1 inhibitors.
- Important clinical features allowing distinction of UCRP from RCC are listed in Table 1.29.

References: [17, 129–133].

Table 1.29 Clinically significant differences between UCRP and RCC

Parameter	UCRP	RCC
Tumor location	Hilar/pelvic region	Renal cortex or medulla
Clinical presentation	Hematuria common and occur at the early tumor stage	Hematuria is a sign of late stage with invasion into renal pelvis
CT/MRI	Pelvic mass if large enough	Renal mass
Ureteroscopy	Mass lesion	Negative
Intravenous pyelogram/ retrograde pyelography (IVP/ RPG)	Positive filling defect	Negative
Urine cytology	Positive	Negative
Preoperative diagnosis	Ureteroscopic biopsy	CT-guided percutaneous needle core biopsy
Cystoscopy	Necessary before and after nephrectomy to rule out lower tract urothelial carcinoma	Unnecessary; no risk of coexisting urothelial carcinoma
Ureter margin	Often need evaluation on frozen section	Not evaluated on frozen section
Surgery	Radical nephrectomy + ureterectomy + bladder cuff	Partial or radical nephrectomy
Chemotherapy	Gemcitabine-, cisplatin-, or carboplatin-based therapy	Required only in advanced disease
Targeted therapy	Not established	Tyrosine kinase inhibitors, mTOR inhibitors, immune therapy

Table 1.30 Distinction of UCRP from RCC by pathology and immunohistochemistry

Parameter/marker	UCRP	RCC
Origin	Pelvic urothelium	Renal parenchyma (epithelium of proximal and distal nephron)
Surface histology	Low- or high-grade papillary UC, carcinoma-in-situ	Normal urothelial mucosa
Gross	White friable mass in renal pelvis extending into the renal parenchyma	Bright yellow or tan mass of renal parenchyma rarely extending into the renal pelvis
Tumor border	Poorly defined	Well defined
Histology of invasive component	Small and large irregular nests of cells with mixed low- and high-grade nuclei	Alveoli, solid, or tubulo-papillary architecture with clear to oncocytic cytoplasm; variable nuclear grade
Desmoplastic response	Quite common	Rarely present
Glandular differentiation	Occasional	Always present
Squamous differentiation	Occasional	Extremely rare
GATA3	Positive	Negative
S100P; Uroplakin II/III	Positive	Negative
p63	Positive	Negative
HMWCK	Positive	Negative
CK20	Positive in 50–70% cases	Negative
CK7	Positive	Positive in PRCC, clear cell papillary RCC, and chromophobe
PAX8	Occasionally positive	Uniformly positive
CD10, vimentin, RCC	Negative	Positive
CAIX	Negative	Positive in CCRCC
AMACR	Negative/weakly positive	Strongly positive in PRCC; focally positive in CCRCC

How to Distinguish Urothelial Carcinoma of the Renal Pelvis (UCRP) from RCC by Histopathology and Immunohistochemistry?

- Both UCRP and RCC can have similar clinical presentation mimicking each other. Due to significant differences in surgical and oncologic treatments for these two cancers, it is very important to distinguish UCRP from RCC on pathology diagnosis.
- With limited material from needle core biopsy or fine needle aspirate, it can be difficult to differentiate UCRP from RCC. Moreover, intraoperative frozen section diagnosis to distinguish UCRP from RCC is not accurate and should be avoided if possible. In such a situation, immunohistochemistry can be particularly useful.
- UCRP will be positive for GATA3, S100P, Uroplakin II/III, high molecular weight cytokeratins (HMWCK), p63, and CK7/CK20. RCC will be positive for PAX8, CD10, RCC, vimentin, and other subtype specific markers (i.e., CAIX for clear cell RCC, AMACR and CK7 for papillary RCC, CD117 and CK7 for chromophobe RCC). However, it should be noted that approximately 18% of UCRP may be positive for PAX8, and a small percentage of RCC could express GATA3. Therefore, utilization of immunohistochemical panels is beneficial in difficult cases. The differential immunohistochemical profiles of these two morphologically overlapping tumors are summarized in Table 1.30 and Fig. 1.30.

References: [17, 129, 130, 134–136].

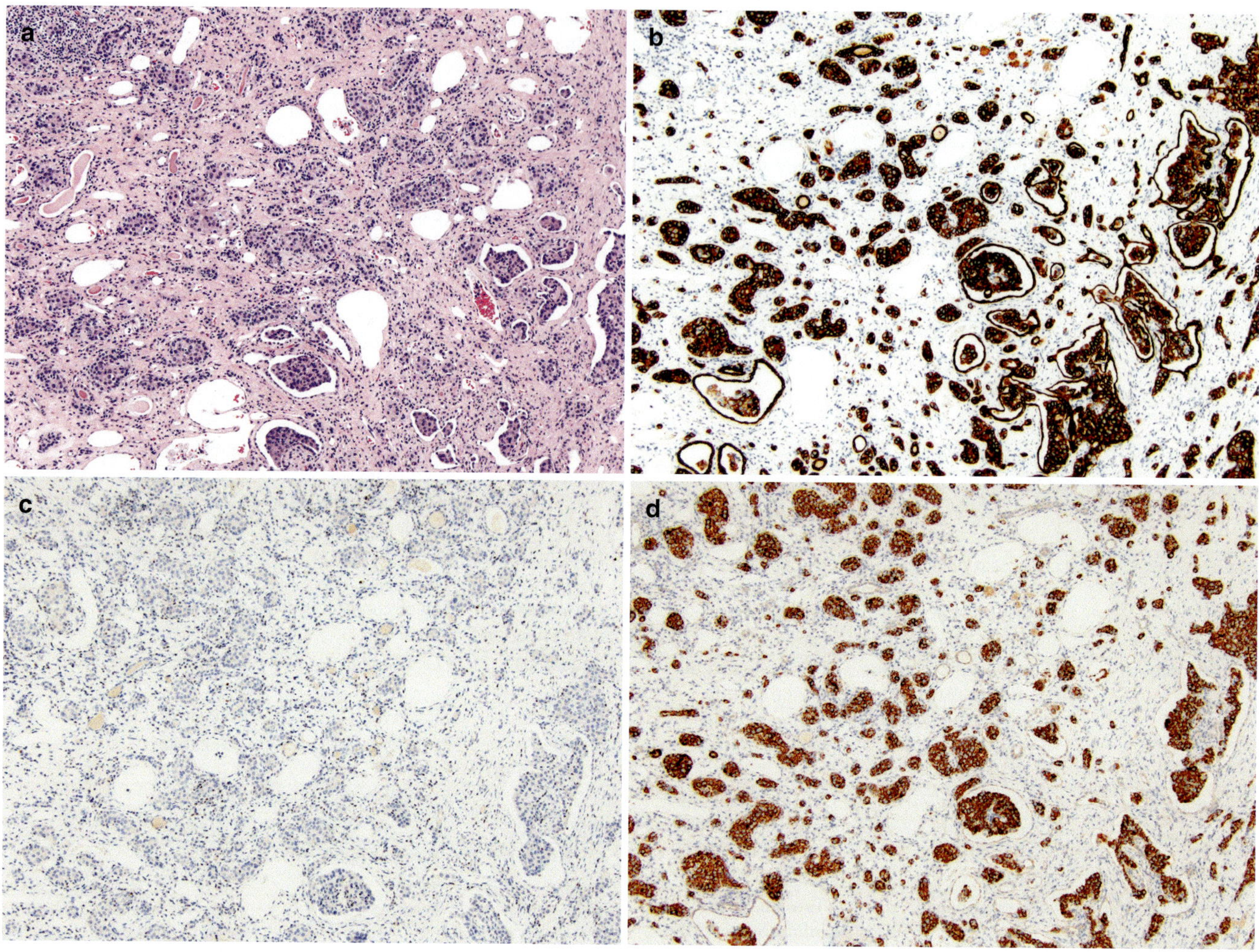

Fig. 1.30 (**a**) This medulla-centered tumor was composed of variably sized tumor nests infiltrating between benign kidney tubules and filling collecting ducts thus closely resembling urothelial carcinoma. (**b**) Strong expression of cytokeratin 7 in this case favors the following differentiation diagnosis: urothelial carcinoma vs. collecting duct carcinoma vs. papillary renal cell carcinoma. (**c**) Negative GATA3 expression in this case in inconsistent with urothelial origin. (**d**) Diffuse and strong expression of AMACR/P504 antibody supports papillary RCC diagnosis

Differential Diagnosis of Small Round Blue Cell Tumors

- "Small round blue cell tumor" (SRBCT) is a descriptive term referring to a large heterogeneous group of highly aggressive neoplasms, composed exclusively/predominantly of undifferentiated, small-sized cells with scant cytoplasm and round hyperchromatic nuclei. Due to their relative rarity in kidneys, similar morphology, and often overlapping immunohistochemical profiles, these tumors may be problematic to diagnose and classify. Moreover, the increasing use of small biopsies in daily practice makes correct diagnosis of these neoplasms even more challenging.
- The main differential diagnoses for SRBCT in pediatric population include Wilms tumor (nephroblastoma), neuroblastoma, clear cell sarcoma of the kidney (CCSK), and desmoplastic small round cell tumor (DSRCT), which are compared in Table 1.31a.
- The main differential diagnoses of SRBCT in adult patients include Ewing sarcoma/primitive neuroectodermal tumor (Ewing/PNET), small cell carcinoma (SmCC), lymphoma, and monophasic synovial sarcoma (SS), which are compared in Table 1.31b and Fig. 1.31a–c.

References: [137–147].

Wilms Tumor vs. Neuroblastoma

- Wilms tumor (nephroblastoma) and neuroblastoma (peripheral neuroblastic tumor) are among the most common childhood malignancies. Both tumors affect the same age group of patients often with similar clinical presentation and mor-

Table 1.31a Differential diagnosis of pediatric SRBCT

Parameter/marker	Wilms tumor	Neuroblastoma	CCSK	DSRCT
Mean age	2–3 years	1–2 years	3 years	10–20 years
Gross	Circumscribed and encapsulated, nodular, rounded, soft friable tan or gray mass	Solitary mass with necrosis, cysts, and hemorrhage	Large (11 cm), unifocal, soft, mucoid with necrosis	Bulky (>10 cm) firm multinodular mass with necrosis and hemorrhage
Histology	Sheets of undifferentiated, small, closely packed, blastemal cells with nuclear molding	Sheets and rosettes of primitive cells, fibrillary matrix, and rare ganglion cells	Nests, cords, trabeculae of small blue cells with fine chromatin	Solid nests of round-to-oval cells, small blue cells within dense desmoplastic stroma
Survival	>90%	~70%	70%	2 years (median)
WT1	Positive nuclear	Cytoplasmic	Negative	Positive (C-term)
PAX8	Positive	Negative	Some positive	Negative
CD99	Often positive	Some positive	Negative	Some positive
NB84	Negative	Positive	Negative	Negative
Chromogranin	Negative	Positive	Negative	May be focal
Synaptophysin	Negative	Positive	Negative	May be focal
Cytokeratin/EMA	Some positive	Negative	Negative	Positive
Desmin	Some positive	Negative	Negative	Positive, dot-like
Translocation	None	None	t(10;17) 10%	t(11;22)(p13;q12)
Genetic alterations	*WT1* mutations; *WT2, IGF2, CTNNB1, SIX1/2*; LOH 1p,16q	*N-myc* amplification; LOH 1p and 11q	*YWHAE-NUTM2B*; 85% *BCOR* duplication	*EWS-WT1*

Table 1.31b Differential diagnosis of adult SRBCT

Tumor type	Ewing/PNET	SmCC	Lymphoma	SS
Mean age	27 years	59 years	50–60 years	36 years
Gross	16 cm (mean) yellow lobulated infiltrating mass	Solid, soft, whitish gritty necrotic mass	Diffuse kidney enlargement or solid mass	11 cm (mean), necrotic cystic mass
Histology	Sheets of primitive small round cells and occasional rosettes	Small blue cells with molding, lots of mitoses and no visible nucleoli	Diffusely infiltrating or large sheets of discohesive cells	Monomorphic, highly cellular neoplasm with plump growing in short fascicles
Survival	2 years (median)	1–2 years	2 years	3 years (median)
FLI1	Positive nuclear	Negative	Negative	Negative
CD99	Positive diffusely	Negative	Some positive	Positive
BCL2	Negative	Negative	Positive	Positive
TLE1	Negative	Negative	Negative	Positive
CD45/CD3/CD20	Negative	Negative	Positive	Negative
Chromogranin	Some positive	Positive	Negative	Negative
Synaptophysin	Some positive	Positive	Negative	Negative
Pan-cytokeratin	Focally positive	Dot-like	Negative	Positive focally
Translocation	t(11;22)(q24;q12)	None	Variable	t(X;18)(p11;q11)
Gene fusion	*EWS-FLI1*	None	Variable	*SYT-SSX*

phological features of undifferentiated small blue cells phenotype making their differential diagnosis challenging, especially on small biopsies. This is particularly true in case of blastemal predominant Wilms tumor and undifferentiated neuroblastoma, which are considered high-risk malignancies and require more aggressive treatment (Fig. 1.32a, b).

- Table 1.32 highlights significant differences in epidemiology, presentation, pathology, molecular findings, and ancillary studies of these tumors.

References: [148–153].

Wilms Tumor vs. Clear Cell Sarcoma

- Both Wilms tumor and clear cell sarcoma of the kidney (CCSK) arise in pediatric patients with peak incidence at 2–3 years, similar presentation, and overlapping morphology.

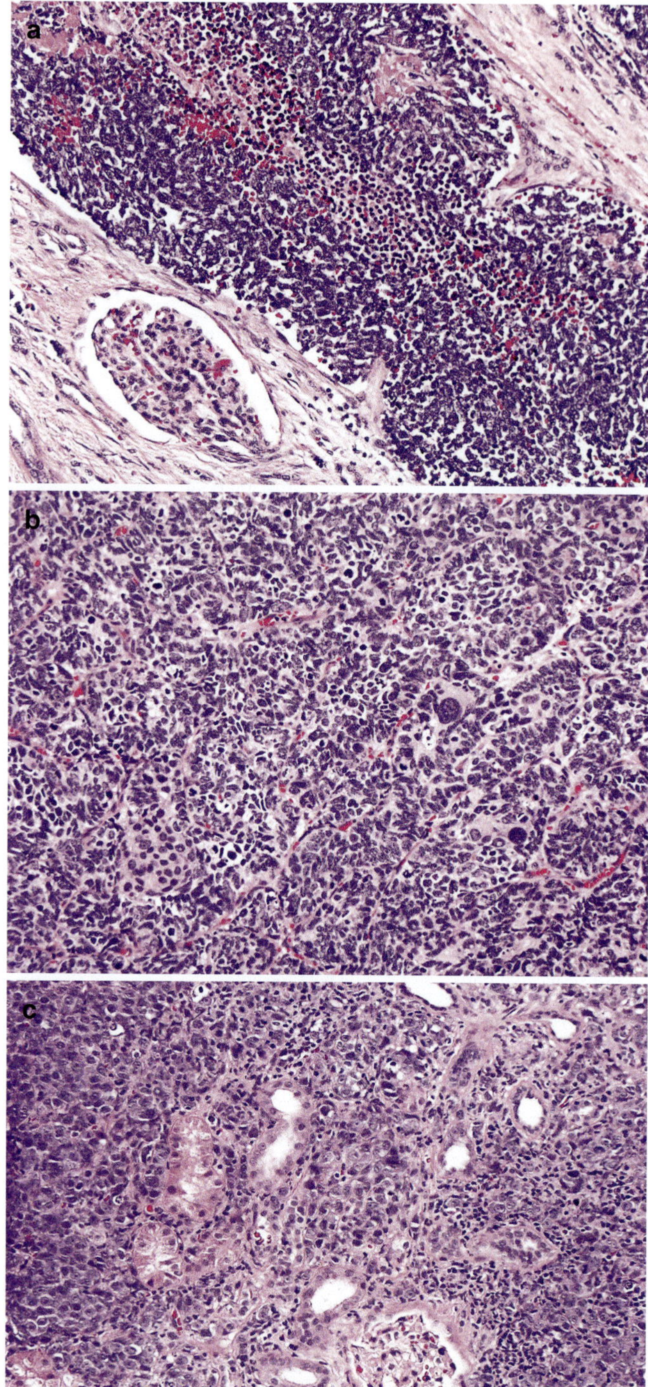

Fig. 1.31 (**a**) Primitive neuroectodermal tumor (PNET) of the kidney. (**b**) Small cell carcinoma with cell molding, lack of nucleoli, and abundant apoptotic debris. (**c**) Diffuse large B-cell lymphoma infiltrating between tubules and glomeruli

- In the National Wilms Tumor Study Group (NWTSG), CCSK is listed as a renal tumor with "unfavorable histology." Historically, CCSK was considered "Bone-metastasizing Wilms tumor," although this term is outdated since CCSK and Wilms tumor are unrelated.
- CCSK classically has three components: (1) small round-to-oval streaming (cord) cells with bland cytology and cytoplasmic clearing, (2) branching chicken-wire vessels forming fibrovascular septa (hallmark feature), and (3) intercellular mucoid matrix. Depending on cellularity and matrix prominence, CCSK could mimic either predominantly blastemal (more cellular) or predominantly stromal (less cellular) monophasic Wilms tumor (Fig. 1.33a, b).
- Table 1.33 highlights distinctive features of these two tumors.

References: [142, 147, 154–156].

Wilms Tumor vs. Rhabdoid Tumor

- Renal malignancies are quite common in children and a leader among them is Wilms tumor (nephroblastoma), representing ~85% of all diagnoses. Fortunately, Wilms tumor also has the best prognosis with overall survival exceeding 90%. Despite advances in treatment achieved with Wilms tumor, other pediatric renal tumors still have overall survival less than 70%. The most aggressive of all pediatric tumors is rhabdoid tumor with overall survival of 15–30%.
- Rhabdoid tumor was initially classified as a possible rhabdomyosarcomatoid variant of Wilms and historically included in the treatment protocols of the National Wilms Tumor Study (NWTS) Group. Absence of muscular differentiation coined the term rhabdoid tumor of the kidney (RTK), which is now recognized as a distinct tumor type of uncertain origin.
- RTK and Wilms tumor could share similar radiologic and morphologic features, especially with blastemal and anaplastic variant. In contrast to Wilms, RTK is characterized by an early onset of local and distant metastases (stage IV), and resistance to chemotherapy.
- Classic RTK exhibit cytological triad of vesicular chromatin, prominent cherry-red nucleoli, and hyaline pink cytoplasmic inclusions. However, many rhabdoid tumors lack characteristic cytologic triad and have the appearance of undifferentiated polyphenotypic tumor (Fig. 1.34a, b).
- A key to the RTK diagnosis is negative immunostaining for SWI/SNF-related, matrix-associated, actin-dependent regulator of chromatin, subfamily B, member 1 INI1.
- In Table 1.34, we outline the most important distinctive features of RTK vs. Wilms tumor, which should raise concern of this aggressive tumor and prompt diagnostic immunostaining.

References: [142, 154, 157–161].

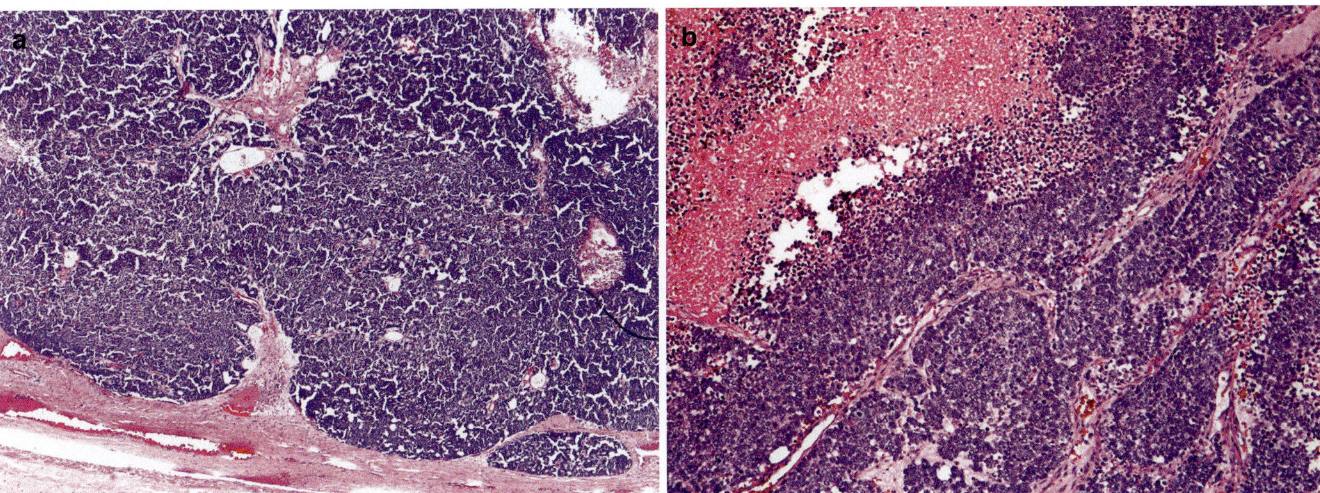

Fig. 1.32 (**a**) Wilms tumor (nephroblastoma) of predominantly blastemal morphology showing sheets of slightly spindled small blue cells. (**b**) Neuroblastoma with geographic necrosis and sheets of undifferentiated small blue cells

Table 1.32 Differential diagnosis of nephroblastoma (Wilms tumor) and neuroblastoma

Parameter/marker	Wilms, blastemal predominant	Neuroblastoma
Frequency	Most common renal pediatric cancer; 6% of pediatric cancers	Most common extracranial pediatric solid cancer
Peak incidence	Slightly older: 2–4 years	1–2 years; 25% congenital
Syndromic associations	10% syndromic: i.e., trisomies 13 and 18, Beckwith-Wiedemann, WAGR, Denys-Drash, bloom syndromes	Sporadic; 1% autosomal dominant familial cases
Presentation	Hematuria, hypertension, and often painless palpable abdominal mass with mass effect	Nonspecific (fever, weight loss, anemia, HTN) plus painful palpable mass
Prognosis	>90% survival, depends on histologic category (favorable or unfavorable) and stage	>70% survival; depends on age, subclass (level of differentiation), histologic category, *N-myc* status, mitosis-karyorrhexis index, etc.
Cell of origin	Nephrogenic blastema	Neural crest cells, primordial
Location	Kidney-centered; unifocal (88%), bilateral (5%), multifocal (7%)	Abdominal (54%), adrenal-centered (36%), extra-adrenal (18%)
Gross	Circumscribed and encapsulated, nodular, rounded, soft friable tan or gray kidney mass	Solitary mass with necrosis and hemorrhage, 80% with calcifications; adrenal-centered, displacing kidney
Histology	Blastemal predominant composed of sheets of undifferentiated closely packed small cells with nuclear molding; rare rosette-like tubules	Sheets of small round blue cells; Homer Wright rosettes or pseudorosettes; fibrillary neutrophil matrix, rare ganglionic cells
WT1	Positive nuclear	Some cytoplasmic only
PAX8	Positive	Negative
NB84	Negative	Positive
PGP9.5	Negative	Positive
Chromogranin	Negative	Positive
Synaptophysin	Negative	Positive
NSE	Negative	Positive
Cytokeratin/EMA	Some positive	Negative
Genetic alterations	*WT1* mutations (11p13); *WT2, IGF2, CTNNB1, SIX1/2*; LOH 1p,16q; 1q gain, p53 mutations	*N-myc* amplification (advanced stage); DNA ploidy, LOH 1p and 11q; *ALK* and *PHOX2B* mutations

Cystic Partially Differentiated Nephroblastoma vs. Pediatric Cystic Nephroma

- Unilateral multilocular cystic tumors in pediatric patients are represented by two different entities: cystic partially differentiated nephroblastoma and pediatric cystic nephroma. Both tumors affect young children, and have similar clinical presentation and undistinguishable radiologic and gross features causing significant diagnostic and therapeutic challenge. Definitive discrimination of these two entities should be based on detailed histologic assessment after rigorous tumor sampling.

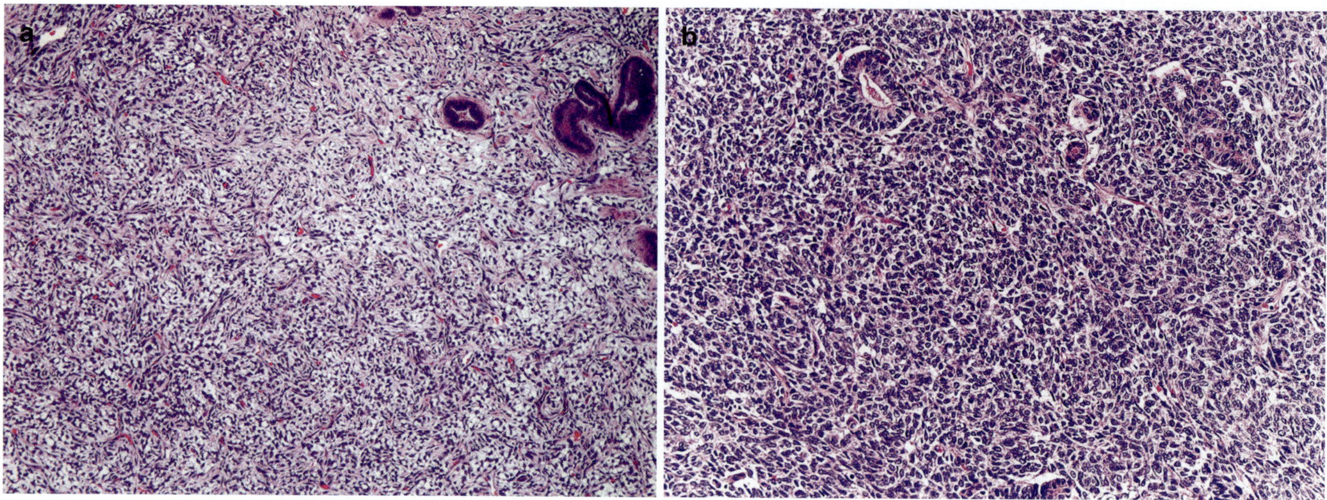

Fig. 1.33 (**a**) Clear cell sarcoma of the kidney composed of spindled clear cells embedded into intercellular mucoid matrix with chicken-wire vascular network and few entrapped tubules. (**b**) Wilms tumor of predominantly blastemal type composed of sheets of spindled hyperchromatic cells with scant cytoplasm and coarse chromatin and few epithelial-like tubules

Table 1.33 Differential diagnosis of Wilms tumor and clear cell sarcoma

Parameter/marker	Wilms tumor (nephroblastoma)	Clear cell sarcoma of the kidney
Frequency	Common: ~85% of all pediatric renal malignancies	Uncommon: 3–5% of all pediatric renal malignancies
Cell origin	Nephrogenic blastema	Unknown, probably mesenchymal
Syndromic associations	10% syndromic: i.e., trisomies 13 and 18, Beckwith-Wiedemann, WAGR, Denys-Drash, bloom syndromes, etc.	None
Prognosis	>90% survival, depends on histologic category (favorable or unfavorable) and stage	~ 70% survival; more aggressive tumor with pelvic lymph node metastasis in 1/3 patients and propensity to distant metastasis to bone, lung, brain, and liver
Location	Kidney-centered; unifocal (88%), bilateral (5%), multifocal (7%)	Unifocal, initially medulla-centered
Gross	Circumscribed and encapsulated, nodular, rounded, soft friable tan or gray kidney mass	Large (11 cm), unifocal, soft, yellow, mucoid with necrosis; often distorting or replacing kidney
Histology	Blastemal, small, closely packed, hyperchromatic cells with molding, coarse chromatin, scant cytoplasm, or stromal component with nondescript spindled cells	Lobular architecture with thin fibrovascular septa separating nests, cords, and trabeculae of small blue spindled cells with bland cytological features; chicken-wire vessels
Patterns/variants	Triphasic (>50%); predominantly blastemal, epithelial (tubular, rosette-like, papillary, glomeruloid), and predominantly stromal	Classic (~90%); also myxoid, sclerosing, cellular, epithelioid, palisading, storiform, spindle cell, and sinusoidal patterns
Other	Nephrogenic rests often present	No associated lesions
Anaplasia	~5% tumors	2–3% of primary or recurrent tumors
WT1	Positive nuclear, except stroma	Negative
PAX8	Positive	Some positive
CD99	Often positive	Negative
Cytokeratin/EMA	Some positive	Negative
Desmin	Blastema often positive	Negative
Genetic alterations	*WT1* mutations (11p13); *WT2, IGF2, CTNNB1, SIX1/2*; LOH 1p,16q; 1q gain, p53 mutations (anaplastic cells)	85% *BCOR* duplication; *YWHAE- NUTM2B*; t(10:17) and −14q; p53 mutation in anaplastic variant

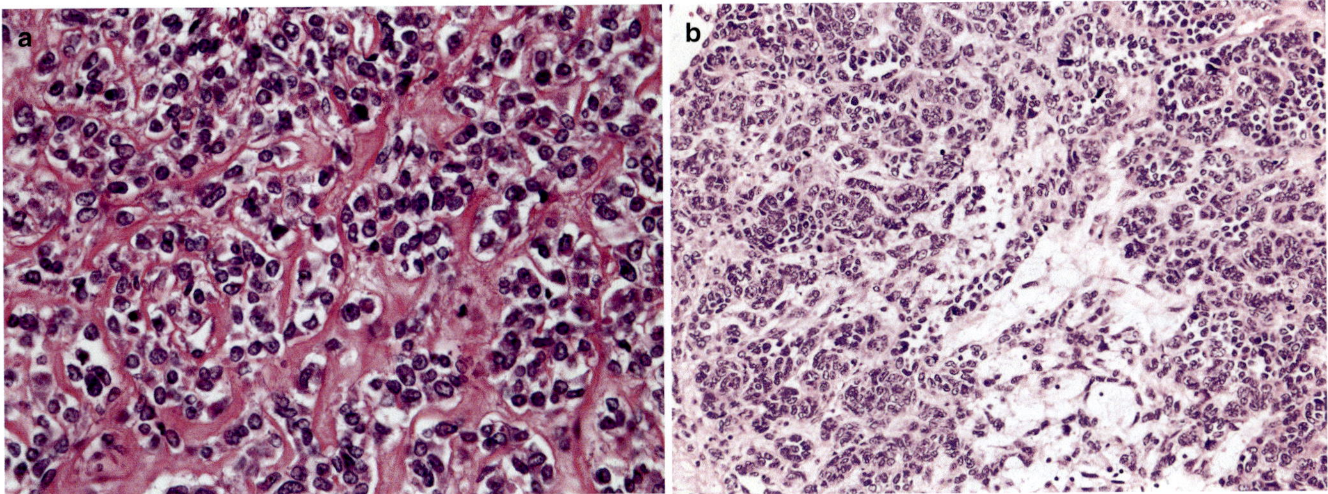

Fig. 1.34 (**a**) Rhabdoid tumor of the kidney composed of nests of undifferentiated cells with irregular nuclei and vesicular chromatin. (**b**) Wilms tumor of blastemal type with anaplastic features composed of pleomorphic cells with coarse chromatin and scant cytoplasm

Table 1.34 Differential diagnosis of nephroblastoma (Wilms tumor) and rhabdoid tumor

Parameter/marker	Wilms tumor (nephroblastoma)	Rhabdoid tumor
Frequency	~85% of pediatric renal tumors	~2% of pediatric renal tumors
Peak incidence	2–3 years of age	1 year
Cell origin	Nephrogenic blastema	Unknown
Syndromic associations	10% syndromic: i.e., trisomies 13 and 18, Beckwith-Wiedemann, WAGR, Denys-Drash, bloom syndromes, etc.	30% have rhabdoid predisposition syndrome with *hSNF5/INI1* germline mutation
Symptoms	Palpable painless abdominal mass, hematuria, hypertension	Hematuria plus symptoms of widespread metastatic disease
Location	Kidney-centered; unifocal (88%), bilateral (5%), multifocal (7%)	Renal mass plus often concurrent brain/CNS or soft tissue mass
Gross	Circumscribed and encapsulated, nodular, rounded, soft friable tan or gray kidney mass	Large (9.6 cm) irregular infiltrative unencapsulated mass with extensive hemorrhages and necrosis
Histology	Blastemal, small, closely packed, hyperchromatic cells with molding, coarse chromatin, and scant cytoplasm; larger anaplastic cells (3x) with hyperchromasia and multipolar mitoses	Discohesive sheets of polygonal cells with occasional globular or hyaline inclusions and eccentric nuclei ("rhabdoid"); nuclei usually pleomorphic, with vesicular chromatin and large cherry-red nucleoli
Associated lesions	Nephrogenic rests often present	15% patients with synchronous PNET-like brain mass
WT1	Positive nuclear: 75% blastema, 44% stroma	Cytoplasmic, but reported nuclear with C-terminus antibody
INI1/BAF47	Intact nuclear expression	Loss of nuclear expression
Cytokeratin/EMA	Some positive	Positive, but focal
Desmin	Blastema could be positive	Often positive
Genetic alterations	*WT1* mutations (11p13); *WT2, IGF2, CTNNB1, SIX1/2*; LOH 1p,16q; 1q gain, p53 mutations (anaplastic cells)	Biallelic inactivation of *hSNF5/INI/SMARCB1* tumor suppressor gene (mutation or deletion of 22q11.2)
Prognosis	>90% survival, depends on histologic category (favorable or unfavorable) and stage	Dismal: 15–30% survival; 80% patients die within 2 years from diagnosis (improved with combined surgical/radio−/chemo−/autologous stem cell transplant treatment)

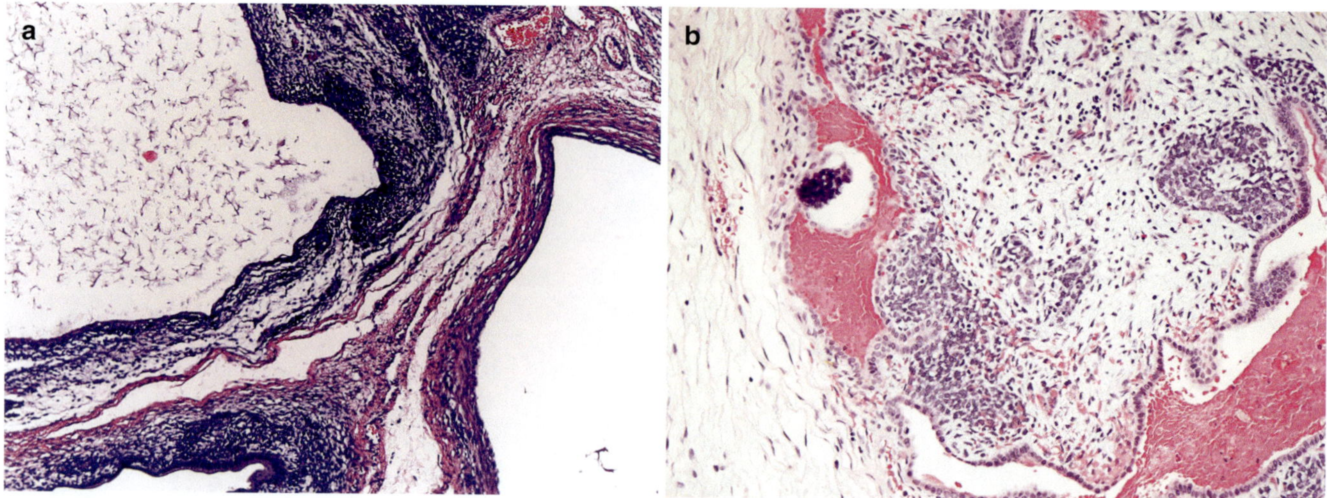

Fig. 1.35 Cystic partially differentiated nephroblastoma (CPDN) is characterized by multilocular architecture lacking expansile solid nodules (**a**) with fibrovascular septa containing immature nephroblastic elements (**b**)

- Cystic partially differentiated nephroblastoma (CPDN) is an indolent variant of Wilms tumor with pure multilocular architecture lacking discernible expansile nodules. Thin fibrovascular septa contain immature blastemal or differentiating epithelial elements that are not distorting septal contours or form expansile nodular areas (Fig. 1.35a, b). Due to low tumor burden, CPDN is characterized by indolent behavior with only two reported recurrences after incomplete resection or tumor spillage.
- Pediatric cystic nephroma (PCN) is a benign pediatric neoplasm composed of multilocular cysts with flattened, cuboidal, or hobnailed epithelium and fibrous septa with entrapped well-differentiated tubules lacking immature nephroblastic elements.
- PCN and CPDN have been regarded as part of the spectrum of Wilms tumor for a long time. However, recent molecular studies showed that *DICER1* mutations are the major genetic event in the development of PCN, which could be rarely detected in conventional Wilms tumors (0.4% cases), but not in CPDN.
- *DICER1* is mapped to chromosome 14q and function as a haplo-insufficient tumor suppressor gene. *DICER1* gene loss of function and hotspot missense mutations were seen respectively in 70% and 90% of PCN cases. Approximately, 30% of PCN cases arise in a syndromic setting with germline-inactivating *DICER1* mutations. These patients also develop more aggressive tumors including malignant pleuropulmonary blastoma (PPB), ovarian Sertoli–Leydig cell tumor, and urogenital embryonal rhabdomyosarcomas. Therefore, accurate diagnosis of PCN is crucial and should prompt further testing for *DICER1* mutations.
- Detailed differential diagnosis between CPDN and PCN is summarized in Table 1.35.

References: [162–170].

Table 1.35 Differential diagnosis of cystic partially differentiated nephroblastoma vs. pediatric cystic nephroma

Parameter/ marker	Cystic partially differentiated nephroblastoma	Pediatric cystic nephroma
Frequency	Rare	Rare
Peak incidence	12 months	18 months
Cell origin	Nephrogenic blastema	Urogenital sinus cells
Syndromic associations	10% syndromic: i.e., trisomies 13 and 18, Beckwith-Wiedemann, WAGR, Denys-Drash, bloom syndromes, etc.	30% with *DICER1* pleuropulmonary blastoma (PPB) familial tumor predisposition syndrome
Presentation	Usually asymptomatic abdominal mass; could be pain, hematuria	Usually asymptomatic abdominal mass; could be pain, hematuria
Gross	Entirely cystic well-circumscribed multiloculated mass; could be large (18 cm); no apparent solid expansile nodules; cysts with clear fluid	Entirely cystic well-circumscribed (9 cm mean size); thin septa (< 5 mm), translucent, uniform; cysts with clear or hemorrhagic fluid
Histology	Thin septations with clusters of immature blastemal cells, epithelial or mesenchymal derivates; no expansile nodules altering shape of septa; luminal papulonodular protrusions acceptable	Flattened, cuboidal, or hobnailed epithelial cyst lining; thin fibrous septa with areas of increased cellularity; entrapped well-differentiated tubules lacking immature nephroblastic elements
WT1	Positive nuclear, except stroma	Negative
ER/PR	Negative	50% cases positive
Cytokeratin/ EMA	Focal positivity only	Uniform strong positivity
Genetic alterations	*WT1* mutations (11p13); *WT2, IGF2, CTNNB1, SIX1/2*; LOH 1p,16q; 1q gain, p53 mutations (anaplastic cells)	*DICER1* gene loss of function (70%) and hotspot missense (90%)
Prognosis	Low-risk tumor, with local recurrence reported in few cases	Benign, but progression to renal sarcoma has been described

Rhabdoid Tumor vs. Rhabdomyosarcoma

- Malignant rhabdoid tumor of the kidney is a highly aggressive neoplasm that occasionally demonstrates phenotypic overlap with other soft tissue malignancies. This tumor was recognized as a distinct type in 1978 and characterized by large polygonal cells with eosinophilic cytoplasmic inclusions and eccentric nuclei suggestive of rhabdomyoblastic differentiation. However, ultrastructural examination revealed the filamentous nature of the cytoplasmic inclusions. Because of its striking microscopic resemblance to rhabdomyosarcoma but lack of acceptable rhabdomyoblastic features, this tumor was termed malignant rhabdoid tumor of the kidney (RTK) in 1981. Follow-up immunohistochemical studies also showed no expression of true myogenic markers in RTK.
- Pediatric rhabdomyosarcomas with exclusive/predominant solid growth pattern may be morphologically confused with RTK (Fig. 1.36). Both tumors are characterized by a frequent metastatic spread and poor prognosis, but their accurate distinction has important prognostic and treatment implications.
- The hallmark molecular feature of RTK is in biallelic inactivation of tumor suppressor gene *hSNF5/INI1/SMARCB1* from SWI/SNF chromatin remodeling complex. Resulting loss of INI1 protein nuclear expression is a key immunohistochemical finding.
- The most important distinctive features of rhabdoid tumor vs. rhabdomyosarcoma are summarized in Table 1.36.

References: [142, 158, 161, 171–174].

Mesoblastic Nephroma vs. Wilms Tumor

- Congenital mesoblastic nephroma (CMN) is a mesenchymal renal tumor that was distinguished from Wilms tumor in 1967. CMN is the most frequent renal tumor in the neonates and infants comprising 3–10% of all childhood renal tumors (Fig. 1.37a, b). Three pathological variants of CMN are described: classic CMN (~25%), the more aggressive cellular CMN (~65%), and the mixed variant (~10%). Classic CMN has a good overall prognosis, but cellular CMN is associated with the potential for malignancy, and is capable of recurrence and metastasis. However, surgical resection with nephrectomy is considered an adequate therapy for all subtypes, provided that a complete resection is achieved.
- A differential diagnosis between CMN and Wilms tumor is critical to develop the most effective therapeutic approach. The examination of clinical symptoms, imaging characteristics, and histologic features shows that

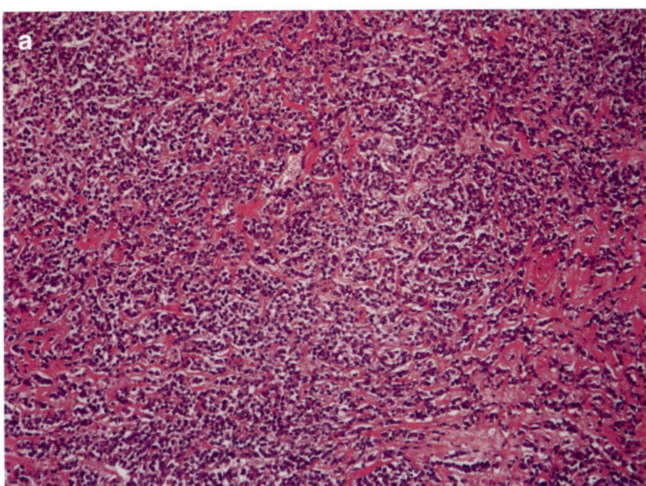
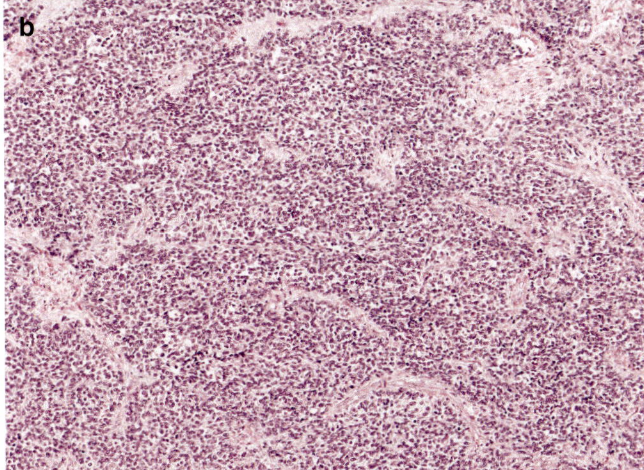
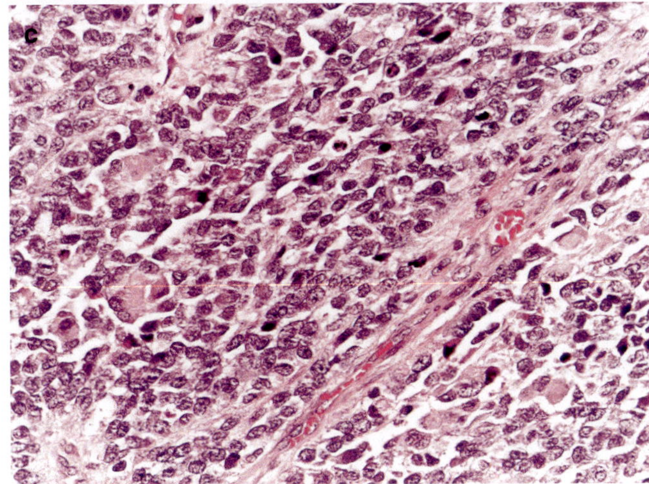

Fig. 1.36 (**a**) Malignant rhabdoid tumor (RTK) of the kidney with sheet-like architecture comprised of loosely cohesive ovoid-to-polygonal cells surrounded by a network of fibrovascular septa. (**b**) Embryonal rhabdomyosarcoma case with very similar to RTK morphology of highly cellular tumor with sheets of monotonous loosely cohesive cells. (**c**) The same tumor at higher magnification composed of spindle, ovoid, and polygonal eosinophilic cells representing rhabdomyoblasts at different stages of differentiation

Table 1.36 Differential diagnosis of rhabdoid tumor vs. rhabdomyosarcoma

Parameter/ marker	Rhabdoid tumor	Rhabdomyosarcoma
Frequency	~2% of pediatric renal tumors	5–8% of all pediatric tumors
Peak incidence	1 year of age	Bimodal peak: 2–4 and 14 years of age
Cell origin	Unknown	Mesenchymal stem cell
Syndromic associations	30% have rhabdoid predisposition syndrome with *hSNF5/ INI1* germline mutation	None
Symptoms	Hematuria plus symptoms of widespread metastatic disease	Suddenly enlarging mass with local symptoms at site of origin
Location	Originally described in kidney, but could be extrarenal in CNS and soft tissue	Deep mass (retroperitoneum, pelvis, genitourinary, etc.); widespread dissemination
Gross	Large (9.6 cm), irregular, infiltrative, unencapsulated mass with extensive hemorrhages and necrosis	Fleshy mass with infiltrative borders, tan cut surface, frequent necrosis and hemorrhage
Histology	Discohesive sheets of polygonal cells with occasional globular or hyaline inclusions and eccentric nuclei ("rhabdoid"); nuclei usually pleomorphic, with vesicular chromatin and large cherry-red nucleoli	Solid variant with sheets of medium-sized cells; vague alveolar architecture and variable degree of rhabdomyoblastic differentiation with cross-striations at higher power; nuclei round-to-oval with hyperchromasia
INI1/BAF47	Loss of nuclear expression	Intact nuclear expression
Myogenin	Negative	Positive
MyoD1	Negative	Positive
Desmin	Often positive (trapped in hyaline globule)	Positive, diffuse and strong
Genetic alterations	Biallelic inactivation of *hSNF5/INI/SMARCB1* tumor suppressor gene (mutation or deletion of 22q11.2)	Balanced translocation: *PAX3/7-FOXO1*: t(2;13), t(1;13); complex karyotypes and frequent LOH
Prognosis	Dismal: 15–30% survival; 80% patients die within 2 years from diagnosis (improved with combined surgical/radio–/ chemo–/autologous stem cell transplant treatment)	Variable, depending on disease stage, site, and histologic type (alveolar much worse than embryonal); overall 5-year survival 64.5%

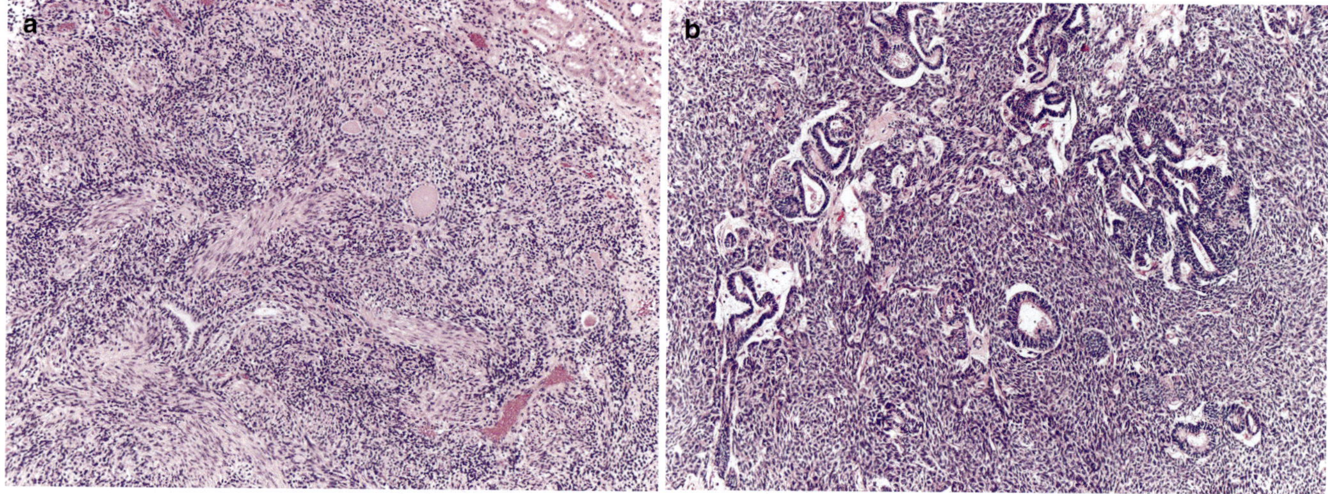

Fig. 1.37 (**a**) Classic variant of congenital mesoblastic nephroma with fascicles and bundles of spindle cells infiltrating between entrapped benign tubules. (**b**) Biphasic nephroblastoma (Wilms tumor) with blastemal and epithelial components

Wilms tumor has a lot of similarities with CMN, particularly the cellular variant. On the other hand, fewer than 2% patients with Wilms tumor (WT) present at under 3 months of age. Tumors with congenital syndromes or anomalies, and the presence of bilateral tumors are more suggestive of Wilms. These and other important characteristics allowing distinction of these two tumors are highlighted in Table 1.37.

References: [153, 159, 175–180].

Metanephric Adenoma vs. Congenital Mesoblastic Nephroma

- Metanephric kidney develops between fifth and ninth weeks of gestation and is derived from two main embryonic structures: nephrogenic blastema and embryonic bud. Nephrogenic blastema is composed of primitive tubules surrounded by cellular condensations developing into the glomeruli. The embryonic bud forms collecting system with cortical and medul-

Table 1.37 Mesoblastic nephroma vs. Wilms tumor

Parameter/marker	Congenital mesoblastic nephroma	Wilms tumor
Frequency	Most common tumor of infancy	~85% of all pediatric renal tumors
Peak incidence	3 months; >90% occur in first year	2–3 years of age
Cell origin	Embryonic bud stem cells	Nephrogenic blastema
Syndromic associations	Rare association with Beckwith-Wiedemann syndrome	10% syndromic: i.e., trisomies 13 and 18, Beckwith-Wiedemann, WAGR, Denys-Drash, bloom syndromes, etc.
Location	Medulla-centric; infiltrating and extensively involving renal sinus	Kidney-centered; unifocal (88%), bilateral (5%), multifocal (7%)
Symptoms	Abdominal mass, polyhydramnios, premature delivery, hypertension	Abdominal mass, pain, hematuria, hypertension, acute abdominal crisis
Gross	Solitary, unilateral, whorled or trabeculated with gray-white or fleshy surface and indistinct borders; necrosis, cysts, hemorrhage common, but no prognostic significance	Sharply demarcated and often encapsulated, nodular, bulging, soft friable tan or gray kidney mass; could be whorled and firm if contains prominent stromal component
Typical histology	Cellular (2/3): Pushing borders, dense cellularity of spindly small blue myofibroblastic cells growing in fascicles, intersecting bundles, and showing high mitotic activity	Predominantly blastemal: Sheets of small, closely packed, mitotically active cells with scant cytoplasm and overlapping nuclei; admixed epithelial and stroma components
Stroma-rich variants	Classic (1/3): Infiltrating spindle cells resembling fibromatosis with minimal pleomorphism and mitoses; lobular architecture with finger-like extensions and entrapped tubules, glomeruli, islands of cartilage	Predominantly stromal: Nondescript spindled cells with minimal pleomorphism and mitoses within loose, myxoid background; could show rhabdomyoblastic, fibroblastic, or smooth muscle differentiation
WT1	Negative	Positive nuclear expression: 75% blastema, 44% stroma
PAX8	Entrapped tubules only	Positive
Desmin	Negative	Blastema could be positive
Genetic alterations	t(12;15)(p13;q25) *ETV6-NTRK3* (cellular); aneuploidy 11,8,17 (classic)	*WT1* mutations (11p13); *WT2, IGF2, CTNNB1, SIX1/2;* LOH 1p,16q; 1q gain, p53 mutations
Prognosis	Excellent	>90% survival, depends on stage and histology (favorable or unfavorable)

lary ducts, rudimentary calyces and pelvis embedded into supporting mesoblastic stroma. These two components of metanephric kidney are morphologically recapitulated in metanephric tumors including metanephric adenoma (MA), metanephric adenofibroma (MAF), and metanephric stromal tumor (MST), as well as in congenital mesoblastic nephroma (CMN; see Fig. 1.38a, b).

Table 1.38 shows metanephric adenoma vs. congenital mesoblastic nephroma.
References: [68, 177–179, 181, 182].

What Are the Most Common Syndromes Associated with Renal Tumors?

Approximately, 4–5% of all renal tumors are associated with heritable autosomal dominant syndromes. In general, these renal tumors have an earlier age of onset, often multifocal and bilateral. Knowledge of molecular abnormalities, pathogenesis, specifics of renal pathology, and characteristic of extrarenal manifestations is important for early recognition of individuals and families at risk for early screening, active surveillance, and timely management (see Tables 1.39, 1.40, 1.41, 1.42, 1.43, and 1.44).

- Von Hippel-Lindau (VHL) Syndrome.
- Hereditary papillary renal cell carcinoma (PRCC).
- Birt-Hogg-Dube (BDH) syndrome.
- Hereditary leiomyomatosis renal cell carcinoma (HLRCC).
- Tuberous sclerosis complex (TSC).
- Hereditary paraganglioma-pheochromocytoma syndrome or
- Succinate Dehydrogenase (SDH) Complex deficiency syndrome.

References: [183–189].

Case Presentations

Case 1

Learning Objectives

1. To understand differential diagnostic considerations for renal mass biopsy.
2. To become familiar with the immunohistochemical profile of the tumor.
3. To generate a relevant differential diagnosis.

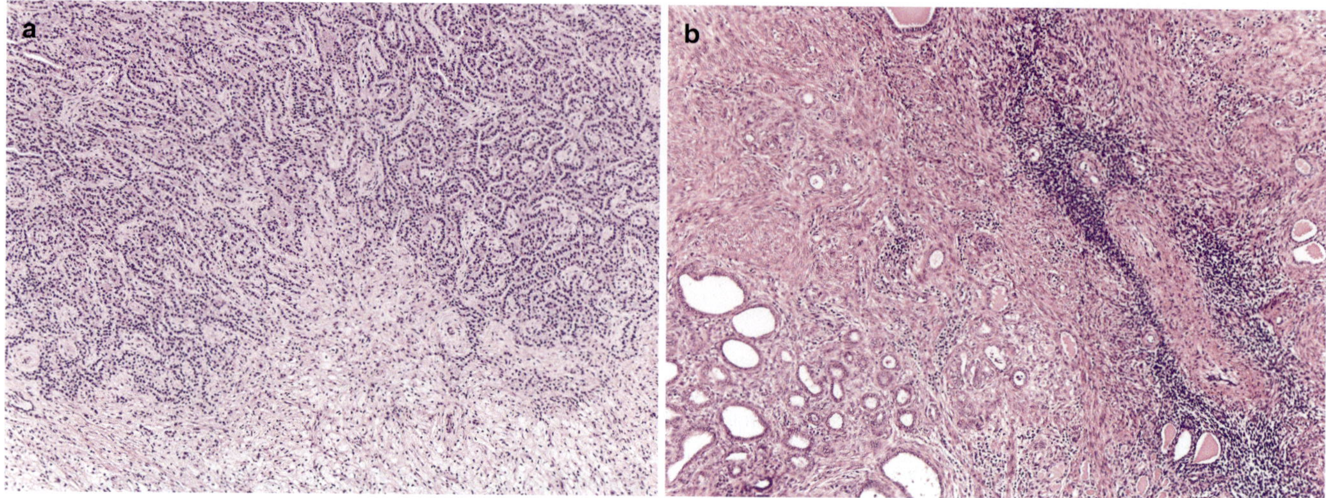

Fig. 1.38 (**a**) Metanephric adenofibroma composed of small blue cells arranged in tubules and papillary structures admixed with sheets of spindled cells within myxoid stroma. (**b**) Classic variant of congenital mesoblastic nephroma composed of tubules embedded into the cellular stroma with intersecting fascicles and bundles of spindle cells with minimal atypia

Table 1.38 Metanephric adenoma vs. congenital mesoblastic nephroma

Parameter/ marker	Metanephric tumors	Congenital mesoblastic nephroma
Frequency	Most common benign tumor in children, but could be seen in any age (range 1–83 years)	Most common tumor of infancy: >90% occur in first year
Location	Renal cortex (MA) or medulla-centric (MAF, MST)	Medulla-centric; infiltrating and extensively involving renal sinus
Symptoms	Usually asymptomatic incidental (>50%); 12% with polycythemia; pain, hematuria, hypertension	Abdominal mass, polyhydramnios, premature delivery, hypertension; Beckwith-Wiedemann syndrome
Cell origin	Persistent blastema cells	Embryonic bud stem cells
Gross	Unilateral, solitary, variable sizes (1–22 cm, mean 3.8–5.5 cm); well-circumscribed, unencapsulated, solid fleshy mass; calcifications in 20%; necrosis, hemorrhage, cysts <15%	Solitary, unilateral, whorled or trabeculated with gray-white or fleshy surface and indistinct borders; necrosis, cysts, hemorrhage common, but no prognostic significance
Typical histology	MA: Tightly packed tubules; papillary and glomeruloid structures; small blue crowded cells with scant cytoplasm; grooved nuclei without discernible nuclei	Cellular (2/3): Pushing borders, dense cellularity of spindly small blue myofibroblastic cells growing in fascicles, intersecting bundles, and showing high mitotic activity
Rare stroma-rich variants	MAF/MST: Spindled stellate cells forming collarets and concentric stromal rings around epithelium and vessels; angiodysplasia, myxoid stroma, hyalinization, calcifications, cysts, or heterologous elements	Classic (1/3): Infiltrating spindle cells resembling fibromatosis with minimal pleomorphism and mitoses; frequently lobular architecture with finger-like extensions and entrapped tubules, glomeruli, islands of cartilage
WT1	Positive in epithelium	Negative
CD57	Positive in epithelium	Negative
BRAF	Positive in epithelium	Negative
AMACR/CK7	Negative	Entrapped tubules
CD34	Positive in stroma	Usually negative
Genetic alterations	*BRAF V600E* mutation in 90% cases; 2p13 alteration in 56% cases	t(12;15)(p13;q25) *ETV6-NTRK3* (cellular); aneuploidy 11,8,17 (classic)
Prognosis	Benign; excellent	Benign; excellent

Case History

A 55-year-old man with history of pancreatic cancer is found to have multiple renal masses. Core biopsy is performed to evaluate for metastasis vs. primary renal neoplasm.

Gross

Core biopsy fragments of 1 mm diameter and 0.5–1.2 cm length are received.

Table 1.39 Von Hippel-Lindau (VHL) Syndrome

Parameter	Description
Gene	*VHL* (tumor suppressor), 3p25–26 3p loss plus *VHL* point mutations/deletions, LOH, hypermethylation
Pathogenesis	Absence of pVHL protein causes accumulation and overexpression of HIF-1α/HIF-2α and increased transcription of hypoxia-inducible genes and proteins: VEGF, PDGF, GLUT1, erythropoietin, CAIX, TGF-α, CXCR4
Renal involvement	Mean age 37 years; high penetrance (70% with RCC by age 70)
Renal tumors	Clear cell RCC (cystic and solid) in a background of numerous renal cysts
Extrarenal lesions	CNS hemangioblastomas, pheochromocytomas, pancreatic tumors and cysts, epididymal cystadenomas, endolymphatic sac tumors of ear
Treatment/ prognosis	Multiple nephron-sparing surgeries to reduce tumor burden and preserve kidney function; rare development of metastatic RCC

Table 1.40 Hereditary papillary renal cell carcinoma (PRCC)

Parameter	Description
Gene	*c-MET* (protooncogene), 7q31
Pathogenesis	Activating mutations/amplification of *c-MET* gene, accumulation of oncoprotein MET with tyrosine kinase function, inducing cell proliferation, stimulating tumor growth and invasion
Renal involvement	Mean age ~55 years; high penetrance (67% develop PRCC by age 60)
Renal tumors	Enumerable bilateral papillary adenomas (<1.5 cm) and PRCCs, type 1
Extrarenal lesions	None
Treatment/ prognosis	*c-MET*-inhibitors; nephron-sparing surgeries to reduce tumor burden and preserve kidney function; rare development of metastatic PRCC

Table 1.41 Birt-Hogg-Dube (BDH) syndrome

Parameter	Description
Gene	*Folliculin (FLCN),* tumor suppressor, 17p12-q11.2
Pathogenesis	Inherited germline mutation of 1 allele followed by frameshift and missense mutations in exons 4–14, hotspot exon 11; activation of mTOR pathway via loss of negative regulation of *FLCN*; cause abnormal differentiation of distal renal tubular cells
Renal involvement	Renal tumors at 50–54 years; low penetrance (~20% of BHD patients)
Renal tumors	Chromophobe RCC, oncocytoma, and hybrid oncocytoma/chromophobe tumors (HOCT) in a background of oncocytosis
Extrarenal lesions	Skin lesions (90%): Fibrofolliculomas, acrochordones, and trichodiscomas; lung cysts (83%) with spontaneous pneumothorax in 23–40%
Treatment/ prognosis	Nephron-sparing surgery; radiologic follow-up; >85% indolent tumors

Table 1.42 Hereditary leiomyomatosis renal cell carcinoma (HLRCC)

Parameter	Description
Gene	*FH* (tumor suppressor gene), 1q42.3–43
Pathogenesis	FH point mutations/deletions or whole gene mutations lead to loss of fumarate hydratase function in Krebs cycle; accumulation of fumarate and 2-succino-cysteine (2SC) with further activation of HIF-1 and its target genes stimulating tumor growth
Renal involvement	Mean age 36–46 years; low penetrance (2–20% of HLRCC patients)
Renal tumors	Unilateral and solitary high-grade and high-stage tumors with heterogeneous solid, papillary, tubular, and cystic architecture; most often morphology similar to papillary RCC, type 2. Hallmark feature: Prominent CMV-like large eosinophilic nucleoli
Extrarenal lesions	Uterine and cutaneous leiomyomas at young age
Treatment/ prognosis	Poor prognosis; most patients develop widely metastatic disease

Table 1.43 Tuberous sclerosis complex (TSC)

Parameter	Description
Gene	*TSC1* (encodes tumor suppressor hamartin), 9q34 *TSC2* (encodes tumor suppressor tuberin), 16p13.3
Pathogenesis	Germline mutations of *TSC1* or *TSC2* lead to activation of mTOR pathway and increased cell proliferation, metabolism, and cytoskeletal abnormalities
Renal involvement	Mean age 30–42 years; variable penetrance (80% for AML and 2.4% for RCC)
Renal tumors	Multiple and bilateral angiomyolipomas with variant histologies (triphasic, fat-rich, fat-poor, sclerosing, AMLEC, epithelioid); polycystic change. Heterogeneous group of RCC: Chromophobe RCC-like, clear cell RCC with smooth muscle stroma, or eosinophilic solid and cystic RCC
Extrarenal lesions	Brain: Cortical tubers, subependymal nodules, and giant cell astrocytoma; Skin: Shagreen patch, hypopigmented macules, facial angiofibroma, forehead plaque, ungula fibromas, retinal hamartomas; Lungs: Lymphangioleiomyomatosis; heart: Rhabdomyomas
Treatment/ prognosis	mTOR inhibitors; death from RCC uncommon

Table 1.44 Hereditary paraganglioma-pheochromocytoma syndrome or succinate dehydrogenase (SDH) complex deficiency syndrome

Parameter	Description
Gene	*SDHA* (5q15), *SDHB* (1p36), *SDHC* (1q21), *SDHD* (11q23)
Pathogenesis	75% mutations affect *SDHB*; germline mutations of SDH-genes plus LOH lead to loss of Krebs cycle related succinate-dehydrogenase enzyme in the inner mitochondrial membrane and loss of efficient electron transport; SDH-complex deficiency causes HIF overexpression and shift of cell metabolism toward anaerobic glycolysis and fatty acid synthesis
Renal involvement	Mean age 37 years; low penetrance (14% RCC by age 70)
Renal tumors	SDH-deficient RCC characterized by solid architecture, eosinophilic cells with pale vacuolated cytoplasm, and flocculent cytoplasmic inclusions
Extrarenal lesions	Pheochromocytomas, paragangliomas, carotid body tumors, GIST
Treatment/ prognosis	Surgical treatment; 2/3 tumors indolent

Histologic Findings

- Sections demonstrate cells with clear cytoplasm forming glands and tubular structures with a somewhat branched configuration in edematous, loose stroma (Fig. 1.39a).
- At higher magnification, there is a suggestion that nuclei are aligned at a similar height within the cytoplasm (Fig. 1.39b).

Differential Diagnosis

- Clear cell RCC.
- Clear cell papillary RCC.
- Papillary RCC with clear cell changes.
- Metastatic pancreatic cancer.

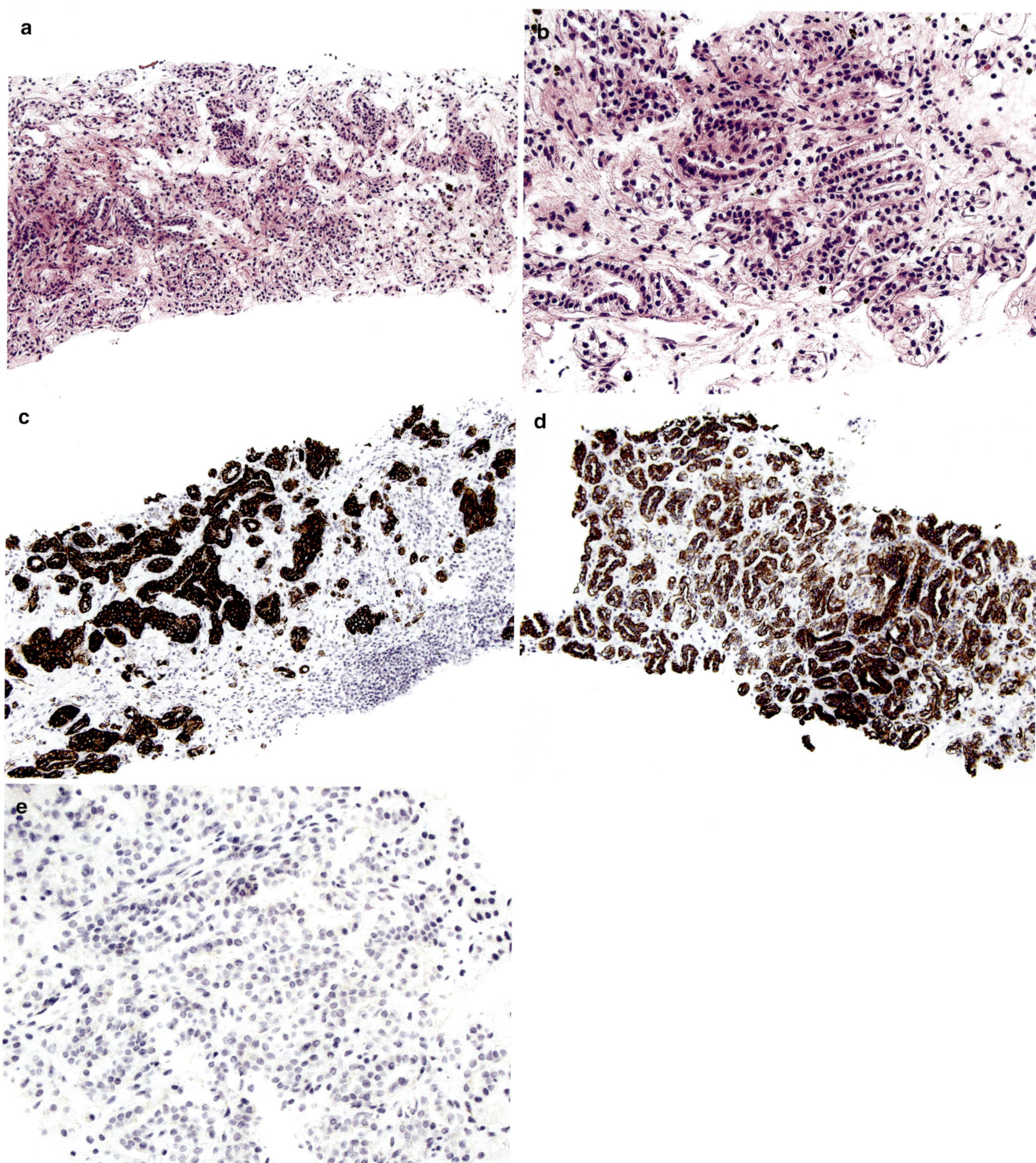

Fig. 1.39 (**a**) Renal mass biopsy shows a neoplasm composed of glandular structures in loose stroma. (**b**) Higher magnification demonstrates some alignment of nuclei at a uniform height in the cytoplasm. (**c**) Immunohistochemistry shows diffuse strong positivity for cytokeratin 7. (**d**) Immunohistochemistry also shows substantial positivity for high molecular weight cytokeratin. (**e**) Immunohistochemistry is negative for alpha-methylacyl-CoA racemase (AMACR)

IHC and Other Ancillary Studies

- Carbonic anhydrase IX diffusely positive with cup-shaped pattern.
- Cytokeratin 7 is diffusely positive (Fig. 1.39c).
- High molecular weight cytokeratin is diffusely positive (Fig. 1.39d).
- AMACR is negative (Fig. 1.39e).
- GATA3 is patchy positive.
- CD10 is negative.

Final Diagnosis

Clear cell papillary (tubulopapillary) RCC.

Take-Home Messages

1. Clear cell papillary RCC is a nonaggressive subtype of RCC that accounts for 3–4% of adult renal neoplasms.
2. Despite similarity to clear cell RCC morphologically, the immunohistochemical profile is distinctive (cytokeratin 7 positive, carbonic anhydrase IX positive, high molecular weight cytokeratin often positive, GATA3 often positive, AMACR negative, CD10 negative).
3. Aggressive behavior from a prototypical case has not been described to date, suggesting this may be reclassified as a low malignant potential or benign neoplasm in the future.
4. Some cases may have multifocal or bilateral tumors, for unknown reasons.
5. This entity is associated with end-stage renal disease; however, most cases likely occur in non-end-stage kidneys.

References: [4, 17, 29].

Case 2

Learning Objectives

1. To understand the differential diagnosis of renal cancers with clear cell and papillary features.
2. To apply relevant immunohistochemical profiles.
3. To understand the role of molecular testing in RCC.

Case History

A 40-year-old man presents for resection of a 5.5 cm renal mass.

Gross

Sectioning reveals a solid, yellow-tan renal mass that bulges from the normal contour of the kidney.

Histologic Findings

- Sections demonstrate a renal cancer composed of cells with clear cytoplasm, arranged in tubulopapillary structures with prominent nuclear alignment (Fig. 1.40a).
- Other areas demonstrate more papillary architecture with psammoma bodies (Fig. 1.40b).

Differential Diagnosis

- Clear cell RCC.
- Papillary RCC.
- Translocation-associated RCC.
- Clear cell papillary RCC.
- Unclassified RCC.

IHC and Other Ancillary Studies

- Cytokeratin 7 negative.
- Carbonic anhydrase IX negative.
- PAX8 positive.
- Melan-A focal positive.
- Break-apart FISH for *TFE3* shows a split signal pattern with small gaps between the signals.

Final Diagnosis

Translocation-associated RCC with *NONO-TFE3* fusion.

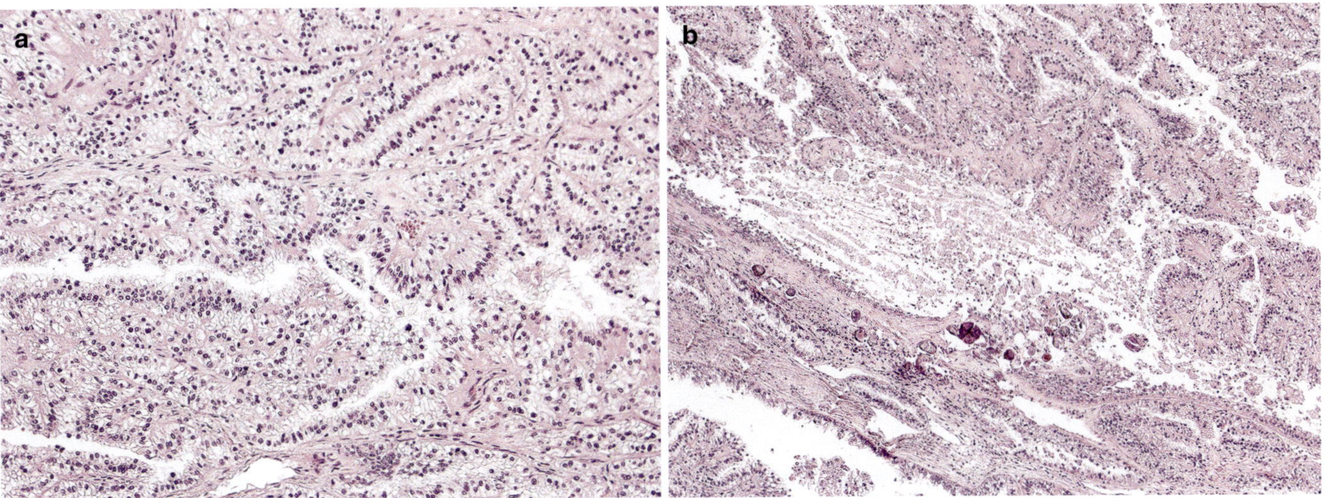

Fig. 1.40 (**a**) Histology demonstrates a renal cell carcinoma with clear to eosinophilic cells and papillary architecture with nuclear alignment. (**b**) More prominent papillary architecture and psammoma bodies are evident in other areas

Take-Home Messages

1. Translocation RCC is a relatively rare subtype of renal cancer.
2. Although children and young adults with RCC are more likely to have translocation tumors, there are likely more cases that occur in older adults in the conventional age range for renal cancer (>55).
3. Translocation tumors are consistently negative for carbonic anhydrase IX, positive for PAX8, and often have positivity for melanocytic markers or cathepsin-K.
4. Translocations *NONO-TFE3* and *RBM10-TFE3* can be difficult to detect with FISH, as both are caused by intra-chromosomal fusions on the X chromosome, which may yield a small gap in the split signal, or a false-negative result.
5. *NONO-TFE3* and *SFPQ-TFE3* fusion tumors often have nuclear alignment resembling clear cell papillary RCC; however, psammoma bodies are not typical of the latter.

References: [35, 47, 49, 190].

Case 3

Learning Objectives

1. To recognize morphologic clues for diagnosis of oncocytic renal tumors.
2. To be familiar with immunohistochemistry for diagnosis of oncocytic neoplasms.
3. Integrate genetic findings in the differential diagnosis of oncocytic tumors.

Case History

A 58-year-old woman presented for resection of a 5.5 cm renal mass.

Gross

Sectioning reveals a circumscribed, solid, tan-brown renal mass with a pushing border.

Histologic Findings

- Some areas exhibit nests of oncocytic cells, reminiscent of oncocytoma (Fig. 1.41a).

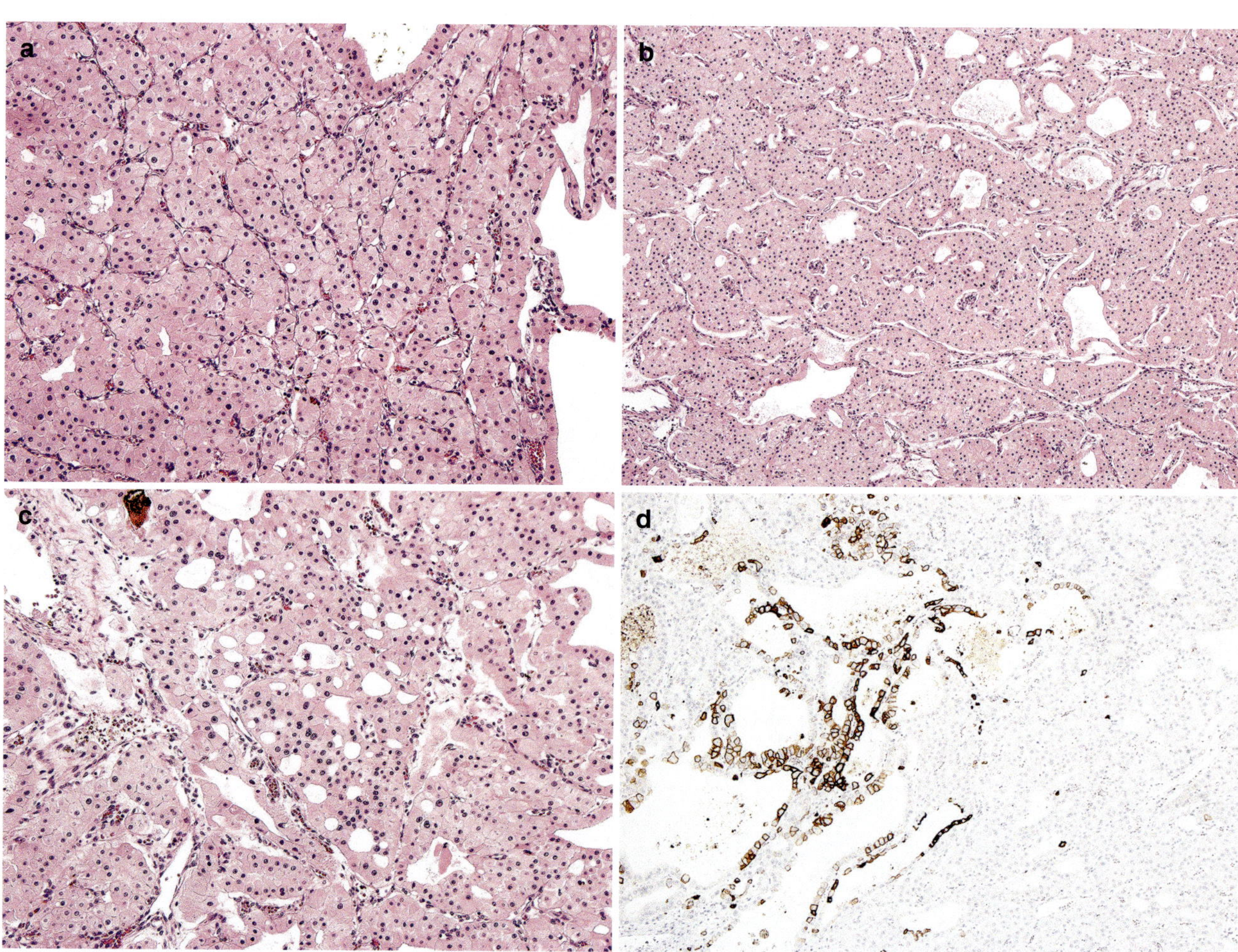

Fig. 1.41 (**a**) Histology demonstrates an oncocytic neoplasm with relatively round, regular nuclei. (**b**) Other areas of the same neoplasm show trabecular architecture. (**c**) Cribriform architecture and some nuclear size variation are also present. (**d**) Immunohistochemistry shows patchy confluent staining for cytokeratin 7

- Other areas contain large trabecular solid and microscystic structures (Fig. 1.41b).
- Higher magnification includes cribriform nests of cells with some nuclear irregularity and nuclear size variation (Fig. 1.41c).

Differential Diagnosis
- Oncocytoma.
- Chromophobe RCC.
- Succinate dehydrogenase-deficient RCC.
- Papillary RCC with oncocytic features.
- Unclassified RCC.

IHC and Other Ancillary Studies
- Cytokeratin 7 shows variable patchy staining with some confluent areas (Fig. 1.41d).
- Vimentin immunohistochemistry is negative.
- KIT (CD117) demonstrates positive membrane staining.
- FISH demonstrates losses of several chromosomes, including 1, 6, and 10.

Final Diagnosis
Eosinophilic variant chromophobe RCC.

Take-Home Messages
1. Distinguishing oncocytoma from chromophobe RCC remains challenging even today, despite numerous immunohistochemical and molecular markers that have been explored.
2. The most commonly used immunohistochemical method for distinguishing oncocytoma from chromophobe RCC is cytokeratin 7 staining, although a precise threshold of positivity that excludes oncocytoma is not well defined.
3. Oncocytoma generally should demonstrate only rare cells and small clusters of cells positive for cytokeratin 7.
4. Oncocytoma and chromophobe RCC are consistently negative for vimentin (except in central scar areas of oncocytoma) and usually positive for KIT.
5. Chromophobe RCC often exhibits losses of multiple chromosomes, particularly Y, 1, 2, 6, 10, 13, 17, and 21.

References: [21, 36, 84, 85].

Case 4

Learning Objectives
1. To understand the differential diagnosis of renal cancers with clear cell and papillary features.
2. To apply relevant immunohistochemical profiles.
3. To be able to counsel clinical colleagues regarding the behavior of RCC variants.

Case History
A 59-year-old man presents for resection of a 5.7 cm renal mass with invasion of the renal sinus.

Gross
Sectioning reveals a circumscribed renal mass with finger-like extensions into the renal sinus. The cut surface is golden-yellow.

Histologic Findings
- The neoplasm is composed of cells with clear cytoplasm lining branched glandular structures (Fig. 1.42a).
- Some areas have small formations of branched papillae (Fig. 1.42b).

Differential Diagnosis
- Clear cell RCC.
- Clear cell papillary RCC.
- Translocation RCC.
- Unclassified RCC.

IHC and Other Ancillary Studies
- Cytokeratin 7 demonstrates patchy (partial) positivity (Fig. 1.42c).
- Carbonic anhydrase IX exhibits diffuse membrane positivity (Fig. 1.42d).
- CD10 demonstrates substantial apical membrane positivity (Fig. 1.42e).
- AMACR demonstrates moderate to strong cytoplasmic positivity (Fig. 1.42f).

Final Diagnosis
Clear cell RCC (with areas mimicking clear cell papillary RCC).

Take-Home Messages
1. Some clear cell RCC tumors can demonstrate morphology overlapping with clear cell papillary RCC.
2. Although these tumors may have partial or substantial positivity for cytokeratin 7, they typically have an otherwise imperfect immunohistochemical profile for clear cell papillary subtype, such as with substantial positivity for AMACR and/or CD10.
3. High molecular weight cytokeratin, which is often positive in clear cell papillary tumors, is usually negative or focal in clear cell RCC, and GATA3 is typically negative.
4. Tumors with these overlapping features have been found to have chromosome 3p abnormalities, necrosis, high-stage parameters, and aggressive behavior, supporting exclusion from the diagnosis of clear cell papillary RCC.

References: [29, 60, 61].

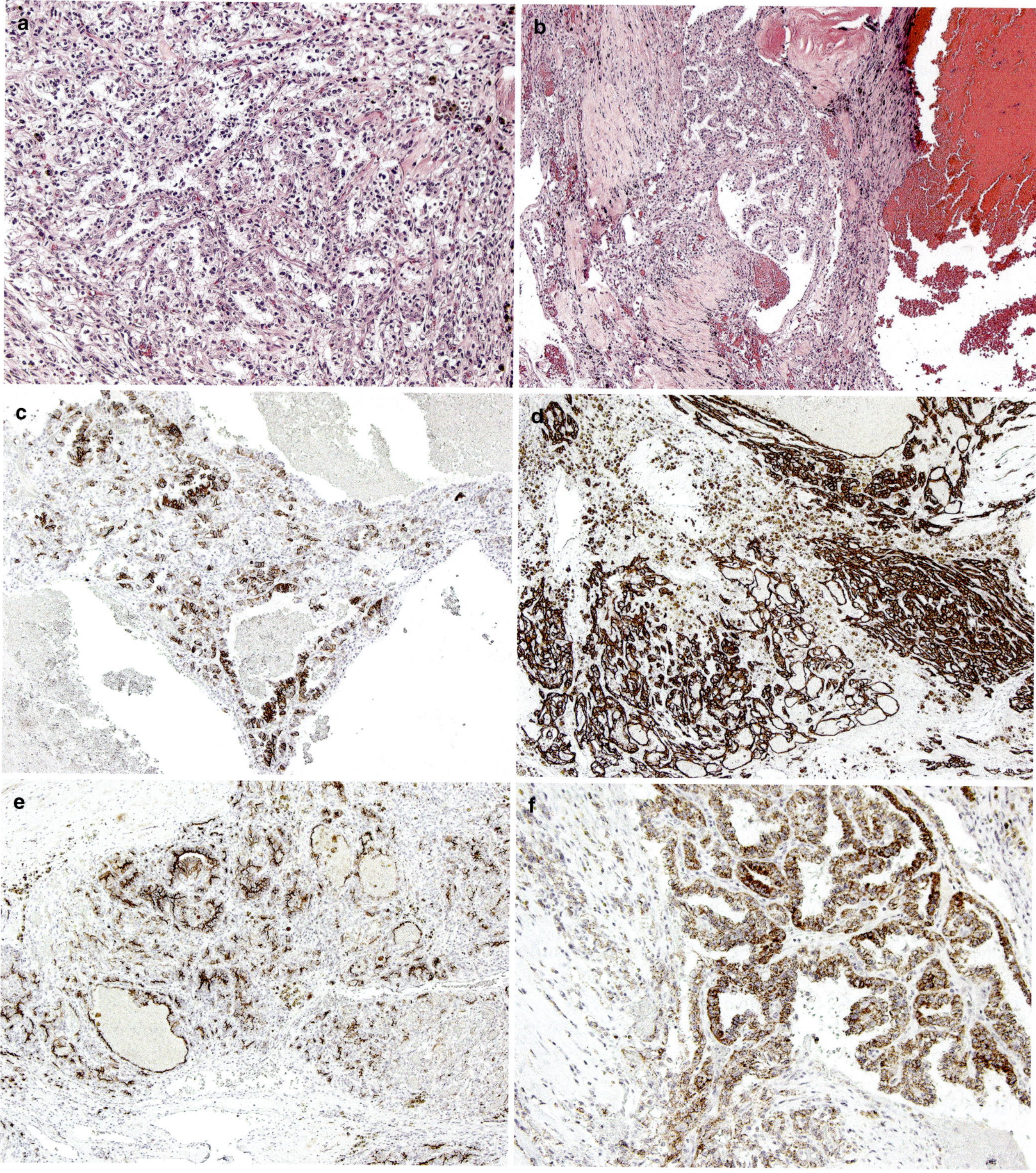

Fig. 1.42 (**a**) Histology demonstrates a neoplasm composed of clear cells arranged in glandular/papillary formations. (**b**) Other areas show small, branched papillary tufts protruding into small cystic spaces. (**c**) Immunohistochemical staining for cytokeratin 7 demonstrates partial but not diffuse positivity. (**d**) Carbonic anhydrase IX demonstrates diffuse positivity. (**e**) Substantial apical membrane positivity for CD10 is also present. (**f**) There is moderate to strong cytoplasmic staining for alpha-methylacyl-CoA racemase (AMACR)

Case 5

Learning Objectives
1. To become familiar with the histologic features of the tumor.
2. To become familiar with the immunohistochemical profile of the tumor.
3. To generate a relevant differential diagnosis.

Case History
A 45-year-old woman presented with polycythemia and a 2.5 cm renal mass. Partial nephrectomy was performed.

Gross
Sectioning reveals a solid, white-tan mass with homogeneous cut surface.

Histologic Findings
- Histology demonstrates a well-circumscribed but unencapsulated neoplasm composed of crowded basophilic cells (Fig. 1.43a).
- Higher magnification demonstrates crowded nests of basophilic cells (Fig. 1.43b).
- Other areas contain edematous stroma with small, tight clusters of basophilic cells with bland nuclei (Fig. 1.43c).

Differential Diagnosis
- Papillary RCC.
- Metanephric adenoma.
- Wilms tumor (nephroblastoma).

IHC and Other Ancillary Studies
- WT1 demonstrates diffuse nuclear positivity (Fig. 1.43d).
- CD57 demonstrates diffuse positivity.
- AMACR, cytokeratin 7, and epithelial membrane antigen are negative.

Final Diagnosis
Metanephric adenoma.

Take-Home Messages
1. Metanephric adenoma is a rare benign renal neoplasm composed of compact clusters of basophilic cells with bland nuclei.
2. Papillary architecture and psammoma bodies can be present.

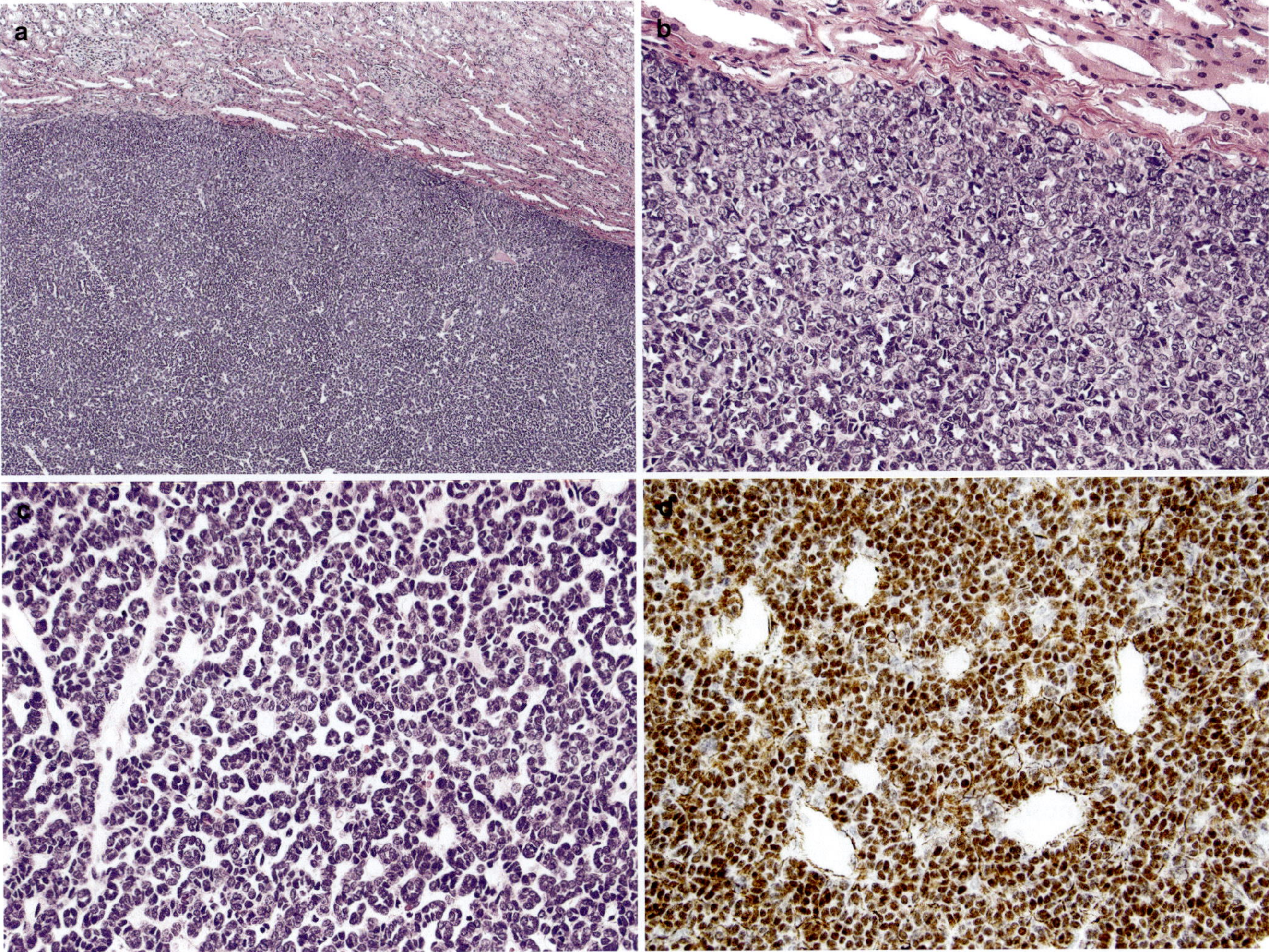

Fig. 1.43 (**a**) Histology demonstrates a circumscribed neoplasm composed of crowded basophilic cells. (**b**) Higher magnification reveals small nests reminiscent of solid papillary renal cell carcinoma. (**c**) Other areas are composed of cells with small, bland nuclei in edematous stroma. (**d**) Diffuse nuclear positivity with WT1 antibody

3. Morphologic features can overlap with papillary RCC and nephroblastoma; however, the immunohistochemical profile is helpful to distinguish these tumors.
4. Metanephric adenoma is typically positive for WT1 and CD57 and negative for AMACR and cytokeratin 7, whereas papillary RCC usually shows the opposite pattern.
5. The majority of metanephric adenomas harbor *BRAF* mutations and immunohistochemistry for the mutant BRAF protein often correlates with mutation.

References: [68–70].

Case 6

Learning Objectives

1. To become familiar with the histologic features of the tumor.
2. To become familiar with the immunohistochemical profile of the tumor.
3. To generate the differential diagnosis.

Case History

A 51-year-old female presented with history of long-standing diabetes and hypertension, with status post renal transplant. She developed hematuria, ureteral stricture, and hydronephrosis in her native kidney. Due to severe stricture and non-functioning kidney, the patient elected to have a right nephrectomy.

Gross

A nephrectomy specimen weighing 144 g is bivalved showing dilated renal pelvis and calyces with tan-white smooth and glistening urothelial mucosa. Renal parenchyma is markedly atrophic, pale brown with blurred corticomedullary junction and areas of vague nodularity.

Histologic Findings

- Urothelial lining of renal calyces overlies highly atypical cellular areas of spindled pleomorphic cells with numerous mitoses and discohesive growth (Fig. 1.44a).
- Haphazardly arranged sarcomatoid cells embedded into myxoid stroma and undermine urothelium without any obvious in situ urothelial carcinoma (UC). No low-grade or high-grade renal cell carcinoma (RCC) or invasive UC are identified (Fig. 1.44b).

Differential Diagnosis

- Sarcomatoid UC.
- Sarcomatoid RCC.
- Renal sarcoma.

IHC and Other Ancillary Studies

- CK7 strongly positive (Fig. 1.44c).
- GATA3 variably positive: strong in benign overlying urothelium and variable in sarcomatoid cells (Fig. 1.44d).
- PAX8 negative.

Final Diagnosis

Pure sarcomatoid urothelial carcinoma of the renal pelvis.

Take-Home Messages

1. Carcinomas with pure sarcomatoid morphology of kidney are extremely rare aggressive tumors and pose significant morphologic challenge.
2. Distinction between sarcomatoid RCC and sarcomatoid UC is very important due to different prognosis and patient management. This patient received additional surgical treatment with removal of the entire right ureter with bladder cuff.
3. Immunohistochemistry with pan-cytokeratins, urothelial markers, markers of RCC, or markers of sarcoma histogenesis is important in making this diagnosis.

References: [8, 93].

Case 7

Learning Objectives

1. To become familiar with the histologic and immunohistochemical features of the tumor.
2. To generate the differential diagnosis.

Case History

A 50-year-old male presented with back pain, weight loss, and hematuria.

Gross

Radical nephrectomy specimen with renal mass measuring 20.5 cm × 18 × 8 cm. On cut surface the tumor is partly cystic and partly solid with yellow-maroon variegated cut surface and friable necrotic hemorrhagic areas.

Histologic Findings

The neoplasm consists of sheets and nests of epithelioid cells with clear cytoplasm and well-defined cytoplasmic borders. Focal perinuclear clearing and nuclear wrinkling are seen. Other areas have a more prominent oncocytic appearance, in which the nuclei are round with prominent nucleoli and coarsely granular eosinophilic cytoplasm. There are also multiple entrapped benign renal tubules (Fig. 1.45a).

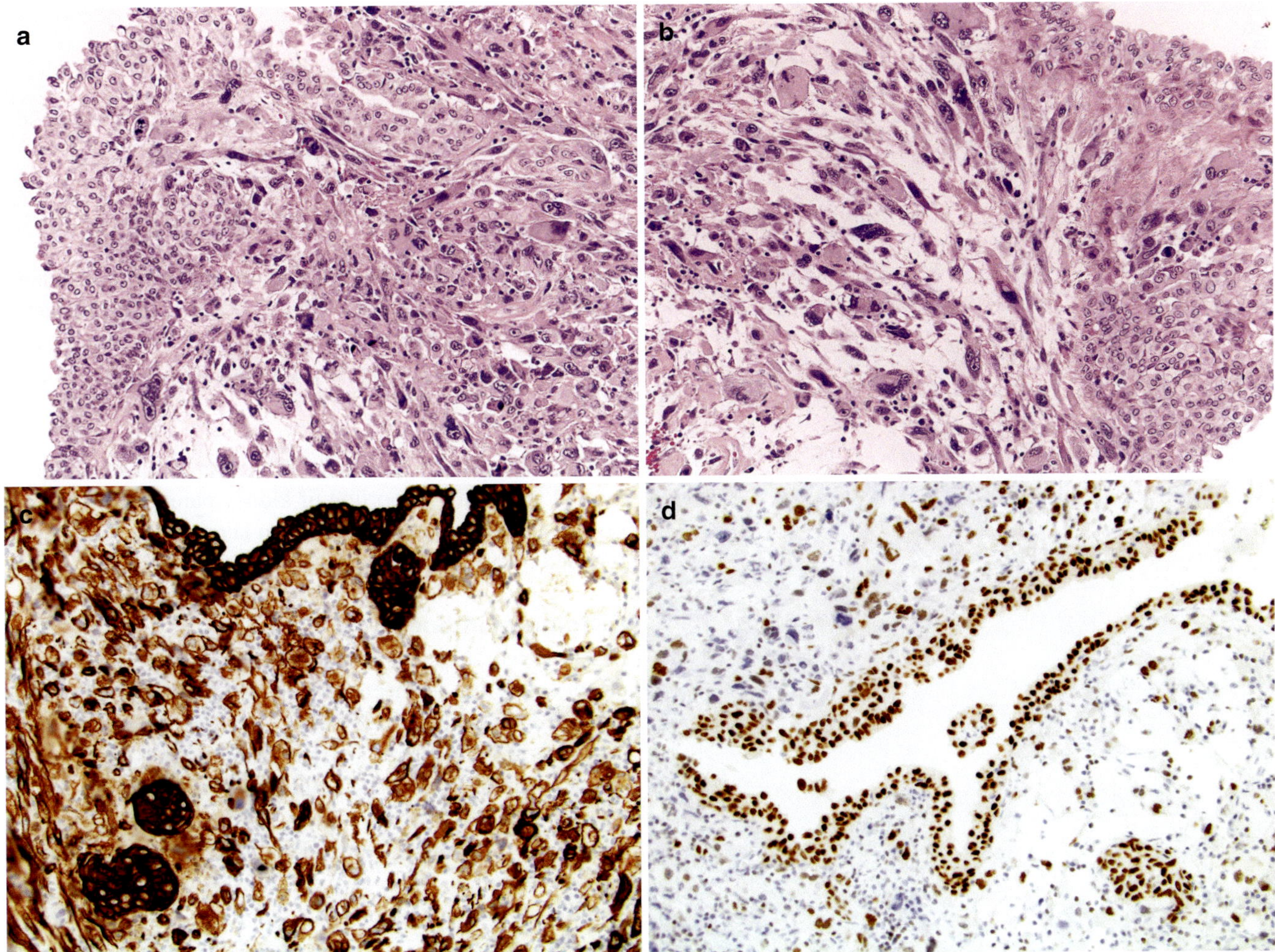

Fig. 1.44 (**a**) Histology shows high-grade pleomorphic cells undermining benign appearing surface urothelium of the renal pelvis. (**b**) Higher magnification reveals spindled malignant cells with multinucleation, hyperchromasia, and bizarre atypical nuclei. (**c**) Strong CK7 immunoreactivity in both infiltrating malignant tumor cells and urothelium. (**d**) GATA3 nuclear positivity is variable in sarcomatoid cells in contrast to strong expression in benign urothelium

Differential Diagnosis
- Clear cell renal cell carcinoma with eosinophilic features.
- Chromophobe renal cell carcinoma, eosinophilic variant.
- Oncocytoma.
- Epithelioid angiomyolipoma.

First Round of IHC Studies
- Positive immunostains: Vimentin, CAIX (focally), Cytokeratin 7 (focally).
- Negative immunostains: CD10, CKIT, TFE3.

Second Round of IHC Studies
- Positive immunostains: HMB45 (Fig. 1.45b), Melan-A (Fig. 1.45c).
- Negative immunostains: Smooth muscle actin (SMA).

Final Diagnosis
Epithelioid angiomyolipoma.

Take-Home Messages
1. Epithelioid angiomyolipomas (AMLs) show substantial morphologic overlap with oncocytoma and various subtypes of renal cell carcinoma posing diagnostic difficulties.
2. AMLs are always negative for PAX8, mostly negative for cytokeratins while positive for vimentin, SMA, and melanocytic markers.
3. Expression of melanocytic markers and SMA in epithelioid AML could be very focal or even negative; therefore, a panel of 3–4 markers may be necessary for definitive diagnosis.

References: [116, 117].

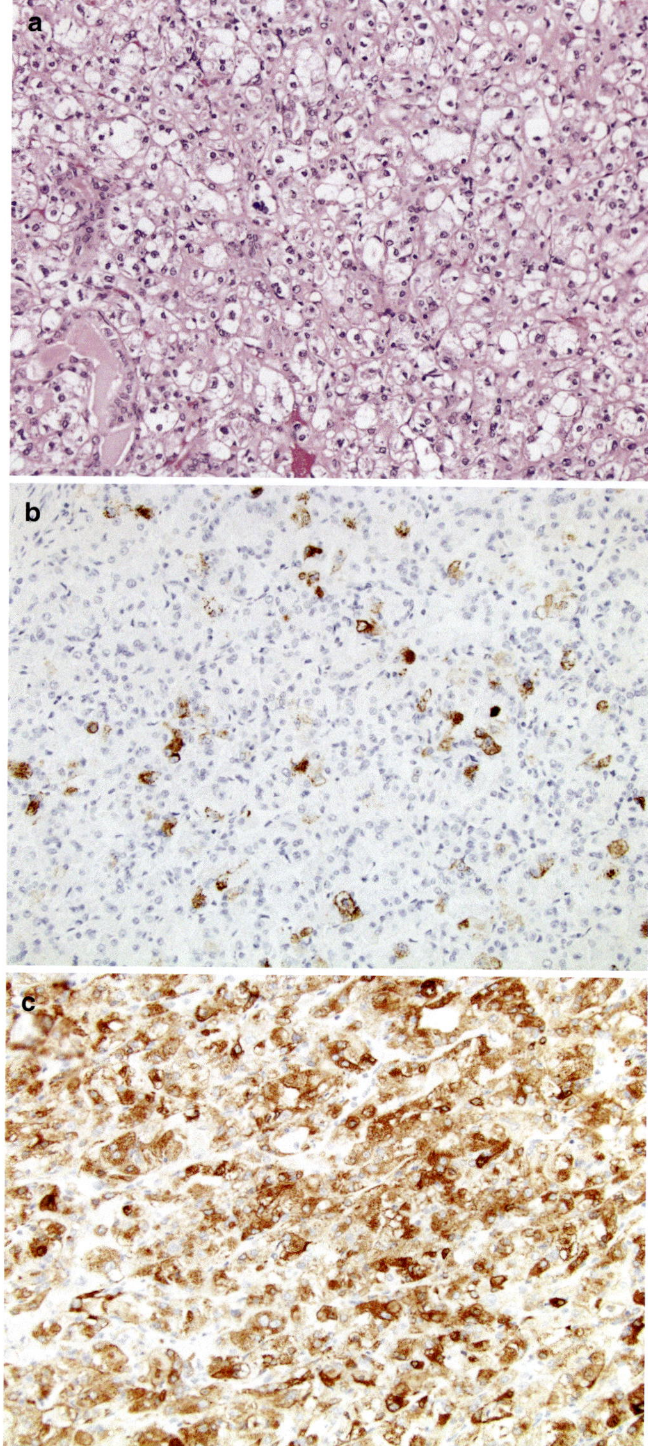

Fig. 1.45 (**a**) Histologically clear cell tumor composed of nests of epithelioid cells with sharp cell borders. (**b**) Immunohistochemistry demonstrates scattered HMB45 positivity. (**c**) Expression of another melanocytic marker Melan-A is more diffuse and uniform

Case 8

Learning Objectives

1. To become familiar with the histologic and immunohistochemical features of the tumor.
2. To generate the differential diagnosis.

Case History

The patient is a healthy 34-year-old female, former marathon-runner with two little children, who presented with acute flank pain and hematuria. Abdominal CT revealed a renal fatty mass with central density, consistent with hemorrhage.

Gross

Partial nephrectomy specimen with extrarenal 11.5 cm mass loosely attached to a portion of kidney parenchyma. On cut surface the mass has a central 7 cm hemorrhagic cavity surrounded by areas of brightly yellow discoloration.

Histologic Findings

At low power, this mass appears to be pure lipomatous neoplasm consisting of sheets of variably sized adipocytes with areas of hemorrhage (Fig. 1.46a). At higher power, the central portion of tumor shows extensive fat necrosis (Fig. 1.46b). At the periphery, tumor contains a few irregular thickened vessels and vascular channels surrounded by elongated plump smooth muscle cells (Fig. 1.46c). No obvious lipoblasts and pleomorphic atypical cells are identified. Renal parenchyma is unremarkable.

Differential Diagnosis

- Lipoma.
- Well-differentiated liposarcoma.
- Fat-rich angiomyolipoma.

Ancillary IHC Studies

- Positive immunostains: HMB45 (rare cells), Melan-A (focally positive).
- Negative immunostains: MDM2, CDK4.

Final Diagnosis

Lipomatous angiomyolipoma (AML).

Take-Home Messages

1. Angiomyolipomas can be fat-rich and predominantly extrarenal when arising from kidney capsule, thus mimicking retroperitoneal well-differentiated lipomatous tumors or even normal perinephric fat.
2. Presence of necrosis and hemorrhage raises concern for malignancy; however, vascular rupture and subsequent

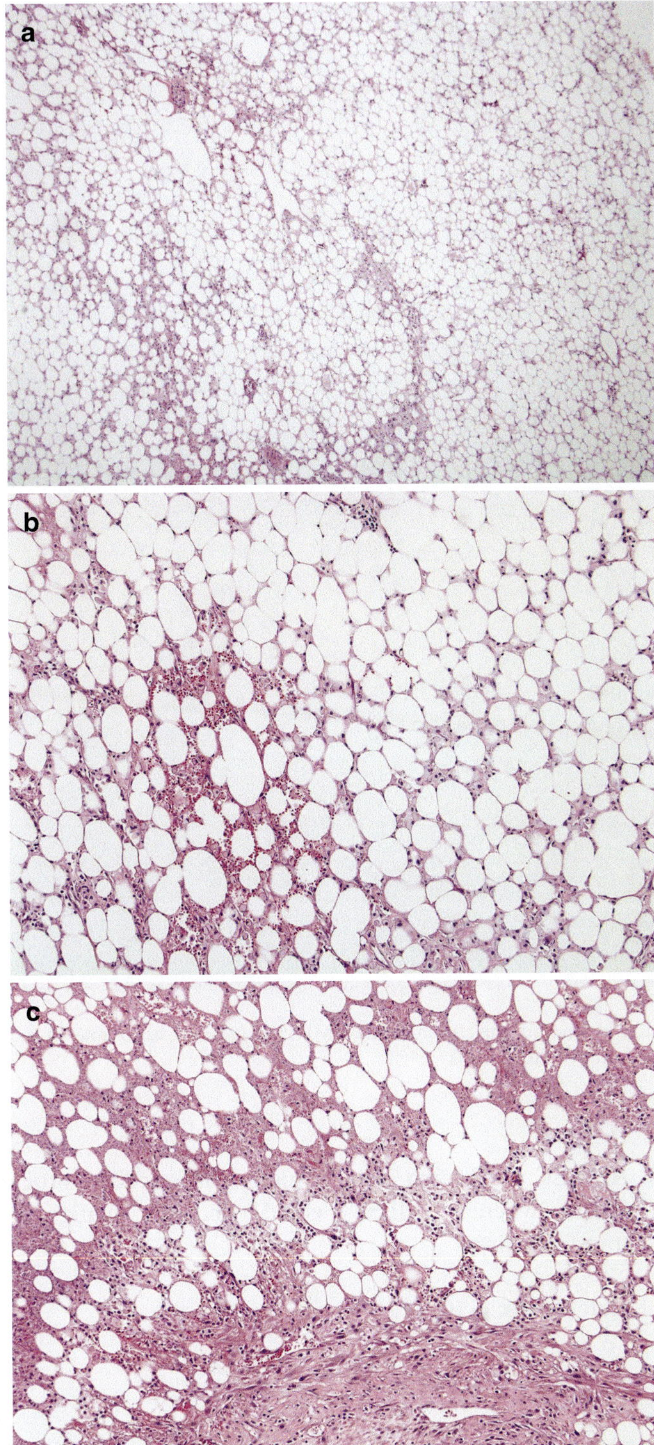

Fig. 1.46 (**a**) Large mass comprised of sheets of variably sized adipocytes. (**b**) Hemorrhage and fat necrosis were apparent at higher magnification. (**c**) Scant stroma represented by spindled plump eosinophilic cells surrounding dysmorphic vessels

ischemic necrosis are well-known complications in larger AMLs.

3. Expression of melanocytic markers and presence of dysmorphic vessels are critical in making a diagnosis of fat-rich AML, whereas smooth muscle actin and MDM2 could be nonspecific (expressed in both AML and well-differentiated liposarcoma).

References: [191, 192].

Case 9

Learning Objectives

1. To become familiar with the histologic and immunohistochemical features of the tumor.
2. To generate the differential diagnosis.

Case History

The patient is a 55-year-old female presented with a left upper quadrant pain after a mild body injury. Radiologic examination revealed a 2.1 cm solid mass with focal cystic change concerning for renal cell carcinoma, which was removed.

Gross

Partial nephrectomy specimen contains a 2.1 x 1.9 x 1.7 cm subcapsular mass with scattered cystic spaces and unremarkable adjacent renal parenchyma.

Histologic Findings

Low-grade mesenchymal neoplasm composed of fascicles and whorls of plump spindle cells surrounding small capillary channels and slit-like vascular spaces with nested, anastomosing pattern (Fig. 1.47a). Other histologic findings include a few cysts within a solid component lined by a single layer of flattened to cuboidal epithelium with hobnailing. These bland cells show eosinophilic cytoplasm, round nuclei, fine chromatin, and inconspicuous nucleoli (Fig. 1.47b).

Differential Diagnosis

- Leiomyoma with entrapped cystically dilated renal tubules.
- Angiomyolipoma with epithelial cysts (AMLEC).
- Mixed epithelial and stromal tumor (MEST).

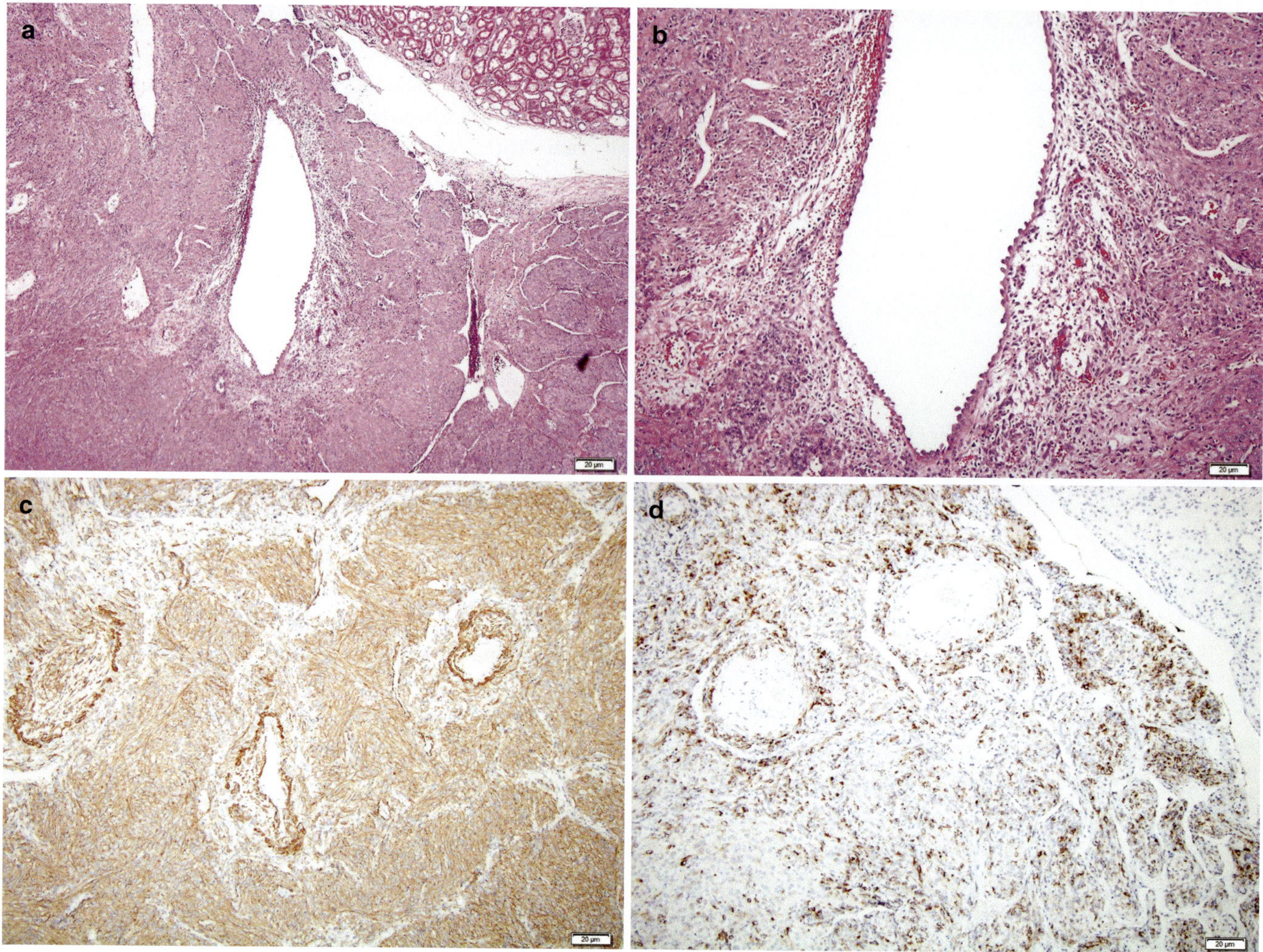

Fig. 1.47 (**a**) Histology demonstrated a smooth muscle neoplasm with scattered cystic spaces. (**b**) Cyst lined by a single layer of eosinophilic cells with hobnailing. (**c**) Immunohistochemistry shows diffuse expression of smooth muscle actin. (**d**) HMB45 expression is obvious in the majority of tumor cells

Ancillary IHC Studies
- Positive immunostains: stromal component positive for SMA (Fig. 1.47c) and HMB45 (Fig. 1.47d), as well as CD10, ER/PR, and vimentin; cyst lining positive for PAX8 and pan-cytokeratin.
- Negative immunostains: Melan-A, CD34, S100.

Final Diagnosis
AML with epithelial cysts (AMLEC).

Take-Home Messages
1. AMLEC is a rare variant of muscle-predominant AML mimicking MEST, but lacking ovarian-type stroma, stromal luteinization, and harboring abnormal vasculature.
2. Panel of melanocytic markers HMB45, Melan-A, and MITF is the most helpful ancillary study to diagnose AMLEC since other markers (SMA, caldesmon, CD10, ER/PR, vimentin) are shared by MEST.

3. AMLEC is a benign indolent tumor with excellent prognosis, whereas MEST could undergo malignant transformation.

References: [110, 113].

Case 10

Learning Objectives
1. To become familiar with the histologic and immunohistochemical features of the tumor.
2. To generate the differential diagnosis.

Case History
The patient is a 55-year-old male who presented with hematuria and acute abdominal pain. He was found to have an extremely large mass in the left kidney, small lesions in the

right kidney, and lymphadenopathy. The patient underwent left radical nephrectomy after embolization and regional lymph node dissection with a plan of subsequent potential second operation of right kidney exploration at a later date. His medical history is significant for pigmented cutaneous lesions, recent acute heart attack, aortic stenosis, and aortic valve replacement.

Gross

Radical nephrectomy specimen weighing 2813 gm is sectioned revealing a 14 × 13.5 × 10 cm tumor extending from the interpolar region into the pelvic fat. The tumor is 60% necrotic with large areas of hemorrhage. A second mass, measuring 5.0 × 4.0 × 2.5 cm, extends from the cortex of the superior pole anteriorly. This smaller mass is firm, tan, and somewhat fleshy. There is marked hydronephrosis. Additionally, a large aggregate of at least eight lymph node candidates was submitted.

Histologic Findings

The dominant tumor mass widely invasive into the hilar fat has variable morphology including intimately admixed epithelioid and mesenchymal areas with hemorrhagic background (Fig. 1.48a). The epithelioid component is composed of nests and sheets of round-to-cuboidal uniform cells with eosinophilic and vacuolated cytoplasm. These tumor nests are separated by abundant stroma with clusters of vessels with eccentrically thickened walls, adipocytes, and plump spindle cells (Fig. 1.48b). In some areas, tumor cells are forming large sheets of clear cells with prominent plant-like membranes, irregular wrinkled nuclei, and prominent perinuclear halos (Fig. 1.48c). Regional lymph nodes contain several areas of extensive spindle cell proliferations (Fig. 1.48d) splitting and invading into the sinusoidal spaces (Fig. 1.48e).

Differential Diagnosis

- Multifocal chromophobe renal cell carcinoma (RCC), suspicious for Birt-Hogg-Dube syndrome.
- Chromophobe RCC with sarcomatoid dedifferentiation and lymph node metastases.
- Multiple angiomyolipomas (AML) and RCC, suggestive of tuberous sclerosis syndrome.
- Clear cell RCC with abundant smooth muscle stroma.

Ancillary Studies

- Positive immunostains: PAX8 and CK7 in epithelioid areas (spindle cell areas negative).
- Negative immunostains: CAIX, AMACR, CD10.

Final Diagnosis

Chromophobe-like RCC and multiple angiomyolipomas (AMLs) involving kidney and lymph nodes, suggestive of tuberous sclerosis (later confirmed clinically).

Take-Home Messages

1. Multiple bilateral tumors including AML and RCC with AML-like stroma (Fig. 1.48a–c) are hallmark features of tuberous sclerosis complex.
2. Rare metastasis of RCC to regional lymph nodes has been reported, but death from RCC in patients with tuberous sclerosis is extremely uncommon.
3. Presence of AML in the lymph node is not considered a metastasis.

References: [188, 193].

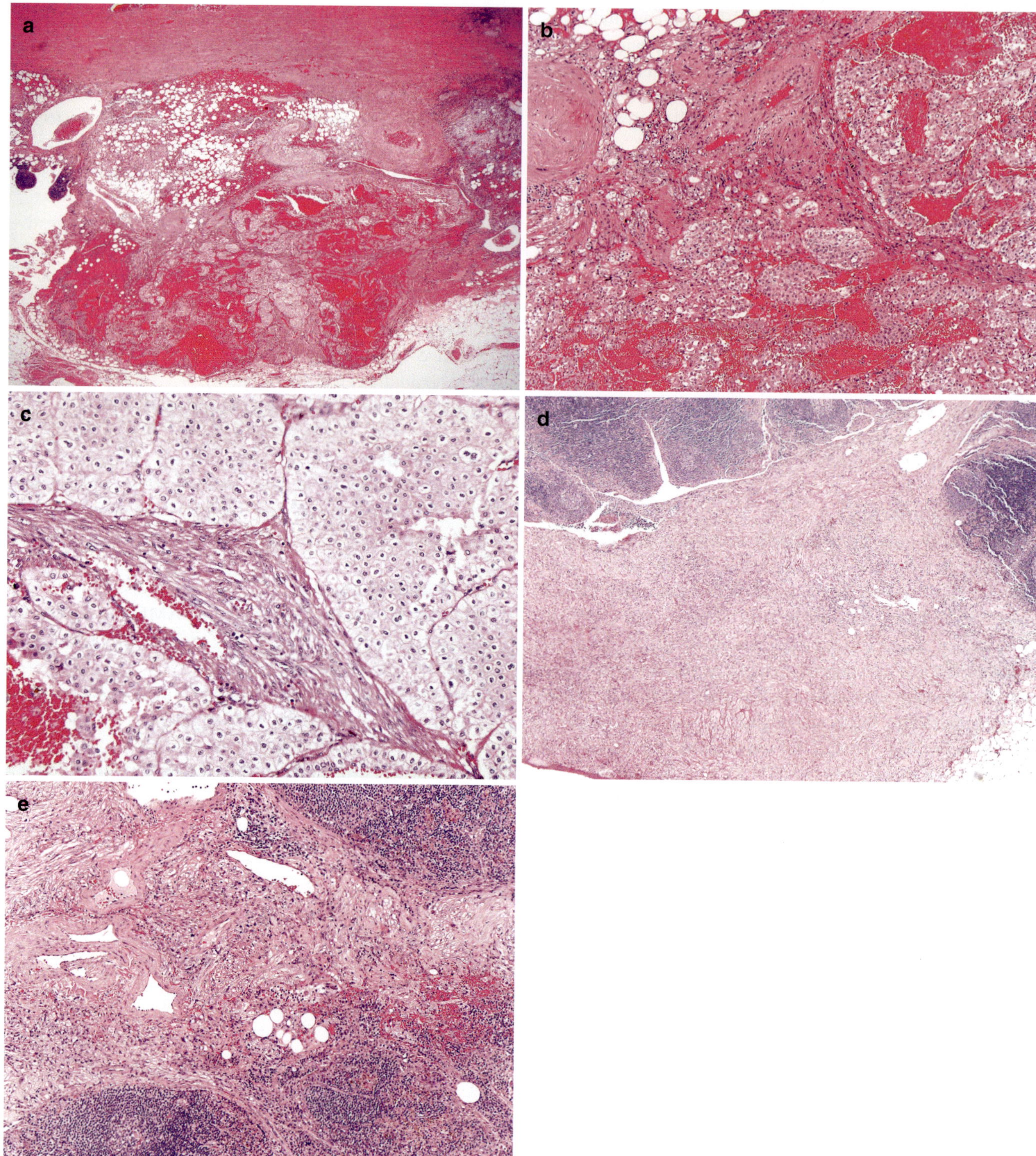

Fig. 1.48 (**a**) Renal hilum contains hemorrhagic tumor. (**b**) Clusters of clear to eosinophilic tumor cells infiltrate hilar fat and stroma. (**c**) Large confluent solid sheets are composed of cells with sharp borders and hyperchromatic raisinoid nuclei surrounded by clear halos. (**d**) Lymph node histology demonstrates pink area of spindle cell proliferation arising from capsule and extending into the extranodal adipose tissue. (**e**) Spindle cells with plump eosinophilic cytoplasm expand sinusoidal spaces of the lymph node

References

1. Halverson SJ, Kunju LP, Bhalla R, Gadzinski AJ, Alderman M, Miller DC, et al. Accuracy of determining small renal mass management with risk stratified biopsies: confirmation by final pathology. J Urol. 2013;189:441–6.
2. Evans AJ, Delahunt B, Srigley JR. Issues and challenges associated with classifying neoplasms in percutaneous needle biopsies of incidentally found small renal masses. Semin Diagn Pathol. 2015;32:184–95.
3. Richard PO, Jewett MA, Bhatt JR, Evans AJ, Timilsina N, Finelli A. Active surveillance for renal neoplasms with oncocytic features is safe. J Urol. 2016;195:581–6.
4. Williamson SR, Eble JN, Cheng L, Grignon DJ. Clear cell papillary renal cell carcinoma: differential diagnosis and extended immunohistochemical profile. Mod Pathol. 2013;26:697–708.
5. Kuroda N, Agatsuma Y, Tamura M, Martinek P, Hes O, Michal M. Sporadic renal hemangioblastoma with CA9, PAX2 and PAX8 expression: diagnostic pitfall in the differential diagnosis from clear cell renal cell carcinoma. Int J Clin Exp Pathol. 2015;8:2131–8.
6. Ohe C, Smith SC, Sirohi D, Divatia M, de Peralta-Venturina M, Paner GP, et al. Reappraisal of morphologic differences between renal medullary carcinoma, collecting duct carcinoma, and fumarate hydratase-deficient renal cell carcinoma. Am J Surg Pathol. 2018;42:279–92.
7. Wu AJ, Mehra R, Hafez K, Wolf JS Jr, Kunju LP. Metastases to the kidney: a clinicopathological study of 43 cases with an emphasis on deceptive features. Histopathology. 2015;66:587–97.
8. Chang A, Brimo F, Montgomery EA, Epstein JI. Use of PAX8 and GATA3 in diagnosing sarcomatoid renal cell carcinoma and sarcomatoid urothelial carcinoma. Hum Pathol. 2013;44:1563–8.
9. Klatte T, Said JW, Seligson DB, Rao PN, de Martino M, Shuch B, et al. Pathological, immunohistochemical and cytogenetic features of papillary renal cell carcinoma with clear cell features. J Urol. 2011;185:30–5.
10. Trpkov K, Grignon DJ, Bonsib SM, Amin MB, Billis A, Lopez-Beltran A, et al. Handling and staging of renal cell carcinoma: the International Society of Urological Pathology Consensus (ISUP) conference recommendations. Am J Surg Pathol. 2013;37:1505–17.
11. Bonsib SM. The renal sinus is the principal invasive pathway: a prospective study of 100 renal cell carcinomas. Am J Surg Pathol. 2004;28:1594–600.
12. Bonsib SM. T2 clear cell renal cell carcinoma is a rare entity: a study of 120 clear cell renal cell carcinomas. J Urol. 2005;174:1199–202; discussion 202
13. Bonsib SM. Renal lymphatics, and lymphatic involvement in sinus vein invasive (pT3b) clear cell renal cell carcinoma: a study of 40 cases. Mod Pathol. 2006;19:746–53.
14. Williamson SR, Rao P, Hes O, Epstein JI, Smith SC, Picken MM, et al. Challenges in pathologic staging of renal cell carcinoma: a study of interobserver variability among urologic pathologists. Am J Surg Pathol. 2018;42:1253–61.
15. Taneja K, Arora S, Rogers CG, Gupta NS, Williamson SR. Pathological staging of renal cell carcinoma: a review of 300 consecutive cases with emphasis on retrograde venous invasion. Histopathology. 2018;73:681–91.
16. Thompson RH, Blute ML, Krambeck AE, Lohse CM, Magera JS, Leibovich BC, et al. Patients with pT1 renal cell carcinoma who die from disease after nephrectomy may have unrecognized renal sinus fat invasion. Am J Surg Pathol. 2007;31:1089–93.
17. Srigley JR, Delahunt B, Eble JN, Egevad L, Epstein JI, Grignon D, et al. The International Society of Urological Pathology (ISUP) Vancouver classification of renal neoplasia. Am J Surg Pathol. 2013;37:1469–89.
18. Amin MB, Crotty TB, Tickoo SK, Farrow GM. Renal oncocytoma: a reappraisal of morphologic features with clinicopathologic findings in 80 cases. Am J Surg Pathol. 1997;21:1–12.
19. Perez-Ordonez B, Hamed G, Campbell S, Erlandson RA, Russo P, Gaudin PB, et al. Renal oncocytoma: a clinicopathologic study of 70 cases. Am J Surg Pathol. 1997;21:871–83.
20. Trpkov K, Yilmaz A, Uzer D, Dishongh KM, Quick CM, Bismar TA, et al. Renal oncocytoma revisited: a clinicopathological study of 109 cases with emphasis on problematic diagnostic features. Histopathology. 2010;57:893–906.
21. Wobker SE, Williamson SR. Modern pathologic diagnosis of renal Oncocytoma. J Kidney Cancer VHL. 2017;4:1–12.
22. Hes O, Michal M, Sima R, Vanecek T, Brunelli M, Martignoni G, et al. Renal oncocytoma with and without intravascular extension into the branches of renal vein have the same morphological, immunohistochemical, and genetic features. Virchows Arch. 2008;452:193–200.
23. Wobker SE, Przybycin CG, Sircar K, Epstein JI. Renal oncocytoma with vascular invasion: a series of 22 cases. Hum Pathol. 2016;58:1–6.
24. Xiao GQ, Ko HB, Unger P. Telangiectatic oncocytoma: a previously undescribed variant of renal oncocytoma. Am J Clin Pathol. 2013;140:103–8.
25. Williamson SR, Halat S, Eble JN, Grignon DJ, Lopez-Beltran A, Montironi R, et al. Multilocular cystic renal cell carcinoma: similarities and differences in immunoprofile compared with clear cell renal cell carcinoma. Am J Surg Pathol. 2012;36:1425–33.
26. Tran T, Jones CL, Williamson SR, Eble JN, Grignon DJ, Zhang S, et al. Tubulocystic renal cell carcinoma is an entity that is immunohistochemically and genetically distinct from papillary renal cell carcinoma. Histopathology. 2016;68:850–7.
27. Calio A, Eble JN, Grignon DJ, Delahunt B. Mixed epithelial and stromal tumor of the kidney: a clinicopathologic study of 53 cases. Am J Surg Pathol. 2016;40:1538–49.
28. Park HS, Lee K, Moon KC. Determination of the cutoff value of the proportion of cystic change for prognostic stratification of clear cell renal cell carcinoma. J Urol. 2011;186:423–9.
29. Mantilla JG, Antic T, Tretiakova M. GATA3 as a valuable marker to distinguish clear cell papillary renal cell carcinomas from morphologic mimics. Hum Pathol. 2017;66:152–8.
30. Park JJ, Jeong BC, Kim CK, Seo SI, Carriere KC, Kim M, et al. Postoperative outcome of cystic renal cell carcinoma defined on preoperative imaging: a retrospective study. J Urol. 2017;197:991–7.
31. Hartman DS, Davis CJ Jr, Johns T, Goldman SM. Cystic renal cell carcinoma. Urology. 1986;28:145–53.
32. Liu L, Qian J, Singh H, Meiers I, Zhou X, Bostwick DG. Immunohistochemical analysis of chromophobe renal cell carcinoma, renal oncocytoma, and clear cell carcinoma: an optimal and practical panel for differential diagnosis. Arch Pathol Lab Med. 2007;131:1290–7.
33. Miettinen M, McCue PA, Sarlomo-Rikala M, Rys J, Czapiewski P, Wazny K, et al. GATA3: a multispecific but potentially useful marker in surgical pathology: a systematic analysis of 2500 epithelial and nonepithelial tumors. Am J Surg Pathol. 2014;38:13–22.
34. Gonzalez-Roibon N, Faraj SF, Munari E, Bezerra SM, Albadine R, Sharma R, et al. Comprehensive profile of GATA binding protein 3 immunohistochemical expression in primary and metastatic renal neoplasms. Hum Pathol. 2014;45:244–8.
35. Camparo P, Vasiliu V, Molinie V, Couturier J, Dykema KJ, Petillo D, et al. Renal translocation carcinomas: clinicopathologic, immunohistochemical, and gene expression profiling analysis of 31 cases with a review of the literature. Am J Surg Pathol. 2008;32:656–70.

36. Williamson SR, Gadde R, Trpkov K, Hirsch MS, Srigley JR, Reuter VE, et al. Diagnostic criteria for oncocytic renal neoplasms: a survey of urologic pathologists. Hum Pathol. 2017;63:149–56.

37. Brugarolas J. Molecular genetics of clear-cell renal cell carcinoma. J Clin Oncol. 2014;32:1968–76.

38. Favazza L, Chitale DA, Barod R, Rogers CG, Kalyana-Sundaram S, Palanisamy N, et al. Renal cell tumors with clear cell histology and intact VHL and chromosome 3p: a histological review of tumors from the Cancer genome atlas database. Mod Pathol. 2017;30:1603–12.

39. Cancer Genome Atlas Research Network. Comprehensive molecular characterization of clear cell renal cell carcinoma. Nature. 2013;499:43–9.

40. Sato Y, Yoshizato T, Shiraishi Y, Maekawa S, Okuno Y, Kamura T, et al. Integrated molecular analysis of clear-cell renal cell carcinoma. Nat Genet. 2013;45:860–7.

41. Green WM, Yonescu R, Morsberger L, Morris K, Netto GJ, Epstein JI, et al. Utilization of a TFE3 break-apart FISH assay in a renal tumor consultation service. Am J Surg Pathol. 2013;37:1150–63.

42. Rao Q, Williamson SR, Zhang S, Eble JN, Grignon DJ, Wang M, et al. TFE3 break-apart FISH has a higher sensitivity for Xp11.2 translocation-associated renal cell carcinoma compared with TFE3 or cathepsin K immunohistochemical staining alone: expanding the morphologic spectrum. Am J Surg Pathol. 2013;37:804–15.

43. Williamson SR, Grignon DJ, Cheng L, Favazza L, Gondim DD, Carskadon S, et al. Renal cell carcinoma with chromosome 6p amplification including the TFEB gene: a novel mechanism of tumor pathogenesis? Am J Surg Pathol. 2017;41:287–98.

44. Argani P, Reuter VE, Zhang L, Sung YS, Ning Y, Epstein JI, et al. TFEB-amplified renal cell carcinomas: an aggressive molecular subset demonstrating variable melanocytic marker expression and morphologic heterogeneity. Am J Surg Pathol. 2016;40:1484–95.

45. Gupta S, Johnson SH, Vasmatzis G, Porath B, Rustin JG, Rao P, et al. TFEB-VEGFA (6p21.1) co-amplified renal cell carcinoma: a distinct entity with potential implications for clinical management. Mod Pathol. 2017;30:998–1012.

46. Sukov WR, Ketterling RP, Lager DJ, Carlson AW, Sinnwell JP, Chow GK, et al. CCND1 rearrangements and cyclin D1 overexpression in renal oncocytomas: frequency, clinicopathologic features, and utility in differentiation from chromophobe renal cell carcinoma. Hum Pathol. 2009;40:1296–303.

47. Argani P, Zhang L, Reuter VE, Tickoo SK, Antonescu CR. RBM10-TFE3 renal cell carcinoma: a potential diagnostic pitfall due to cryptic intrachromosomal Xp11.2 inversion resulting in false-negative TFE3 FISH. Am J Surg Pathol. 2017;41:655–62.

48. Xia QY, Wang XT, Zhan XM, Tan X, Chen H, Liu Y, et al. Xp11 translocation renal cell carcinomas (RCCs) with RBM10-TFE3 gene fusion demonstrating melanotic features and overlapping morphology with t(6;11) RCC: interest and diagnostic pitfall in detecting a paracentric inversion of TFE3. Am J Surg Pathol. 2017;41:663–76.

49. Xia QY, Wang Z, Chen N, Gan HL, Teng XD, Shi SS, et al. Xp11.2 translocation renal cell carcinoma with NONO-TFE3 gene fusion: morphology, prognosis, and potential pitfall in detecting TFE3 gene rearrangement. Mod Pathol. 2017;30:416–26.

50. Delahunt B, Cheville JC, Martignoni G, Humphrey PA, Magi-Galluzzi C, McKenney J, et al. The International Society of Urological Pathology (ISUP) grading system for renal cell carcinoma and other prognostic parameters. Am J Surg Pathol. 2013;37:1490–504.

51. Delahunt B, McKenney JK, Lohse CM, Leibovich BC, Thompson RH, Boorjian SA, et al. A novel grading system for clear cell renal cell carcinoma incorporating tumor necrosis. Am J Surg Pathol. 2013;37:311–22.

52. Delahunt B, Sika-Paotonu D, Bethwaite PB, William Jordan T, Magi-Galluzzi C, Zhou M, et al. Grading of clear cell renal cell carcinoma should be based on nucleolar prominence. Am J Surg Pathol. 2011;35:1134–9.

53. Paner GP, Amin MB, Alvarado-Cabrero I, Young AN, Stricker HJ, Moch H, et al. A novel tumor grading scheme for chromophobe renal cell carcinoma: prognostic utility and comparison with Fuhrman nuclear grade. Am J Surg Pathol. 2010;34:1233–40.

54. Renshaw AA, Cheville JC. Quantitative tumour necrosis is an independent predictor of overall survival in clear cell renal cell carcinoma. Pathology. 2015;47:34–7.

55. Sengupta S, Lohse CM, Leibovich BC, Frank I, Thompson RH, Webster WS, et al. Histologic coagulative tumor necrosis as a prognostic indicator of renal cell carcinoma aggressiveness. Cancer. 2005;104:511–20.

56. Williamson SR, MacLennan GT, Lopez-Beltran A, Montironi R, Tan PH, Martignoni G, et al. Cystic partially regressed clear cell renal cell carcinoma: a potential mimic of multilocular cystic renal cell carcinoma. Histopathology. 2013;63:767–79.

57. Kryvenko ON, Jorda M, Argani P, Epstein JI. Diagnostic approach to eosinophilic renal neoplasms. Arch Pathol Lab Med. 2014;138:1531–41.

58. Kryvenko ON, Roquero L, Gupta NS, Lee MW, Epstein JI. Low-grade clear cell renal cell carcinoma mimicking hemangioma of the kidney: a series of 4 cases. Arch Pathol Lab Med. 2013;137:251–4.

59. Williamson SR, Kum JB, Goheen MP, Cheng L, Grignon DJ, Idrees MT. Clear cell renal cell carcinoma with a syncytial-type multinucleated giant tumor cell component: implications for differential diagnosis. Hum Pathol. 2014;45:735–44.

60. Dhakal HP, McKenney JK, Khor LY, Reynolds JP, Magi-Galluzzi C, Przybycin CG. Renal neoplasms with overlapping features of clear cell renal cell carcinoma and clear cell papillary renal cell carcinoma: a clinicopathologic study of 37 cases from a single institution. Am J Surg Pathol. 2016;40:141–54.

61. Williamson SR, Gupta NS, Eble JN, Rogers CG, Michalowski S, Zhang S, et al. Clear cell renal cell carcinoma with borderline features of clear cell papillary renal cell carcinoma: combined morphologic, immunohistochemical, and cytogenetic analysis. Am J Surg Pathol. 2015;39:1502–10.

62. Williamson SR, Zhang S, Eble JN, Grignon DJ, Martignoni G, Brunelli M, et al. Clear cell papillary renal cell carcinoma-like tumors in patients with von Hippel-Lindau disease are unrelated to sporadic clear cell papillary renal cell carcinoma. Am J Surg Pathol. 2013;37:1131–9.

63. Gobbo S, Eble JN, Maclennan GT, Grignon DJ, Shah RB, Zhang S, et al. Renal cell carcinomas with papillary architecture and clear cell components: the utility of immunohistochemical and cytogenetical analyses in differential diagnosis. Am J Surg Pathol. 2008;32:1780–6.

64. Tickoo SK, Amin MB, Zarbo RJ. Colloidal iron staining in renal epithelial neoplasms, including chromophobe renal cell carcinoma: emphasis on technique and patterns of staining. Am J Surg Pathol. 1998;22:419–24.

65. Li L, Parwani AV. Xanthogranulomatous pyelonephritis. Arch Pathol Lab Med. 2011;135:671–4.

66. Eble JN, Moch H, Amin MB, Argani P, Cheville J, Delahunt B, et al. Papillary adenoma. In: Moch H, Humphrey PA, Ulbright TM, Reuter VE, editors. WHO classification of tumours of the urinary system and male genital organs. 4th ed. Lyon: International Agency for Research on Cancer; 2016. p. 42–3.

67. Umbreit EC, Shimko MS, Childs MA, Lohse CM, Cheville JC, Leibovich BC, et al. Metastatic potential of a renal mass according to original tumour size at presentation. BJU Int. 2012;109:190–4; discussion 4

68. Kinney SN, Eble JN, Hes O, Williamson SR, Grignon DJ, Wang M, et al. Metanephric adenoma: the utility of immunohistochemical and cytogenetic analyses in differential diagnosis, including solid

variant papillary renal cell carcinoma and epithelial-predominant nephroblastoma. Mod Pathol. 2015;28:1236–48.

69. Choueiri TK, Cheville J, Palescandolo E, Fay AP, Kantoff PW, Atkins MB, et al. BRAF mutations in metanephric adenoma of the kidney. Eur Urol. 2012;62:917–22.

70. Udager AM, Pan J, Magers MJ, Palapattu GS, Morgan TM, Montgomery JS, et al. Molecular and immunohistochemical characterization reveals novel BRAF mutations in metanephric adenoma. Am J Surg Pathol. 2015;39:549–57.

71. Delahunt B, Eble JN. Papillary renal cell carcinoma: a clinicopathologic and immunohistochemical study of 105 tumors. Mod Pathol. 1997;10:537–44.

72. Trpkov K, Hes O, Agaimy A, Bonert M, Martinek P, Magi-Galluzzi C, et al. Fumarate hydratase-deficient renal cell carcinoma is strongly correlated with fumarate hydratase mutation and hereditary leiomyomatosis and renal cell carcinoma syndrome. Am J Surg Pathol. 2016;40:865–75.

73. Cancer Genome Atlas Research Network, Linehan WM, Spellman PT, Ricketts CJ, Creighton CJ, Fei SS, et al. Comprehensive molecular characterization of papillary renal-cell carcinoma. N Engl J Med. 2016;374:135–45.

74. Cossu-Rocca P, Eble JN, Delahunt B, Zhang S, Martignoni G, Brunelli M, et al. Renal mucinous tubular and spindle carcinoma lacks the gains of chromosomes 7 and 17 and losses of chromosome Y that are prevalent in papillary renal cell carcinoma. Mod Pathol. 2006;19:488–93.

75. Eble JN. Mucinous tubular and spindle cell carcinoma and postneuroblastoma carcinoma: newly recognised entities in the renal cell carcinoma family. Pathology. 2003;35:499–504.

76. Fine SW, Argani P, DeMarzo AM, Delahunt B, Sebo TJ, Reuter VE, et al. Expanding the histologic spectrum of mucinous tubular and spindle cell carcinoma of the kidney. Am J Surg Pathol. 2006;30:1554–60.

77. Mehra R, Vats P, Cieslik M, Cao X, Su F, Shukla S, et al. Biallelic alteration and dysregulation of the Hippo pathway in mucinous tubular and spindle cell carcinoma of the kidney. Cancer Discov. 2016;6:1258–66.

78. Peckova K, Martinek P, Sperga M, Montiel DP, Daum O, Rotterova P, et al. Mucinous spindle and tubular renal cell carcinoma: analysis of chromosomal aberration pattern of low-grade, high-grade, and overlapping morphologic variant with papillary renal cell carcinoma. Ann Diagn Pathol. 2015;19:226–31.

79. Ren Q, Wang L, Al-Ahmadie HA, Fine SW, Gopalan A, Sirintrapun SJ, et al. Distinct genomic copy number alterations distinguish mucinous tubular and spindle cell carcinoma of the kidney from papillary renal cell carcinoma with overlapping histologic features. Am J Surg Pathol. 2018;42:767–77.

80. Wang L, Zhang Y, Chen YB, Skala SL, Al-Ahmadie HA, Wang X, et al. VSTM2A overexpression is a sensitive and specific biomarker for mucinous tubular and spindle cell carcinoma (MTSCC) of the kidney. Am J Surg Pathol. 2018;42(12):1571–84.

81. Gunia S, Erbersdobler A, Koch S, Otto W, Staibano S, D'Alterio C, et al. Protein gene product 9.5 is diagnostically helpful in delineating high-grade renal cell cancer involving the renal medullary/sinus region from invasive urothelial cell carcinoma of the renal pelvis. Hum Pathol. 2013;44:712–7.

82. Davis CF, Ricketts CJ, Wang M, Yang L, Cherniack AD, Shen H, et al. The somatic genomic landscape of chromophobe renal cell carcinoma. Cancer Cell. 2014;26:319–30.

83. Sperga M, Martinek P, Vanecek T, Grossmann P, Bauleth K, Perez-Montiel D, et al. Chromophobe renal cell carcinoma--chromosomal aberration variability and its relation to Paner grading system: an array CGH and FISH analysis of 37 cases. Virchows Arch. 2013;463:563–73.

84. Ng KL, Morais C, Bernard A, Saunders N, Samaratunga H, Gobe G, et al. A systematic review and meta-analysis of immunohistochemical biomarkers that differentiate chromophobe renal cell carcinoma from renal oncocytoma. J Clin Pathol. 2016;69:661–71.

85. Ng KL, Rajandram R, Morais C, Yap NY, Samaratunga H, Gobe GC, et al. Differentiation of oncocytoma from chromophobe renal cell carcinoma (RCC): can novel molecular biomarkers help solve an old problem? J Clin Pathol. 2014;67:97–104.

86. Zhou C, Urbauer DL, Fellman BM, Tamboli P, Zhang M, Matin SF, et al. Metastases to the kidney: a comprehensive analysis of 151 patients from a tertiary referral centre. BJU Int. 2016;117:775–82.

87. Pal SK, Choueiri TK, Wang K, Khaira D, Karam JA, Van Allen E, et al. Characterization of clinical cases of collecting duct carcinoma of the kidney assessed by comprehensive genomic profiling. Eur Urol. 2016;70:516–21.

88. Amin MB, Smith SC, Agaimy A, Argani P, Comperat EM, Delahunt B, et al. Collecting duct carcinoma versus renal medullary carcinoma: an appeal for nosologic and biological clarity. Am J Surg Pathol. 2014;38:871–4.

89. Calderaro J, Masliah-Planchon J, Richer W, Maillot L, Maille P, Mansuy L, et al. Balanced translocations disrupting SMARCB1 are hallmark recurrent genetic alterations in renal medullary carcinomas. Eur Urol. 2016;69:1055–61.

90. Calderaro J, Moroch J, Pierron G, Pedeutour F, Grison C, Maille P, et al. SMARCB1/INI1 inactivation in renal medullary carcinoma. Histopathology. 2012;61:428–35.

91. Carlo MI, Chaim J, Patil S, Kemel Y, Schram AM, Woo K, et al. Genomic characterization of renal medullary carcinoma and treatment outcomes. Clin Genitourin Cancer. 2017;15:e987–e94.

92. Liu Q, Galli S, Srinivasan R, Linehan WM, Tsokos M, Merino MJ. Renal medullary carcinoma: molecular, immunohistochemistry, and morphologic correlation. Am J Surg Pathol. 2013;37:368–74.

93. Shuch B, Bratslavsky G, Linehan WM, Srinivasan R. Sarcomatoid renal cell carcinoma: a comprehensive review of the biology and current treatment strategies. Oncologist. 2012;17:46–54.

94. Merrill MM, Wood CG, Tannir NM, Slack RS, Babaian KN, Jonasch E, et al. Clinically nonmetastatic renal cell carcinoma with sarcomatoid dedifferentiation: natural history and outcomes after surgical resection with curative intent. Urol Oncol. 2015;33:166.e21–9.

95. Zhang L, Wu B, Zha Z, Zhao H, Feng Y. The prognostic value and clinicopathological features of sarcomatoid differentiation in patients with renal cell carcinoma: a systematic review and meta-analysis. Cancer Manag Res. 2018;10:1687–703.

96. Wang Z, Kim TB, Peng B, Karam J, Creighton C, Joon A, et al. Sarcomatoid renal cell carcinoma has a distinct molecular pathogenesis, driver mutation profile, and transcriptional landscape. Clin Cancer Res. 2017;23:6686–96.

97. Dotan ZA, Tal R, Golijanin D, Snyder ME, Antonescu C, Brennan MF, et al. Adult genitourinary sarcoma: the 25-year memorial Sloan-Kettering experience. J Urol. 2006;176:2033–8; discussion 8–9

98. Shuch B, Bratslavsky G, Shih J, Vourganti S, Finley D, Castor B, et al. Impact of pathological tumour characteristics in patients with sarcomatoid renal cell carcinoma. BJU Int. 2012;109:1600–6.

99. Tan PH, Cheng L, Rioux-Leclercq N, Merino MJ, Netto G, Reuter VE, et al. Renal tumors: diagnostic and prognostic biomarkers. Am J Surg Pathol. 2013;37:1518–31.

100. Fatima N, Canter DJ, Carthon BC, Kucuk O, Master VA, Nieh PT, et al. Sarcomatoid urothelial carcinoma of the bladder: a contemporary clinicopathologic analysis of 37 cases. Can J Urol. 2015;22:7783–7.

101. Fatima N, Osunkoya AO. GATA3 expression in sarcomatoid urothelial carcinoma of the bladder. Hum Pathol. 2014;45:1625–9.

102. Martignoni G, Pea M, Zampini C, Brunelli M, Segala D, Zamboni G, et al. PEComas of the kidney and of the genitourinary tract. Semin Diagn Pathol. 2015;32:140–59.

103. Lane BR, Aydin H, Danforth TL, Zhou M, Remer EM, Novick AC, et al. Clinical correlates of renal angiomyolipoma subtypes in 209 patients: classic, fat poor, tuberous sclerosis associated and epithelioid. J Urol. 2008;180:836–43.

104. Fine SW, Reuter VE, Epstein JI, Argani P. Angiomyolipoma with epithelial cysts (AMLEC): a distinct cystic variant of angiomyolipoma. Am J Surg Pathol. 2006;30:593–9.

105. Martignoni G, Pea M, Bonetti F, Brunelli M, Eble JN. Oncocytoma-like angiomyolipoma. A clinicopathologic and immunohistochemical study of 2 cases. Arch Pathol Lab Med. 2002;126:610–2.

106. Matsuyama A, Hisaoka M, Ichikawa K, Fujimori T, Udo K, Uchihashi K, et al. Sclerosing variant of epithelioid angiomyolipoma. Pathol Int. 2008;58:306–10.

107. Chowdhury PR, Tsuda N, Anami M, Hayashi T, Iseki M, Kishikawa M, et al. A histopathologic and immunohistochemical study of small nodules of renal angiomyolipoma: a comparison of small nodules with angiomyolipoma. Mod Pathol. 1996;9:1081–8.

108. Calio A, Warfel KA, Eble JN. Renomedullary interstitial cell tumors: pathologic features and clinical correlations. Am J Surg Pathol. 2016;40:1693–701.

109. Gatalica Z, Lilleberg SL, Koul MS, Vanecek T, Hes O, Wang B, et al. COX-2 gene polymorphisms and protein expression in renomedullary interstitial cell tumors. Hum Pathol. 2008;39:1495–504.

110. Wei J, Li Y, Wen Y, Li L, Zhang R. Renal angiomyolipoma with epithelial cysts: a rare entity and review of literature. Int J Clin Exp Pathol. 2015;8:11760–5.

111. Zhou M, Kort E, Hoekstra P, Westphal M, Magi-Galluzzi C, Sercia L, et al. Adult cystic nephroma and mixed epithelial and stromal tumor of the kidney are the same disease entity: molecular and histologic evidence. Am J Surg Pathol. 2009;33:72–80.

112. Lane BR, Campbell SC, Remer EM, Fergany AF, Williams SB, Novick AC, et al. Adult cystic nephroma and mixed epithelial and stromal tumor of the kidney: clinical, radiographic, and pathologic characteristics. Urology. 2008;71:1142–8.

113. Michal M, Hes O, Bisceglia M, Simpson RH, Spagnolo DV, Parma A, et al. Mixed epithelial and stromal tumors of the kidney. A report of 22 cases. Virchows Arch. 2004;445:359–67.

114. Jung SJ, Shen SS, Tran T, Jun SY, Truong L, Ayala AG, et al. Mixed epithelial and stromal tumor of kidney with malignant transformation: report of two cases and review of literature. Hum Pathol. 2008;39:463–8.

115. Aydin H, Magi-Galluzzi C, Lane BR, Sercia L, Lopez JI, Rini BI, et al. Renal angiomyolipoma: clinicopathologic study of 194 cases with emphasis on the epithelioid histology and tuberous sclerosis association. Am J Surg Pathol. 2009;33:289–97.

116. Aron M, Aydin H, Sercia L, Magi-Galluzzi C, Zhou M. Renal cell carcinomas with intratumoral fat and concomitant angiomyolipoma: potential pitfalls in staging and diagnosis. Am J Clin Pathol. 2010;134:807–12.

117. He W, Cheville JC, Sadow PM, Gopalan A, Fine SW, Al-Ahmadie HA, et al. Epithelioid angiomyolipoma of the kidney: pathological features and clinical outcome in a series of consecutively resected tumors. Mod Pathol. 2013;26:1355–64.

118. Martignoni G, Cheville J, Fletcher CDM, Pea M, Reuter VE, Ro JY, et al. Epithelioid angiomyolipoma. In: Moch A, Humphrey PA, Ulbright TM, Reuter VE, editors. World Health Organization classification of tumours the urinary system and male genital organs. 4th ed. Lyon: IARC Press; 2016. p. 65–6.

119. Brimo F, Robinson B, Guo C, Zhou M, Latour M, Epstein JI. Renal epithelioid angiomyolipoma with atypia: a series of 40 cases with emphasis on clinicopathologic prognostic indicators of malignancy. Am J Surg Pathol. 2010;34:715–22.

120. Nese N, Martignoni G, Fletcher CD, Gupta R, Pan CC, Kim H, et al. Pure epithelioid PEComas (so-called epithelioid angiomyolipoma) of the kidney: a clinicopathologic study of 41 cases: detailed assessment of morphology and risk stratification. Am J Surg Pathol. 2011;35:161–76.

121. Varma S, Gupta S, Talwar J, Forte F, Dhar M. Renal epithelioid angiomyolipoma: a malignant disease. J Nephrol. 2011;24:18–22.

122. Konosu-Fukaya S, Nakamura Y, Fujishima F, Kasajima A, McNamara KM, Takahashi Y, et al. Renal epithelioid angiomyolipoma with malignant features: histological evaluation and novel immunohistochemical findings. Pathol Int. 2014;64:133–41.

123. Zheng S, Bi XG, Song QK, Yuan Z, Guo L, Zhang H, et al. A suggestion for pathological grossing and reporting based on prognostic indicators of malignancies from a pooled analysis of renal epithelioid angiomyolipoma. Int Urol Nephrol. 2015;47:1643–51.

124. Lei JH, Liu LR, Wei Q, Song TR, Yang L, Yuan HC, et al. A four-year follow-up study of renal epithelioid angiomyolipoma: a multicenter experience and literature review. Sci Rep. 2015;5:10030.

125. Park JH, Lee C, Suh JH, Kim G, Song B, Moon KC. Renal epithelioid angiomyolipoma: histopathologic review, immunohistochemical evaluation and prognostic significance. Pathol Int. 2016;66:571–7.

126. Miller JS, Zhou M, Brimo F, Guo CC, Epstein JI. Primary leiomyosarcoma of the kidney: a clinicopathologic study of 27 cases. Am J Surg Pathol. 2010;34:238–42.

127. Mayes DC, Fechner RE, Gillenwater JY. Renal liposarcoma. Am J Surg Pathol. 1990;14:268–73.

128. Matsushita M, Ito A, Ishidoya S, Endoh M, Moriya T, Arai Y. Intravenous extended liposarcoma arising from renal sinus. Int J Urol. 2007;14:769–70.

129. Olgac S, Mazumdar M, Dalbagni G, Reuter VE. Urothelial carcinoma of the renal pelvis: a clinicopathologic study of 130 cases. Am J Surg Pathol. 2004;28:1545–52.

130. Gupta R, Paner GP, Amin MB. Neoplasms of the upper urinary tract: a review with focus on urothelial carcinoma of the pelvicalyceal system and aspects related to its diagnosis and reporting. Adv Anat Pathol. 2008;15:127–39.

131. Lughezzani G, Jeldres C, Isbarn H, Sun M, Shariat SF, Alasker A, et al. Nephroureterectomy and segmental ureterectomy in the treatment of invasive upper tract urothelial carcinoma: a population-based study of 2299 patients. Eur J Cancer. 2009;45:3291–7.

132. Cha EK, Shariat SF, Kormaksson M, Novara G, Chromecki TF, Scherr DS, et al. Predicting clinical outcomes after radical nephroureterectomy for upper tract urothelial carcinoma. Eur Urol. 2012;61:818–25.

133. Gupta R, Billis A, Shah RB, Moch H, Osunkoya AO, Jochum W, et al. Carcinoma of the collecting ducts of Bellini and renal medullary carcinoma: clinicopathologic analysis of 52 cases of rare aggressive subtypes of renal cell carcinoma with a focus on their interrelationship. Am J Surg Pathol. 2012;36:1265–78.

134. Higgins JP, Kaygusuz G, Wang L, Montgomery K, Mason V, Zhu SX, et al. Placental S100 (S100P) and GATA3: markers for transitional epithelium and urothelial carcinoma discovered by complementary DNA microarray. Am J Surg Pathol. 2007;31:673–80.

135. Albadine R, Schultz L, Illei P, Ertoy D, Hicks J, Sharma R, et al. PAX8 (+)/p63 (−) immunostaining pattern in renal collecting duct carcinoma (CDC): a useful immunoprofile in the differential diagnosis of CDC versus urothelial carcinoma of upper urinary tract. Am J Surg Pathol. 2010;34:965–9.

136. Williams PA, Mai KT. Primary carcinoma of renal calyx. Pathol Res Pract. 2013;209:654–61.

137. Perlman EJ. Pediatric renal tumors: practical updates for the pathologist. Pediatr Dev Pathol. 2005;8:320–38.

138. Parham DM, Roloson GJ, Feely M, Green DM, Bridge JA, Beckwith JB. Primary malignant neuroepithelial tumors of the kidney: a clinicopathologic analysis of 146 adult and pediatric cases from the National Wilms' Tumor Study Group Pathology Center. Am J Surg Pathol. 2001;25:133–46.

139. Ellison DA, Parham DM, Bridge J, Beckwith JB. Immunohistochemistry of primary malignant neuroepithelial tumors of the kidney: a potential source of confusion? A study of 30 cases from the National Wilms Tumor Study Pathology Center. Hum Pathol. 2007;38:205–11.

140. Argani P, Faria PA, Epstein JI, Reuter VE, Perlman EJ, Beckwith JB, et al. Primary renal synovial sarcoma: molecular and morphologic delineation of an entity previously included among embryonal sarcomas of the kidney. Am J Surg Pathol. 2000;24:1087–96.

141. Arnold MA, Schoenfield L, Limketkai BN, Arnold CA. Diagnostic pitfalls of differentiating desmoplastic small round cell tumor (DSRCT) from Wilms tumor (WT): overlapping morphologic and immunohistochemical features. Am J Surg Pathol. 2014;38:1220–6.

142. Magro G, Longo FR, Angelico G, Spadola S, Amore FF, Salvatorelli L. Immunohistochemistry as potential diagnostic pitfall in the most common solid tumors of children and adolescents. Acta Histochem. 2015;117:397–414.

143. da Silva RC, Medeiros Filho P, Chioato L, Silva TR, Ribeiro SM, Bacchi CE. Desmoplastic small round cell tumor of the kidney mimicking Wilms tumor: a case report and review of the literature. Appl Immunohistochem Mol Morphol. 2009;17:557–62.

144. Gustafson S, Medeiros LJ, Kalhor N, Bueso-Ramos CE. Anaplastic large cell lymphoma: another entity in the differential diagnosis of small round blue cell tumors. Ann Diagn Pathol. 2009;13:413–27.

145. Thyavihally YB, Tongaonkar HB, Gupta S, Kurkure PA, Amare P, Muckaden MA, et al. Primitive neuroectodermal tumor of the kidney: a single institute series of 16 patients. Urology. 2008;71:292–6.

146. Lane BR, Chery F, Jour G, Sercia L, Magi-Galluzzi C, Novick AC, et al. Renal neuroendocrine tumours: a clinicopathological study. BJU Int. 2007;100:1030–5.

147. Argani P, Perlman EJ, Breslow NE, Browning NG, Green DM, D'Angio GJ, et al. Clear cell sarcoma of the kidney: a review of 351 cases from the National Wilms Tumor Study Group Pathology Center. Am J Surg Pathol. 2000;24:4–18.

148. Dumba M, Jawad N, McHugh K. Neuroblastoma and nephroblastoma: a radiological review. Cancer Imaging. 2015;15:5.

149. Shimada H. The international neuroblastoma pathology classification. Pathologica. 2003;95:240–1.

150. Campbell K, Gastier-Foster JM, Mann M, Naranjo AH, Van Ryn C, Bagatell R, et al. Association of MYCN copy number with clinical features, tumor biology, and outcomes in neuroblastoma: a report from the Children's Oncology Group. Cancer. 2017;123:4224–35.

151. Sharma S, Kamala R, Nair D, Ragavendra TR, Mhatre S, Sabharwal R, et al. Round cell tumors: classification and immunohistochemistry. Indian J Med Paediatr Oncol. 2017;38:349–53.

152. Morgenstern BZ, Krivoshik AP, Rodriguez V, Anderson PM. Wilms' tumor and neuroblastoma. Acta Paediatr Suppl. 2004;93:78–84; discussion -5

153. Dome SJ, Millen EM, Argani P. Pediatric renal tumors. In: Orkin SH, Nathan DG, Ginsburg D, Look AT, Fisher DE, Lux SE, editors. Nathan and Oski's hematology and oncology of infancy and childhood. 8th ed. Philadelphia: Elsevier/Saunders; 2015. p. 1714–46.

154. Al-Hussain T, Ali A, Akhtar M. Wilms tumor: an update. Adv Anat Pathol. 2014;21:166–73.

155. Jet Aw S, Hong Kuick C, Hwee Yong M, Wen Quan Lian D, Wang S, Liang Loh AH, et al. Novel karyotypes and cyclin D1 immunoreactivity in clear cell sarcoma of the kidney. Pediatr Dev Pathol. 2015;18:297–304.

156. Karlsson J, Valind A, Gisselsson D. BCOR internal tandem duplication and YWHAE-NUTM2B/E fusion are mutually exclusive events in clear cell sarcoma of the kidney. Genes Chromosomes Cancer. 2016;55:120–3.

157. Franckevica I, Kleina R, Voika O. Originally misdiagnosed rhabdoid tumour of the kidney. A case report and differential diagnosis. Pol J Pathol. 2011;62:163–7.

158. Lee JS, Sanchez TR, Wootton-Gorges S. Malignant renal tumors in children. J Kidney Cancer VHL. 2015;2:84–9.

159. Goyal S, Mishra K, Sarkar U, Sharma S, Kumari A. Diagnostic utility of Wilms' tumour-1 protein (WT-1) immunostaining in paediatric renal tumours. Indian J Med Res. 2016;143:S59–s67.

160. Hong CR, Kang HJ, Ju HY, Lee JW, Kim H, Park SH, et al. Extracranial malignant rhabdoid tumor in children: a single institute experience. Cancer Res Treat. 2015;47:889–96.

161. Geller JI, Roth JJ, Biegel JA. Biology and treatment of Rhabdoid tumor. Crit Rev Oncog. 2015;20:199–216.

162. Delahunt B, Thomson KJ, Ferguson AF, Neale TJ, Meffan PJ, Nacey JN. Familial cystic nephroma and pleuropulmonary blastoma. Cancer. 1993;71:1338–42.

163. Eble JN, Bonsib SM. Extensively cystic renal neoplasms: cystic nephroma, cystic partially differentiated nephroblastoma, multilocular cystic renal cell carcinoma, and cystic hamartoma of renal pelvis. Semin Diagn Pathol. 1998;15:2–20.

164. van den Hoek J, de Krijger R, van de Ven K, Lequin M, van den Heuvel-Eibrink MM. Cystic nephroma, cystic partially differentiated nephroblastoma and cystic Wilms' tumor in children: a spectrum with therapeutic dilemmas. Urol Int. 2009;82:65–70.

165. Bahubeshi A, Bal N, Rio Frio T, Hamel N, Pouchet C, Yilmaz A, et al. Germline DICER1 mutations and familial cystic nephroma. J Med Genet. 2010;47:863–6.

166. Doros LA, Rossi CT, Yang J, Field A, Williams GM, Messinger Y, et al. DICER1 mutations in childhood cystic nephroma and its relationship to DICER1-renal sarcoma. Mod Pathol. 2014;27:1267–80.

167. Stout TE, Au JK, Hicks JM, Gargollo PC. A case of bilateral cystic partially differentiated nephroblastoma vs cystic Wilms' tumor: highlighting a diagnostic dilemma. Urology. 2016;92:106–9.

168. Irtan S, Ehrlich PF, Pritchard-Jones K. Wilms tumor: "state-of-the-art" update, 2016. Semin Pediatr Surg. 2016;25:250–6.

169. Faure A, Atkinson J, Bouty A, O'Brien M, Levard G, Hutson J, et al. DICER1 pleuropulmonary blastoma familial tumour predisposition syndrome: what the paediatric urologist needs to know. J Pediatr Urol. 2016;12:5–10.

170. Schultz KAP, Williams GM, Kamihara J, Stewart DR, Harris AK, Bauer AJ, et al. DICER1 and associated conditions: identification of at-risk individuals and recommended surveillance strategies. Clin Cancer Res. 2018;24:2251–61.

171. Haas JE, Palmer NF, Weinberg AG, Beckwith JB. Ultrastructure of malignant rhabdoid tumor of the kidney. A distinctive renal tumor of children. Hum Pathol. 1981;12:646–57.

172. Hoot AC, Russo P, Judkins AR, Perlman EJ, Biegel JA. Immunohistochemical analysis of hSNF5/INI1 distinguishes renal and extra-renal malignant rhabdoid tumors from other pediatric soft tissue tumors. Am J Surg Pathol. 2004;28:1485–91.

173. Egas-Bejar D, Huh WW. Rhabdomyosarcoma in adolescent and young adult patients: current perspectives. Adolesc Health Med Ther. 2014;5:115–25.

174. Keller C, Guttridge DC. Mechanisms of impaired differentiation in rhabdomyosarcoma. FEBS J. 2013;280:4323–34.

175. Bolande RP, Brough AJ, Izant RJ Jr. Congenital mesoblastic nephroma of infancy. A report of eight cases and the relationship to Wilms' tumor. Pediatrics. 1967;40:272–8.

176. Glick RD, Hicks MJ, Nuchtern JG, Wesson DE, Olutoye OO, Cass DL. Renal tumors in infants less than 6 months of age. J Pediatr Surg. 2004;39:522–5.

177. Sebire NJ, Vujanic GM. Paediatric renal tumours: recent developments, new entities and pathological features. Histopathology. 2009;54:516–28.

178. Ranganathan S. Pediatric renal neoplasms. Surg Pathol Clin. 2009;2:27–60.

179. England RJ, Haider N, Vujanic GM, Kelsey A, Stiller CA, Pritchard-Jones K, et al. Mesoblastic nephroma: a report of the United Kingdom Children's Cancer and Leukaemia Group (CCLG). Pediatr Blood Cancer. 2011;56:744–8.

180. Wang ZP, Li K, Dong KR, Xiao XM, Zheng S. Congenital mesoblastic nephroma: clinical analysis of eight cases and a review of the literature. Oncol Lett. 2014;8:2007–11.

181. Davis CJ Jr, Barton JH, Sesterhenn IA, Mostofi FK. Metanephric adenoma. Clinicopathological study of fifty patients. Am J Surg Pathol. 1995;19:1101–14.

182. Chami R, Yin M, Marrano P, Teerapakpinyo C, Shuangshoti S, Thorner PS. BRAF mutations in pediatric metanephric tumors. Hum Pathol. 2015;46:1153–61.

183. Adeniran AJ, Shuch B, Humphrey PA. Hereditary renal cell carcinoma syndromes: clinical, pathologic, and genetic features. Am J Surg Pathol. 2015;39:e1–e18.

184. Przybycin CG, Magi-Galluzzi C, McKenney JK. Hereditary syndromes with associated renal neoplasia: a practical guide to histologic recognition in renal tumor resection specimens. Adv Anat Pathol. 2013;20:245–63.

185. Kim E, Zschiedrich S. Renal cell carcinoma in von Hippel-Lindau disease-from tumor genetics to novel therapeutic strategies. Front Pediatr. 2018;6:16.

186. Wadt KA, Gerdes AM, Hansen TV, Toft BG, Friis-Hansen L, Andersen MK. Novel germline c-MET mutation in a family with hereditary papillary renal carcinoma. Familial Cancer. 2012;11:535–7.

187. Chen YB, Brannon AR, Toubaji A, Dudas ME, Won HH, Al-Ahmadie HA, et al. Hereditary leiomyomatosis and renal cell carcinoma syndrome-associated renal cancer: recognition of the syndrome by pathologic features and the utility of detecting aberrant succination by immunohistochemistry. Am J Surg Pathol. 2014;38:627–37.

188. Guo J, Tretiakova MS, Troxell ML, Osunkoya AO, Fadare O, Sangoi AR, et al. Tuberous sclerosis-associated renal cell carcinoma: a clinicopathologic study of 57 separate carcinomas in 18 patients. Am J Surg Pathol. 2014;38:1457–67.

189. Gill AJ. Succinate dehydrogenase (SDH)-deficient neoplasia. Histopathology. 2018;72:106–16.

190. Argani P, Zhong M, Reuter VE, Fallon JT, Epstein JI, Netto GJ, et al. TFE3-fusion variant analysis defines specific Clinicopathologic associations among Xp11 translocation cancers. Am J Surg Pathol. 2016;40:723–37.

191. Asch-Kendrick RJ, Shetty S, Goldblum JR, Sharma R, Epstein JI, Argani P, et al. A subset of fat-predominant angiomyolipomas label for MDM2: a potential diagnostic pitfall. Hum Pathol. 2016;57:7–12.

192. Seyam RM, Alkhudair WK, Kattan SA, Alotaibi MF, Alzahrani HM, Altaweel WM. The risks of renal angiomyolipoma: reviewing the evidence. J Kidney Cancer VHL. 2017;4:13–25.

193. Yang P, Cornejo KM, Sadow PM, Cheng L, Wang M, Xiao Y, et al. Renal cell carcinoma in tuberous sclerosis complex. Am J Surg Pathol. 2014;38:895–909.

Ximing J. Yang and Jenny Ross

Can Urothelial Inverted Papillomas Be Seen in the Upper Urinary Tract? How to Distinguish Inverted Papilloma from Urothelial Carcinoma?

Yes. Inverted papilloma can be seen in the upper tract. The inverted papilloma are benign urothelial proliferations, which can be distinguished from urothelial carcinoma (UCa) in the following features: (1) inverted papilloma will show inverted growth pattern, while urothelial carcinoma may show invasive features; (2) inverted papilloma is expansile, while urothelial carcinoma is destructive; (3) grossly, an inverted papilloma is dome-shaped, while carcinomas can be dome-shaped but more often present as papillary or mass lesions; (4) microscopically, the inverted nests are small and regular with jigsaw puzzle configurations, while carcinoma nests are irregular; (5) inverted papilloma nests often display palisading cells in the periphery of the nest (Fig. 2.1), while carcinoma does not; (6) inverted papilloma will exhibit minimal cytological atypia, while carcinoma will show various degrees of cytological atypia; finally, (7) inverted papillary typically demonstrates negative CK20 staining, weak and patchy p53 staining (wild-type p53), and very low Ki67 proliferative activity, contrary to urothelial carcinoma, which is typically positive for CK20 and p53, and has high Ki67 proliferative activity (Jones, Sun). The differences are summarized in Table 2.1.

If diagnostic criteria are strictly followed, this is a benign condition. However, inverted papilloma in the upper tract may lead to urinary obstruction or—rarely—intussusception. In such cases, surgical resection will be necessary. Finally, due to reported cases of increased association of inverted papilloma with urothelial carcinoma, long-term follow-up is prudent. The differences of these two conditions are summarized in Table 2.1.

References: [1–4].

Can a Nephrogenic Adenoma Be Seen in the Upper Urinary Tract?

Yes.

Nephrogenic adenoma (NA) is defined as renal tubules implanted into injured urothelial mucosa. NA may develop in any part of the urinary tract, including the renal pelvis and ureter. However, NA is more commonly seen in the bladder than the upper tract. Typically, there is a history of instrumentation, calculi, or biopsy, which all lead to disruption of urothelial integrity. Similar to the counterpart in the bladder, NA in the upper tract is histologically characterized by the presence of small clusters of proliferative tubules of epithelial cells (Fig. 2.2). These tubules very much resemble renal tubules, but they may display many different patterns such as papillary, capillary, thyroid-like, signet ring-like, tubular, or even flat appearance. One lesion often displays multiple patterns. Hobnail cells may occasionally be seen, which can be confused with urothelial carcinoma. The following are several key features of NA distinguishing from other lesions.

1. Granulation tissue background often associated with acute and chronic inflammation.
2. Single layer of cuboidal epithelial cells with clear or eosinophilic cytoplasm, mostly without cytologic atypia.
3. Hyalinized base membrane around epithelial cells.

X. J. Yang (✉) · J. Ross
Department of Pathology, Northwestern Memorial Hospital,
Northwestern University Feinberg School of Medicine,
Chicago, IL, USA
e-mail: xyang@northwestern.edu

© Springer Nature Switzerland AG 2021
X. J. Yang, M. Zhou (eds.), *Practical Genitourinary Pathology*, Practical Anatomic Pathology,
https://doi.org/10.1007/978-3-030-57141-2_2

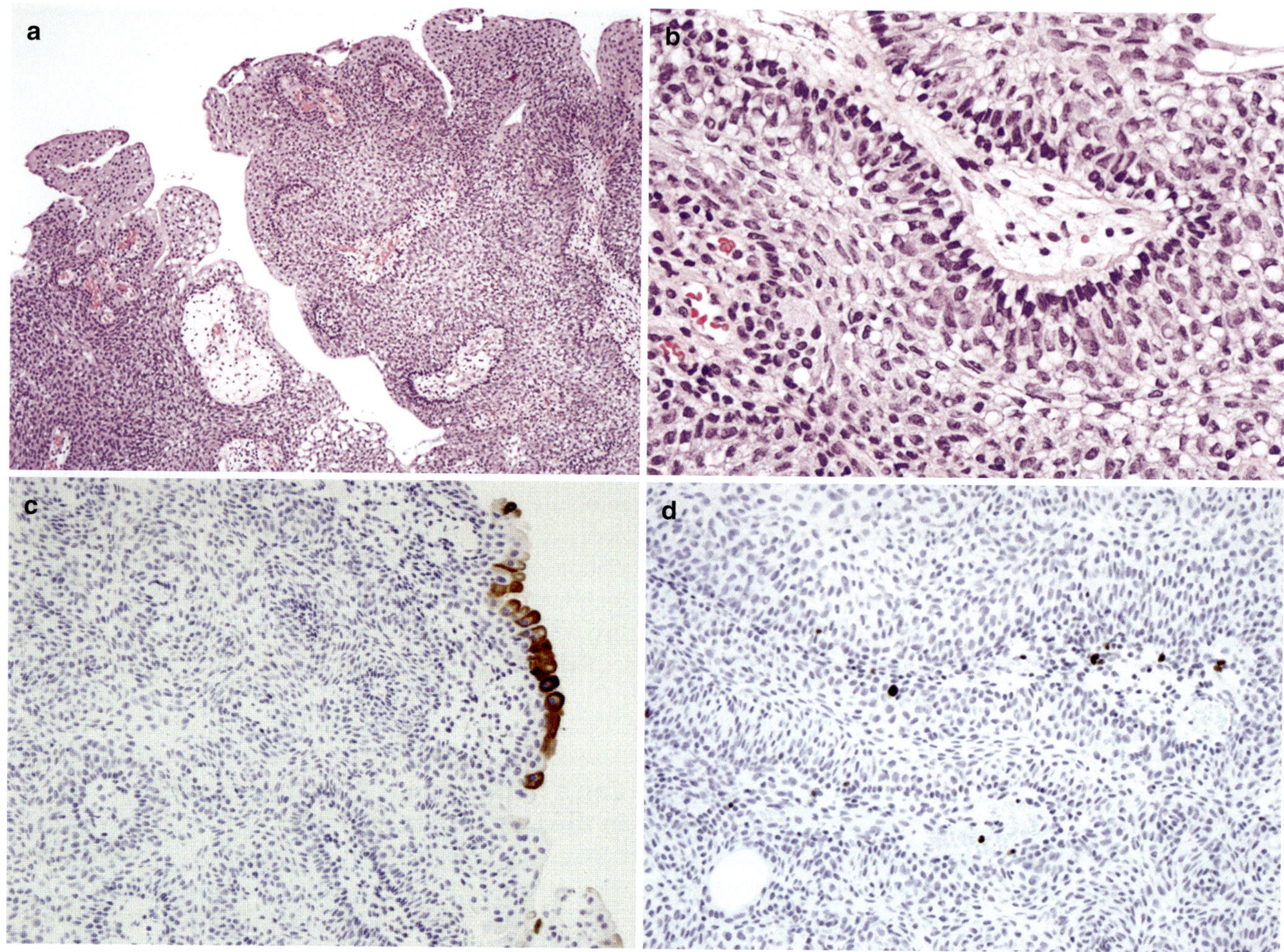

Fig. 2.1 Inverted papilloma. An inverted papilloma in the upper urinary tract, which is composed of large islands of benign urothelial cells (**a**). High magnification shows the presence of palisading cells in the periphery of the cell nest (**b**). Ck20 is negative in the lesional cells but positive in umbrella cells (**c**), and KI67 is very low in the lesional cells (**d**)

Table 2.1 Comparison of inverted urothelial papilloma and urothelial carcinoma

	Inverted papilloma	Urothelial carcinoma
Behavior	Benign	Malignant
Growth pattern	Inverted or inward	Typically exophytic
Destruction	No, expansile	Yes, infiltrative
Macroscopically	Dome-shaped	Papillary, mass, flat; occasionally dome-shaped
Microscopically	Jigsaw puzzle configuration of small nests	Irregular or invasive nests
Peripheral palisading cells	Present	Not present
Cytological atypia	None or minimal	Mild to severe
Desmoplastic stromal reaction	Absent	Can be present
CK20	Negative	Positive
P53	Weak and patchy (wild type)	Negative or positive (mutant)
Ki67	Very low	Low to high
Treatment	Local resection or conservative	Radical resection

4. Finally, if there is any doubt, immunostains can be applied. NA cells will be positive for PAX8 and negative for GATA3 and p63.

References: [5–7].

What Are the Features of Amyloidosis of the Upper Tract?

Amyloidosis may affect the upper urinary tract often as a part of systemic disease. Clinically, the patient with upper tract amyloidosis may present with urinary obstruction or hemorrhage. The key histologic feature is the presence of amyloid material in the renal pelvis or the wall of the ureter. The deposit can be seen in the vascular wall or in lamina propria (Fig. 2.3). This should be distinguished from the hyalinized fibrosis. Congo red stain will help to confirm the diagnosis when it shows apple green staining under

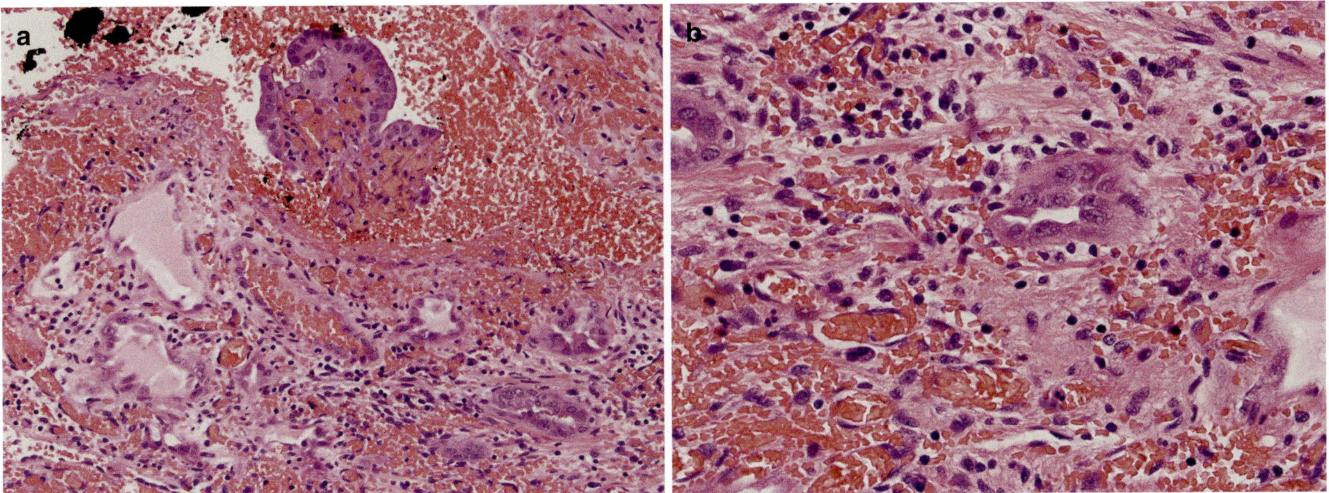

Fig. 2.2 Nephrogenic adenoma in the renal pelvis. The nephrogenic adenoma is characterized by the presence of glandular structures lined by cuboidal or hobnail epithelial cells (**a**). Sometimes the lesional cells may show nuclear enlargement and prominent nucleoli (**b**)

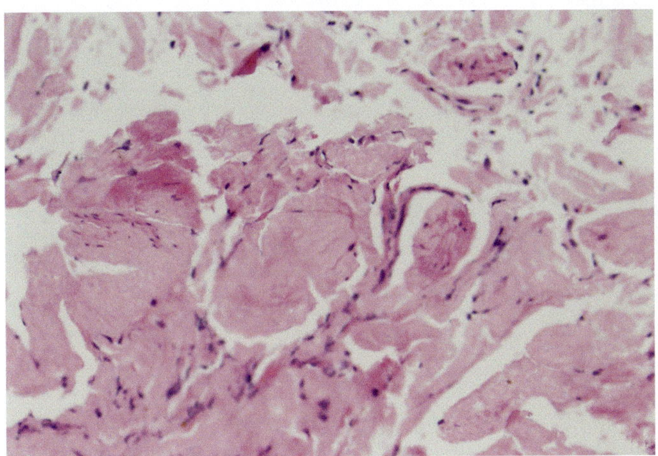

Fig. 2.3 Amyloidosis of the ureter is characterized by the presence of eosinophilic homogenous material—amyloid deposit—in the stroma

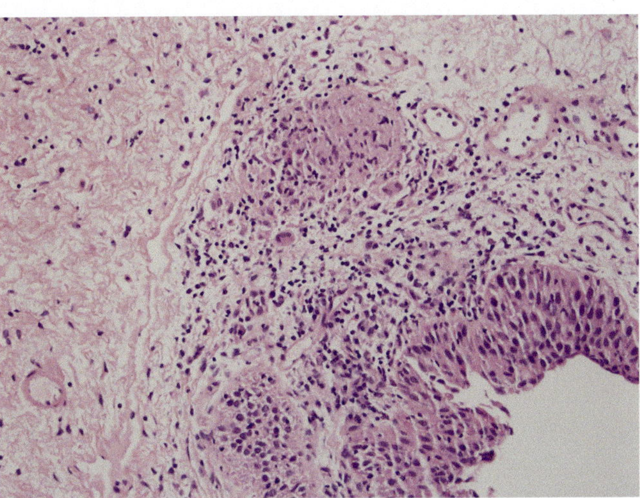

Fig. 2.4 Bacillus Calmette-Guérin (BCG) granuloma. BCG-induced granulomas of the ureter in a patient who received BCG treatment for bladder cancer. The granuloma is well defined with predominantly histiocytes, lymphocytes, and occasional multinuclear giant cells

polarized light. The patients may have systemic disease such as multiple myeloma or chronic inflammatory processes.

References: [8–11].

Granulomas due to various substances used to remove stones have also been reported.

References: [12–15].

What Is the Differential Diagnosis of Granulomatous Inflammation of the Upper Tract?

Granulomatous inflammation is far less common in the upper tract than the lower tract.

Generally, it may occur as a consequence of Bacillus Calmette-Guérin (BCG) exposure (Fig. 2.4), or rarely after long-term impaction of ureteral stones, although rare cases of sarcoidosis involving the ureter have been reported.

What Are the Histological Features of Endometriosis in the Upper Tract?

Endometriosis may develop in the upper tract, which can cause hematuria, mass lesion, urinary obstruction, or rarely pyelonephritis. Endometriosis is characterized by the presence of endometrial glands and/or endometrial stroma in the upper tract (Fig. 2.5a). Areas of hemorrhage or hemosiderin-laden macrophages are commonly associated with endometrial tissue. Sometimes, the epithelial component is not obvious, but dense endometrial stromal cells can be seen (Fig. 2.5b). Confirmation of endometriosis can be easily done with positive immunostaining for CD10 (stromal cells), PAX8 (epithelial cells), or estrogen and progesterone receptors in both epithelial and stromal cells (Fig. 2.5c, d).

The involvement of the ureter by endometriosis may have non-specific symptoms or no symptoms at all. When the diagnosis is delayed, endometriosis may lead to persistent hydronephrosis and eventually loss of renal function. Ultrasonography is the first-line technique for the assessment of the upper tract endometriosis; alternatively, magnetic resonance imaging provides an evaluation of ureteral-type involvement. In addition to hormonal treatment, the surgical treatment of endometriosis aims to relieve ureteral obstruction and avoid disease recurrence. It includes conservative ureterolysis or radical approaches, such as ureterectomy with end-to-end anastomosis or ureteroneocystostomy performed in relation to the type of ureteral involvement. Fertility and pregnancy outcomes are in line with those observed after surgical treatment of deep infiltrating endometriosis. Current evidence does not support the potential risk of malignant transformation of endometriosis.

References: [16, 17].

What Kind of Pathologic Change Can a Stone Cause in the Upper Tract?

A renal calculus (stone), which is more common in the upper tract than the lower tract, can cause urinary obstruction in the upper tract and lead to hydronephrosis and infection

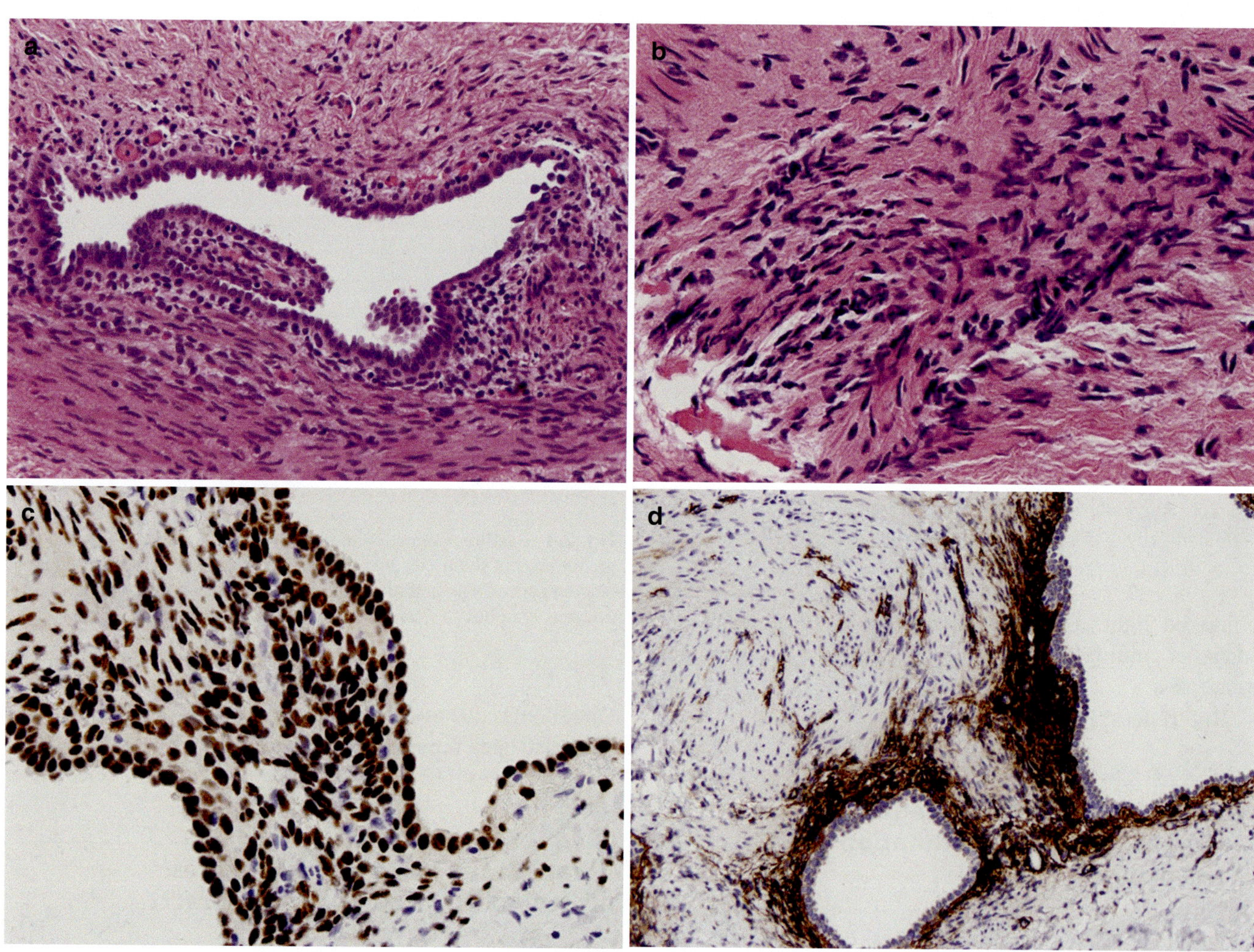

Fig. 2.5 Endometriosis of the ureter. Endometriosis is characterized by the presence of endometrial glands and endometrial stroma (**a**). Sometimes, there is only dense endometrial stroma without glandular component (**b**). Both glandular and stromal components are positive for the estrogen receptor (**c**), while stromal component is positive for CD10 (**d**)

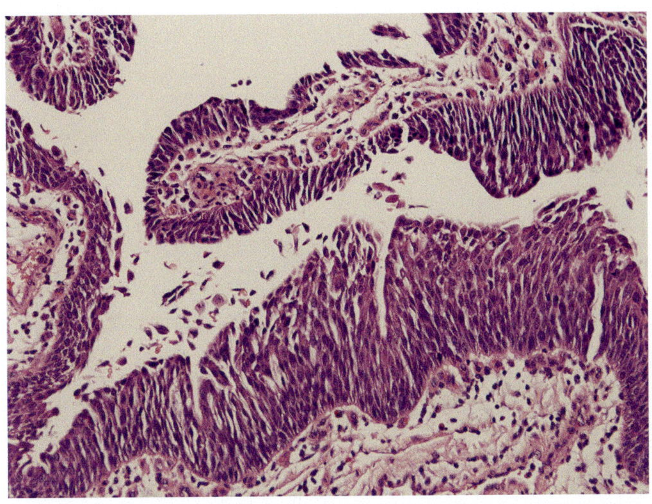

Fig. 2.6 The reactive urothelium in the renal pelvis in a patient with renal stone. The urothelium shows papillary configuration and thickened reactive urothelium

upstream. Locally, a calculus lodged in the renal pelvis or ureter will cause inflammation and subsequent ulceration of urothelium. Papillary hyperplasia with non-branching pseudopapillae may develop. In many cases of long-standing lithiasis, marked reactive changes in involved urothelium may exhibit prominent cytological atypia (Fig. 2.6). In this situation, it can be difficult to distinguish from neoplastic conditions, particularly the upper tract biopsy material, which is generally very small and limited.

When the upper tract biopsy material is small, it is imperative to rule out reactive changes. A false positive diagnosis can result in radical surgery including nephroureterectomy, ureterectomy, and partial resection of bladder cuff for upper tract urothelial carcinoma regardless of grade and depth invasion.

References: [18–20].

What Are the Pathologic Features of Hydronephrosis?

Literally, hydronephrosis means water in the kidney. In reality, the cause of the enlarged kidney is not a disease of renal parenchyma, but it is usually caused by accumulation of urine in the renal pelvic system. The hydronephrosis is resulted from downstream obstruction in the urinary tract, including kidney or ureter stones, tumors of urinary tract, benign prostatic hyperplasia, prostatic adenocarcinoma, infection, and fibrosis. Grossly, the renal pelvis and its

branches (renal calyces) are dilated (Fig. 2.7) and dilatation can involve the ureter, if the obstruction site is lower. The dilated renal pelvis is filled with clear fluid (urine). If there is secondary infection, the fluid can be milky or full of pus. Gross diagnosis is key for hydronephrosis, since its histological features are not specific, although calyceal dilatation may sometimes be appreciated microscopically. Under microscope, the urothelium underlying the hydronephrosis will be thinner and often associated with chronic inflammation. Urothelial atypia is often present in addition to chronic inflammation.

References: [21].

What Are the Histological Features of Xanthogranulomatous Pyelonephritis?

Xanthogranulomatous pyelonephritis (XGPN) is defined as a granulomatous inflammation with numerous foamy macrophages. Often XGPN starts from the renal pelvis and calyces. Typically, initial inflammation induces focal renal tissue necrosis, which attracts a large number of macrophages to repair the tissue damage. XGPN is uncommon. Clinically, it is presented with a destructive mass-like lesion involving renal parenchyma. It is commonly associated with infection due to *Escherichia coli* or other Gram-negative bacteria. Clinically, it is difficult to distinguish XGPN from renal cell carcinoma (RCC) by imaging studies.

Grossly, XGPN can be diffuse or focal. It features presence of yellow spots (collection of foamy macrophages) distributed throughout the entire kidney (diffuse form) or a yellow spot in the center of a mass lesion (focal). Histologically, XGPN is characterized by the accumulation of a large number of lipid-laden macrophages, surrounded by other chronic inflammatory cells (Fig. 2.8). Sometimes, necrosis can be seen in the middle of the lesion associated with the macrophages. Foamy macrophages can be confused with RCC cells, particularly with those with clear cell RCC. It can be especially difficult when available tissue is limited, such as needle core biopsy. And in extremely rare cases, XGPN may coexist with malignancy.

When necessary, a panel of antibodies including renal epithelial markers such as AE1/AE3, PAX8, and CA-IX as well as macrophage markers such as CD68 and CD163 may be used to distinguish XGPN from RCC. As a note, CA-IX may be positive in benign renal epithelial cells adjacent to necrosis.

References: [22–24].

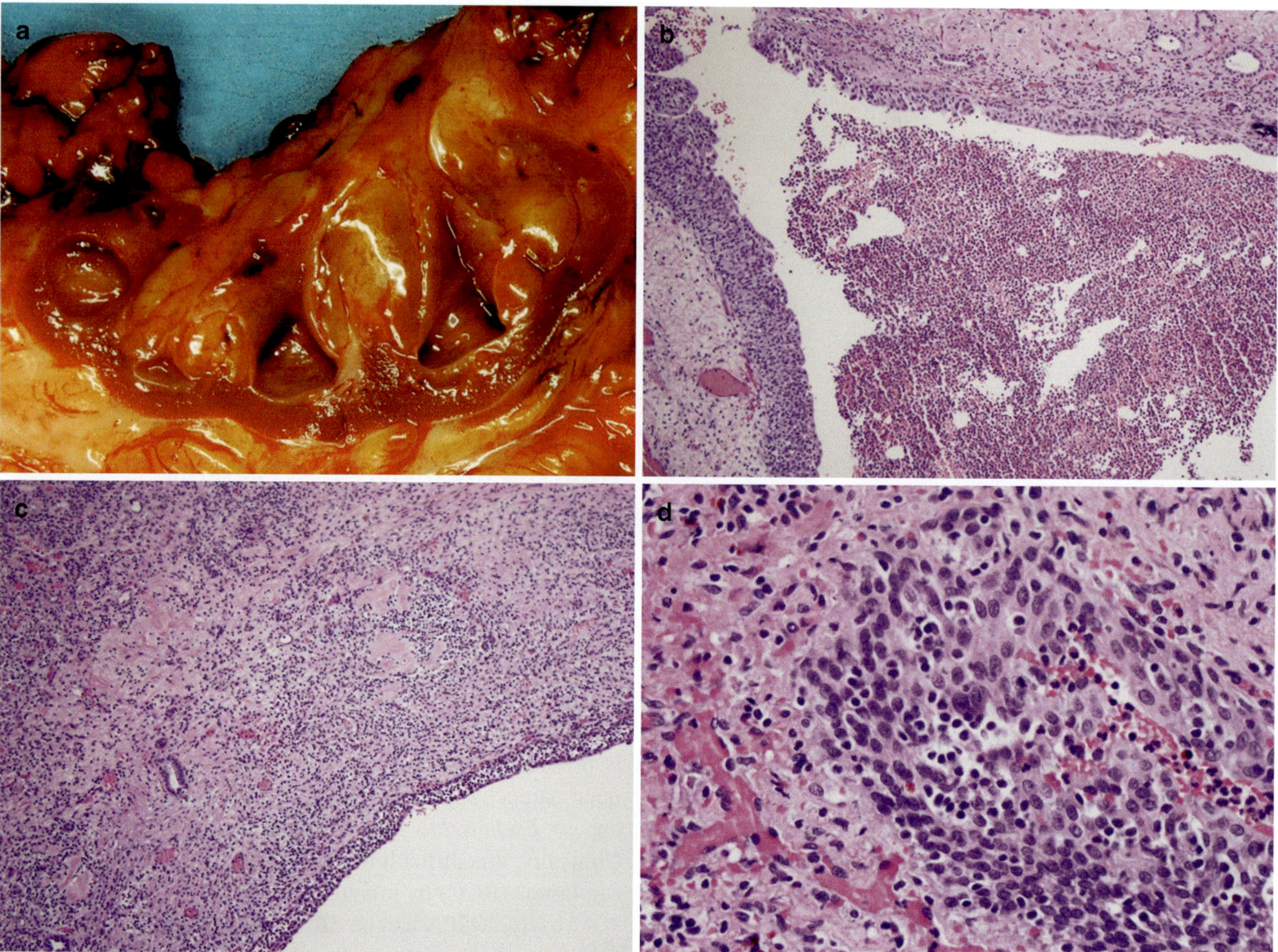

Fig. 2.7 Macroscopically, hydronephrosis shows the dilated renal pelvis and atrophic renal cortex (**a**). Dilated renal pelvis filled with puss (**B**) and chronic inflammation (**c**). The overlaying urothelium shows presence of intraepithelial lymphocytes and significant reactive atypia (**d**)

What Is Perirenal Fibrosis?

Periureteral fibrosis and perirenal (retroperitoneal) fibrosis are rare conditions that may have a wide range of causes or unknown etiology. Although it is a benign condition, the extensive fibrosis may lead to urinary obstruction and upper tract infection, eventually resulting in hydronephrosis and renal failure. Clinically, this condition may mimic a malignancy obstructing the upper urinary tract. However, an endoscopic biopsy typically shows normal urothelial mucosa. Only resection specimens will demonstrate extensive subepithelial fibrosis, narrowing of the ureteral lumen, and distortion of the ureter (Fig. 2.9) or the renal pelvis. The fibrosis may be associated with chronic inflammation.

References: [25–28].

Can Adenoma of Intestinal Type Be Found in the Upper Tract?

Intestinal type adenoma, such as tubular adenoma or villous adenoma, is uncommon in the upper tract. It is believed that most adenomas are derived from the intestinal metaplasia that develops in the urothelium. There are only a handful case reports of adenoma of intestinal types in the upper tract. These tumors may undergo malignant transformation to adenocarcinoma similar to the progression pathway of adenoma-adenocarcinoma in the colon.

Clinically, the patient may present with hematuria, urinary obstruction, and hydronephrosis. In rare cases, muconephrosis can develop if the tumor is extensive and producing a large amount of mucin.

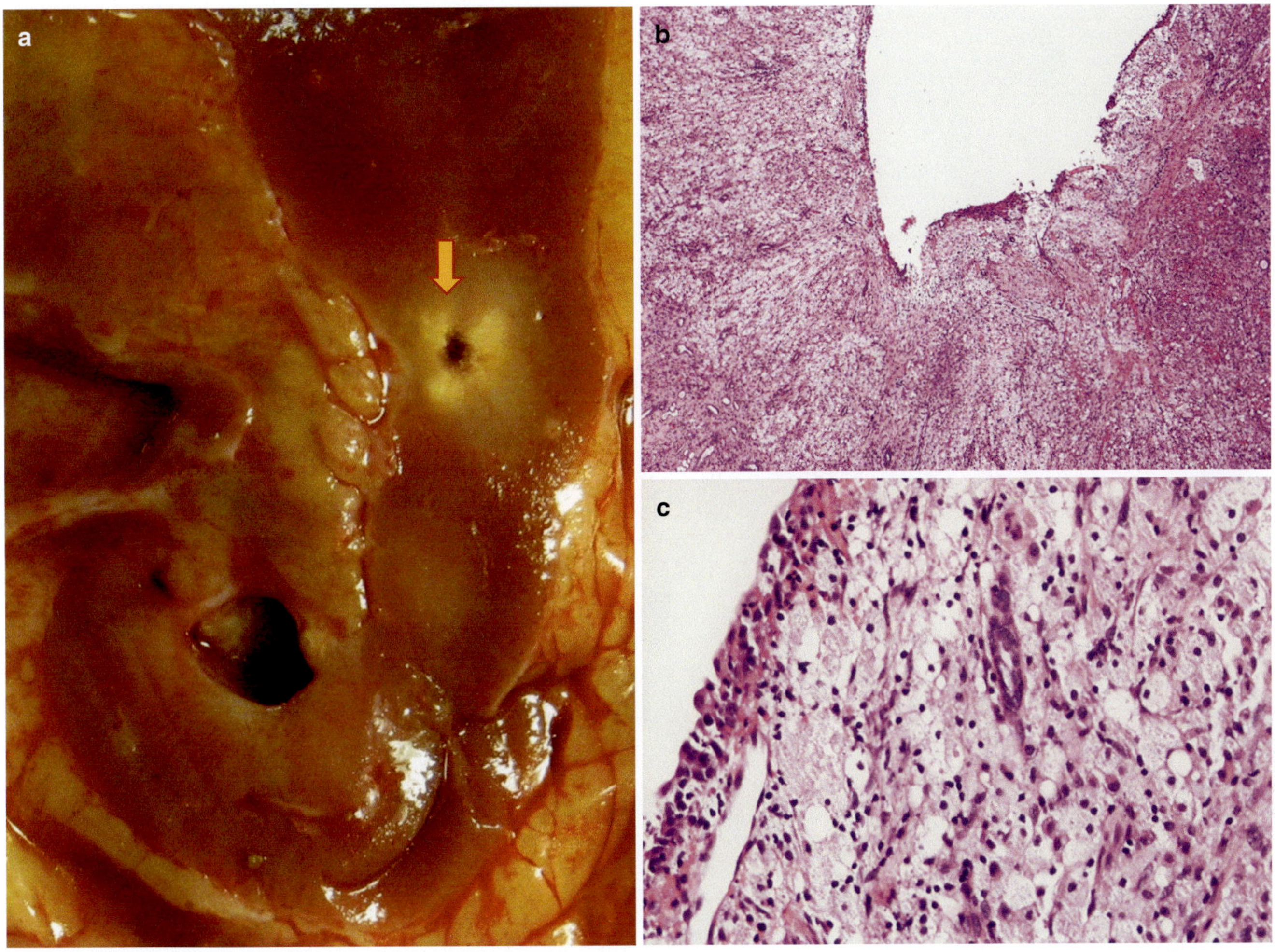

Fig. 2.8 Xanthogranulomatous pyelonephritis (XGPN). Grossly, XGPN (**a**, arrow) appears to be a lesion in the kidney with bright yellow cut surface mimicking clear cell renal cell carcinoma (RCC). Microscopically, XGPN is composed of predominant histiocytes that replaced the renal parenchyma (**b**). High magnification shows the numerous histiocytes (**c**) underneath the urothelium. The histiocytes contain abundant foamy cytoplasm, which can also be confused with clear cell RCC

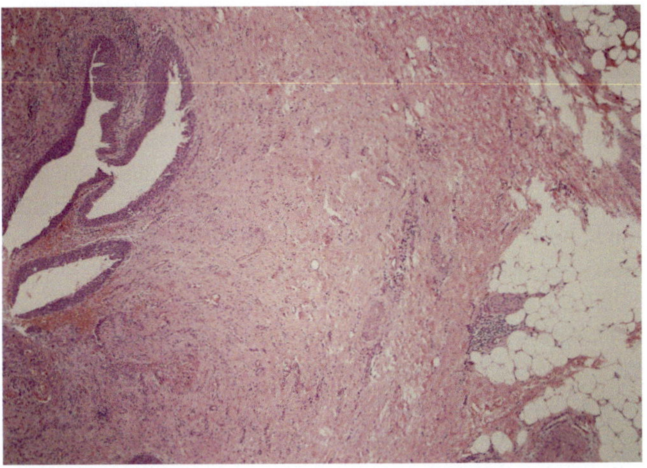

Fig. 2.9 Periureteral fibrosis. A cross section of the ureter showing the ureteral muscularis propria has been replaced by extensive fibrosis with focal chronic inflammation. The ureteral lumen is pushed aside

Grossly, the tumor is a polypoid lesion protruding into the lumen of ureter or renal pelvis. In some cases, tumor involves the entire renal pelvis/ureter as superficial growth on the urothelial surface leading to muconephrosis (Fig. 2.10a). Microscopically, similar to the colon counterpart, adenoma is polypoid with tubular (tubular adenoma) or villous (villous adenoma) pattern. Tumor cells are tall columnar with cigar-shaped nuclei. Some tumors may produce abundant mucin (Fig. 2.10b, c). It is important to determine whether there is any evidence of high-grade dysplasia (loss of polarity, cribriform arrangement, or significant cytological atypia) as present in the tubular/villous adenoma of the colon.

Although adenoma is a benign lesion, it should be surgically or endoscopically removed since it has potential to undergo malignant transformation. In cases of extensive disease with muconephrosis, nephroureterectomy can be considered.

References: [29–31].

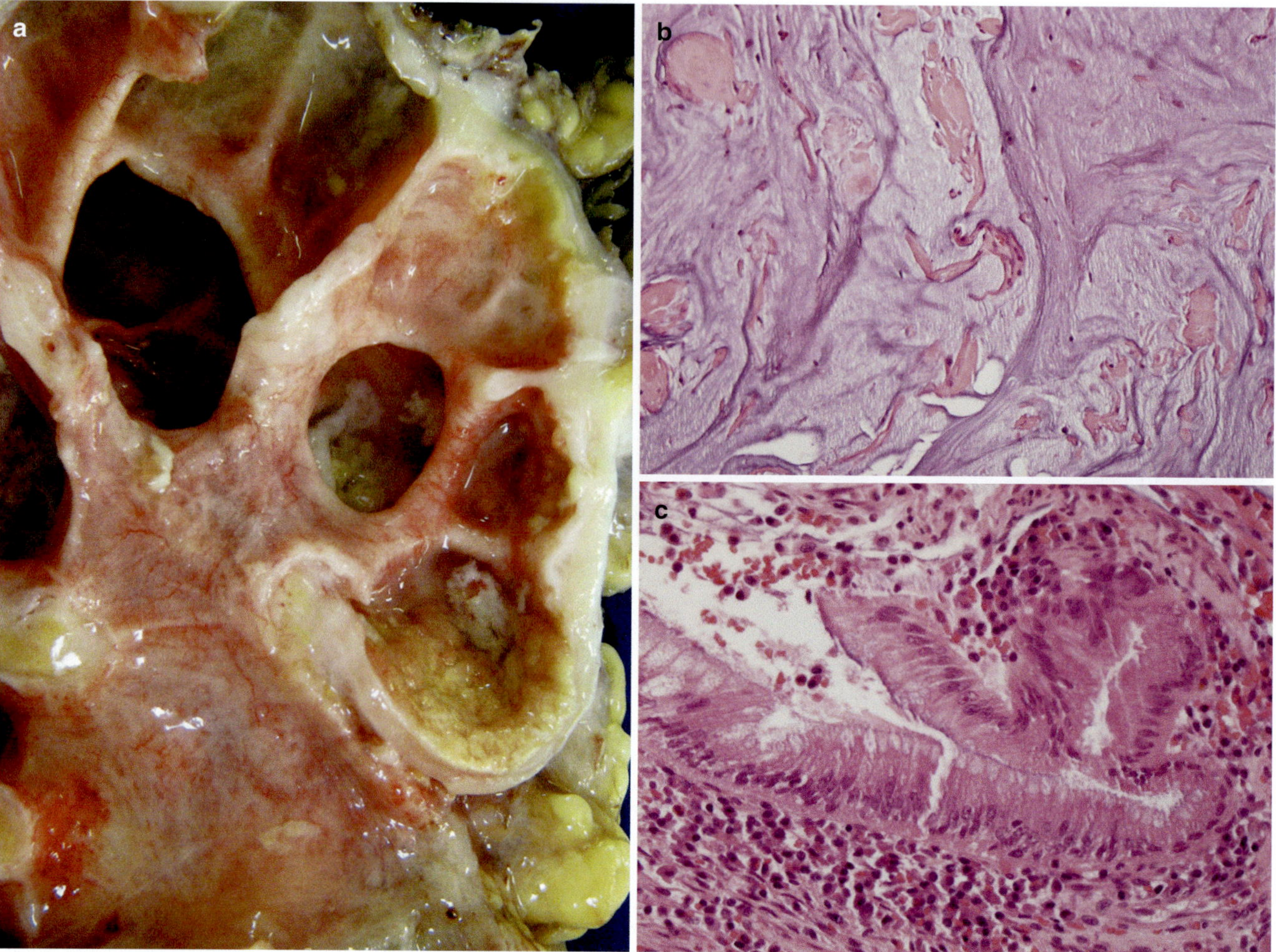

Fig. 2.10 Mucinous adenoma involving the surface of the renal pelvis and ureter. Grossly, the renal pelvis and ureter are dilated, smooth, and covered by mucinous secretions (**a**). Microscopically, there is a large amount of acellular mucin (**b**). The neoplastic cells are tall columnar with cigar-shaped nuclei (**c**), similar to tubular adenoma of the colon. No invasion is identified

What Is the Difference in Biological Behavior Between Upper Tract Cancer and Lower Tract (Including Bladder) Cancer?

Generally speaking, urothelial carcinoma that develops in the upper urinary tract is more aggressive than the one in the bladder and other lower urinary tract. The main reason for the aggressiveness of upper tract cancer is the anatomic characteristics of the renal pelvis and ureter; however, there is increasing evidence for differences at the genetic level as well.

First, the ureter is a much smaller muscular tubular structure than the bladder with a much thinner and less well-organized muscularis propria, and is therefore weaker in providing a barrier to tumor invasion. With respect to the renal pelvis, while the parietal side has somewhat thicker muscularis propria than the ureter, the visceral side of renal pelvis/calyces is in direct contact with renal papilla, which does not have muscularis propria.

Second, the upper tract tumors are more difficult to detect than the ones in the lower tract. By the time the symptoms appear, the tumor is often at an advanced stage. Endoscopic biopsy of the upper tract is also more difficult and usually results in just one or two small tissue fragments, only 0.1–0.2 cm in diameter, often with crush artifact. These limitations pose major challenge for definitive diagnosis and classification of material provided.

Third, there are major vessels and vital organs such as liver, spleen, and bowel, in close proximity to the upper urinary tract. Tumor invasion into these organs often leads to major mortality and morbidity.

Finally, the upper tract tumors may have different molecular genetic differences contributing to their aggressiveness. However, this notion needs further investigation to be fully accepted.

Because of their rapacious nature, the upper urinary tract tumors will generally be treated more aggressively.

References: [32–36].

What Is the Difference in Treatment Between Upper Tract Cancer and Bladder Cancer?

There is a major difference in the surgical treatment of the upper tract cancer vs bladder cancer. Majority of bladder cancer cases will be treated with local resection with or without BCG. For bladder cancer, carcinoma in situ (CIS) will be treated with intravesical BCG or intravesical chemotherapy such as Mitomycin installation. Papillary urothelial carcinoma with or without lamina propria invasion will be subject to transurethral resection with or without BCG. Urothelial carcinoma with muscular propria invasion will make the patient a candidate for radical cystectomy. However, majority of the upper tract UCa will be treated with radical resections, although on rare occasions BCG may be tried for upper tract CIS, and partial ureterectomy may be used for some patients with early and limited ureteral UCa.

Therefore, the implication of diagnosis of urothelial carcinoma in the upper tract is very different from the one in the bladder. Typically, indication for radical cystectomy is urothelial carcinoma invading muscularis propria, which generally happens at a large tumor burden and several years after tumor genesis. However, urothelial carcinomas of the renal pelvis and ureter, including those of high grade and low grade, with or without invasion (including lamina propria invasion and muscularis propria invasion), are all sub-ject to surgical treatment. This surgical procedure is extensive and usually includes resection of kidney, entire ureter, and portion of bladder (bladder cuff) adjacent to the ureter. Therefore, considering the limitations of diagnostic material and resulting challenges to diagnosis, the diagnosis of urothelial carcinoma in the renal pelvic and ureteral biopsy should be made with caution because of its significant surgical implications.

References: [37, 38].

Can PUNLMP Be Identified in the Upper Tract?

This is a controversial topic. Papillary urothelial neoplasm of low malignant potential (PUNLMP) is considered the lower end of a spectrum of papillary urothelial neoplastic lesions, with low risk of progression, but common recurrences—at least from the bladder studies. However, there is no molecular or biochemical marker to distinguish PUNLMP from low-grade urothelial carcinoma. As we discussed earlier in this chapter, the upper tract urothelial carcinoma is more aggressive, because of the different anatomic—and possibly molecular—environment. Therefore, the diagnosis of PUNLMP should be avoided in the upper urinary tract. The lesions in the renal pelvis and ureter that display histological features of PUNLMP will behave as a low-grade urothelial carcinoma (Fig. 2.11), and although attempts at conservative endoscopic resections have been tried, most cases will most likely be treated aggressively.

References: [39–41].

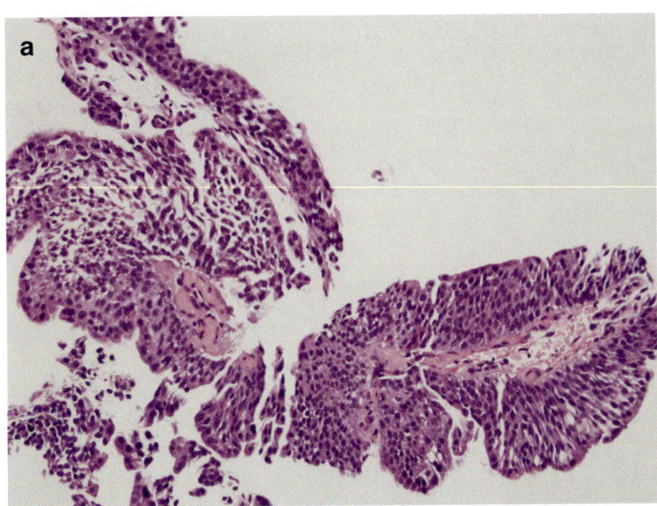
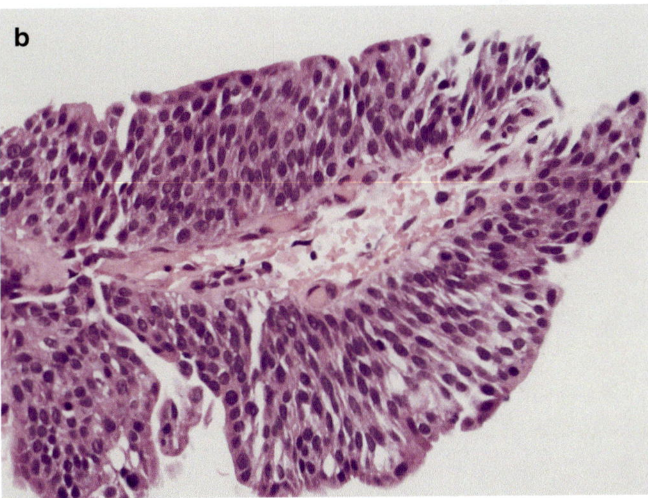

Fig. 2.11 Low-grade papillary urothelial carcinoma in the ureter (**a**) shows papillary configurations with a thin fibrovascular core (**a**). Higher magnification (**b**) shows neoplastic cells with mild cytological atypia, with relatively good polarity retained. Although morphologically similar to papillary urothelial neoplasm of low malignant potential (PUNLMP) in the bladder, we prefer to call this low-grade papillary urothelial carcinoma

How to Distinguish Upper Tract Urothelial Carcinoma from Renal Cell Carcinoma?

Urothelial carcinoma (UCa) may invade renal parenchyma as a mass lesion, while renal cell carcinoma (RCC) may protrude into or invade the renal pelvis, mimicking urothelial carcinoma. Particularly when a tumor is large and high grade, it can be difficult to decide whether it is urothelial or renal cell in origin.

Generally, urothelial carcinoma is centered on the renal pelvis (Fig. 2.12); only a small subset of high-grade invasive urothelial carcinoma will involve renal medulla, and even rarely will UCa invade into renal cortex. When they do, the tumor cells tend to be highly infiltrating with trapping of the glomeruli. To the contrary, high-grade RCC shows expansile growth and destroys the surrounding renal parenchyma without trapping the glomeruli, although as an exception, collecting duct carcinoma may have similar growth patterns as urothelial carcinoma. In most cases, urothelial carcinoma in situ (CIS) or non-invasive papillary urothelial carcinoma will be present in association with the invasive element, and lower-grade component of RCC will be identified when resection specimen is thoroughly examined. Distinction can be difficult on limited biopsy tissue, in which cases a panel of markers including urothelial markers (GATA3, p63, and CK20) and RCC markers (PAX8, CA-IX, AMACR[P504S], CK7, CD10, and vimentin) may be helpful. The differences are summarized in Table 2.2.

References: [42–44].

Can PAX8 Be Expressed in Urothelial Carcinoma of the Upper Tract?

Yes. Although PAX8 is a known renal marker, a small subset of urothelial carcinoma of the upper tract may express PAX8, mimicking renal cell carcinoma; this overlap also covers a

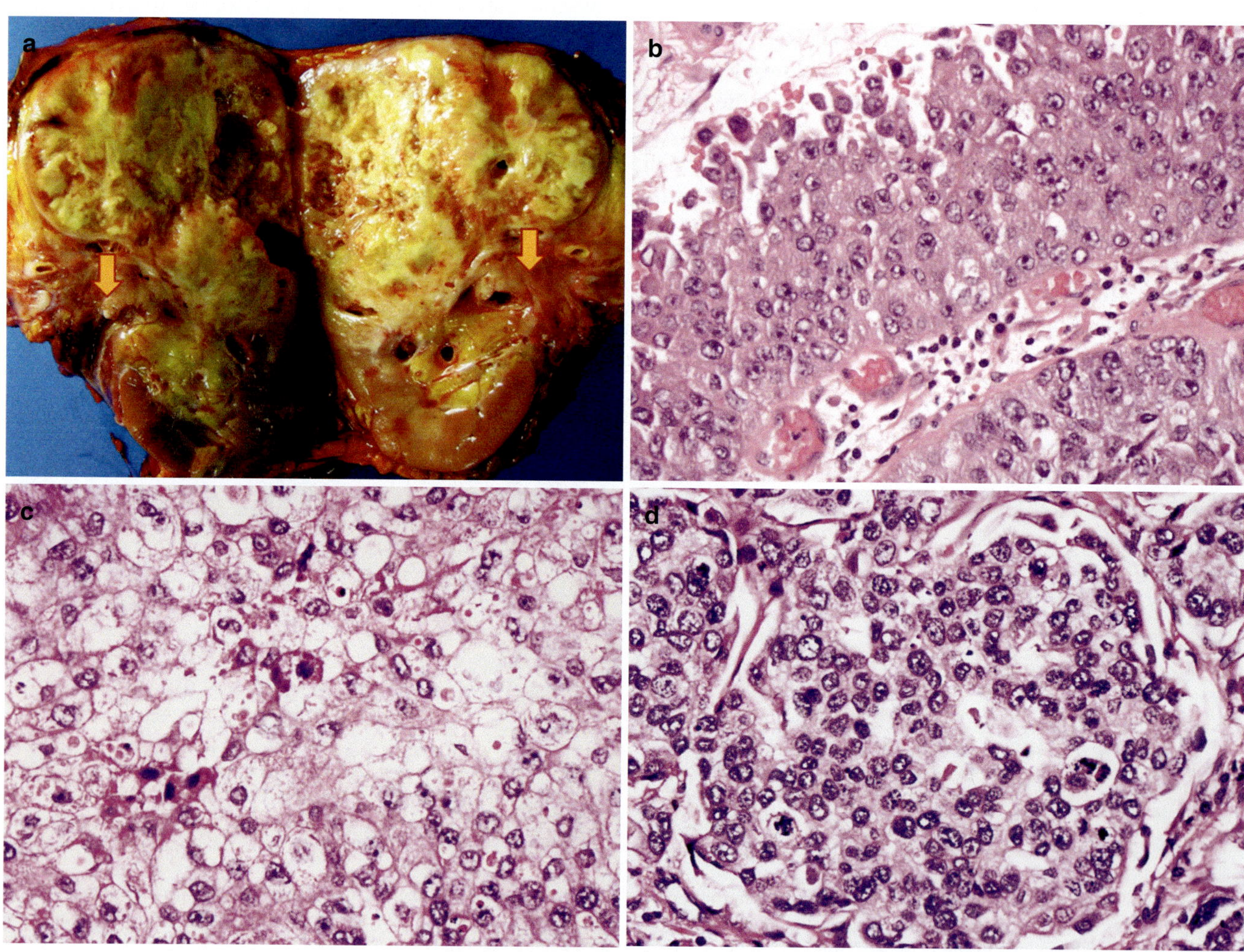

Fig. 2.12 Grossly, urothelial carcinoma of the renal pelvis present as a large mass replacing almost the entire kidney (**a**). It has an appearance of renal cell carcinoma (RCC), but the tumor also involves the surface of renal pelvis (A, arrows). Microscopically, typical urothelial carcinoma can be identified (**b**), although other areas of tumor showed clear cytoplasm (**c**) and pseudoglandular differentiation (**d**) mimicking RCC

Table 2.2 Comparison of urothelial carcinoma of the renal pelvis and renal cell carcinoma

	Urothelial carcinoma of renal pelvis	Renal cell carcinoma (clear cell type and papillary types)
Center of the tumor	Renal pelvis	Renal parenchyma
Involves renal pelvic system	Always	Sometimes protrudes to the renal pelvis
Mass lesion involving renal cortex	Uncommon; only small subset of high-grade invasive tumors	Usual
Tumor growth pattern	Highly infiltrating when involving renal parenchyma	Expansile growth with defined border but no capsule
Urothelial carcinoma in situ	Often present	Not seen
Trapped glomeruli	Yes	Uncommon
PAX8	May be positive	Always positive
GATA3	Positive	Negative
p63, CK20	Positive	Negative (except in rare cases)
CA-IX, AMACR	Usually negative; necrotic areas may show patchy CA-IX expression	CA-IX positive for clear cell RCC; AMACR positive for papillary RCC

portion of sarcomatoid variants of both UCa and RCC. Even benign urothelium in the renal pelvis and ureter may express PAX8, usually to a lesser degree. PAX8-positive urothelial carcinoma can be distinguished from renal cell carcinoma by the following features:

1. Low-grade urothelial carcinoma, although positive for PAX8, still retains features of urothelium, which displays multilayered tumor cells in a papillary configuration (Fig. 2.13a).
2. If urothelial carcinoma in situ is seen, the main tumor is more likely to be urothelial in origin.
3. Urothelial carcinoma, both low grade and high grade, will not show "chicken-wire" vascular pattern characteristic of clear cell RCC.
4. High-grade papillary RCC may have eosinophilic cytoplasm and psammoma bodies, which is unusual for urothelial carcinoma.
5. Finally, urothelial carcinomas of the upper tract may express PAX8, but they will also be positive for urothelial markers,

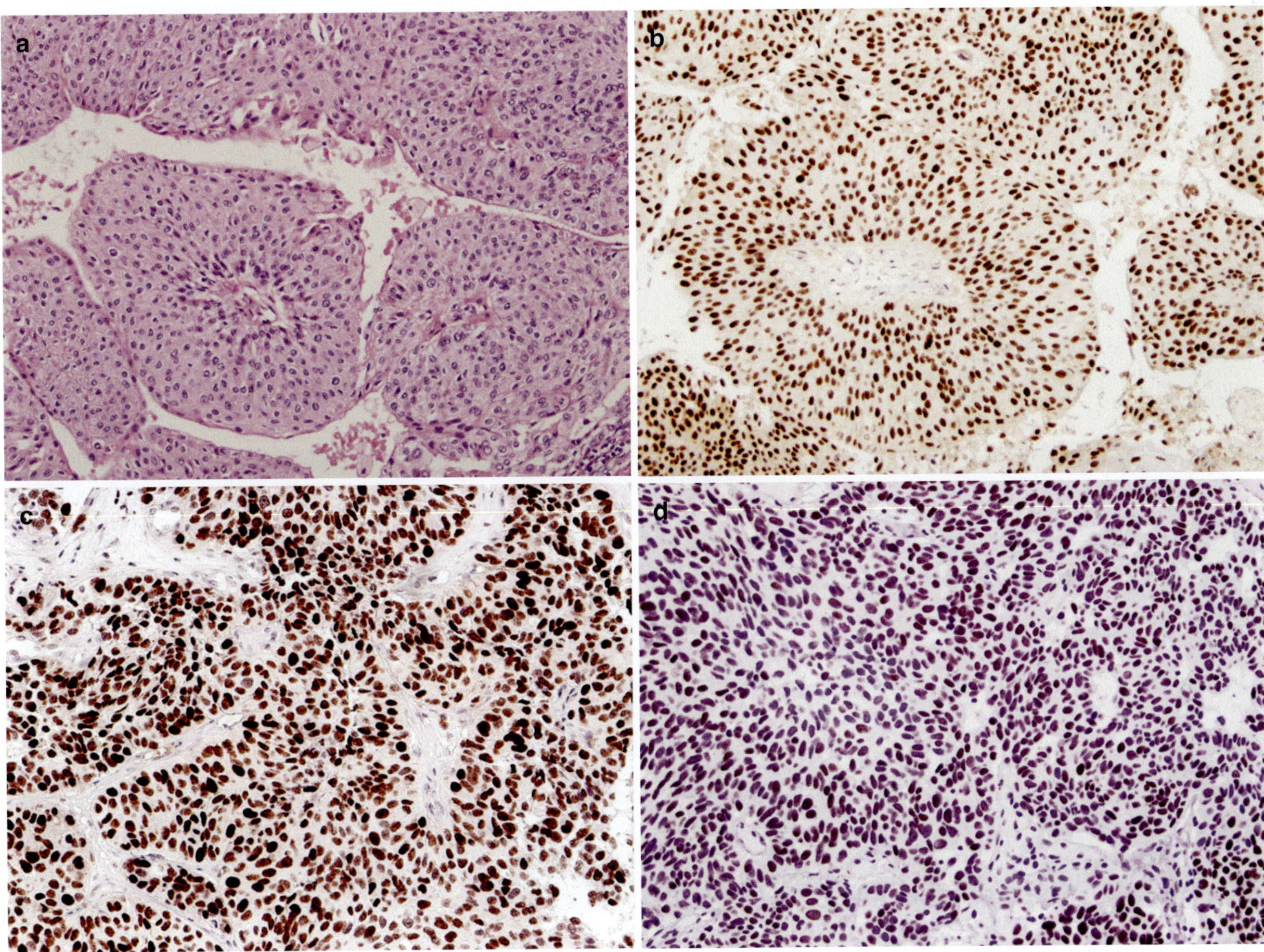

Fig. 2.13 High-grade papillary urothelial carcinoma of the renal pelvis (H&E, **a**) showing PAX8-positive nuclear staining (**b**), but it is also positive for urothelial markers such as GATA3 (**c**) and p63 (**d**)

such as GATA3, p63, and CK20 (Fig. 2.13b–d), with negative or weak staining for other renal cell markers.

References: [45–47].

What Are the Growth Patterns of Upper Tract Urothelial Carcinoma?

The architecture or growth pattern of upper tract urothelial carcinoma is somewhat different from the ones in the bladder. Because of the limited space or relative thinner wall of the upper tract, the urothelial carcinoma appears to have less exophytic papillary growth and more inverted or invasive growth.

There are three major gross growth patterns for these tumors: papillary, flat, and solid mass-forming (Fig. 2.14). The papillary tumors of renal pelvis and ureter have less well-developed papillary fronds and often have grossly dome-shaped appearance. With a flat lesion, there is no obvious papillary tumor; instead, there is a white plaque with markedly thickened urothelial mucosa. With solid mass appearance, a mass lesion centered on the renal pelvis or ureter will be present with a poorly defined infiltrating border mimicking renal cell carcinoma.

References: [48–50].

How to Evaluate Ureteral Margin of a Cystectomy Specimen on Frozen Sections?

Evaluation of ureteral margin on frozen sections, in a patient undergoing radical cystectomy for bladder cancer, may be important for operative and clinical management. The evaluation of ureteral margin is done to identify not only urothelial carcinoma in situ or dysplasia but also invasive disease, which may occur at the periphery of the specimen or in the periureteric fat. Several issues have been associated with this procedure.

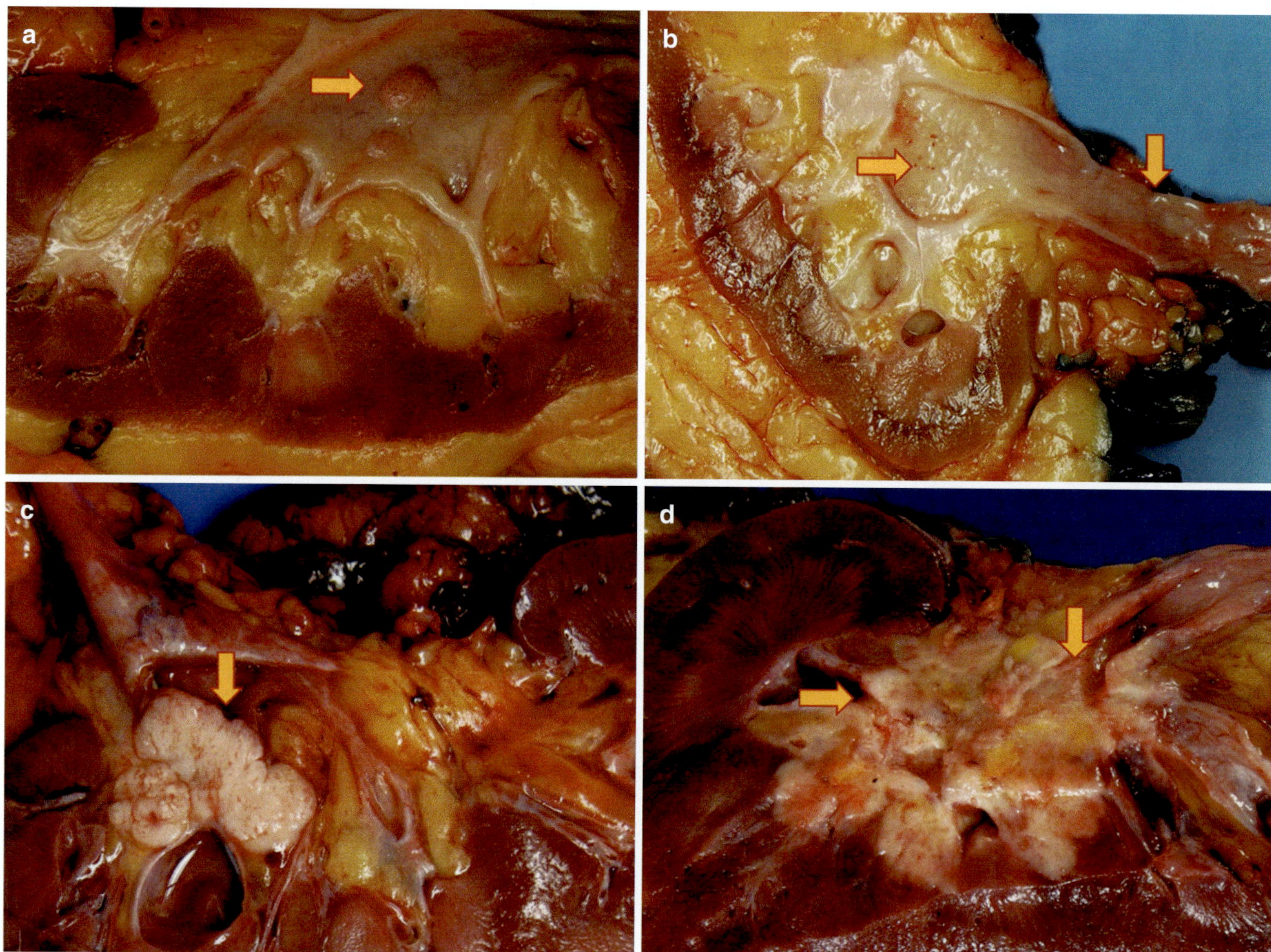

Fig. 2.14 Urothelial carcinoma of the upper urinary tract. Various gross appearances of urothelial carcinoma of the upper urinary tract: tumor with a dome-shaped papillary appearance (**a**, arrow) in the renal pelvis; flat lesions with granular surface and thickened urothelium without obvious tumor mass in the entire renal pelvis and upper ureter (**b**, arrows); mass lesion protruding into the renal pelvis (**c**, arrow) or as an infiltrating mass in the renal hilar region (**d**, arrows)

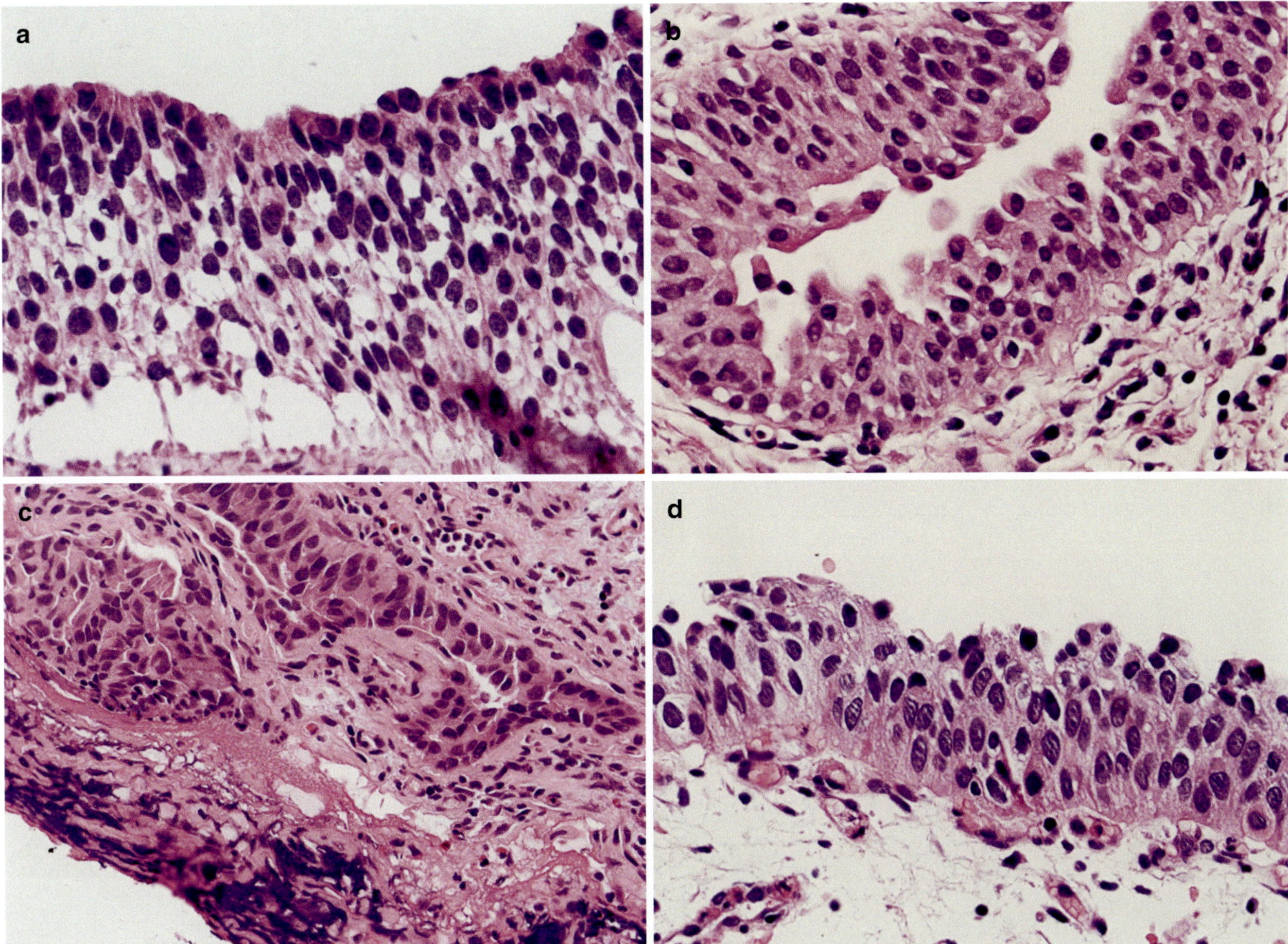

Fig. 2.15 Ureteral margin evaluation. Frozen section evaluation of the ureteral margins. Reactive urothelial cells on frozen section (**a**) appear to be larger, but their nuclear contour is smooth and the cells are well organized, retaining the polarity. Permanent section (**b**) confirms the reactive urothelium from part A. Although there are significant crushing artifacts on frozen section, the urothelial carcinoma in situ display hyperchromasia and lost polarity (**c**). Permanent section (**d**) confirms the presence of urothelial carcinoma in situ

First, there may be difficulty in identification of lumen in the specimen (Fig. 2.15). Frozen section is therefore distorted with no urothelium to be evaluated. In that case, deeper sections should be obtained or the specimen should be rearranged to have a better chance at urothelium. If these measures fail, a request for additional ureteral margin is necessary. On rare occasions, the margin provided is a blind end due to prior surgery. In such cases, the lumen is obliterated by scar and there may be no lumen identified despite proper orientation and multiple deeper levels. Prior operative history obtained from the surgeon will provide a clue.

Second, it is crucial to examine the entire section for invasive or intravascular tumor cells in the lamina propria, muscularis propria, and periureteral tissue, not just to focus on the surface urothelium (Fig. 2.16). Finding invasive carcinoma may impact clinical decision such as additional lymph node dissection.

Finally, on frozen sections, the urothelial cells often look bigger and more atypical than those on the permanent sections. That is because the frozen section has less stringent conditions for dehydration and processing. Unfamiliarity with frozen sections of urothelium may result in misdiagnosis of urothelial carcinoma in situ or dysplasia particularly if urothelium shows reactive changes. We recommend examination of the cryosection first at low power (10× or lower) to evaluate the architecture and orientation of the urothelium. Although benign urothelial cells appear to be bigger than those in the permanent sections, they are well organized with retained polarity. The nuclei have smooth nuclear membrane and mitoses are uncommon. In contrast, CIS will often lose the cell–cell adhesion, and display disorganization, irregular nuclear membrane, and brisk mitotic activity. Finally, if there is urothelial atypia but no certainty for CIS or dysplasia, it may be necessary to request additional margins.

References: [51–53].

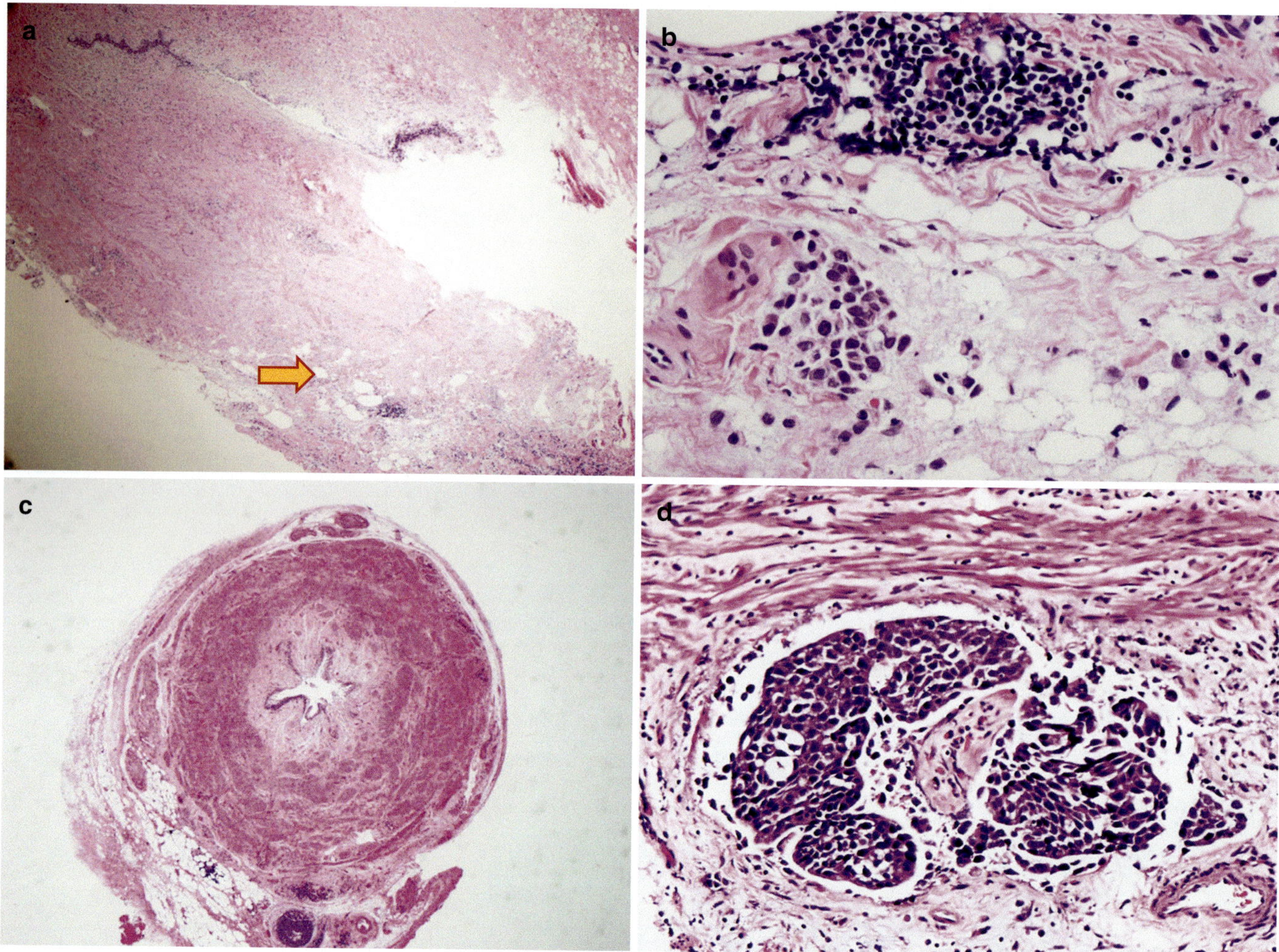

Fig. 2.16 The presence of invasive urothelial carcinoma should be carefully evaluated on ureteral margins. A cross section of the ureter (**a**) with benign surface urothelium, but there are infiltrating cells in the periureteral adipose tissue (**a**, arrow). High magnification confirms the presence of plasmacytoid urothelial carcinoma in the adipose tissue (**b**). Another case of ureter margin (**c**) showing benign surface urothelium, and clusters of tumor cells in the peripheral of the section (**c**). High magnification confirms the presence of lymphovascular invasion of urothelial carcinoma (**d**)

How to Make a Diagnosis of Metastatic Carcinoma Involving the Upper Tract?

Metastatic carcinoma to the renal pelvis and ureter is much less common than to the bladder. Because of the diversity of histological variants of urothelial carcinoma, the diagnosis of a metastatic disease in the upper tract can be difficult, particularly if there is no clinical history. In our experience, the cases of metastatic carcinoma involving the ureters can be from the genitourinary tract such as RCC and prostate cancer (Fig. 2.17), or adjacent organs such as colon or female reproductive organs. The key components of accurate diagnosis are: (1) clinical history of other malignancy; (2) morphological features inconsistent with urothelial carcinoma and its histological variants; and (3) immunohistochemical profile inconsistent with urothelial carcinoma.

References: [54, 55].

Can We See Other Malignant Tumors Involving the Upper Tract?

History and age are important factors to consider when a malignant tumor develops in the upper urinary tract to exclude malignancies other than urothelial carcinoma. Sarcomas and lymphomas can involve the upper tract by direct extension or metastasis (which will be discussed in other chapters). Melanoma may also involve the ureter or renal pelvis as a primary disease or as secondary involvement (metastasis or direct extension). Metastatic prostatic adenocarcinoma should be always considered in the older men, particularly those with a history of high-grade prostatic adenocarcinoma as previously mentioned. Metastatic germ cell tumor from the testis in the pelvic lymph nodes may also involve the ureter. Immunohistochemistry is often necessary to confirm the diagnosis in these situations.

References: [56–59].

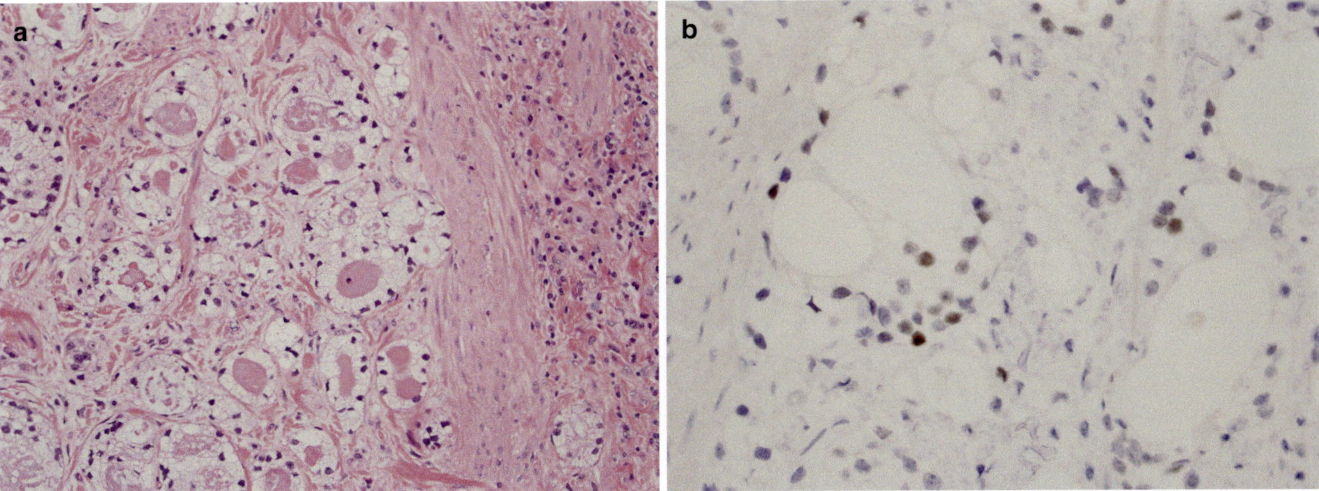

Fig. 2.17 Metastatic prostatic adenocarcinoma in the upper ureter (**a**). Tumor cells, composed of well-formed glands with subtle atypia and occasional cribriform figures, infiltrating muscularis propria of the ureter. They are positive for NKX3.1 (**b**)

Case Discussion

Case 1: Stone-Associated Reactive Urothelial Atypia

A 67-year-old man underwent nephrectomy for a nonfunctional kidney. Grossly, there is prominent hydronephrosis. Numerous calculi can be observed in the dilated renal pelvis and calyces. The renal cortex is atrophic (Fig. 2.18a). Microscopically, papillary urothelial hyperplasia is present in the background of pyelonephritis (Fig. 2.18b). Higher magnification demonstrates disorganization and prominent cytological atypia in the reactive urothelium associated with stones and inflammation (Fig. 2.18c).

Case 2: Urothelial Carcinoma In Situ in the Ureter

An 81-year-old female with ureteral biopsy shows the following morphology.

Although there is only limited material, the presence of significant cytological atypia can be seen in the attached and detached urothelium (Fig. 2.19a). Higher magnification shows the pagetoid tumor cells with high nuclear:cytoplasmic ratio and hyperchromasia (Fig. 2.19b). The tumor cells are positive for p53 (Fig. 2.19c) and CK20 (Fig. 2.19d).

Case 3: Polypoid Ureteritis

A 22-year-old man with obstruction in the ureteropelvic junction (UPJ). The biopsy shows the following histology.

The ureteral mucosa displays prominent edema and focal hemorrhage (Fig. 2.20a). Higher magnification shows numerous von Brunn's nests in edematous stroma and reactive urothelium (Fig. 2.20b). Other areas also show fibrotic stroma (Fig. 2.20c) with reactive urothelial lining (Fig. 2.20d), which may represent a mucosal prolapse causing UPJ obstruction.

Case 4: Metastatic Melanoma in the Ureter

A 78-year-old man with a ureteral lesion underwent biopsy.

The biopsy shows a pigmented lesion with high cellularity (Fig. 2.21a). Tumor cells with prominent nucleoli, dusty cytoplasm, and intracytoplasmic pigment are also visible at higher magnification (Fig. 2.21b). The diagnosis of melanoma is confirmed with HMB-45 immunostaining (Fig. 2.21c) and high Ki-67 proliferative activity (Fig. 2.21d).

Case 5: Florid von Brunn's Nests in the Renal Pelvis

A 70-year-old female underwent nephrectomy for obstructive renal disease. An incidental lesion was found in the renal pelvis. Microscopically, the lesion is under the surface of slightly elevated urothelium, measuring approximately 2 mm in the greatest dimension (Fig. 2.22a). The lesion is composed of small nests of urothelial cells separated with edematous stroma. Higher magnification shows the urothelial cells with low nuclear:cytoplasmic ratio and without nuclear atypia (Fig. 2.22b). This is a relative common finding in nephrectomy specimen not resected for urothelial cancer.

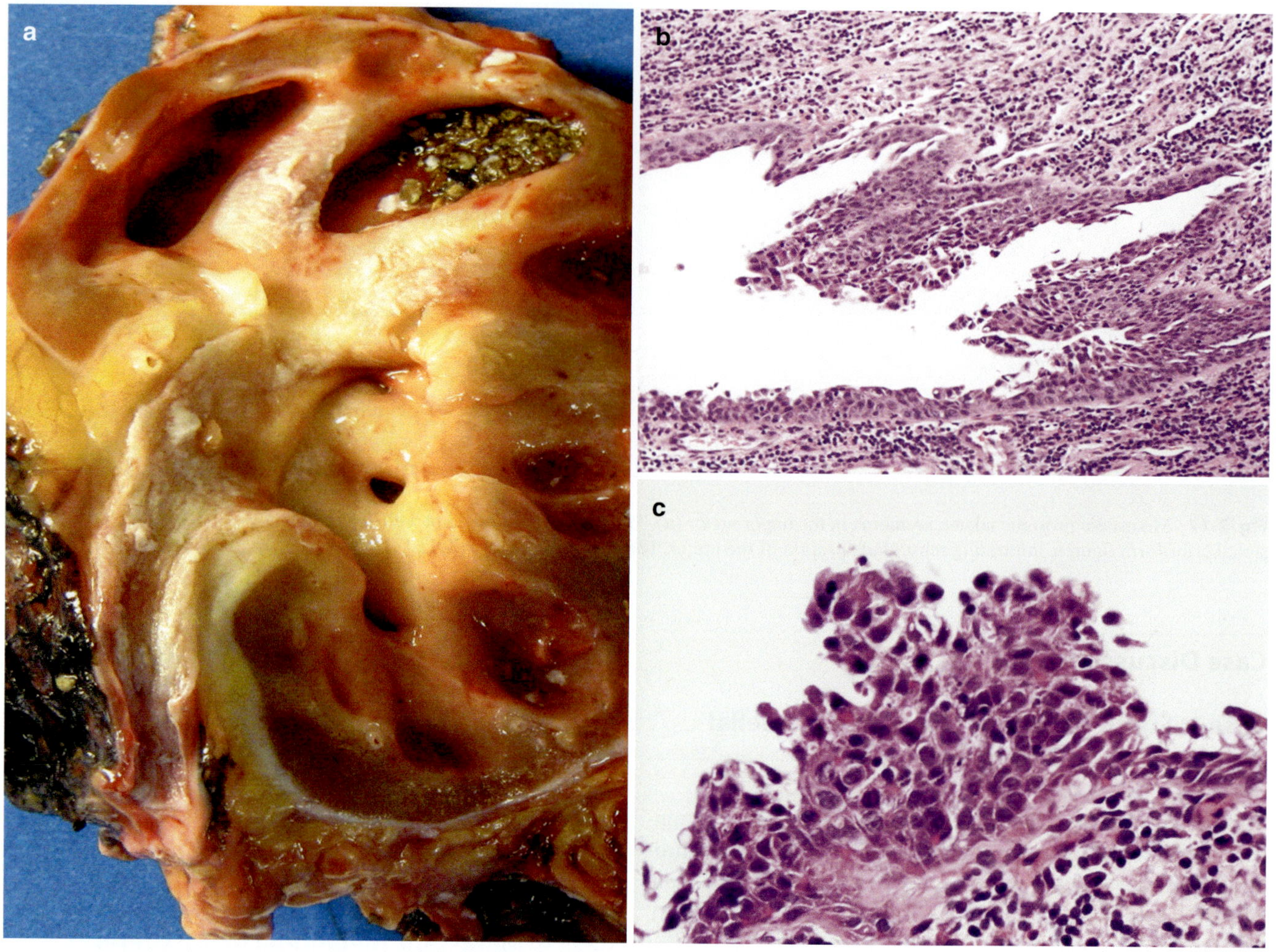

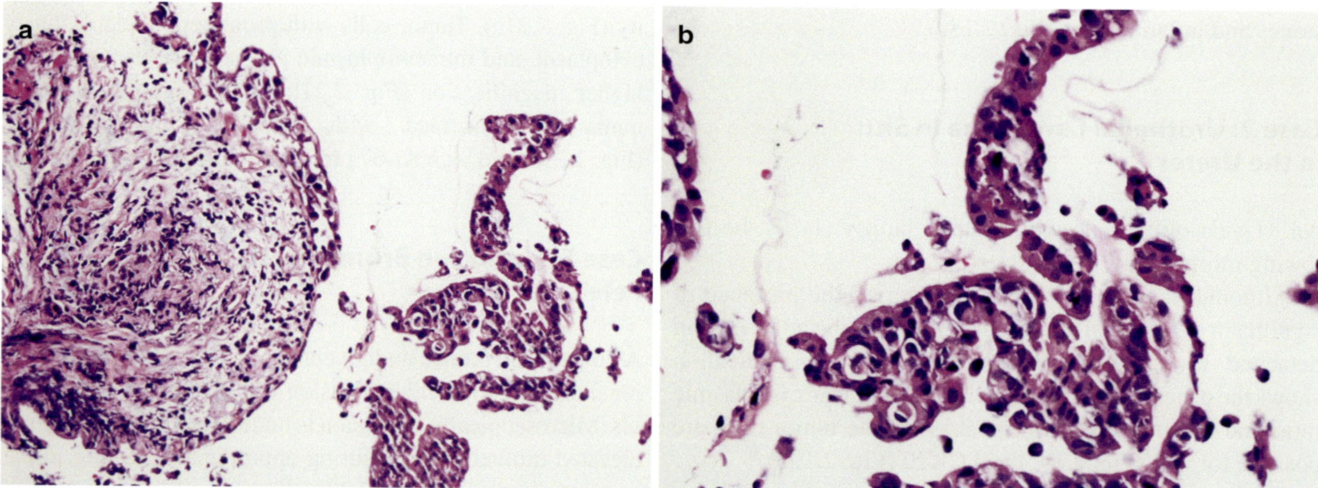

Fig. 2.18 Case 1. Stone-associated reactive urothelial atypia

Fig. 2.19 Case 2. Urothelial carcinoma in situ in the ureter

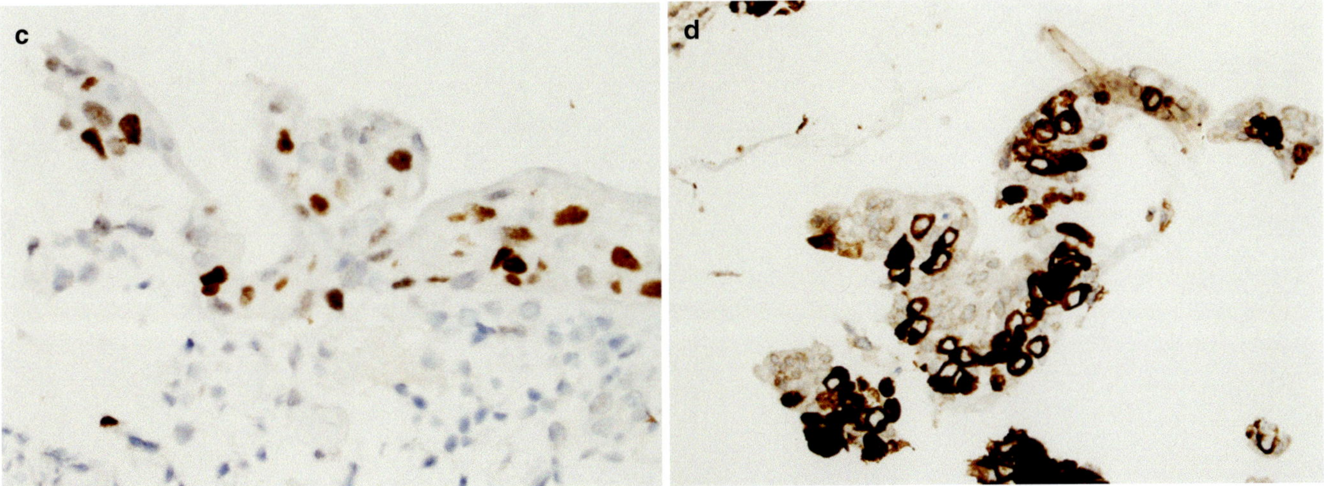

Fig. 2.19   (continued)

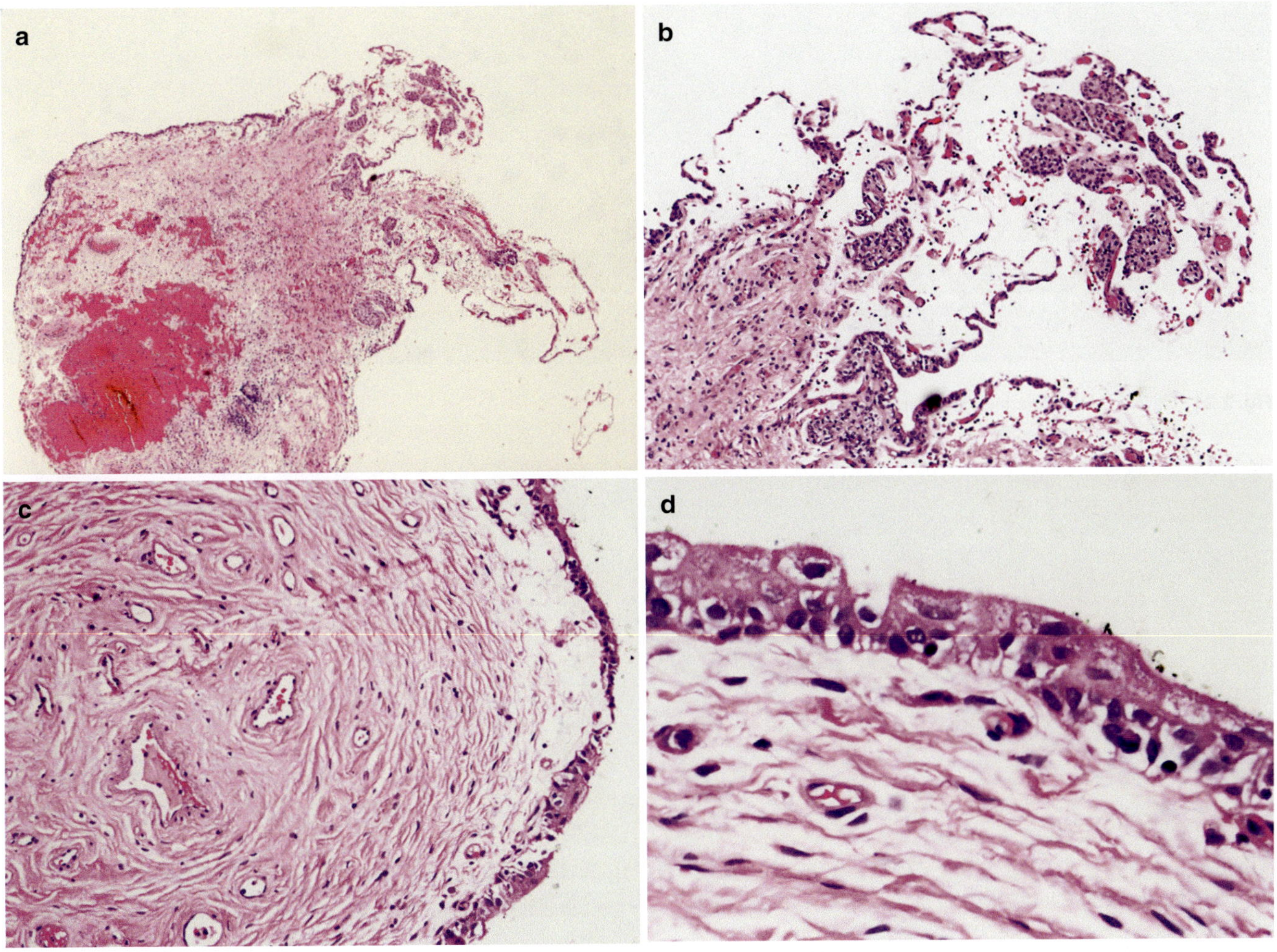

Fig. 2.20   Case 3. Polypoid ureteritis

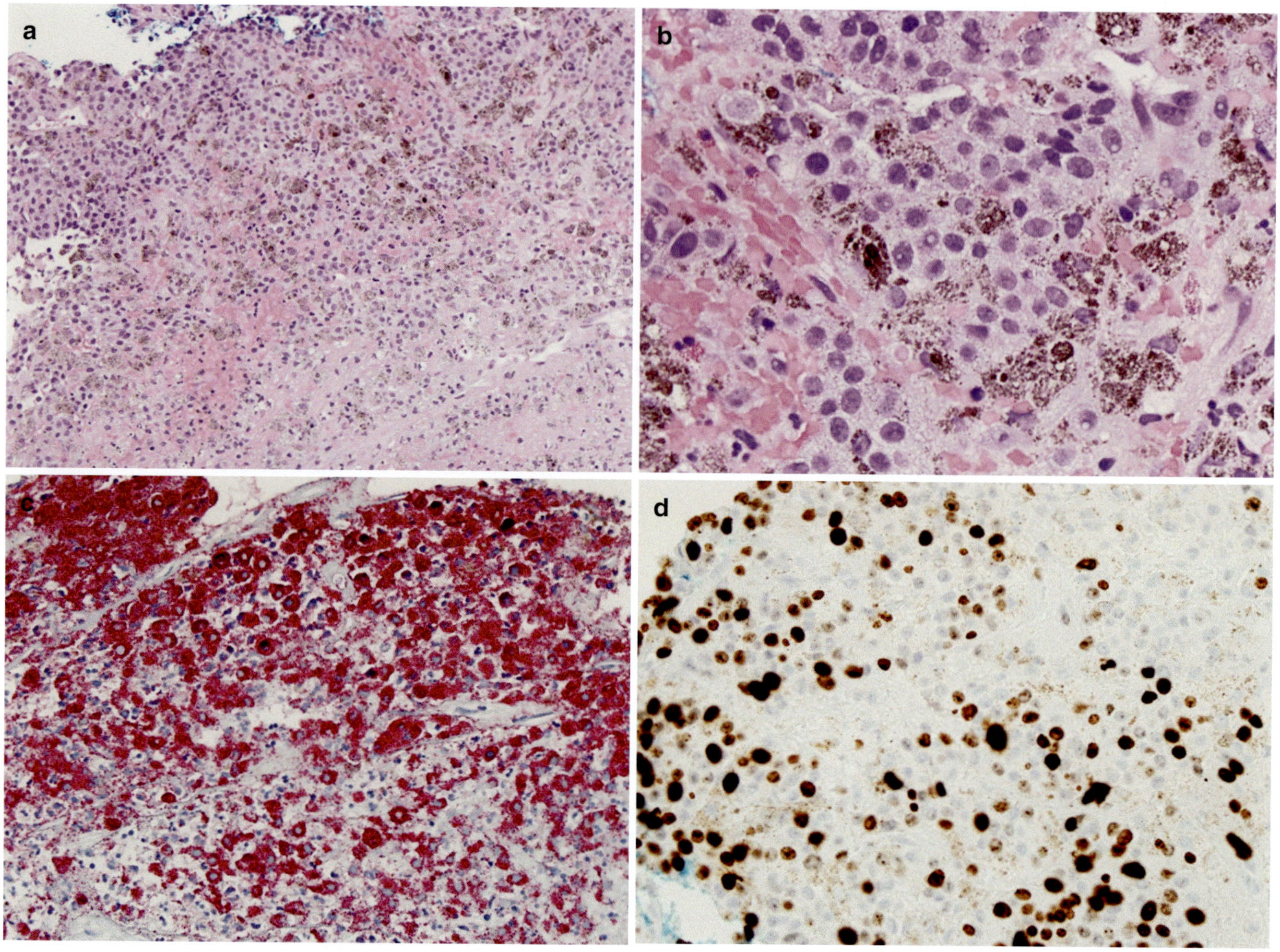

Fig. 2.21 Case 4. Metastatic melanoma in the ureter

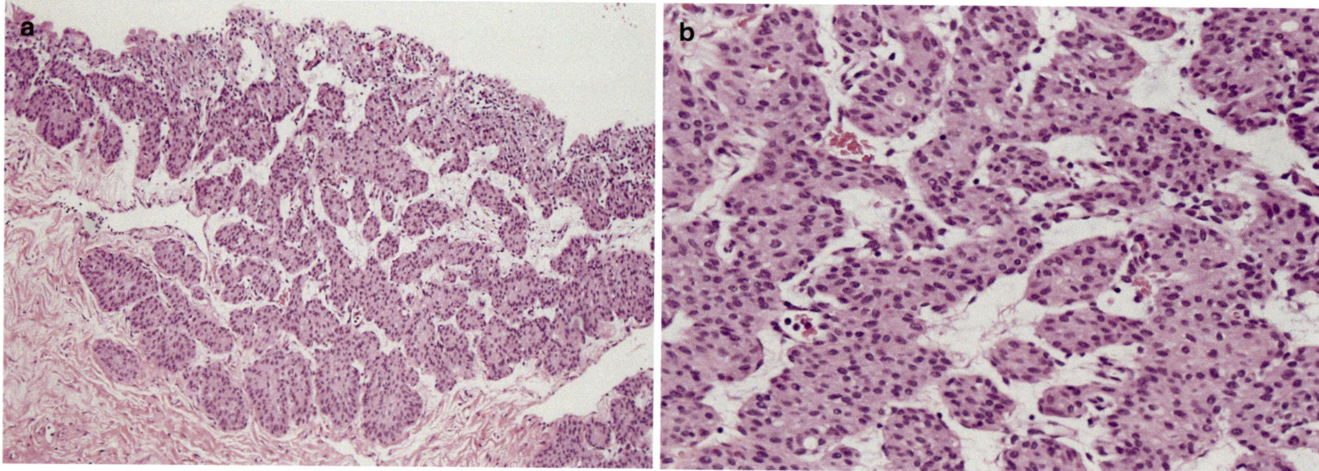

Fig. 2.22 Case 5. Florid von Brunn's nests in the renal pelvis

References

1. Murtaza B, et al. Inverted papilloma of ureter: a rare cause of hydronephrosis. J Coll Physicians Surg Pak. 2012;22(8):542–4.
2. Duchek M, et al. Inverted papilloma with intussusception of the ureter. Case report. Scand J Urol Nephrol. 1987;21(2):147–9.
3. Luo JD, et al. Upper urinary tract inverted papillomas: report of 10 cases. Oncol Lett. 2012;4(1):71–4.
4. Stower MJ, et al. Inverted papilloma of the ureter with malignant change. Br J Urol. 1990;65(1):13–6.
5. Diolombi M, et al. Nephrogenic adenoma: a report of 3 unusual cases infiltrating into perinephric adipose tissue. Am J Surg Pathol. 2013;37(4):532–8.
6. McDaniel AS, et al. Immunohistochemical staining characteristics of nephrogenic adenoma using the PIN-4 cocktail (p63, AMACR, and CK903) and GATA-3. Am J Surg Pathol. 2014;38(12):1664–71.
7. Turcan D, et al. Nephrogenic adenoma of the urinary tract: a 6-year single center experience. Pathol Res Pract. 2017;213(7):831–5.
8. Zhou F, et al. Primary localized amyloidosis of the urinary tract frequently mimics neoplasia: a clinicopathologic analysis of 11 cases. Am J Clin Exp Urol. 2014;2(1):71–5.
9. Mantoo S, et al. A rare case of localised AA-type amyloidosis of the ureter with spheroids of amyloid. Singap Med J. 2012;53(4):e77–9.
10. Ding X, et al. Localized amyloidosis of the ureter: a case report and literature review. Can Urol Assoc J. 2013;7(11–12):E764–7.
11. Hanna DN, Levy JA, Marshall JS. Amyloidosis and acute hemorrhage of the kidney, ureter, and bladder. Can J Urol. 2017;24(4):8934–6.
12. Mugiya S, et al. Endoscopic features of impacted ureteral stones. J Urol. 2004;171(1):89–91.
13. Hashimoto Y, et al. Sarcoidosis of the ureter. Urology. 2012;79(6):e81–2.
14. Perimenis P, Athanasopoulos A, Barbalias G. Sarcoidosis of the ureter. Eur Urol. 1990;18(4):307–8.
15. Albers DD, et al. Oil granuloma of the ureter. J Urol. 1984;132(1):114.
16. Al-Khawaja M, et al. Ureteral endometriosis: clinicopathological and immunohistochemical study of 7 cases. Hum Pathol. 2008;39(6):954–9.
17. Barra F, et al. Ureteral endometriosis: a systematic review of epidemiology, pathogenesis, diagnosis, treatment, risk of malignant transformation and fertility. Hum Reprod Update. 2018;24(6):710–30.
18. Beyer-Boon ME, et al. Cytological changes due to urinary calculi: a consideration of the relationship between calculi and the development of urothelial carcinoma. Br J Urol. 1978;50(2):81–9.
19. Highman W, Wilson E. Urine cytology in patients with calculi. J Clin Pathol. 1982;35(3):350–6.
20. Siddappa S, Mythri K, Kowsalya R. Cytological findings in routine voided urine samples with hematuria from a tertiary care center in South India. J Cytol. 2012;29(1):16–9.
21. Tseng TY, Stoller ML. Obstructive uropathy. Clin Geriatr Med. 2009;25(3):437–43.
22. Li L, Parwani AV. Xanthogranulomatous pyelonephritis. Arch Pathol Lab Med. 2011;135(5):671–4.
23. Ordones FV, et al. High-grade transitional cell carcinoma masquerading as a xanthogranulomatous pyelonephritis and perinephric abscess. Radiol Case Rep. 2017;12(2):281–4.
24. Papadopoulos I, Wirth B, Wand H. Xanthogranulomatous pyelonephritis associated with renal cell carcinoma. Report on two cases and review of the literature. Eur Urol. 1990;18(1):74–6.
25. Alberti C. About a case of unilateral perirenal retroperitoneal fibrosis without aorta involvement. Eur Rev Med Pharmacol Sci. 2015;19(7):1119–20.
26. Corradi D, et al. Idiopathic retroperitoneal fibrosis: clinicopathologic features and differential diagnosis. Kidney Int. 2007;72(6):742–53.
27. Sofiane B, et al. Retroperitoneal fibrosis: an atypical presentation of localized bilateral perirenal fibrosis. Surgery. 2012;151(4):630–1.
28. Vaglio A, Maritati F. Idiopathic retroperitoneal fibrosis. J Am Soc Nephrol. 2016;27(7):1880–9.
29. Bhat S, Chandran V. Villous adenoma of the renal pelvis and ureter. Indian J Urol. 2010;26(4):598–9.
30. Hudson J, et al. Intestinal type villous adenoma of the renal pelvis. Can Urol Assoc J. 2013;7(1–2):E138–42.
31. Karnjanawanichkul W, et al. Renal pelvic villous adenoma presented with mucusuria: report of a case and literature review. Int J Urol. 2013;20(2):247–9.
32. Lee JY, et al. Molecular characterization of urothelial carcinoma of the bladder and upper urinary tract. Transl Oncol. 2018;11(1):37–42.
33. Lughezzani G, et al. Prognostic factors in upper urinary tract urothelial carcinomas: a comprehensive review of the current literature. Eur Urol. 2012;62(1):100–14.
34. Kammerer-Jacquet SF, et al. Genomics in upper tract urothelial carcinoma. Curr Opin Urol. 2017;27(1):35–40.
35. Sanford T, Porten S, Meng MV. Molecular analysis of upper tract and bladder urothelial carcinoma: results from a microarray comparison. PLoS One. 2015;10(8):e0137141.
36. Yates DR, Catto JW. Distinct patterns and behaviour of urothelial carcinoma with respect to anatomical location: how molecular biomarkers can augment clinico-pathological predictors in upper urinary tract tumours. World J Urol. 2013;31(1):21–9.
37. Mandalapu RS, et al. Update of the ICUD-SIU consultation on upper tract urothelial carcinoma 2016: treatment of low-risk upper tract urothelial carcinoma. World J Urol. 2017;35(3):355–65.
38. Verges DP, et al. Endoscopic treatment of upper tract urothelial carcinoma. Curr Urol Rep. 2017;18(4):31.
39. Fujii Y, et al. Long-term outcome of bladder papillary urothelial neoplasms of low malignant potential. BJU Int. 2003;92(6):559–62.
40. Kim JK, et al. Papillary urothelial neoplasm of low malignant potential (PUNLMP) after initial TUR-BT: comparative analyses with noninvasive low-grade papillary urothelial carcinoma (LGPUC). J Cancer. 2017;8(15):2885–91.
41. Ercil H, et al. Papillary ureteral neoplasm of low malignant potential in the upper urinary tract: endoscopic treatment. Clin Genitourin Cancer. 2014;12(6):451–4.
42. Albadine R, et al. PAX8 (+)/p63 (−) immunostaining pattern in renal collecting duct carcinoma (CDC): a useful immunoprofile in the differential diagnosis of CDC versus urothelial carcinoma of upper urinary tract. Am J Surg Pathol. 2010;34(7):965–9.
43. Gonzalez-Roibon N, et al. The role of GATA binding protein 3 in the differential diagnosis of collecting duct and upper tract urothelial carcinomas. Hum Pathol. 2013;44(12):2651–7.
44. Lin XY, et al. Expression and diagnostic implications of carbonic anhydrase IX in several tumours with predominantly clear cell morphology. Histopathology. 2015;66(5):685–94.
45. Chang A, et al. Use of PAX8 and GATA3 in diagnosing sarcomatoid renal cell carcinoma and sarcomatoid urothelial carcinoma. Hum Pathol. 2013;44(8):1563–8.
46. Gailey MP, Bellizzi AM. Immunohistochemistry for the novel markers glypican 3, PAX8, and p40 (DeltaNp63) in squamous cell and urothelial carcinoma. Am J Clin Pathol. 2013;140(6):872–80.
47. Laury AR, et al. A comprehensive analysis of PAX8 expression in human epithelial tumors. Am J Surg Pathol. 2011;35(6):816–26.
48. Fan B, et al. Impact of tumor architecture on disease recurrence and cancer-specific mortality of upper tract urothelial carcinoma treated with radical nephroureterectomy. Tumour Biol. 2017;39(7):1010428317710822.
49. Hartmann A, et al. Urothelial carcinoma of the upper urinary tract: inverted growth pattern is predictive of microsatellite instability. Hum Pathol. 2003;34(3):222–7.
50. Hashimoto T, et al. Prognostic implication of infiltrative growth pattern and establishment of novel risk stratification model for sur-

vival in patients with upper urinary tract urothelial carcinoma. Int J Clin Oncol. 2014;19(2):373–8.

51. Masson-Lecomte A, et al. Predictive factors for final pathologic ureteral sections on 700 radical cystectomy specimens: implications for intraoperative frozen section decision-making. Urol Oncol. 2017;35(11):659.e1–6.

52. Reder NP, et al. Diagnostic accuracy of intraoperative frozen sections during radical cystectomy does not affect disease-free or overall survival: a study of 364 patients with urothelial carcinoma of the urinary bladder. Ann Diagn Pathol. 2015;19(3):107–12.

53. Satkunasivam R, et al. Utility and significance of ureteric frozen section analysis during radical cystectomy. BJU Int. 2016;117(3):463–8.

54. Inoue S, et al. GATA3 immunohistochemistry in urothelial carcinoma of the upper urinary tract as a urothelial marker and a prognosticator. Hum Pathol. 2017;64:83–90.

55. Wilkerson ML, et al. The application of immunohistochemical biomarkers in urologic surgical pathology. Arch Pathol Lab Med. 2014;138(12):1643–65.

56. Zhang Z, et al. Primary osteosarcoma of the ureter. Am J Med Sci. 2012;343(6):504–6.

57. Sreenivas J, et al. Ureteric lymphoma as a rare cause of right lower ureteric obstruction. BMJ Case Rep. 2016;2016:2015213613.

58. Sutton B, et al. Primary malignant melanoma of the genitourinary tract with upper and lower tracts involvement. Case Rep Urol. 2013;2013:217254.

59. Macneil J, Hossack T. A case of metastatic melanoma in the ureter. Case Rep Urol. 2016;2016:1853015.

Bladder Pathology

3

Xunda Luo, Ngoentra Tantranont, and Steven Shen

List of Frequently Asked Questions

What Are the Most Common Presenting Symptoms of Bladder Cancer?

The most common presentation is painless gross hematuria, followed by urgency, nocturia, and dysuria. If a tumor is present at the bladder neck, irritative urinary symptoms may be prominent. Obstructive symptoms or palpable mass can be found in advanced and severe disease. Rarely, in patients who present with metastatic disease, weight loss, and bone pain can be the initial symptoms [1].

What Are the Two Pathogenetic Pathways and Molecular Aberrations in Urothelial Carcinoma?

Hyperplasia and dysplasia are the two essentially mutually exclusive pathogenetic pathways in neoplastic transformation of urothelium. The hyperplasia pathway is characterized by molecular abnormalities in fibroblast growth factor receptor 3 (FGFR3) gene, whereas the dysplasia pathway is characterized by abnormalities in *TP53* gene. Approximately 80% of urothelial carcinoma cases originate from abnormalities in the hyperplasia pathway, which start with urothelial hyperplasia and progress to low-grade papillary urothelial carcinoma. The abnormalities in the dysplasia pathway, however, account for about 20% of urothelial carcinoma cases, starting with dysplasia and progressing to high-grade papillary urothelial carcinoma, urothelial carcinoma in situ, and invasive urothelial carcinoma [2].

What Are the Roles of Cytology in the Diagnosis of Bladder Cancer?

Urine cytology has been used for many years as a tool to screen, diagnose, and monitor bladder cancer. Urine cytology findings allow cytopathologists to identify patients with increased risks of malignancy, and clinicians to choose management options accordingly.

Ancillary studies can be performed on urinary cytology specimens. These studies can be either cell or liquid based. The two commonly used, and FDA-approved cell-based studies are UroVysion (Abbott Laboratories, Abbott Park, IL, USA) and ImmunoCyt/UCyt+ (Diagnocure Inc., Quebec, Canada). UroVysion is a fluorescence in situ hybridization (FISH)-based test that detects numerical and structural abnormalities of chromosomes preferentially seen in urothelial carcinoma, whereas ImmunoCyt/UCyt+, as indicated by the name, is an immunofluorescence-based test at protein expression level. Examples of liquid-based studies are bladder tumor antigen and nuclear matrix protein 22 (NMP22), both of which are dipstick-based tests that can be performed in urologist clinics [3, 4].

What Are the Diagnostic Categories of Urine Cytology?

Diagnostic categories of urine cytology are standard terminologies that label cytology cases based on predefined morphologic criteria. These diagnostic categories distinguish from each other by the likelihood of malignancy and enable clinicians to choose the optimal management options based

X. Luo
Pathology and Laboratory Medicine, Pennsylvania Presbyterian Hospital, Philadelphia, PA, USA

N. Tantranont
Department of Pathology, Siriraj Hospital, Faculty of Medicine, Mahidol University, Bangkok, Thailand

S. Shen (✉)
Department of Pathology and Genomic Medicine, Houston Methodist Hospital, Houston, TX, USA
e-mail: stevenshen@houstonmethodist.org

© Springer Nature Switzerland AG 2021
X. J. Yang, M. Zhou (eds.), *Practical Genitourinary Pathology*, Practical Anatomic Pathology,
https://doi.org/10.1007/978-3-030-57141-2_3

on risk and benefit assessment for individual patients. Prior to the Paris System for Reporting Urinary Cytology, several urine cytology classifications have been proposed and used. These classifications differ in diagnostic categories, diagnostic criteria, and terminology, which have caused inconsistency in reporting and confusion during communication among cytopathologists and clinicians.

The Paris System for Reporting Urinary Cytology is currently recommended by the International Academy of Cytology and the American Society of Cytopathology to report urine cytology. It is evidence and consensus based, incorporates the current understanding on the two pathogenetic pathways in neoplastic transformation of urothelium, acknowledges the suboptimal diagnostic sensitivity of urinary cytology on low-grade urothelial lesions, standardizes the terminology for reporting urinary cytology, and provides "Bethesda" type reference images illustrating definitions and diagnostic criteria for categories [4, 5].

What Are the Categories of Urine Cytology Recommended by the Paris System?

The categories of urine cytology defined in the Paris System are as follows:
- Adequacy.
- Negative for high-grade urothelial carcinoma.
- Atypical urothelial cells.
- Suspicious for high-grade urothelial carcinoma.
- High-grade urothelial carcinoma.
- Low-grade urothelial neoplasm.
- Other malignancies, both primary and secondary [5].

How Can We Distinguish Polypoid/Papillary Cystitis and Papillary Urothelial Carcinoma?

Polypoid/papillary cystitis is an inflammatory/reactive process that may have a similar cystoscopic finding as a papillary urothelial neoplasm. Histologically, it shows a broad frond and is lined by urothelial cells of normal thickness (Fig. 3.1a). Reactive epithelial changes associated with mixed inflammation are normally found (Fig. 3.1b). There may be mild cytologic atypia with uniform nuclear enlargement or small nucleoli. In contrast, papillary urothelial neoplasms have well formed, delicate to complex papillary architecture (Fig. 3.1c), and the cell linings are often markedly thickened and show mild to severe cytologic atypia (Fig. 3.1d). Although inflammatory background can be found in both lesions, it is much more frequently seen and more prominent in polypoid/papillary cystitis. In addition, patients with polypoid/papillary cystitis will often have clinical history of instrumentation, prior therapy, or stone.

What Are the Diagnostic Criteria of Low-Grade Dysplasia?

The diagnosis of low-grade urothelial dysplasia is often difficult. It is unlikely that it will be detected cystoscopically and presented as isolated finding. Generally, there are definitive dysplastic changes characterized by increased epithelial thickness and mild loss of cell polarity, mild nuclear enlargement and pleomorphism, and infrequent mitosis (Fig. 3.2a). Overall, the cytologic atypia is short of urothelial carcinoma in situ (Fig. 3.2b). There may be occasional mitoses, but atypical mitotic figures are not present. It is frequently seen in patients who have prior history or concurrent noninvasive low-grade papillary urothelial carcinoma or urothelial carcinoma in situ.

What Is the Definition of Urothelial Proliferation of Uncertain Malignant Potential?

Urothelial proliferation of uncertain malignant potential is a descriptive term for those lesions that show markedly thickened urothelial lining with no true papillary formation and have no or mild cytologic atypia (Fig. 3.3). This may be found in patients who had a history of papillary urothelial neoplasms or less commonly during work-up for patients presented with microhematuria or urinary obstructive symptoms. Based on the published studies on this not well-defined lesion, it has chromosomal changes similar to that of papillary urothelial neoplasm and occurs frequently in patients with a history of prior, concurrent, and subsequent urothelial neoplasia. Therefore, this lesion most likely represents an early urothelial neoplasia [6].

What Are the Diagnostic Criteria of Urothelial Carcinoma In Situ?

The main diagnostic criteria for urothelial carcinoma in situ (CIS) are severe cytologic atypia characterized by marked nuclear atypia, increased nuclear to cytoplasmic ratio, nuclear enlargement, and pleomorphism as well as hyperchromasia (Fig. 3.4a). Abnormal large nuclei, especially at the base and frequent mitotic figures are helpful features. Cellular discohesion is a frequent finding. The lesion may exhibit loss of cellular polarity and disorganized distribution of cells. Unlike cervical squamous cell carcinoma in situ, the cytologic atypia may not involve the entire thickness

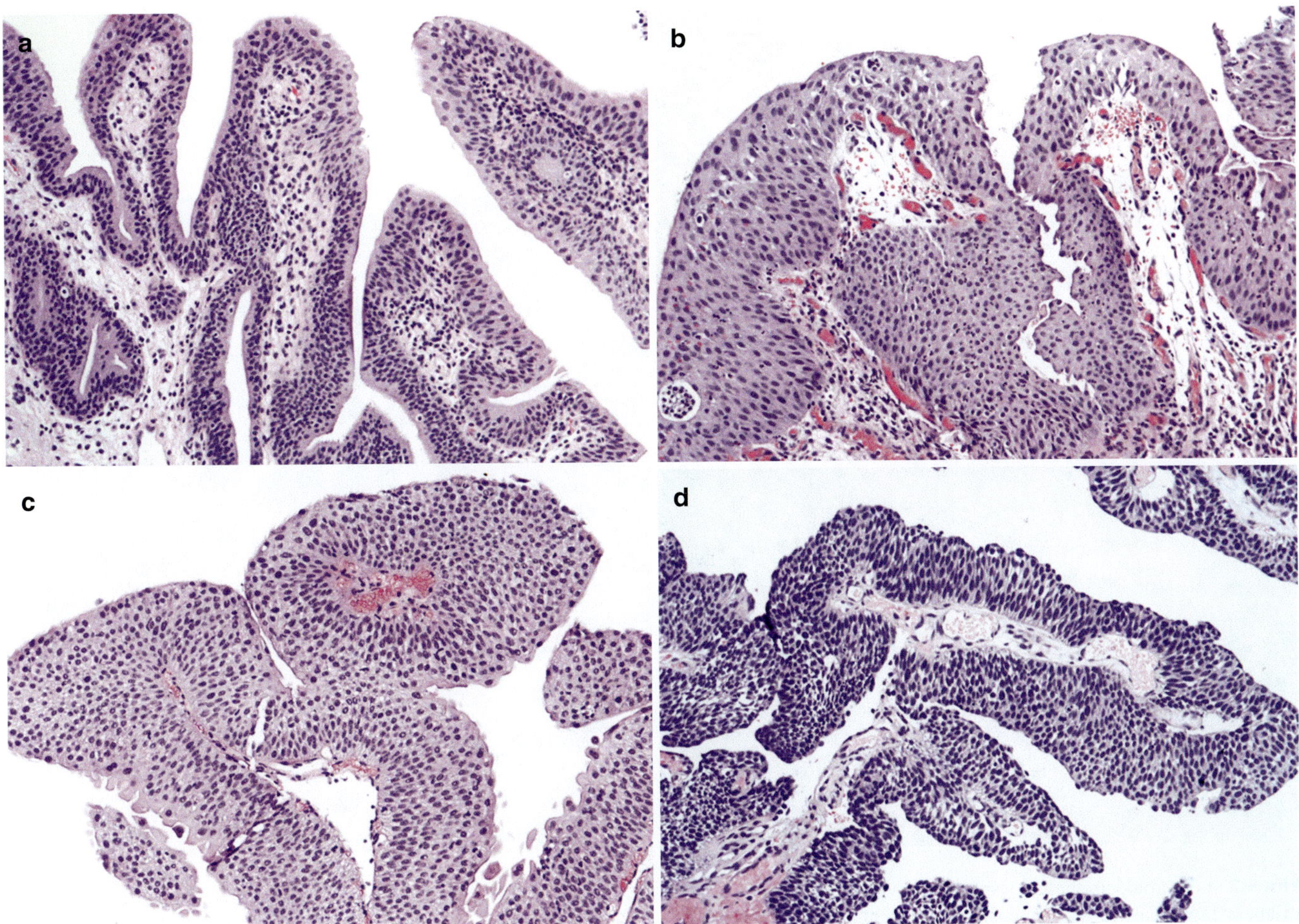

Fig. 3.1 Polypoid/papillary cystitis with broad papillary frond (**a**), edematous stroma, inflammatory infiltrate, and reactive epithelial changes (**b**). In contrast, papillary urothelial neoplasm exhibits well-formed delicate papillae (**c**) and lining cells with variable cytologic atypia (**d**)

of urothelium. In addition, CIS is frequently associated with neovascularization in the subepithelial tissue. It can be seen associated with high-grade papillary urothelial carcinoma. Occasionally, CIS may involve von Brunn nests (Fig. 3.4b), cystitis cystica, and cystitis glandularis, which can be pitfalls in routine practice [7].

What Are the Common Variants of Urothelial Carcinoma In Situ?

The common type of urothelial carcinoma in situ (CIS) is large cell CIS (most common) as described in the above question with large tumor cells (typically 5× size of small stromal lymphocyte). However, a type of small cell CIS has been described. It is composed of smaller neoplastic cells with high N/C ratio, hyperchromasia, and frequent mitoses or apoptosis. A "clinging" or "denuding" CIS is described as flat or isolated large tumor cells attached to the basement membrane (Fig. 3.5a). Pagetoid and undermining (lepidic) CIS is single or clusters of atypical large tumor cells pres-

ent in otherwise normal urothelial cells (Fig. 3.5b). These atypical cells are usually present at the base of the urothelium, but can be present in any levels of urothelium. Urothelial CIS with glandular differentiation (Fig. 3.5c, d) has also been described [8].

What Are the Most Common Diagnostic Features of Reactive Atypia?

The common features of reactive atypia are uniformly enlarged nuclei with vesicular chromatin and prominent nucleoli in almost all cells. The lining cells are of normal thickness and have normal or mildly increased N:C ratio. There is often prominent background of mixed inflammation within the epithelium and/or subepithelial tissue (Fig. 3.6). Other associated changes such as vascular congestion and atypical stromal cells may be seen in patients with clinical history of infection, prior procedure, prior treatments such as intravesical therapy, radiation or chemotherapy, instrumentation, or stone.

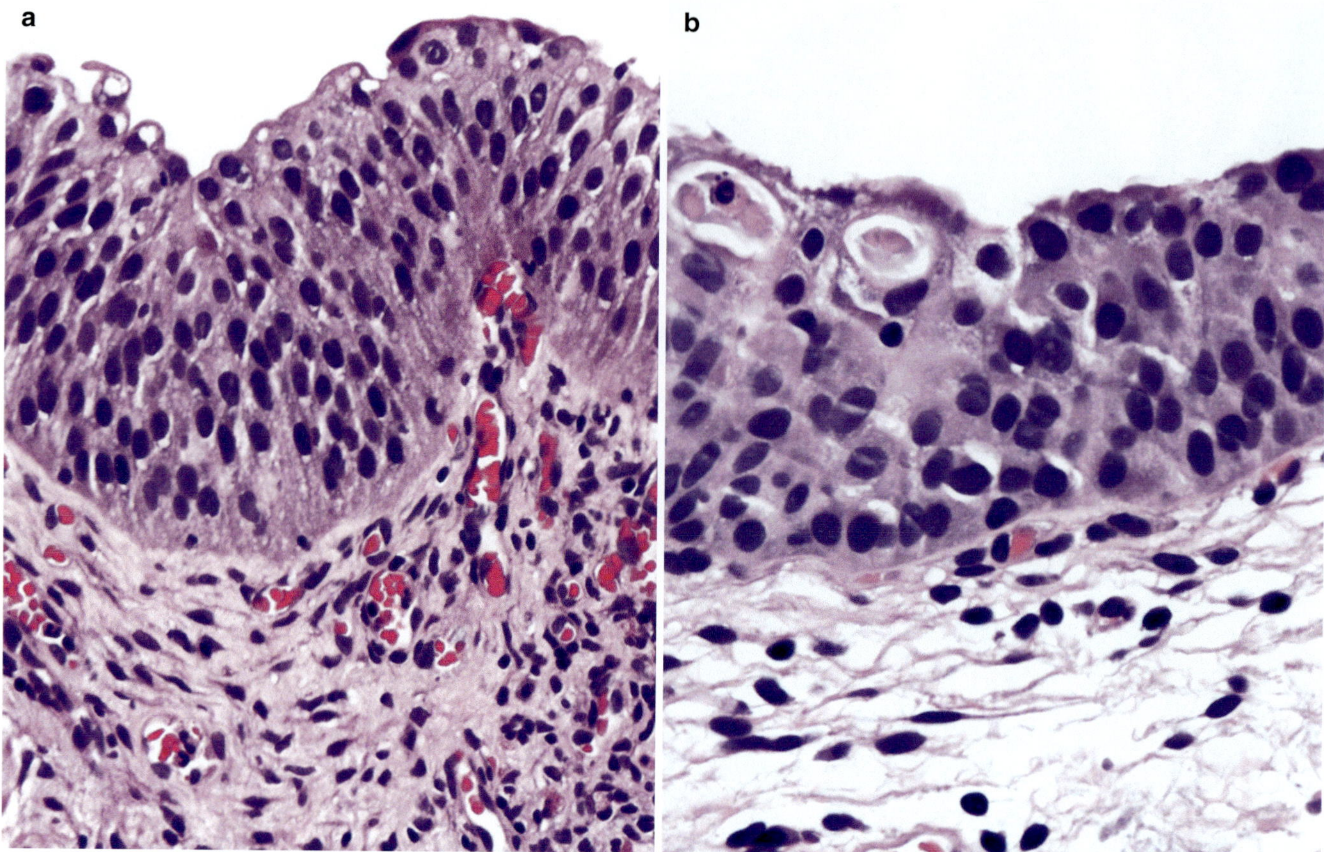

Fig. 3.2 Low-grade urothelial dysplasia showing thickened (**a**) or normal thickness urothelium (**b**) with mild loss of nuclear polarity, increasing of nuclear/cytoplasmic ratio, nuclear enlargement and hyperchromasia

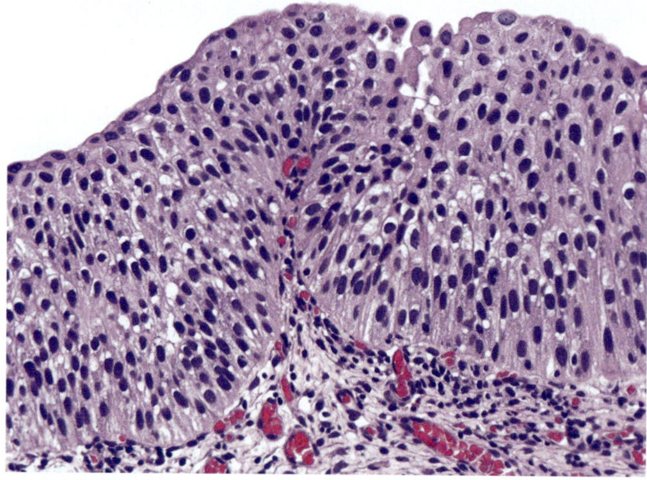

Fig. 3.3 Urothelial proliferation of uncertain malignant potential exhibits marked thickening and focal undulation of urothelium with minimal and mild cytologic atypia

Are There Any Reliable Immunohistochemical Markers that Can Help Diagnose Urothelial Carcinoma In Situ?

There have been some studies exploring the use of immuno-histochemistry with markers such as p53, MIB-1 (Ki-67), CK20, CD44 as an adjunct for the diagnosis of urothelial carcinoma in situ (Fig. 3.7a) and distinction from reactive atypia. Urothelial CIS typically shows diffuse and strong stain for CK20 (Fig. 3.7b), and diffuse nuclear stain for p53 (Fig. 3.7c), but negative stain for CD44 (Fig. 3.7d). In contract, reactive atypia is typically negative for CK20 and p53, but often positive for CD44. However, these results are not uniformly reliable in routine practice, so the diagnosis should still be made primarily based on cytomorphology. Therefore, immunohistochemistry is not recommended by the International Society of Urological Pathology (ISUP) for the diagnosis of urothelial carcinoma in situ.

What Are the Diagnostic Criteria of Urothelial Papilloma?

Diagnostic criteria of urothelial papilloma include delicate, simple papillary architecture, and benign urothelial lining of normal thickness. There is no cytological atypia, architectural atypia, or mitosis. Reactive change, particularly in the umbrella cells, may be seen (Fig. 3.8). Sometimes, the papillary cores may contain dilated lymphatics or foamy histiocytes. The lesion is endoscopically similar to other papillary urothelial neoplasms, but it is usually solitary and small

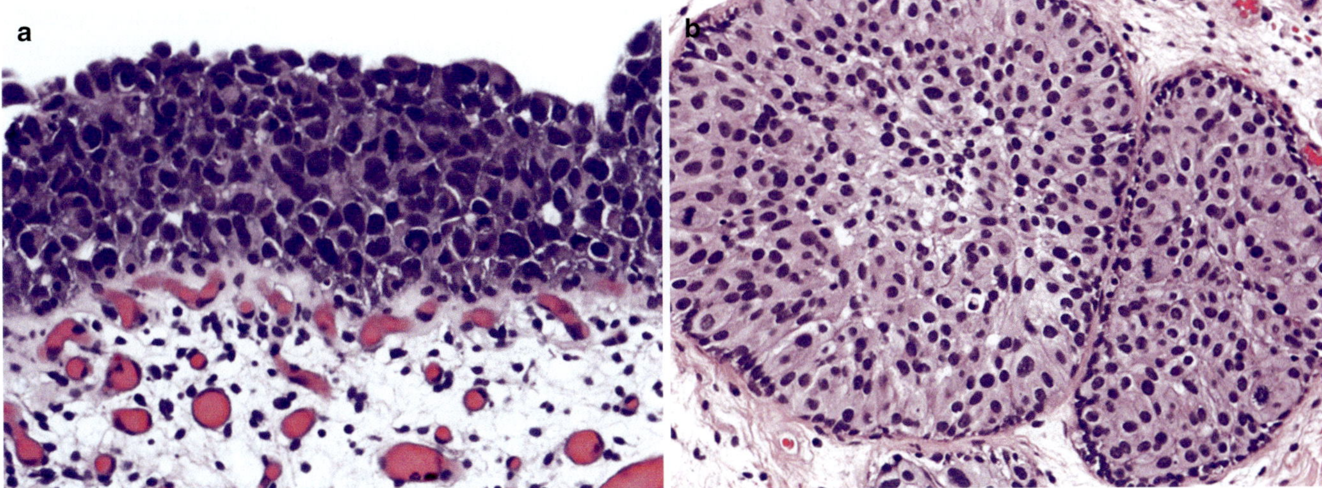

Fig. 3.4 Urothelial carcinoma in situ shows severe cytologic atypia with marked nuclear enlargement and irregularity, hyperchromasia and brisk mitotic figure (**a**). CIS involves von Brunn nests with large rounded nests composed of pleomorphic tumor cells with frequent mitoses (**b**)

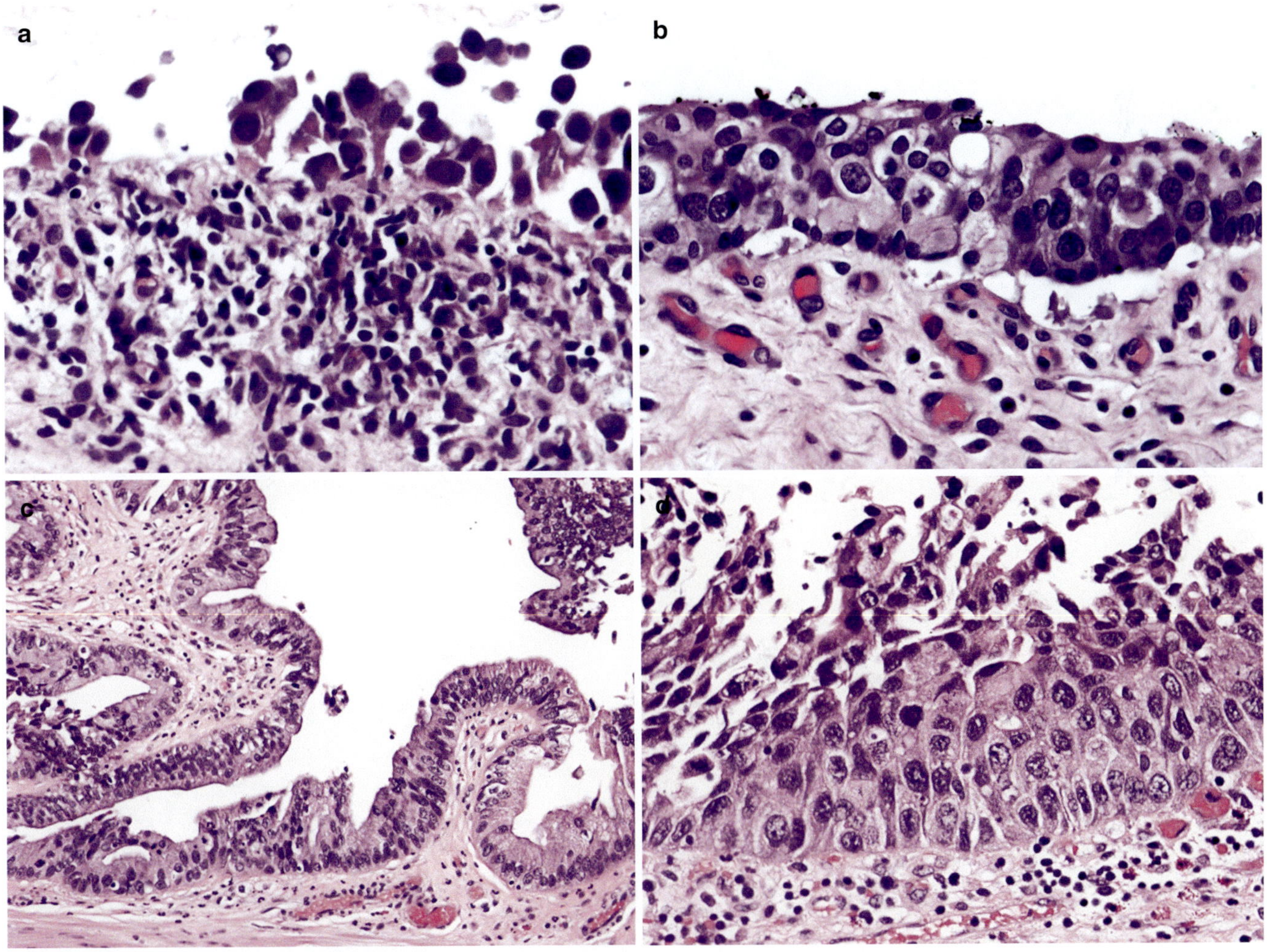

Fig. 3.5 Clinging or denuding urothelial carcinoma in situ (**a**) shows a few clusters of large atypical tumor cells attached to subepithelial basement membrane. An example of urothelial carcinoma in situ with pag-etoid spread of tumor cells (**b**). Urothelial carcinoma in situ with glandular differentiation shows intratumoral tubular or enteric gland-like lumens (**c**, **d**)

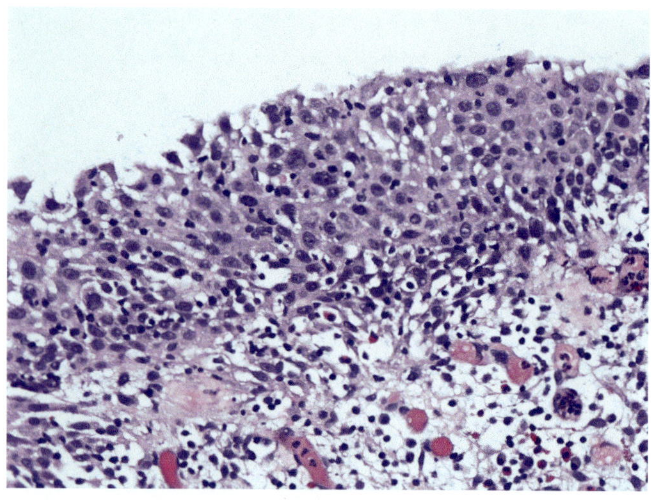

Fig. 3.6 Urothelial reactive atypia with uniform enlargement of nuclei and prominent nucleoli associated with prominent intraepithelial inflammation

lesion. Patients with urothelial papilloma are also typically younger than those with papillary urothelial carcinoma. It is usually an incidental finding and patient does not have prior history or concurrent urothelial carcinoma [6].

What Are the Molecular Subtypes of Urothelial Carcinoma?

Molecular characterization of bladder urothelial tumors shows that they can be subtyped into two major categories— luminal and basal type tumors, similar to those seen in breast carcinomas. Majority molecular subtyping studies focused on muscle-invasive bladder urothelial carcinomas (MIBC). In the protein expression-based, The Cancer Genome Atlas (TCGA) Research Network study, MIBCs were identified as four clusters. Clusters I and II MIBCs express high HER2, elevated estrogen receptor-β signatures, and positive for

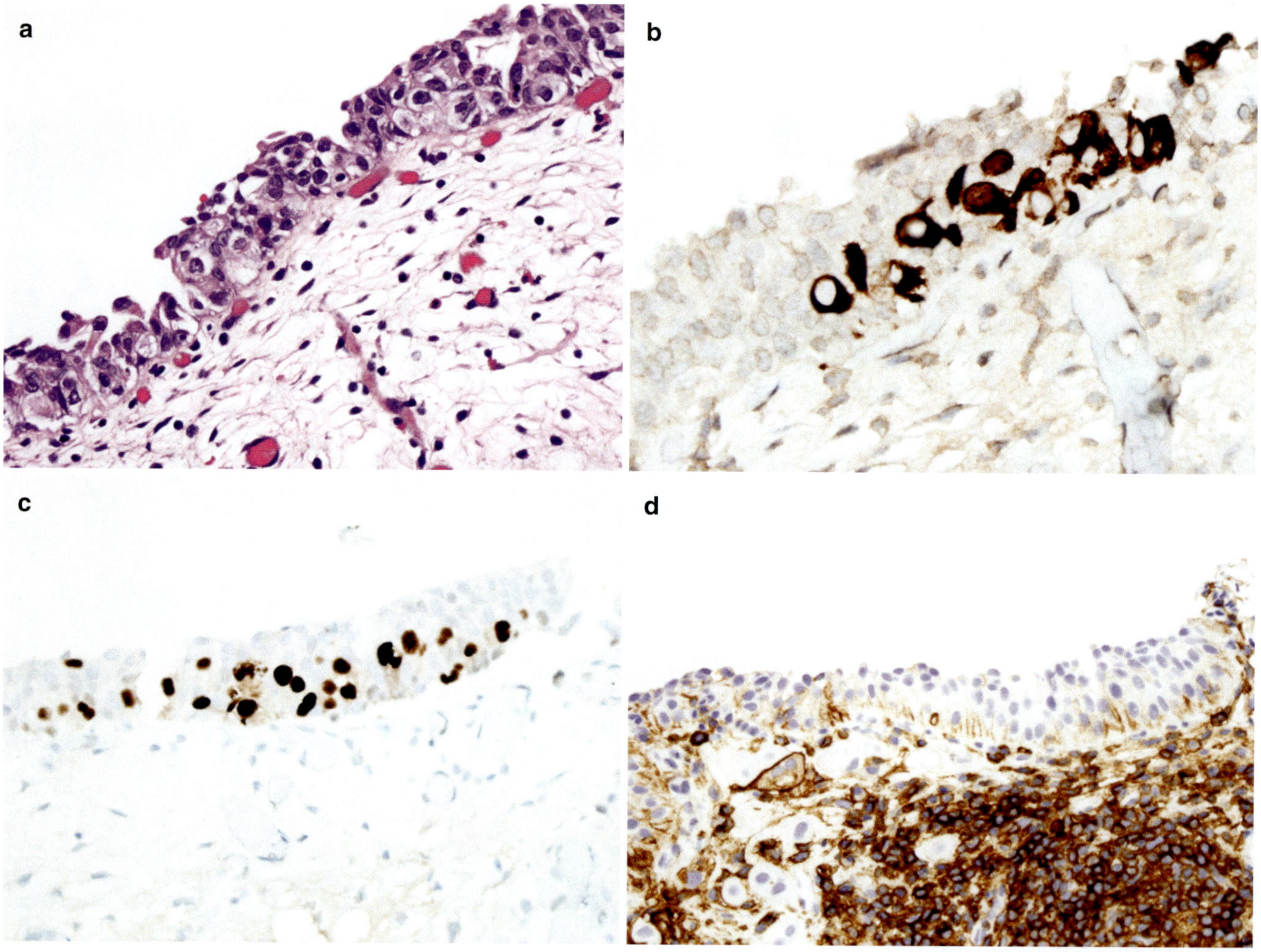

Fig. 3.7 Urothelial carcinoma in situ with pagetoid spread (**a**) showing strong CK20 (**b**) and p53 (**c**) staining patterns and loss of CD44 staining (**d**)

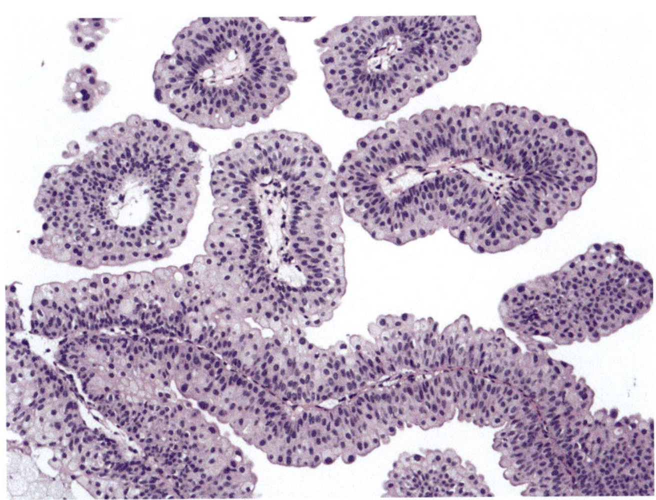

Fig. 3.8 Urothelial papilloma shows delicate papillae lined by normal thickness urothelium lined by normal urothelial cells

GATA3 and FOXA1, consistent with a luminal subtype. Markers for/consistent with urothelial differentiation, such as uroplakins and CK20, are also expressed in luminal tumors. A single study demonstrates that vast majority of micropapillary invasive carcinomas are luminal type tumors. Compared with Cluster II MIBCs, Cluster I MIBCs more commonly present with papillary morphology and harbor *FGFR3* gene alterations. Clusters III and IV MIBCs in the TCGA study, however, do not express high HER2, GATA3, or FOXA1. Cluster III tumors are more likely to present with basal/squamous features and express epithelial lineage-characteristic genes such as *KRT5*, *KRT6A*, *KRT14*, and *EGFR*. They are consistent with a basal subtype. Cluster IV tumors, in contrast, are less likely to present with squamous features or increased *KRT5*, *KRT6A*, *KRT14*, and *EGFR* expression. They could occasionally be papillary in architecture and typically show increased microRNA miR-99a-5p and miR-100-5p expressions.

In addition to TCGA classification for molecular subtypes of urothelial carcinoma, University of North Carolina (UNC), MD Anderson Cancer Center (MDACC), and Lund University (LU) classifications have also been proposed. The UNC classification subtypes urothelial carcinomas into luminal, basal, and claudin-low tumors. The MDACC classification includes luminal, basal, and p53-like subtypes. The LU classification, on the other hand, divides urothelial carcinomas into genomically unstable, urobasal A, infiltrated, urobasal B, and squamous cell carcinoma-like tumors. These classifications overlap more or less with each other.

Molecular subtypes of MIBCs may guide the selection of appropriate targeted therapies. For instance, luminal type (which corresponds to TCGA Cluster I, UNC and MDACC luminal, and Lund genomically unstable) tumors are more likely to respond to FGFR3 and PPARγ inhibitor-based therapies. Molecular subtypes of MIBCs are also of prognostic values. Luminal type carcinomas in general carry a more favorable prognosis compared with nonluminal counterparts [9–14].

What Are the Distinguishing Features of Papillary Urothelial Neoplasm of Low Malignant Potential and Low-Grade Papillary Urothelial Carcinoma?

They are both papillary neoplasms lined by thickened urothelial lining. Most of them show exophytic growth but inverted growth pattern can be present. Papillary urothelial neoplasm of low malignant potential (PUNLMP) typically has delicate papillae without fusion and complexity. Cytologically, and the tumor cells are monotonous and may show very minimal cytologic atypia and preservation of cellular polarity. The nuclei are slightly enlarged and more crowded than benign urothelial lining. Nuclear groove may be seen. Nucleoli are either absent or inconspicuous. The chromatin is uniformly even. Mitoses are very rare and mostly limited to the basal layer (Fig. 3.9a). In contract, low-grade papillary urothelial carcinomas have more complex papillae with branching and fusion. There is mild loss of cellular polarity, mild nuclear irregularity, and pleomorphism (Fig. 3.9b). Mitosis may be present away from the basal layer [6].

What Are the Most Helpful Features that can Distinguish Low-Grade from High-Grade Papillary Urothelial Carcinoma?

Low-grade papillary urothelial carcinoma shows preserved vertical orientation and more monotonous cell population in low power. However, in higher power it can show minimal loss of polarity, mild nuclear crowding, and mild nuclear atypia. Compared to low-grade papillary urothelial carcinoma, high-grade papillary urothelial carcinoma tends to have more fused and more complex papillae. However, the key difference between them is more cytologic atypia in high-grade urothelial carcinoma, including nuclear enlargement and pleomorphism, increased N/C ratio or hypercellularity, hyperchromasia, irregular prominent nucleoli, frequent mitoses including atypical mitoses, and rarely tumor necrosis (Fig. 3.10a). There are situations that a distinction between low and high grade is difficult. One scenario is that the combina-

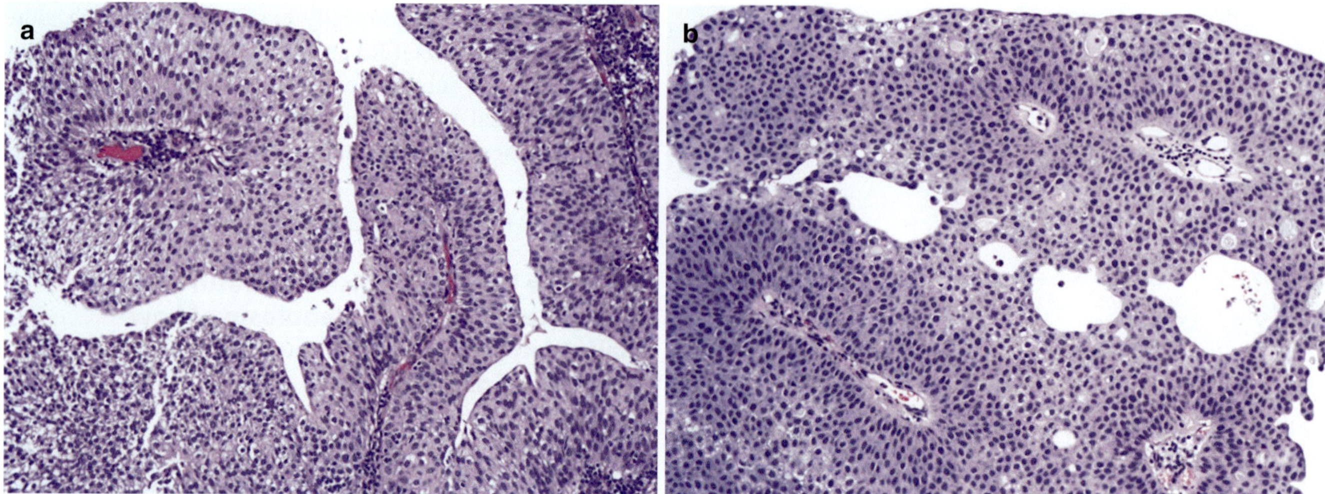

Fig. 3.9 Papillary urothelial neoplasm of low malignant potential (**a**) shows well-formed papillae lined by markedly thickened urothelial cells with minimal cytologic atypia. In contrast, low-grade papillary urothelial carcinoma (**b**) shows papillary complexity and mild cytologic atypia, loss of polarity, and occasional mitoses

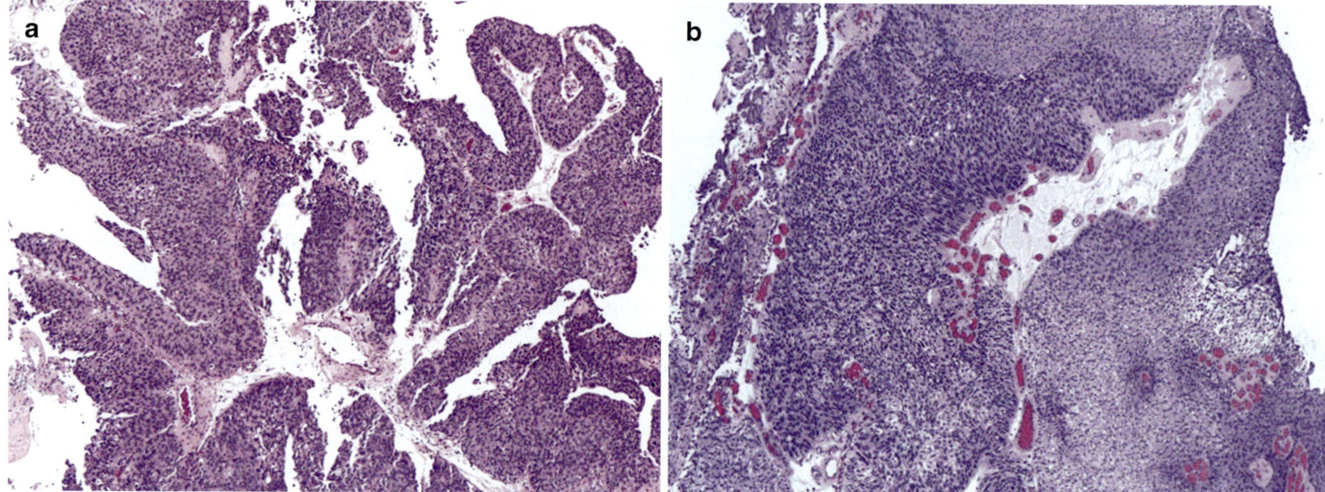

Fig. 3.10 High-grade papillary urothelial carcinoma with marked cytologic atypia which can be easily appreciated at low power magnification (**a**). One example of urothelial carcinoma exhibits low-grade papillary urothelial carcinoma with high-grade area (**b**)

tion of cytologic features in a papillary tumor is truly borderline between a low and high grade. The assignment becomes somewhat subjective depending on the assignment of relative weight of each cytologic and architectural features. The other scenario is that a mixture of distinct low-grade and high areas exist in the same tumor (Fig. 3.10b). It is unlikely that a clear cutoff point exists. A papillary tumor is diagnosed as high-grade urothelial carcinoma if there is more than 5–10% high-grade component. In this situation, a diagnosis of a low-grade papillary urothelial carcinoma with small component of high-grade carcinoma is very reasonable and conveys useful information for the management of patients [15].

What Are the Diagnostic Features and Clinical Significance of Squamous Metaplasia?

There are two types of squamous metaplasia; keratinizing (Fig. 3.11a) and nonkeratinizing (Fig. 3.11b). The diagnostic features of squamous metaplasia are polyhedral-shaped cells and presence of intercellular bridge. Keratinous material can be seen in keratinizing type. Most cases have no significant cytologic atypia. Keratinizing squamous metaplasia is usually a consequence of chronic inflammation result from infection, irritation, or radiation. It is associated with increased risk for squamous cell carcinoma, as well as urothelial carcinoma in urinary mucosa [16].

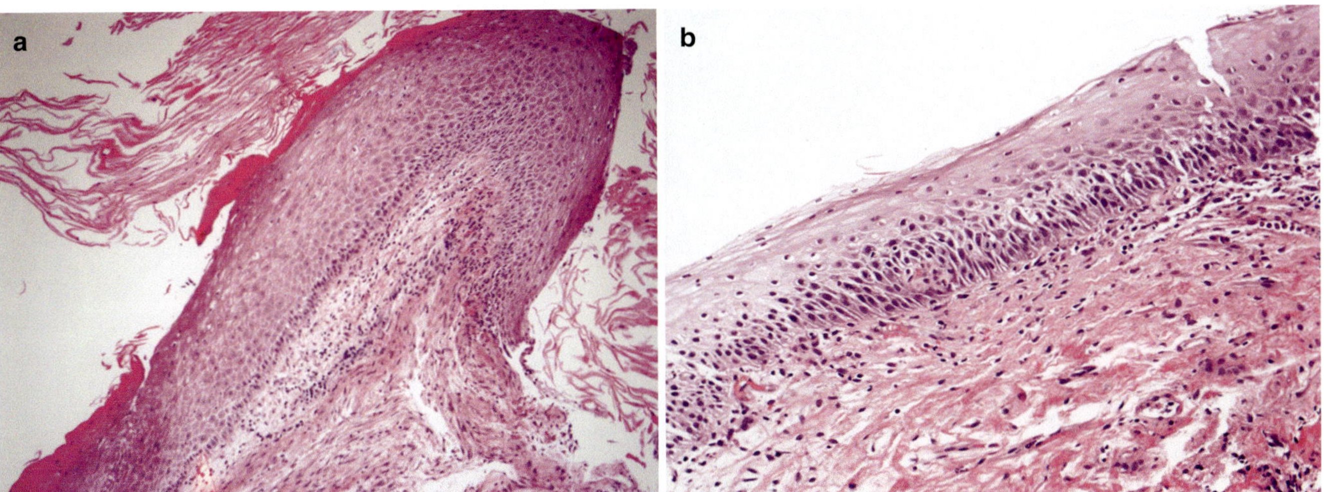

Fig. 3.11 Squamous metaplasia can be categorized into keratinizing (**a**) and nonkeratinizing (**b**) types

What Are the Diagnostic Features of Nephrogenic Adenoma?

Nephrogenic adenoma is typically composed of small compact tubules with or without mucin-like materials. The tubules are lined by monotonous cuboidal cells. The nuclei are centrally located, round, and hyperchromatic. The cells may show marked reactive atypia. The stroma is often very typical and shows granulation tissue with edema, mixed acute and chronic inflammation (Fig. 3.12a). The overlying or adjacent urothelium can range from normal, reactive to rarely urothelial CIS. Nephrogenic adenoma can have variable patterns such as tubular, cystic, polypoid, papillary, fibromyxoid, and diffuse. A mixture of patterns is very commonly seen. When predominantly papillary or polypoid, it may mimic papillary urothelial neoplasm cystoscopically and histologically (Fig. 3.12b). But unlike papillary urothelial neoplasm, papillary nephrogenic adenoma has a single-layer lining. The lining cells can have flat, elongated, or hobnail appearance. Cystic dilatation can be found in 72% of the cases (Fig. 3.12c). Eosinophilic or basophilic secretions can be found in the tubular lumen.

The main differential diagnoses of nephrogenic adenoma include urothelial carcinoma with glandular differentiation, cystitis cystica, or secondary involvement by prostate cancer. Nephrogenic adenoma is positive for Pax 8 (Fig. 3.12d), CK7, and AMACR, whereas urothelial lesion is positive for CK7, negative for Pax8 and AMACR. Prostate cancer would be positive for PSA and AMACR, negative for Pax 8 and CK7 [16].

What Are the Distinguishing Features of Nephrogenic Adenoma and Clear Cell Adenocarcinoma?

The architectural features, including tubular, cystic, and papillary structures and cells with hobnail appearance of nephrogenic adenoma may resemble clear cell carcinoma. However, there are some helpful features to help distinguish between the two lesions. Nephrogenic adenoma is usually small but clear cell adenocarcinoma is often large. Nephrogenic adenoma seldomly has solid growth pattern, clear cell change, glycogen in cytoplasm, nuclear atypia, and mitosis, but these features are common in clear cell adenocarcinoma (Fig. 3.13) [8].

What Are the Diagnostic Criteria of Urachal Carcinoma?

The diagnostic criteria of urachal carcinoma include location of tumor at the dome and/or anterior wall of urinary bladder, absence of cystitis cystica *et* glandularis near the area of tumor, epicenter of the mass in the muscularis propria of bladder with sharp demarcation between urachal tumor and overlying bladder mucosa, and no known primary elsewhere that has spread secondarily to the bladder. Most of the urachal carcinomas are adenocarcinoma which can be enteric, mucinous (colloid) (Fig. 3.14), signet ring, mixed, or not otherwise specified. However, urothelial and squamous cell carcinomas can also arise as urachal carcinoma [8, 17, 18].

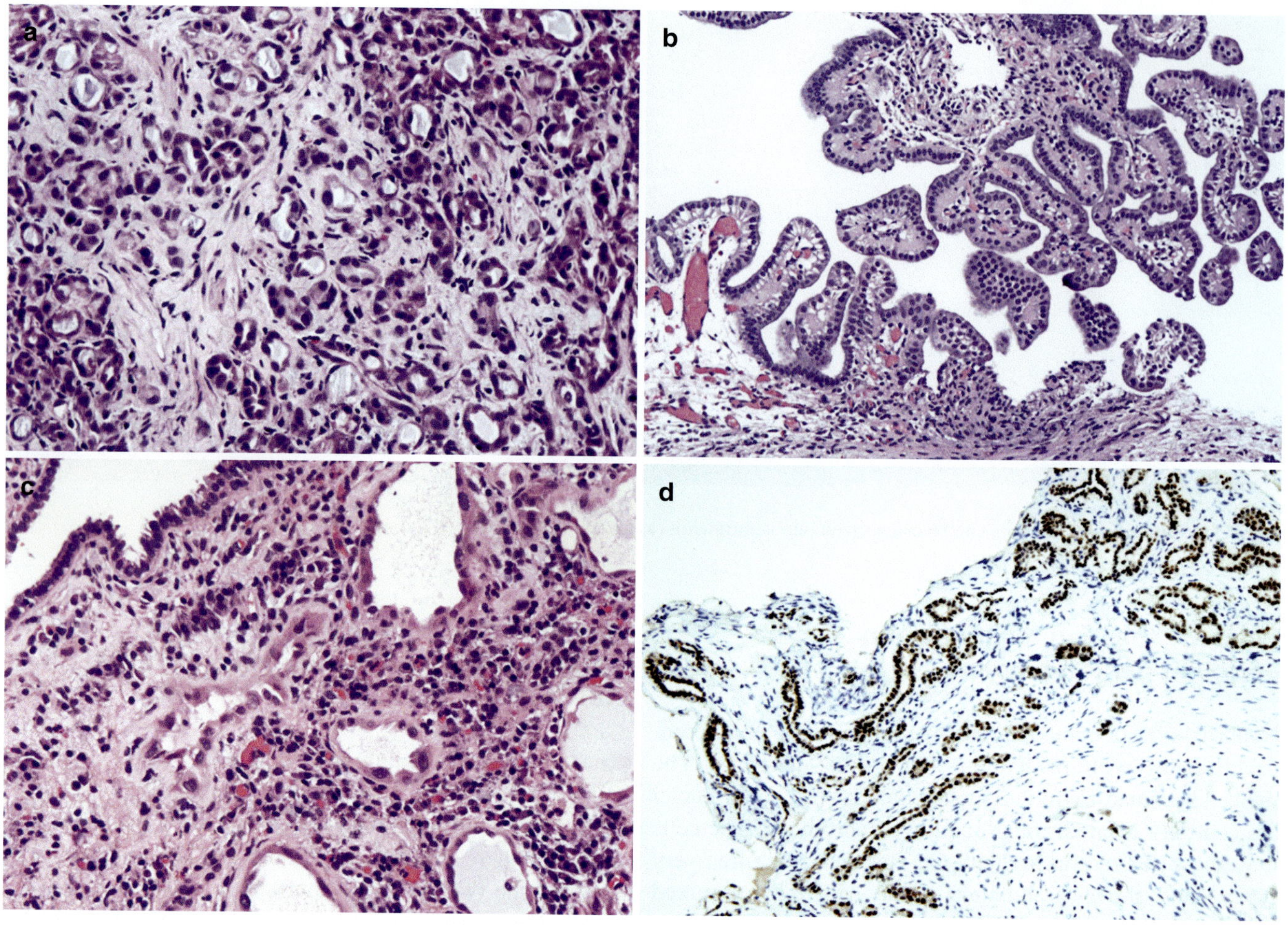

Fig. 3.12 Nephrogenic adenoma shows proliferation of small tubules with single layer of cells with hob nailing and luminal basophilic secretion (**a**), prominent papillary (**b**) or cystic component (**c**), and positivity for Pax8 (**d**)

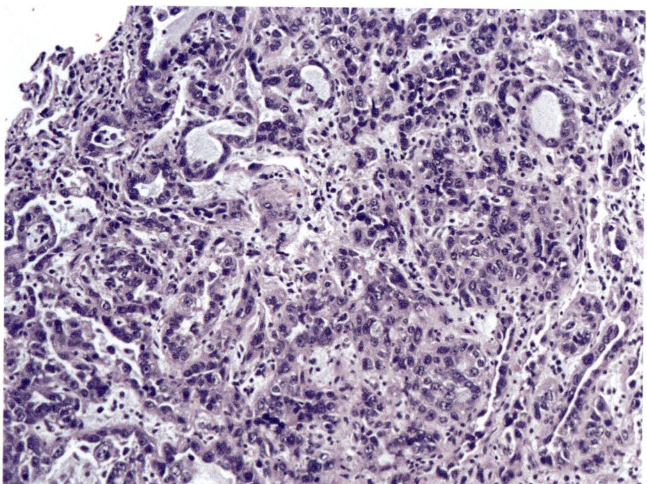

Fig. 3.13 Clear cell adenocarcinoma shows similar morphologic feature as that of nephrogenic adenoma, but more solid growth pattern and marked cytologic atypia and stromal reaction

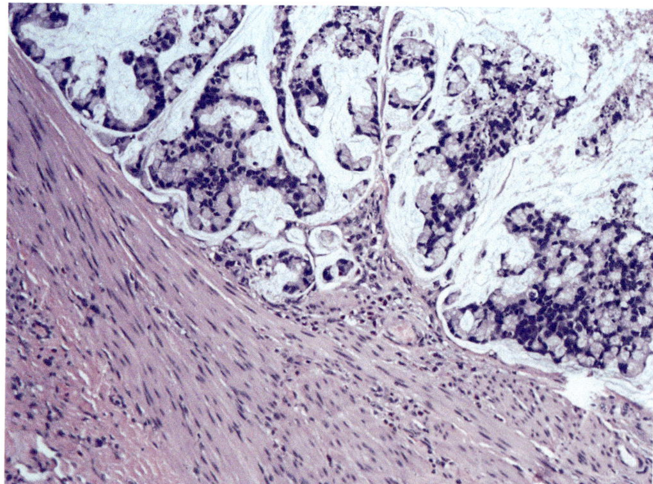

Fig. 3.14 Urachal mucinous adenocarcinoma of bladder shows bladder muscularis propria with infiltrating clusters of poorly formed and cribriform glands and abundant extracellular mucin

What Are the Diagnostic Features of von Brunn Nests, Cystitis Cystica, and Cystitis Glandularis?

von Brunn nests is described as well-circumscribed nests of urothelial cells in the lamina propria which may or may not connect to the surface epithelium. Usually, it presents as a few nests in superficial lamina propria but sometimes the nests can be found in deep lamina propria (Fig. 3.15a). They can be florid and may mimic nested variant urothelial carcinoma. Comparing with nested variant urothelial carcinoma, von Brunn nests have more regular spacing and never involves muscularis propria. Cystitis cystica is characterized by cystic change of von Brunn nests; therefore, the lining cysts are composed of normal urothelial cells. However, the cells can be flattened. Cystitis glandularis has a morphology of cystitis cystica with lining cells undergoing glandular metaplasia (Fig. 3.15b). The luminal cells become columnar with a smooth luminal cytoplasmic border. There are two types of cystitis glandularis: typical type and intestinal type. The typical type is much more common. It has cuboidal or columnar lining cells with minimal mucinous secretion in the lumen. The intestinal type consists of goblet cells and colonic type tall columnar epithelial cells with abundant mucin secretion (Fig. 3.15c). Paneth cells can rarely be present.

von Brunn nests, cystitis cystica, and glandularis are related reactive/proliferative changes and the same lesions occur in entire urinary tracts and are believed to be a local reaction to inflammation or insult [16].

Does Cystitis Glandularis Have Risk for Urothelial Adenocarcinoma?

Focal cystitis glandularis does not increase risk of adenocarcinoma but persistent diffuse cystitis glandularis of intestinal type, so-called "intestinal metaplasia" has association with increased risk of adenocarcinoma [16].

What Are the Most Common Invasive Urothelial Carcinomas with Divergent Differentiation?

Urothelial carcinoma with squamous differentiation (Fig. 3.16a, b) is the most common type, accounting about 40% of invasive urothelial carcinomas. Urothelial carcinoma with glandular differentiation is the second most common type, accounting about 18% of invasive urothelial carcinomas. Uncommonly or rarely, other divergent differentiation includes small cell, trophoblastic and Müllerian differentiation [1].

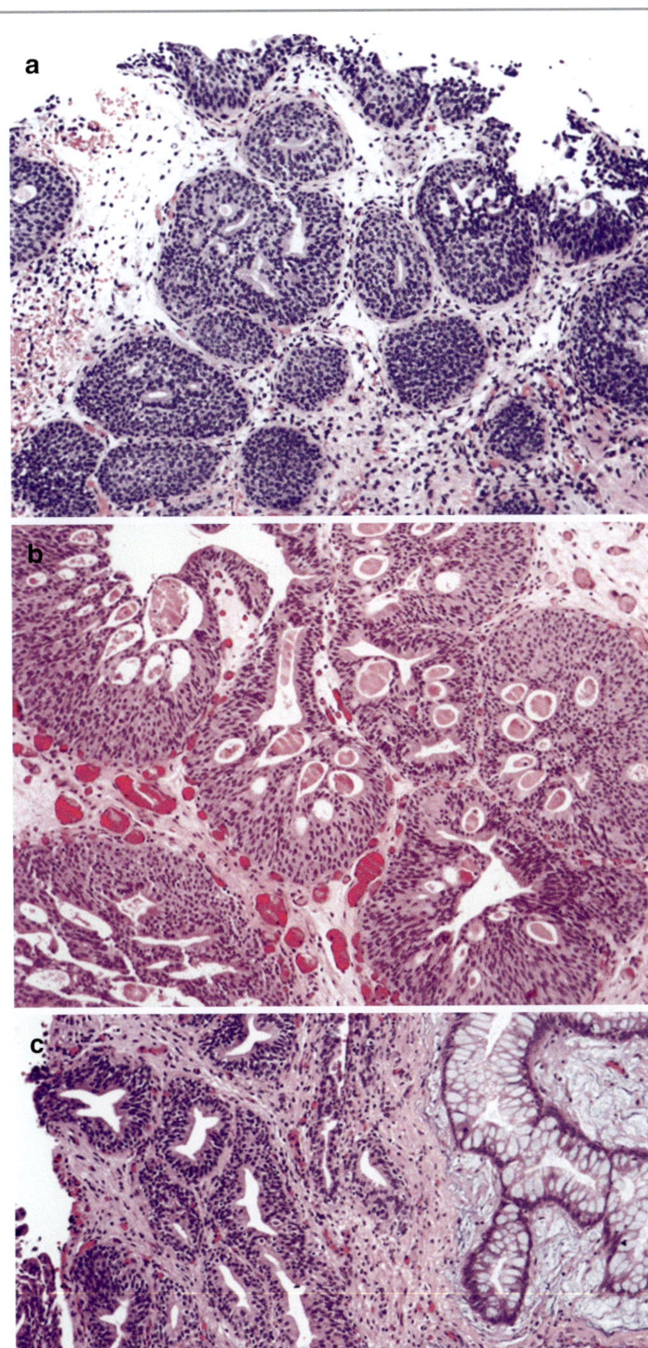

Fig. 3.15 Urothelium with prominent von Brunn nests within subepithelial tissue (**a**), florid cystitis cystica and cystitis glandularis with eosinophilic secretion (**b**), and cystitis glandularis of usual and intestinal type (**c**)

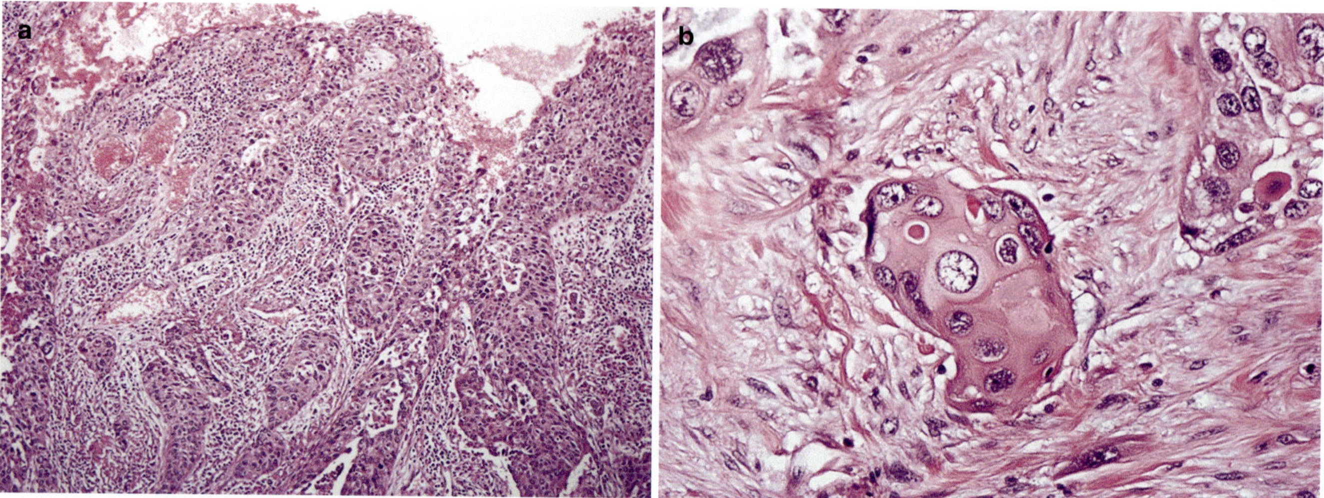

Fig. 3.16 Urothelial carcinoma with squamous differentiation showing intercellular bridges (**a**) and intracellular keratin (**b**)

What Are the Histologic Variants of Invasive Urothelial Carcinoma in 2016 World Health Organization Tumor Classification?

Invasive urothelial carcinoma has been recognized to have diverse morphologic appearances in terms of growth patterns and cytological features. Some of these variations are distinctive enough in terms of their morphologic diagnosis, prognosis, and treatment implication. The following morphologic variants are recognized by 2016 WHO classification.

- Urothelial carcinoma with divergent differentiation [squamous, glandular, trophoblastic (Fig. 3.17a, b), Mullerian differentiation (Fig. 3.17c–f)].
- Nested urothelial carcinoma.
- Microcystic urothelial carcinoma.
- Micropapillary urothelial carcinoma.
- Lymphoepithelioma-like urothelial carcinoma (Fig. 3.17g).
- Plasmacytoid urothelial carcinoma including signet ring cell and diffuse variants.
- Sarcomatoid urothelial carcinoma.
- Giant cell urothelial carcinoma (Fig. 3.17h).
- Poorly differentiated urothelial carcinoma (including those with osteoclast-like giant cells, Fig. 3.17i).
- Clear cell (glycogen-rich) urothelial carcinoma (Fig. 3.17j).
- Lipid-rich urothelial carcinoma (Fig. 3.17k, l) [1].

What Are the Diagnostic Features of Micropapillary Urothelial Carcinoma?

The diagnostic features of micropapillary urothelial carcinoma are small nests or aggregates of cells without vascular core in lacunar spaces resembling lymphovascular invasion by tumor. The most reproducible criteria for the diagnosis are confluent, back-to-back small lacunae, and multiple small nests within lacunar spaces (Fig. 3.18a). Other features include nests with reverse nuclear polarity or peripheral orientation of the nuclei and presence of cytoplasmic vacuoles. This unique variant is frequently mixed together with conventional high grade or urothelial carcinoma with other variant morphologies. Rarely noninvasive papillary urothelial carcinoma may have surface micropapillary component with delicate filiform configuration and lack of fibrovascular core (Fig. 3.18b). It is advisable that the term micropapillary is not used for noninvasive urothelial carcinoma to avoid confusion [1].

What Are the Diagnostic Features of Plasmacytoid Urothelial Carcinoma?

The diagnostic features of plasmacytoid urothelial carcinoma are invasive carcinoma with isolated, discohesive tumor cells with eccentrically placed nuclei and abundant cytoplasm, resembling plasma cells (Fig. 3.19a). The cytoplasm can be eosinophilic, clear, and vacuolated. The stroma is often

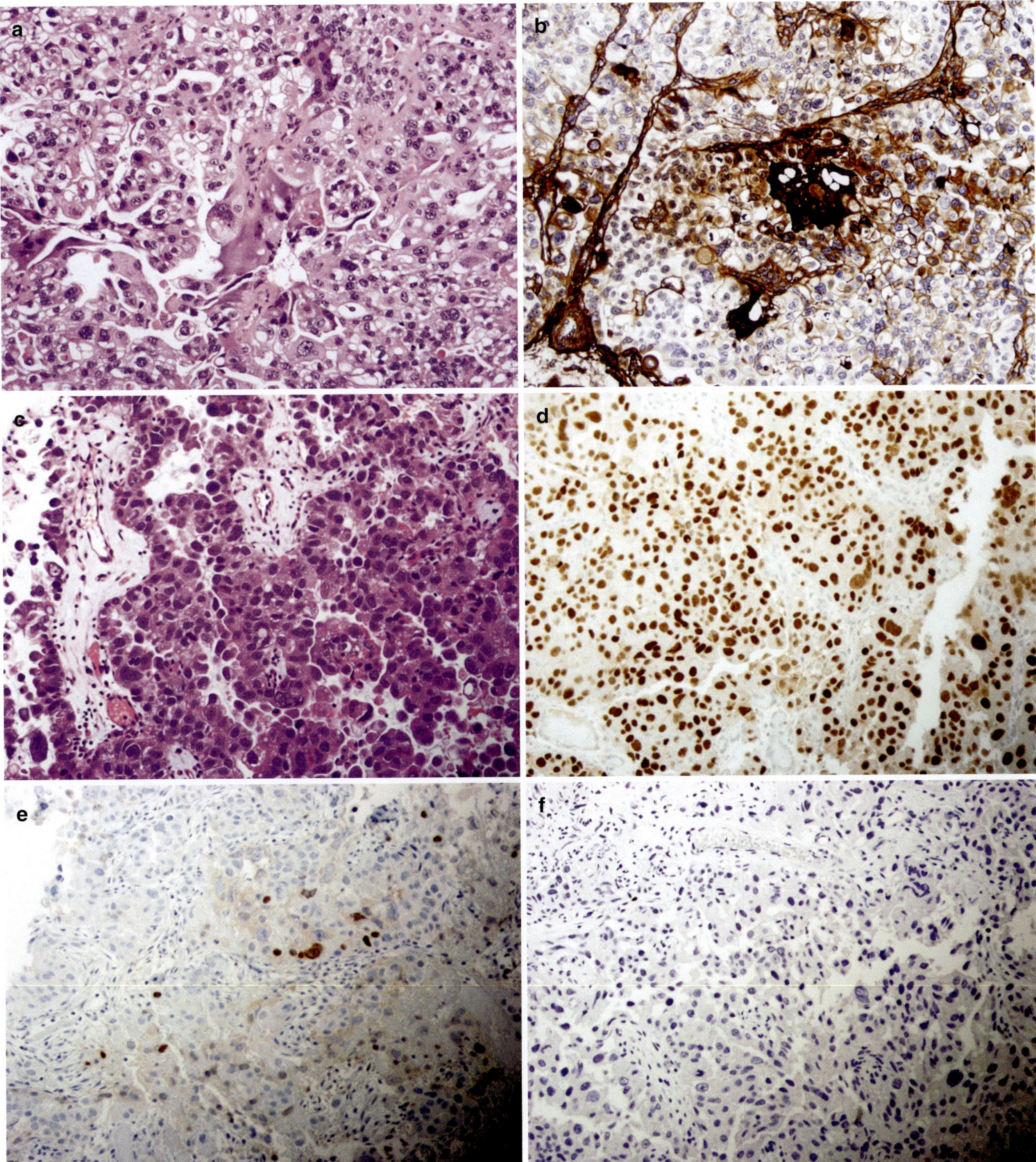

Fig. 3.17 Urothelial carcinoma with trophoblastic differentiation (**a**) is positive for β-HCG (**b**). Urothelial carcinoma with Mullerian differentiation (**c**) is positive for PAX8 (**d**) and p63 (**e**), and negative for GATA3 (**f**). Lymphoepithelioma-like urothelial carcinoma is composed of nests or sheets of pleomorphic cells with large nuclei and prominent nucleoli in a background of abundant mixed lymphoid infiltrate (**g**). Giant cells can be seen in giant cell urothelial carcinoma (**h**) and poorly differenti-ated urothelial carcinoma with osteoclast-like giant cells (**i**). Clear cell (glycogen-rich) urothelial carcinoma is composed of abundant tumor cells with clear cytoplasm secondary to glycogen accumulation (**j**) which are negative for Pax8, excluding the possibility of clear cell renal cell carcinoma. Lipid-rich urothelial carcinoma is characterized by clear cytoplasmic vacuoles (**k**) and lipoblast-like cells (**l**)

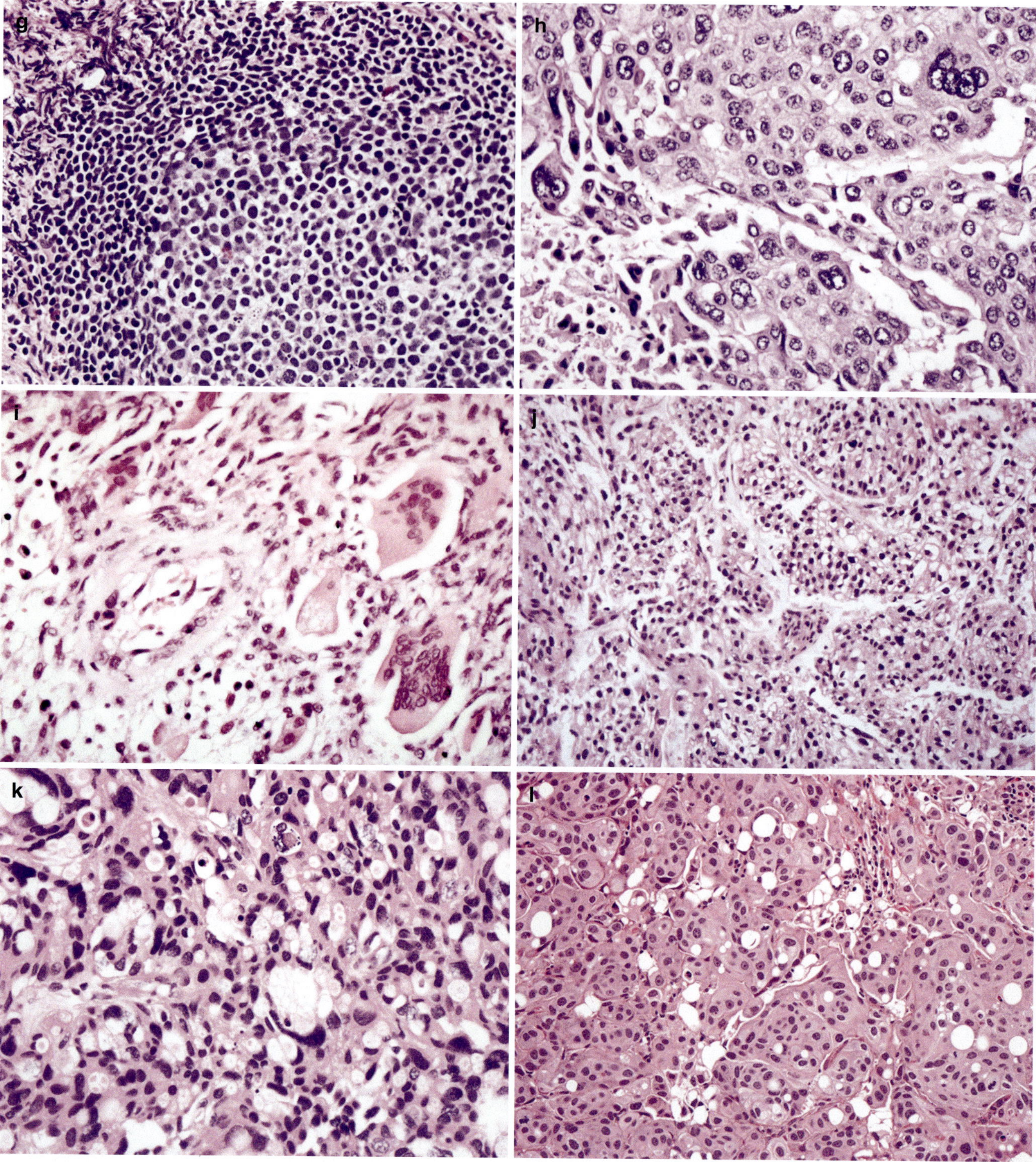

Fig. 3.17 (continued)

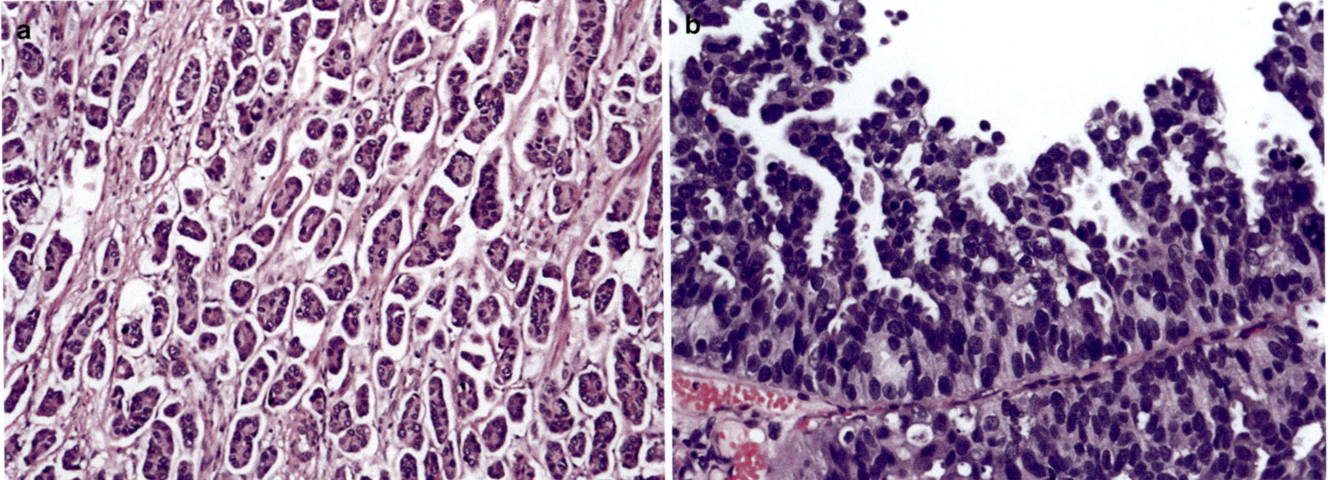

Fig. 3.18 Invasive micropapillary urothelial carcinoma shows exuberant small nests and clusters of tumor cells in lacunar spaces resembling lymphovascular invasion (**a**). Noninvasive papillary urothelial carcinoma exhibits surface micropapillary component composed of delicate filiform papillae with crowded nuclei without fibrovascular cores (**b**)

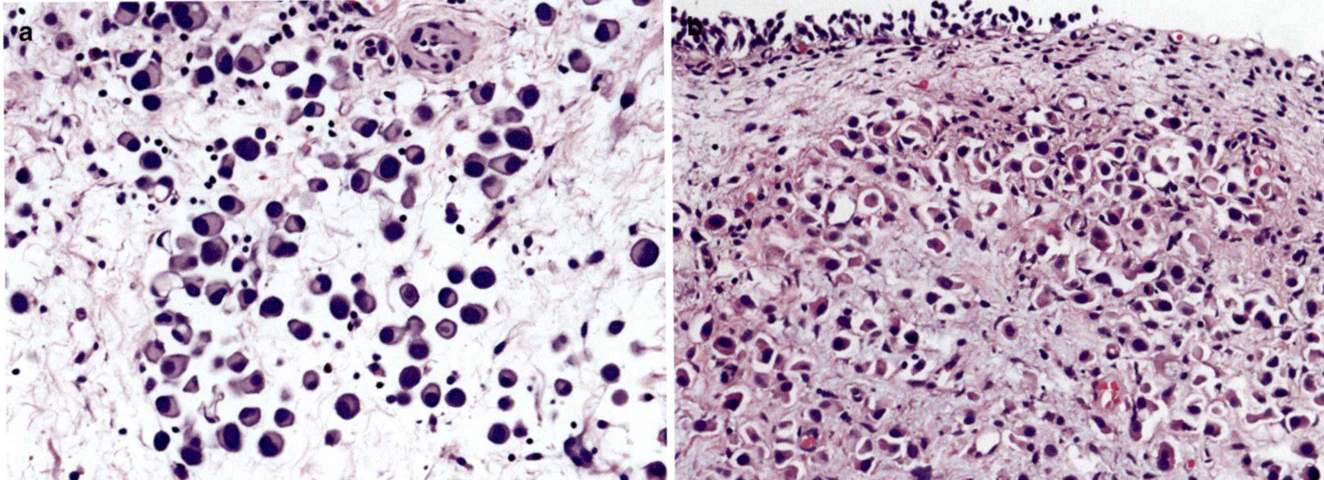

Fig. 3.19 Invasive plasmacytoid urothelial carcinoma shows infiltrating discohesive small cluster and single tumor cells with abundant dense cytoplasm resembling plasma cells (**a**) and rare signet ring cells (**b**)

loosely myxoid. The nuclei range from monotonous to highly pleomorphic. Sometimes, the tumor cells have intracytoplasmic vacuoles with or without intracytoplasmic mucin, giving the appearance of signet-ring cells (Fig. 3.19b). But unlike signet-ring adenocarcinoma, there is no extracellular mucin. Approximately half of the cases are associated with conventional high-grade urothelial carcinoma [1].

What Are the Diagnostic Criteria of Primary Adenocarcinoma of Bladder?

Primary urothelial adenocarcinoma is a malignant neoplasm derived from the urothelium with pure glandular phenotype. To make a diagnosis of primary adenocarcinoma, there should not be a component of urothelial carcinoma or squamous cell carcinoma. Using these strict criteria, primary adenocarcinoma is very rare and accounts for less than 2% of bladder carcinomas. The morphologic can be enteric (intestinal, Fig. 3.20a), mucinous (colloid), or mixed type. The presence of associated intestinal metaplasia or dysplasia or glandular-type carcinoma in situ might increase the possibility of this diagnosis. It is very important to exclude the possibility of direct invasion of prostate adenocarcinoma from prostate, direct extension or metastasis from colorectal adenocarcinoma (Fig. 3.20b–d), or metastatic adenocarcinomas of other primaries, urachal adenocarcinoma, and extensive cystitis glandularis [19].

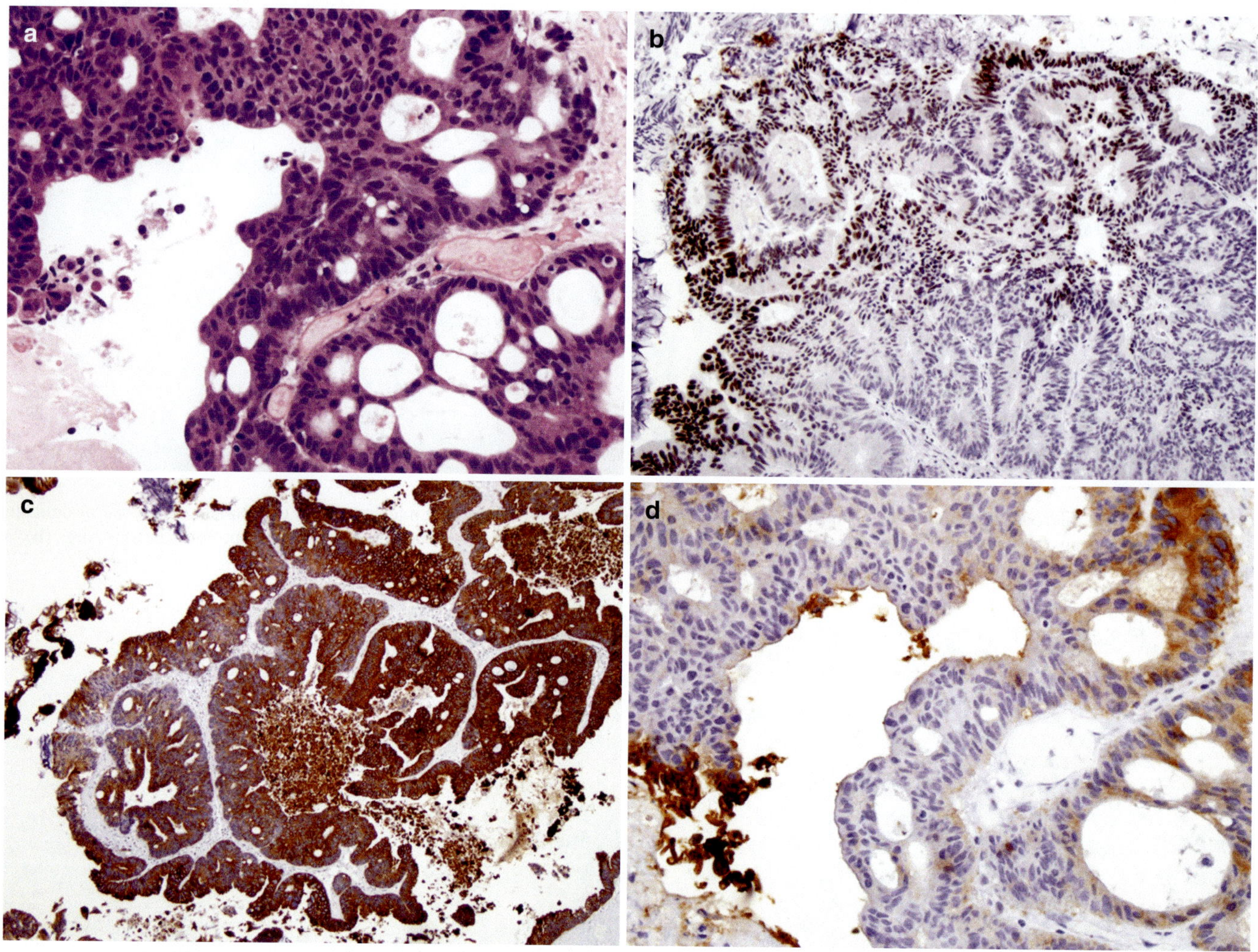

Fig. 3.20 Primary adenocarcinoma of bladder with enteric differentiation (**a**) is positive for CDX2 (**b**) and CK20 (**c**), but negative for β-catenin (**d**)

What Are the Useful Immunohistochemical Markers to Distinguish Bladder Primary Adenocarcinoma from Metastatic Adenocarcinoma?

For enteric-type primary bladder adenocarcinoma, it has overlapping features with colorectal adenocarcinoma. It can also show similar staining patterns with CK7, CK20, and CDX2. Beta-catenin might be helpful as it does not stain with primary bladder adenocarcinoma but frequently shows positive nuclear staining in colorectal adenocarcinoma. NKX3.1 and PSA are helpful when needed to exclude prostatic adenocarcinoma [19].

What Are the Differential Diagnoses of High-Grade Sarcomatoid Neoplasm of the Urinary Bladder?

Major differential diagnoses of spindle cell lesion of urinary bladder encompass malignant epithelial and mesenchymal neoplasms as well as benign tumors. The differential diagnoses of high-grade sarcomatoid neoplasm include mainly sarcomatoid urothelial carcinoma (Fig. 3.21a) and sarcomas including leiomyosarcoma, and rhabdomyosarcoma. The features that favor sarcomatoid carcinoma include history or presence of urothelial CIS or concurrent conventional urothelial carcinoma. Sarcomatoid carcinoma is usually positive for p63, CK5/6, and high-molecular weight cytokeratin and may contain heterologous mesenchymal elements, such as chondrosarcoma or osteosarcoma (Fig. 3.21b). Primary bladder leiomyosarcoma and angiomyosarcoma have the same features as the soft tissue counterparts. Immunohistochemical stains with tissue-specific markers will be helpful for the final diagnosis.

Primary bladder rhabdomyosarcomas occur predominantly in children with an average age of 4 years. Most of them are embryonal and exophytic with or without "botryoid" components. Other histologic subtypes such as small cell, alveolar, and unclassified have also been reported. The diagnosis can be confirmed by immunohistochemical stain

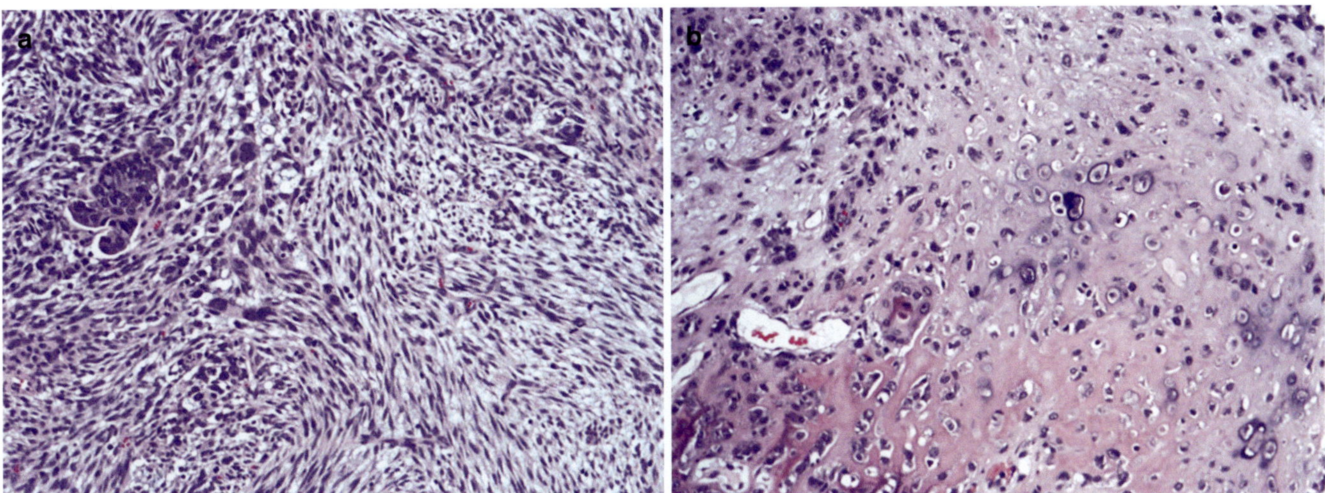

Fig. 3.21 Sarcomatoid urothelial carcinoma shows diffuse spindle cell proliferation with moderately pleomorphic tumor cells and small foci of carcinoma (**a**). Other example of sarcomatoid carcinoma with chondrosarcomatous and osteosarcomatous differentiation is shown (**b**)

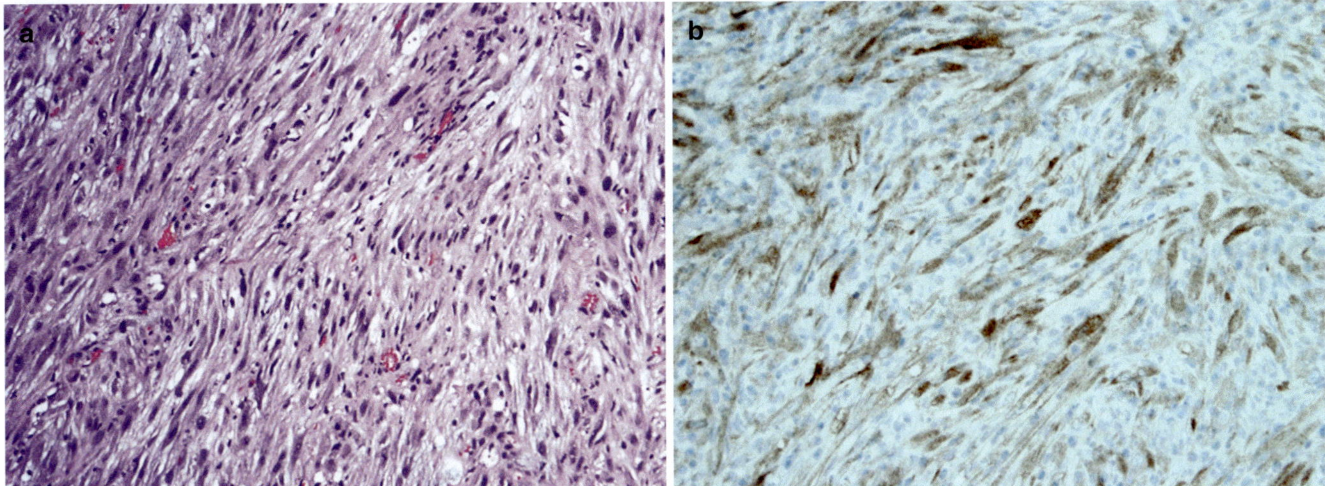

Fig. 3.22 Inflammatory myofibroblastic tumor shows cellular spindle cell proliferation with fascicular growth pattern and inflammatory infiltrate and myxoid stroma (**a**) and is positive for ALK-1 (**b**)

with markers of skeletal muscle differentiation (desmin, myogenin, and MyoD1).

What Are the Differential Diagnoses of Low-Grade Spindle Cell Lesion of Urinary Bladder?

There are a few benign spindle cell tumors that can occur in the urinary bladder. Two morphologically similar tumors are postoperative spindle cell nodule and inflammatory myofibroblastic tumor (IMT). Both tumors show cellular spindle cell proliferation with fascicular growth of plump or elongated cells (Fig. 3.22a). The stroma is edematous or myxoid with delicate vessels. There is viable mitotic activity. No significant pleomorphism or atypical mitotic figure is present. The tumor cells frequently have prominent nucleoli. Patients with postoperative spindle cell nodule has a history of prior bladder surgery or procedure and there may be more prominent extravasation of red blood cells within the stroma. In contract, inflammatory myofibroblastic tumor usually has more prominent inflammatory infiltrate and half of the cases are positive for ALK-1 (Fig. 3.22b).

Other benign mesenchymal tumors (i.e., solitary fibrous tumor (SFT), leiomyoma, and neurofibroma) also occur in urinary bladder and each shows similar features as its counterparts in soft tissue or other visceral organs [20–23].

What Are the Useful Panels of Markers for Diagnosis of Spindle Cell Tumor of Urinary Bladder?

Based on the differential diagnoses of spindle cell lesion of urinary bladder listed in the previous question, a useful panel should include at least following markers: Pan-cytokeratin, CD34, S100, desmin, caldesmon, MyoD1, myogenin, and ALK-1. Additional staining can be ordered based on the results of this basic panel.

What Are the Diagnostic Features of Bladder Paraganglioma? How to Distinguish It from Invasive Urothelial Carcinoma?

For paraganglioma, the tumor nests are typically present as distinctive nests which resemble nested variant urothelial carcinoma. However, paraganglioma cell nests are separated by delicate fibrovascular septa (so-called Zellballen pattern) (Fig. 3.23) while urothelial carcinomatous nests are surrounded by desmoplastic stroma. Unlike urothelial carcinoma, mitosis, hemorrhage, and necrosis are rare in paraganglioma. There is usually no history of bladder cancer and it is not associated with in situ or invasive urothelial carcinoma. In difficult cases, immunostains should be performed to confirm the diagnosis. Paragangliomas are negative for epithelial markers and positive for neuroendocrine markers. Sustentacular cells are highlighted by S100 [24].

What Are the Features that Are Helpful to Diagnose Subepithelial Invasion of Urothelial Carcinoma?

The most helpful feature is small clusters or isolated tumor cells extending beyond the outline of basement membrane with irregular edge and peritumoral retraction spaces (Fig. 3.24a). Look for cytologic differences between the suspicious area and noninvasive carcinoma area, such as greater nuclear atypia or pleomorphism and cytoplasmic eosinophilia or vacuolar changes will support the diagnosis of inva-

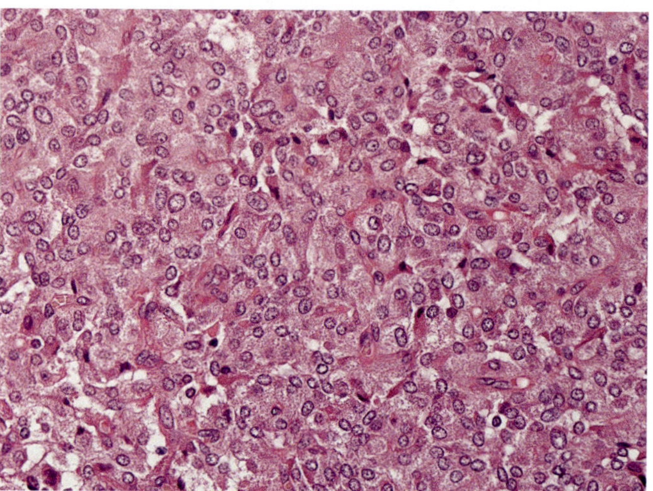

Fig. 3.23 Paraganglioma is composed of nests of polygonal neoplastic cells with abundant eosinophilic granular to clear cytoplasm, central nuclei, and vesicular chromatin

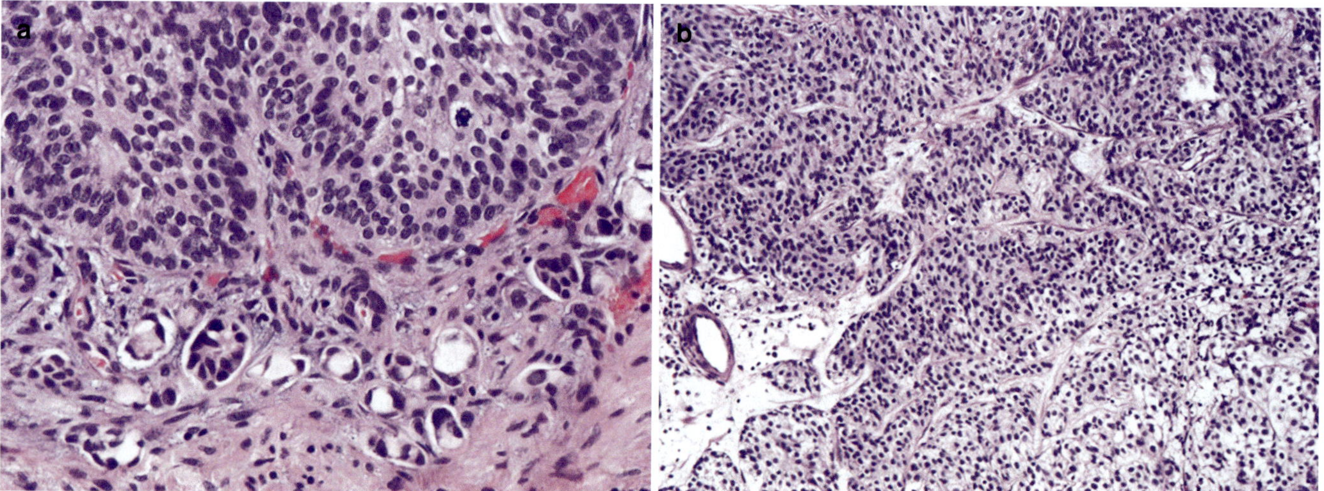

Fig. 3.24 Urothelial carcinoma shows sheets of noninvasive component and subepithelial small clusters tumor cells with pleomorphic nuclei, intracytoplasmic eosinophilia and vacuolization (**a**). Another invasive urothelial carcinoma with confluent growth pattern is shown (**b**)

sion. In addition, confluent tumor growth (Fig. 3.24b) associated with dense stromal desmoplastic reaction is consistent with invasion. Inflammatory infiltrate by itself is not very helpful for diagnosis of invasion.

How to Make a Diagnosis of Muscularis Propria Invasion and What Are the Common Pitfalls?

Muscularis mucosae fibers are usually wispy and discontinuous, whereas muscularis propria usually forms thick muscle bundles (>100 μm in thickness). Tumor cells invading into, surrounded by, and/or immediately adjacent to muscularis propria should be regarded as muscularis propria invasion (Fig. 3.25a). Sometimes, it is difficult to identify muscularis propria invasion when infiltrating tumor cells push apart bundles of muscularis propria widely from each other or destruct muscularis propria extensively which results in a fragmented appearance that may mimic that of muscularis mucosae invasion (Fig. 3.25b). Furthermore, sometimes muscularis mucosae can become hyperplastic so it may be very difficult to distinguish muscularis propria from muscularis mucosa. When associated with undetermined muscle fibers, the following features favor muscularis mucosa: location of muscle fibers near urothelial surface; disorganized, myxoid, and reactive stroma; presence of clusters of large caliber vessels (so called vascular plexuses) and inflammation [25, 26].

What Are the Differential Diagnoses of Urothelial Neoplasm with Endophytic Growth Pattern and What Are Features That Can Be Helpful in Resolving the Diagnosis?

Differential diagnoses of urothelial neoplasm with endophytic growth pattern range from benign inverted papilloma to invasive high-grade urothelial carcinoma. The prototype inverted urothelial neoplasm is benign inverted papilloma. Cystoscopically, it has a raised, pedunculated or rarely polypoid lesion with a smooth surface. Microscopically, it has a normal smooth surface urothelium and is composed of endophytically growing trabeculae or cords of urothelial cell with a smooth pushing border and a peripheral palisading. The tumor cells are bland with no or rare mitoses and there is no stromal reaction (Fig. 3.26a). Rarely, nests of inverted papilloma may show glandular differentiation or nonkeratinizing squamous metaplasia. It is important to differentiate benign inverted papilloma from malignant urothelial neoplasm with inverted growth. Papillary urothelial neoplasm of low-malignant potential (PUNLMP), low-grade and high-grade urothelial carcinoma can have focal or extensive component of inverted growth. The histologic features that can be used to distinguish urothelial neoplasms with inverted growth from benign inverted papilloma are: (1) presence of exophytic component (Fig. 3.26b), (2) thicker endophytically growing cords and more complex architecture, and (3) higher degree of cytologic atypia corresponding to PUNLMP, low- and high-grade urothelial carcinoma.

Occasionally, florid von Brunn nests, cystitis cystica/glandularis may mimic inverted papilloma. However, unlike inverted papilloma, it has more of a lobular architecture with round contour and lacks anastomosing cords or trabeculae [27].

Are There Any Immunohistochemical Markers that Can Help Diagnose Muscularis Propria Invasion?

In cystectomy specimen, distinction between muscularis mucosa and muscularis propria is usually not a problem. The muscularis mucosa is composed of delicate muscle bands often associated with large vessels, whereas muscularis propria consists of compact, thick muscle bundles (Fig. 3.27a).

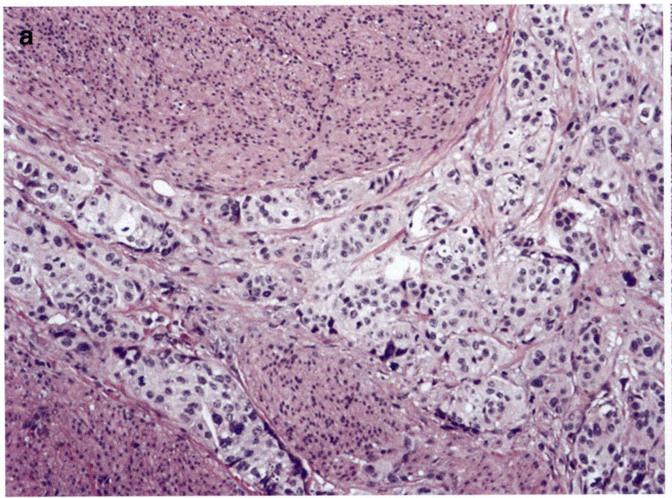
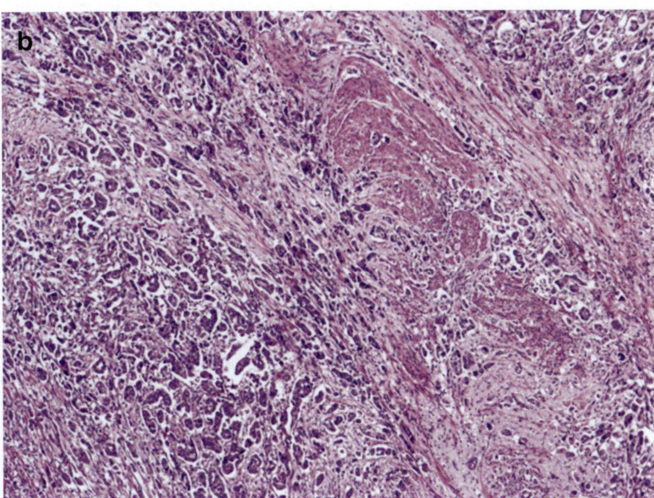

Fig. 3.25 Invasive urothelial carcinoma shows involvement of muscularis propria with nests of tumor cells surrounding large bundles of muscle (**a**). Another example shows invasive urothelial carcinoma destroying bundle of muscle into small fascicles obscuring the outline of muscularis propria bundles (**b**)

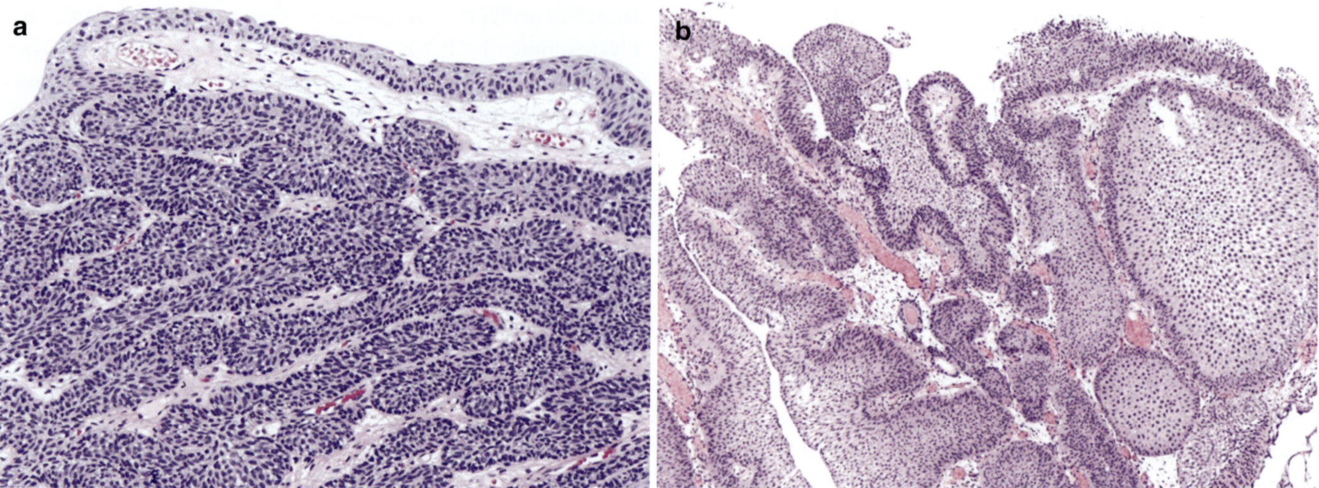

Fig. 3.26 Urothelial inverted papilloma shows a smooth surface with nests, cords and trabeculae of urothelial cells and focal peripheral palisading (**a**). Low-grade urothelial carcinoma with inverted growth pattern and exophytic component (**b**)

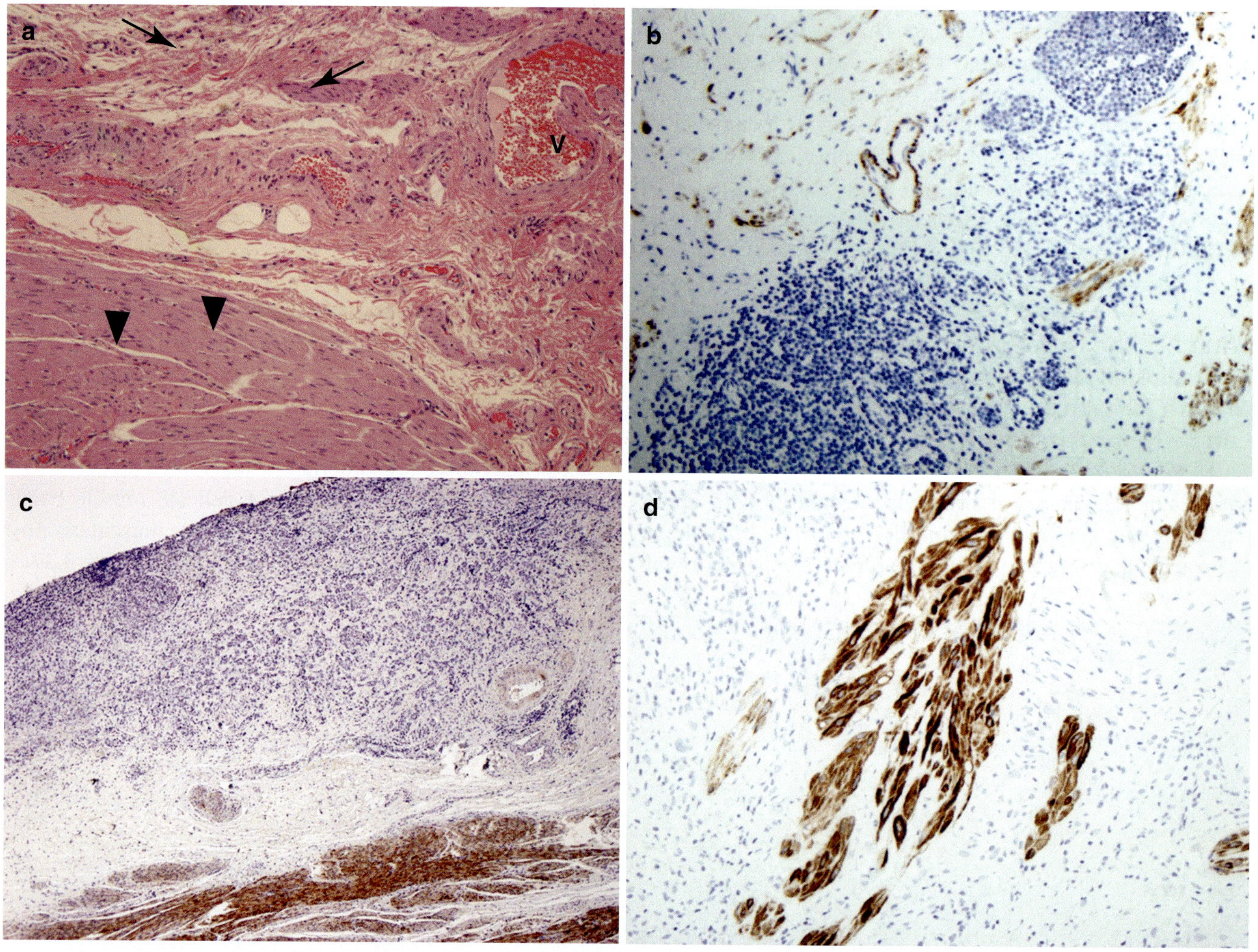

Fig. 3.27 Muscularis mucosae (arrow) consists of delicate muscle bands in close proximity to a large vessel (V), whereas muscularis propria (arrowheads) consists of thick muscle bundles deeper than muscularis mucosae (**a**). Muscularis mucosae is weakly positive for smoothelin (**b**, **c**), whereas muscularis propria is strongly and diffusely positive for smoothelin (**c**, **d**)

However, this distinction can be problematic in transurethral resection specimen. Both smoothelin and vimentin have been studied to aid the diagnosis of muscularis propria invasion, based on the difference in staining pattern of these two markers between muscularis propria and muscularis mucosae. Muscularis mucosae is either negative or stains weakly (occasionally moderately) and focally for smoothelin (Fig. 3.27b, c), and is rarely positive for vimentin. Muscularis propria, however, usually stains strongly and diffusely with smoothelin (Fig. 3.27c, d) and is positive for vimentin. However, one should bear in mind that staining pattern and intensity of smoothelin and vimentin may overlap between muscularis propria and muscularis mucosae [28].

What Are the Most Common Tumors that Secondarily involving the Bladder by Direct Extension or Distant Metastasis?

The most common primary tumor sites for secondary bladder involvement (mostly via direct extension, occasionally via metastasis) are colon (Fig. 3.28) and rectum (40% combined), prostate in men (19%), and cervix in women (11%). The most common primary sites for metastasis to the bladder are stomach, skin, lung, and breast with percentage rates of 4.3%, 3.9%, 2.8%, and 2.5%, respectively [29].

For a Poorly Differentiated Carcinoma, What Are the Best Markers to Establish that Urothelial (Bladder) as a Primary?

There is no great marker that is specific for urothelial carcinoma. However, for poorly differentiated carcinoma, starting with CK7 and CK20 immunostains can be a good option as

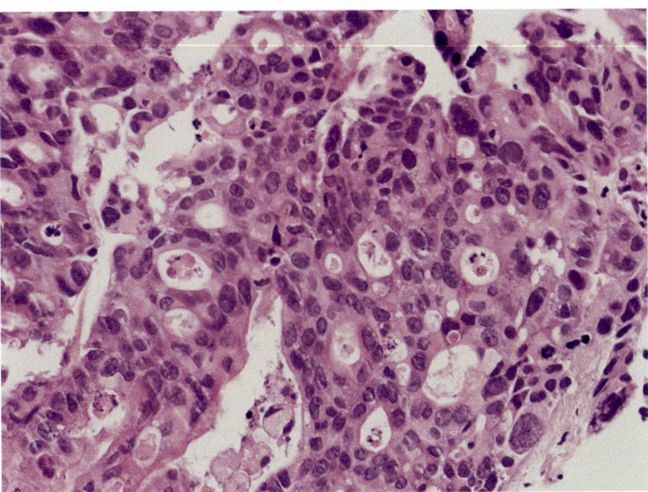

Fig. 3.28 Metastatic colonic adenocarcinoma involves the bladder

65–89% of urothelial carcinoma shows double positive stains for CK7 and CK20, and about 35% of urothelial carcinomas are positive only for CK7, but not for CK20. The other useful markers for urothelial differentiation are GATA-3, 34βE12, p63, CD141, uroplakin II, and uroplakin III.

What Are the Most Useful Morphologic Features to Distinguish Urothelial Carcinoma from High-Grade Prostate Carcinoma?

In general, morphologic features that favor urothelial carcinoma include marked nuclear atypia and pleomorphism, frequent mitoses and tumor cell necrosis, squamous differentiation, and presence of conventional urothelial carcinoma or urothelial carcinoma in situ. In contrast, high-grade prostate carcinoma shows relatively uniform monotonous ovoid to round tumor cells, prominent nucleoli, grows in solid nests (Fig. 3.29a), and shows focal cribriform or glandular differentiation (Fig. 3.29b). In small or poorly preserved specimen, immunohistochemistry with a small panel of markers (GATA3, p63, PSA, PSAP or NKX3.1) will be helpful to confirm the diagnosis.

How to Distinguish Urothelial Carcinoma with Squamous Differentiation from Cervical Squamous Cell Carcinoma?

Squamous differentiation is a very common finding in urothelial carcinoma. In female patients, cervical squamous cell carcinoma may enter the differential diagnosis for urothelial carcinoma with squamous differentiation. In addition to the history of cervical primary or positive cytology, testing of high-risk HPV or p16 immunohistochemistry will indicate cervical squamous cell carcinoma. On the other hand, presence of urothelial carcinoma in situ and conventional papillary urothelial carcinoma strongly support a diagnosis of a urothelial carcinoma with squamous differentiation. Clinical and radiological correlations are necessary for a definitive diagnosis.

What Are the Most Common Patterns of Prostatic Urothelial Carcinoma in Patients with Bladder Cancer?

The most common pattern of prostatic urothelial carcinoma in patients with concomitant bladder cancer is urothelial carcinoma in situ involving prostatic urethra and prostatic ducts (Fig. 3.30a). Other patterns include subepithelial invasion of prostatic urethra (Fig. 3.30b), prostatic stromal invasion (Fig. 3.30c) resulting from either pros-

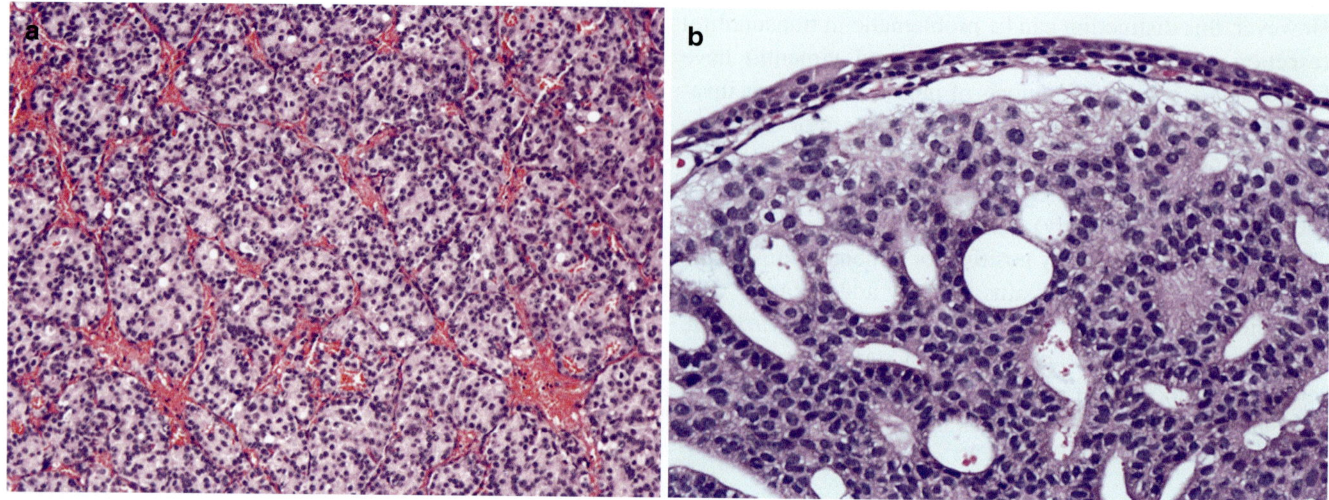

Fig. 3.29 Prostate adenocarcinoma with crowded back to back glandular proliferation of monotonous tumor cells (**a**). Cribriform prostate adenocarcinoma involves in the subepithelial tissue of bladder wall and overlying benign urothelium (**b**)

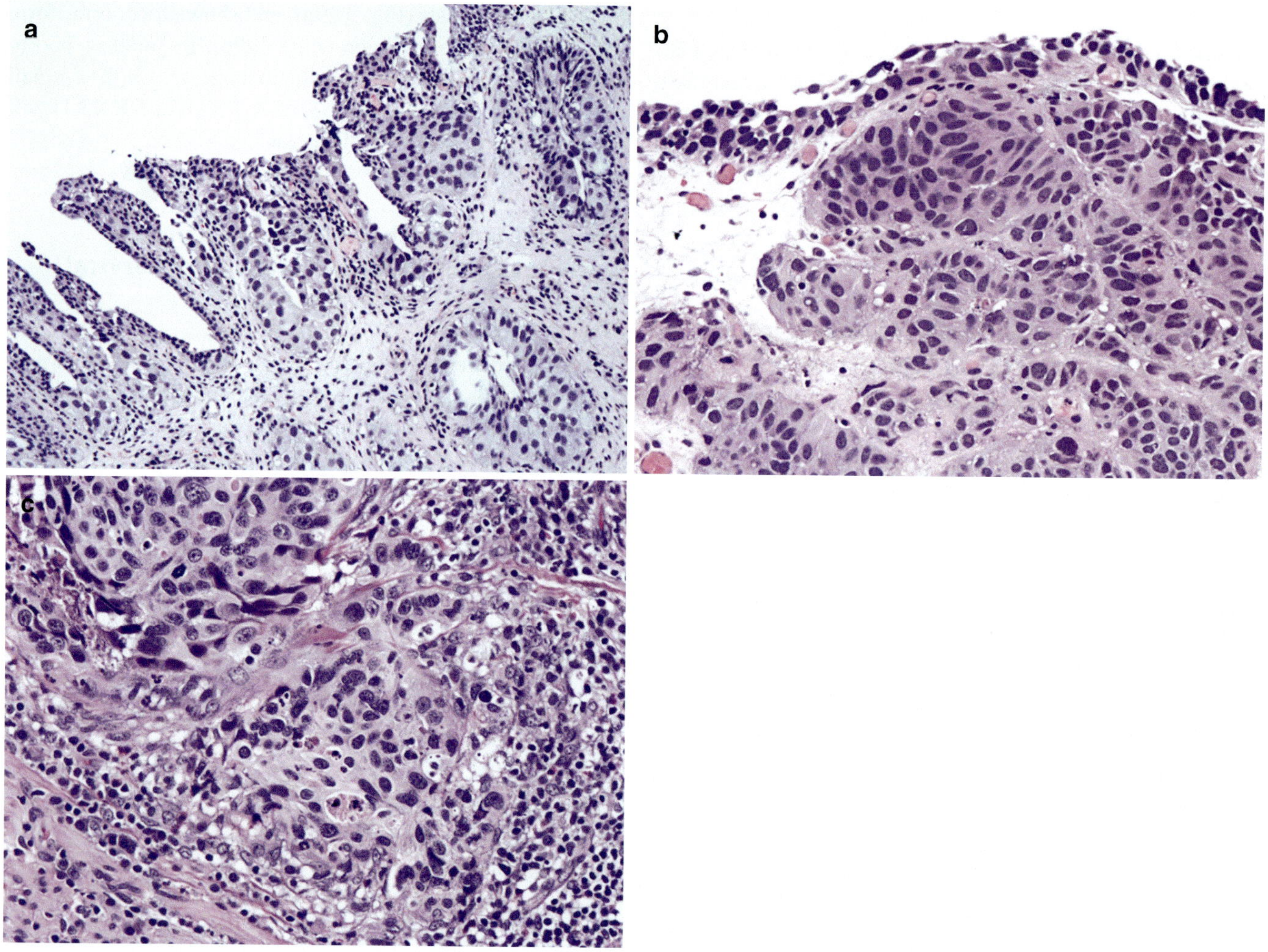

Fig. 3.30 This image shows prostatic urethra with urothelial carcinoma in situ involving prostatic urethra and duct (**a**). Prostatic urethra shows surface urothelial carcinoma in situ and invasive urothelial carcinoma within submucosal tissue (**b**). Urothelial carcinoma next to benign prostatic glands indicates prostatic stromal invasion (**c**)

tatic urethra or duct/acini, or direct transmural invasion of prostate by bladder cancer through bladder neck or extra-prostatic tissue [30].

What Are the Diagnostic Features of Carcinoma of Müllerian Type?

Bladder carcinomas of Müllerian type are newly recognized variants of bladder adenocarcinoma. The two common histo-logic subtypes are clear cell carcinoma and endometrioid carcinoma. While endometrioid carcinoma occurs only in female, clear cell carcinoma is more commonly seen in females, but also in males. It appears that endometrial carci-noma and a small subset of clear cell carcinoma are associ-ated with Müllerian precursors in the bladder such as endometriosis (common) and Müllerianosis (rare). Clear cell carcinoma often represents a specific form of glandular dif-ferentiation in urothelial carcinoma.

Morphologically, both clear cell carcinoma and endome-trioid carcinoma are similar to their counterparts in endome-trium or ovary. Clear cell carcinoma usually has a diverse growth pattern with tubulocystic, papillary, and diffuse solid growth patterns (Fig. 3.31a). The tumor cells are flat, cuboi-dal, or columnar with clear cytoplasm, hobnail appearance, marked cytologic atypia, and frequent mitotic features (Fig. 3.31b). The tumor usually involves bladder lamina propria and most tumors harbor genetic alterations similar to those reported in urothelial carcinoma, although clear cell carcinomas are associated with endometriosis. Immunohistochemically, clear cell carcinoma is positive for CK7, EMA, Pax8, HNF1β, AMACR, and CA-125. In con-trast, endometrioid carcinoma (Fig. 3.17c–f) usually has an epicenter toward the bladder serosa and is frequently associ-ated with adjacent endometriosis. The tumor has a variable histologic appearance ranging from well-formed endometri-oid glands that may show squamous or mucinous differen-tiation to poorly different solid carcinoma and is usually positive for estrogen and progesterone receptors [31].

What Are the most Common Nonurothelial Carcinomas in Urinary Bladder?

Squamous cell carcinoma is the most common nonurothe-lial carcinoma in urinary bladder, accounting for 1.3% of bladder tumor in males and 3.4% of bladder tumor in females. However, in some African countries and Middle East, squamous cell carcinoma is much more common, and the prevalence can be higher than that of urothelial carci-noma, primarily due to *Schistosoma haematobium* infec-tion. Primary adenocarcinoma in bladder is the second most common nonurothelial carcinoma, accounting for 0.5–2% of bladder carcinomas [32].

What Are the Diagnostic Features of Bladder Squamous Cell Carcinoma?

The diagnosis of bladder squamous cell carcinoma is reserved for tumors with purely squamous component and is characterized by the presence of tumor cells with keratin pearls and intercellular bridges (Fig. 3.32a, b). If urothelial CIS or conventional urothelial carcinoma is present, the tumor should be classified as urothelial carcinoma with squamous differentiation. Most bladder squamous cell carci-nomas are moderately and poorly differentiated. Keratinizing squamous metaplasia and dysplasia are present in about half

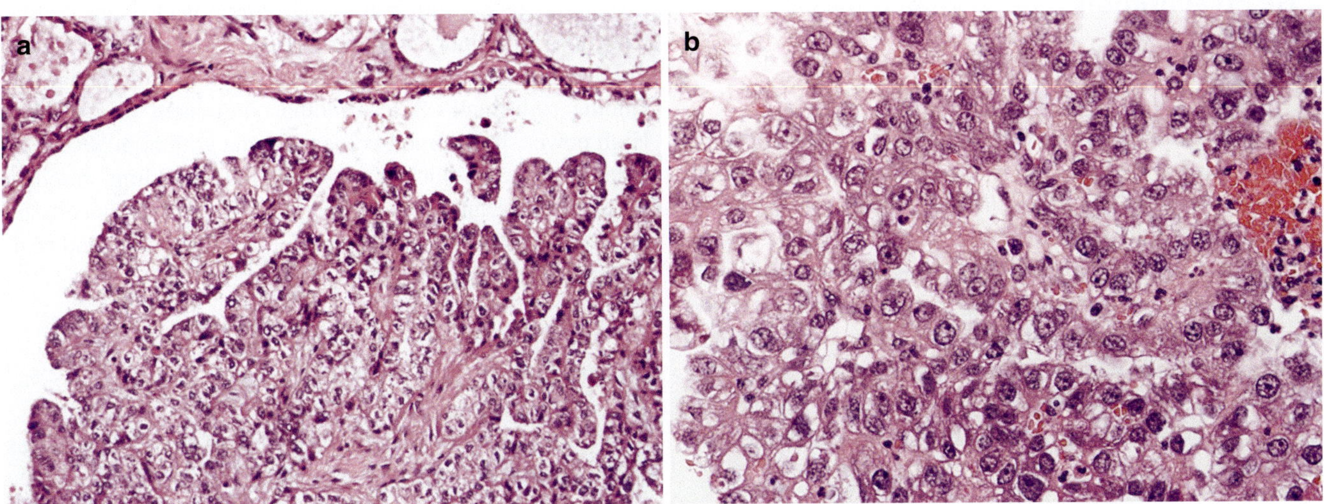

Fig. 3.31 A case of clear cell carcinoma shows papillary architecture (**a**), cells with clear cytoplasm and cytologic atypia (**b**)

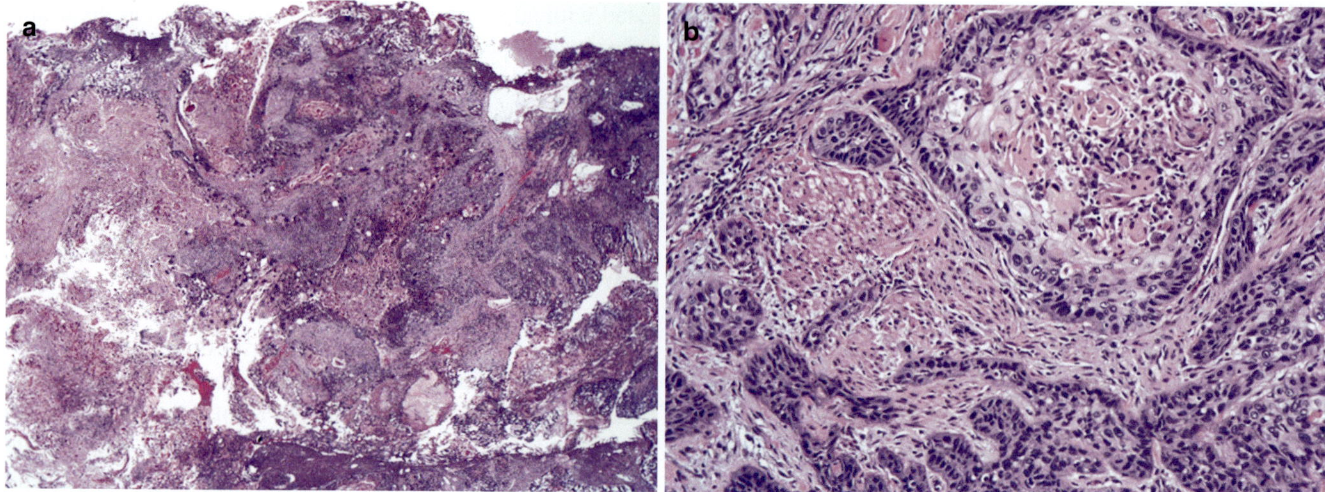

Fig. 3.32 This low power image shows well and moderately differentiated squamous cell carcinoma with prominent keratinization (**a**). An example of invasive moderately differentiated squamous cell carcinoma involving muscularis propria is shown (**b**)

of the cases. Infection of *S. haematobium* is a significant risk factor in some African countries [32].

What Are the Features of Tumors in Bladder Diverticulum?

About one-third of the tumors arising in bladder diverticulum are noninvasive papillary urothelial carcinoma (low or high grade). About half of the invasive carcinomas are conventional invasive urothelial carcinomas. The other histologic subtypes arising in diverticulum include small-cell carcinoma, squamous cell carcinoma, and adenocarcinoma [33].

Case Presentation

Case 1

A 65-year-old man with complicated medical history was found to have a bladder tumor and underwent transurethral resection. Microscopically, at low magnification, the tumor has complex papillary architecture (Fig. 3.33a). The surface noninvasive component shows micropapillary configuration (Fig. 3.33b). Within subepithelial tissue, the tumor shows irregular nests of tumor cells with prominent nuclear atypia and characteristic peritumoral retraction artifact (Fig. 3.33c). In addition, the tumor cells show paradoxical maturation with more abundant cytoplasm with eosinophilia and vacuolization (Fig. 3.33d).

Case 2

A 75-year-old man with biopsy diagnosis of invasive high-grade urothelial carcinoma underwent radical cystoprostatectomy and bilateral pelvic lymph node dissections. The biopsy shows both noninvasive high-grade papillary urothelial carcinoma (Fig. 3.34a) and invasive carcinoma with solid confluent growth (Fig. 3.34b) and focal micropapillary component (Fig. 3.34c). Final diagnose of cystectomy was invasive urothelial carcinoma with perivesical invasion and lymph node metastasis (Fig. 3.34d).

Case 3

An 82-year-old woman with hematuria and a CT scan showed exophytic bladder tumor at the left lateral wall. Transurethral resection of tumor was performed. Microscopically, the tumor is composed of both solid conventional urothelial carcinoma and small-cell carcinoma component (Fig. 3.35a). High power shows small-cell carcinoma with high N/C ratio, scant cytoplasm, nuclear crowding and molding, frequent mitotic figures and apoptosis (Fig. 3.35b). The tumor cells are diffused and strongly positive for CD56 (Fig. 3.35c) and positive for chromogranin (Fig. 3.35d).

Case 4

A 74-year-old man with history of prostate cancer status postradiation therapy and now presented with hematuria.

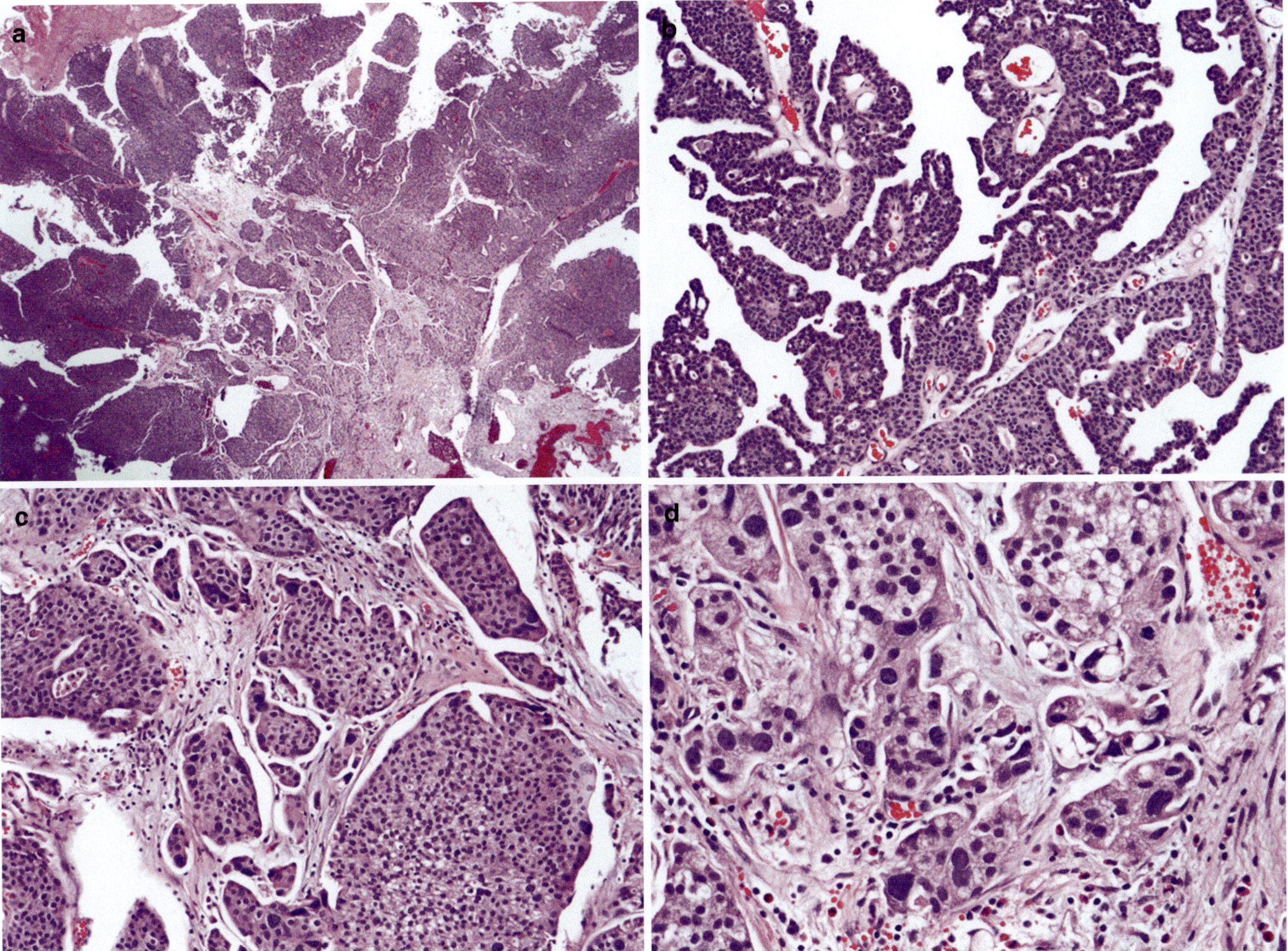

Fig. 3.33 Low power view of a high-grade papillary urothelial carcinoma with prominent exophytic component and subepithelial invasion (**a**). This area shows focal surface micropapillary component with secondary delicate papillae and lack of fibrovascular core (**b**), which is often associated with high-grade invasive urothelial carcinoma. At the interface of noninvasive papillary carcinoma and subepithelial tissue, multiple small irregular nests of tumor cells and retraction artifact are present, indicating invasive carcinoma (**c**). High-power view of small invasive foci with greater nuclear atypia and cytoplasmic vacuolization

He was diagnosed with high-grade papillary urothelial carcinoma and underwent multiple cycles of intravesical BCG therapy. Follow-up cystoscopy and biopsy show focal area of urothelial carcinoma in situ (Fig. 3.36a), and nephrogenic adenoma with denuded urothelium lined by single layer of cuboidal epithelial cells and subepitheliual proliferation of tubules and cysts lined by uniform cuboidal cells, luminal secretion, and a granulation tissue background (Fig. 3.36b). The tubules are positive for cytokeratin 7 (Fig. 3.36c) Pax 8 (Fig. 3.36d) by immunohistochemistry.

Case 5

A 47-year-old man with history of sigmoid colon cancer status post rectosigmoidectomy now presented with bladder cancer 3 years later underwent transurethral resection. Microscopically, the tumor shows a tubulopapillary growth pattern and invasive component within subepithelial tissue (Fig. 3.37a). On high power, the tumor glands are lined by pseudostratified columnar cells and desmoplastic stroma (Fig. 3.37b). By immunohistochemistry, the tumor cells are positive for Cytokeratin 20 (Fig. 3.37c) and CDX-2 (Fig. 3.37d).

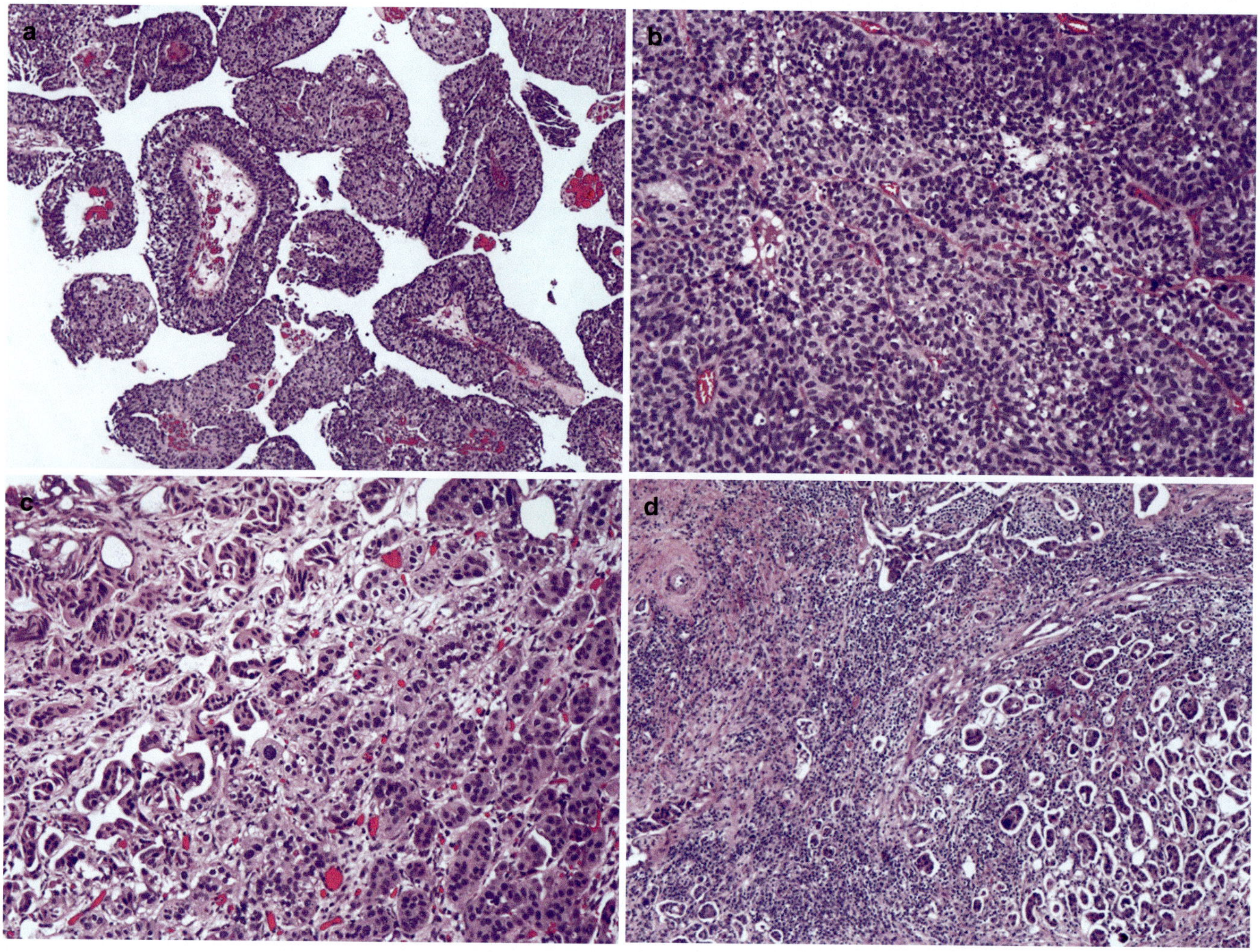

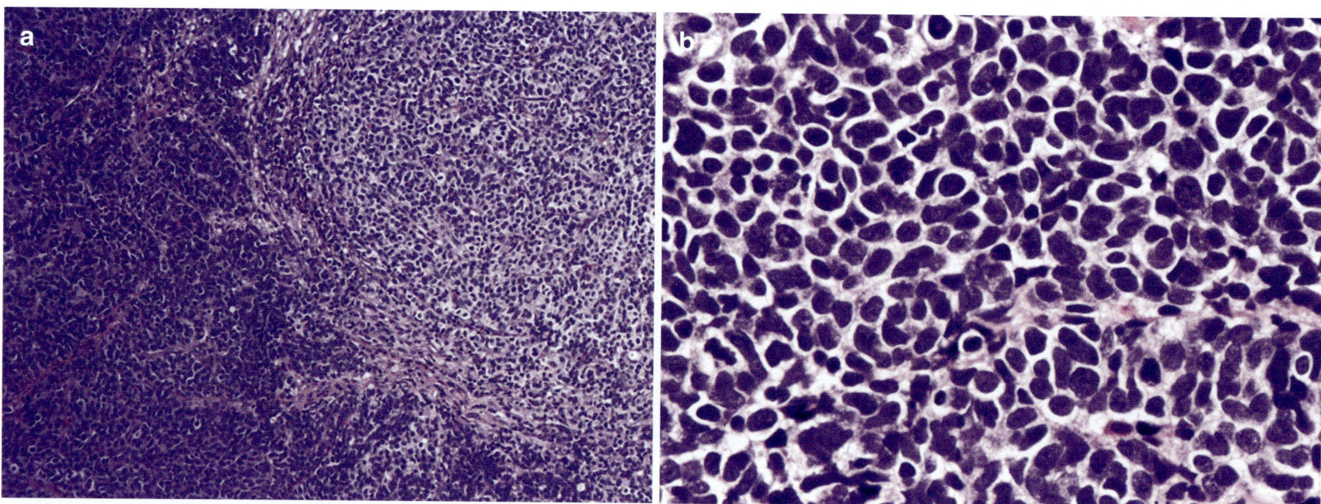

Fig. 3.34 This image shows exophytic noninvasive papillary urothelial carcinoma component (**a**). This area exhibits confluent invasive growth of urothelial carcinoma. Other areas show conventional invasive urothelial carcinoma with focal micropapillary carcinoma component (**c**). Nodal metastasis with micropapillary carcinoma is shown (**d**)

Fig. 3.35 This is an example of conventional high-grade urothelial carcinoma associated with small cell carcinoma (**a**). High power view of small-cell carcinoma exhibits nuclear crowding and molding, high N/C ratio, hyperchromatic nuclei and salt–pepper chromatin (**b**). The tumor cells are diffuse and strongly positive for CD56 (**c**) and chromogranin (**d**)

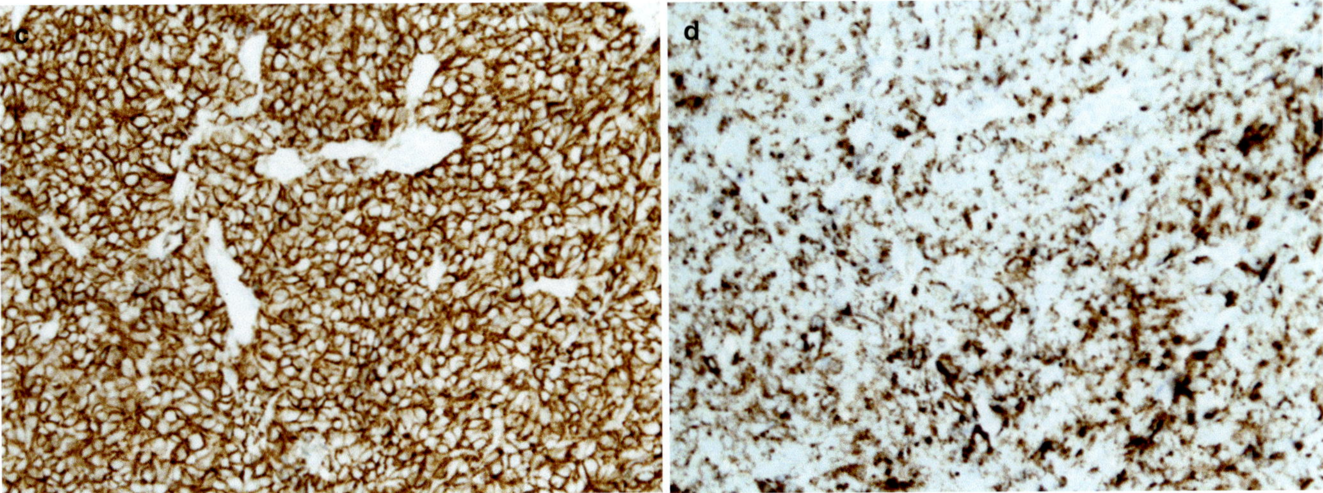

Fig. 3.35 (continued)

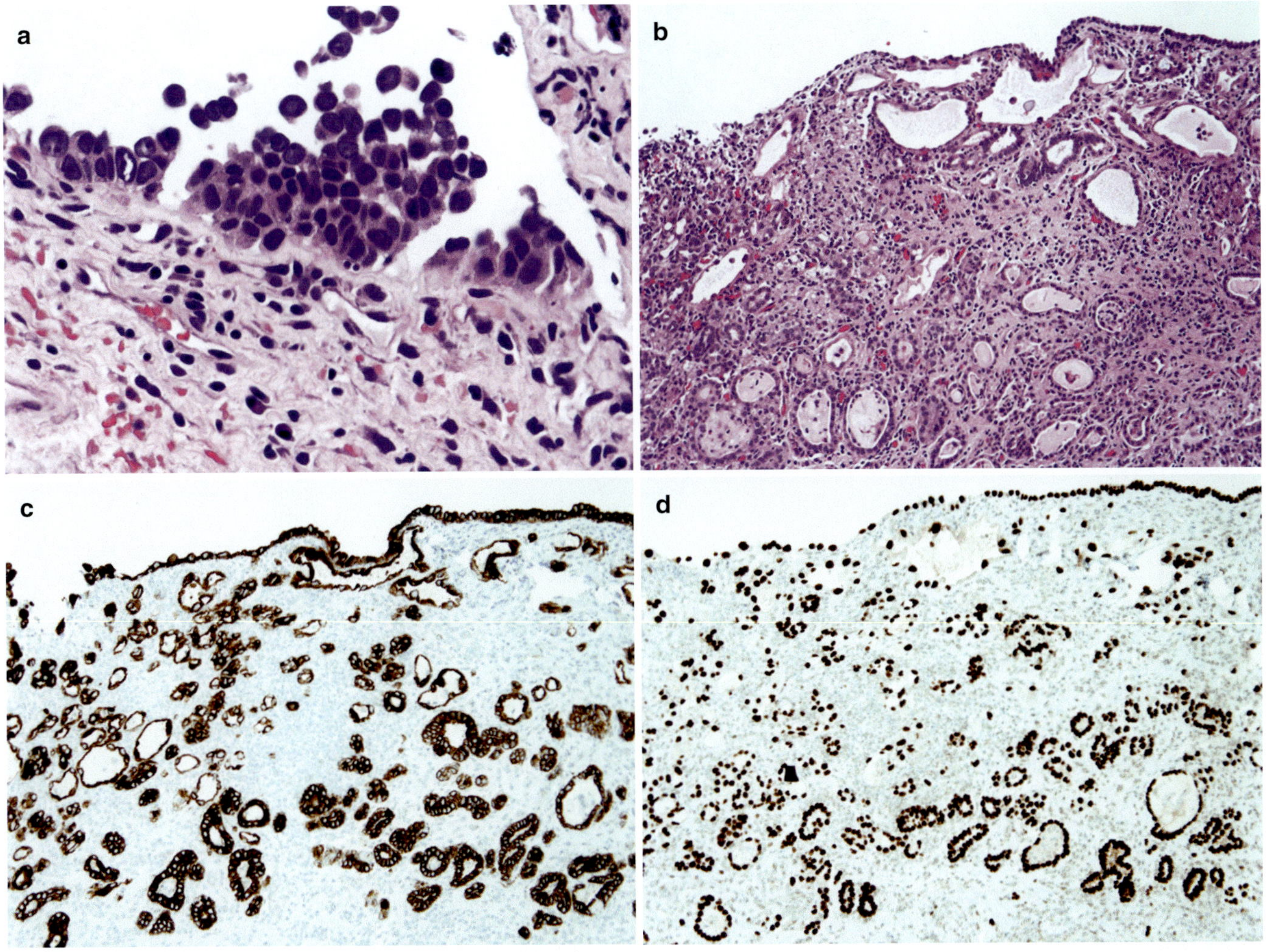

Fig. 3.36 Bladder biopsy shows urothelial carcinoma in situ characterized by nuclear pleomorphism and enlargement, high N/C ratio and hyperchromasia (**a**). This area shows features of nephrogenic adenoma with single layer surface lining, subepithelial proliferation of tubules and cysts lined by uniform cuboidal cells in a granulation tissue background (**b**). The diagnosis of nephrogenic adenoma is confirmed by positive immunoreactivity with CK7 (**c**) and PAX 8 (**d**)

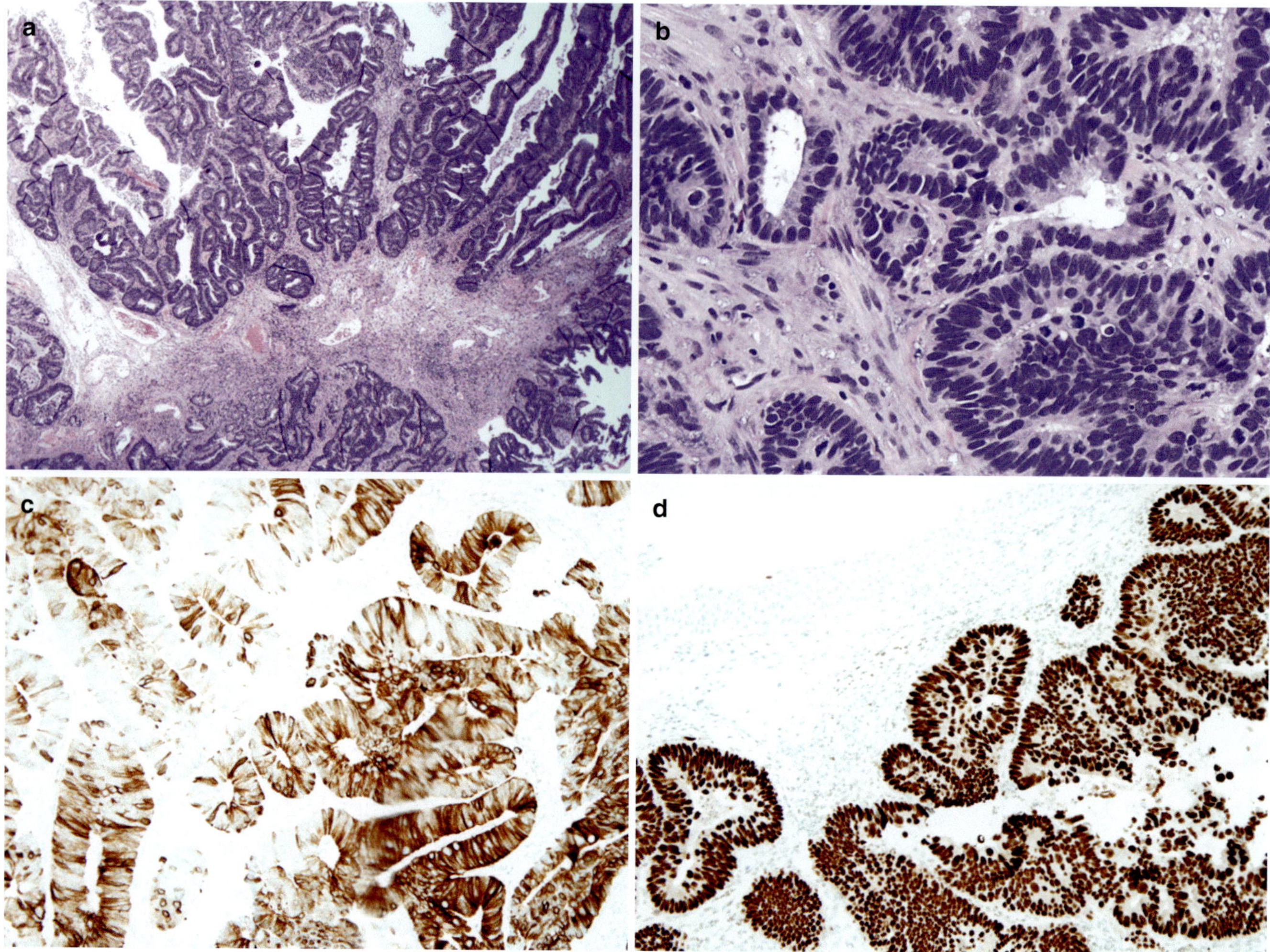

Fig. 3.37 This low power image shows invasive adenocarcinoma with tubulovillous pattern and subepithelial invasion (**a**). High power shows irregular glands lined by pseudostratified columnar cells and desmo-plastic stromal reaction (**b**). The tumor cells are positive for CK20 (**c**) and strongly positive for CDX-2 (**d**)

References

1. Grignon DJ, et al. Infiltrating urothelial carcinoma. In: Moch H, et al., editors. WHO Classification of Tumours of the Urinary System and Male Genital Organs: The International Agency for Research on Cancer (IARC). Lyon:France; 2016. p. 81–98.

2. Knowles MA, Hurst CD. Molecular biology of bladder cancer: new insights into pathogenesis and clinical diversity. Nat Rev Cancer. 2015;15(1):25–41.

3. Bubendorf L, et al. Ancillary studies in urinary cytology. In: Rosenthal DL, Wojcik EM, Kurtycz DFI, editors. The Paris system for reporting urinary cytology: Springer:Newyork; 2016. p. 115–36.

4. Xing J, Reynolds JP. Diagnostic advances in urine cytology. Surg Pathol Clin. 2018;11(3):601–10.

5. The Paris System for reporting urinary cytology, vol. 1: Springer; 2016. p. 159.

6. Reuter VE, et al. Non-invasive urothelial lesions. In: Moch H, et al., editors. WHO classification of tomours of the urinary system and male genital organs: The International Agency for Research on Cancer (IARC); 2016. p. 99–107.

7. Amin MB, et al. Urothelial carcinoma in situ. In: Amin MB, Tickoo SK, editors. Diagnostic pathology: genitourinary. Salk Lake City: Elsevier, Inc.; 2016. p. 332–9.

8. Cheng L, et al. Neoplasms of the urinary bladder. In: Cheng L, MacLennan GT, Bostwick DG, editors. Urologic surgical pathology. China: Elsevier, Inc.; 2020. p. 230–321.

9. Cancer Genome Atlas Research, N. Comprehensive molecular characterization of urothelial bladder carcinoma. Nature. 2014;507(7492):315–22.

10. Choi W, et al. Identification of distinct basal and luminal subtypes of muscle-invasive bladder cancer with different sensitivities to frontline chemotherapy. Cancer Cell. 2014;25(2):152–65.

11. Kardos J, et al. Claudin-low bladder tumors are immune infiltrated and actively immune suppressed. JCI Insight. 2016;1(3):e85902.

12. Sjodahl G, et al. Molecular profiling in muscle-invasive bladder cancer: more than the sum of its parts. J Pathol. 2019;247(5):563–73.

13. Sjodahl G, et al. A molecular taxonomy for urothelial carcinoma. Clin Cancer Res. 2012;18(12):3377–86.

14. Zinnall U, et al. Micropapillary urothelial carcinoma: evaluation of HER2 status and immunohistochemical characterization of the molecular subtype. Hum Pathol. 2018;80:55–64.

15. Epstein JI, Netto GJ. In: Epstein JI, editor. Bladder, in differential diagnoses in surgical pathology: genitourinary system. China: Lippincott Williams & Wilkins; 2014. p. 263–385.

16. Lopez-Beltran A, Young RH. Nonneoplastic disorders of the urinary bladder. In: Cheng L, MacLennan GT, Bostwick DG, editors. Urologic surgical pathology. China: Elsevier, Inc.; 2020. p. 195–229.

17. Amin MB, et al. Tumors of urachus. In: Amin MB, Tickoo SK, editors. Diagnostic pathology: genitourinary. Salk Lake City: Elsevier, Inc.; 2016. p. 522–7.

18. Lopez-Beltran, A., G.P. Paner, and T. Tsuzuki, Urachal carcinoma, in WHO classification of tomours of the urinary system and male genital organs, H. Moch, et al., Editors. 2016, The International Agency for Research on Cancer (IARC). Lyon:France. p. 113–114.

19. Amin MB, et al. Invasive Adenocarcinoma. In: Amin MB, Tickoo SK, editors. Diagnostic pathology: genitourinary. Salk Lake City: Elsevier, Inc.; 2016. p. 410–5.

20. Amin MB, et al. Myofibroblastic proliferations. In: Amin MB, Tickoo SK, editors. Diagnostic pathology: genitourinary. Salk Lake City: Elsevier, Inc.; 2016. p. 432–9.

21. Amin MB, et al. Other mesenchymal tumors. In: Amin MB, Tickoo SK, editors. Diagnostic pathology: genitourinary. Salk Lake City: Elsevier,Inc.; 2016. p. 454–61.

22. Amin MB, et al. Skeletal muscle tumors. In: Amin MB, Tickoo SK, editors. Diagnostic pathology: genitourinary. Salk Lake City: Elsevier, Inc.; 2016. p. 448–53.

23. Amin MB, et al. Smooth muscle tumors. In: Amin MB, Tickoo SK, editors. Diagnostic pathology: genitourinary. Salk Lake City: Elsevier, Inc.; 2016. p. 440–7.

24. Al-Ahmadie H, E C, Epstein JI. Neuroendocrine tumours. In: Moch H, et al., editors. WHO classification of tomours of the urinary system and male genital organs: The International Agency for Research on Cancer (IARC); 2016. p. 117–9.

25. Miyamoto H, et al. Pitfalls in the use of smoothelin to identify muscularis propria invasion by urothelial carcinoma. Am J Surg Pathol. 2010;34(3):418–22.

26. Cheng L, et al. Staging and reporting of urothelial carcinoma of the urinary bladder. Mod Pathol. 2009;22(Suppl 2):S70–95.

27. Epstein JI, Reuter VE, Amin MB. Urothelial neoplasms with inverted growth patterns. In: Biopsy interpretation of the bladder. Lippincott Williams & Wilkins, Philadelphia, PA; 2017. p. 87–103.

28. Wilkerson ML, Cheng L. Urinary bladder and urachus. In: Lin F, Prichard J, editors. Handbook of practical immunohistochemistry: frequently asked questions: Springer:Newyork; 2015. p. 421–37.

29. Bates AW, Baithun SI. The significance of secondary neoplasms of the urinary and male genital tract. Virchows Arch. 2002;440(6):640–7.

30. Grignon DJ. Urothelial carcinoma, in WHO classification of tomours of the urinary system and male genital organs, H. Moch, et al., Editors. 2016, The International Agency for Research on Cancer (IARC). Lyon:France. p. 168–169.

31. Oliva E, Trpkov K. Tumours of Mullerian type. In: Moch H, et al., editors. WHO classification of tomours of the urinary system and male genital organs: The International Agency for Research on Cancer (IARC). Lyon:France; 2016. p. 115–6.

32. Shen, S.S., H. Al-Ahmadie, and S.M. Mahfouz, Squamous cell neoplasms, in WHO Classification of tomours of the urinary system and male genital organs, H. Moch, et al., Editors. 2016, The International Agency for Research on Cancer (IARC). Lyon:France. p. 108–110.

33. Amin MB, et al. Diverticular-associated neoplasia. In: Amin MB, Tickoo SK, editors. Diagnostic pathology: genitourinary. Salk Lake City: Elsevier, Inc.; 2016. p. 482–5.

4

Maria Tretiakova

List of Frequently Asked Questions

What Are the Key Differences between Male and Female Urethra?

The urethra is a muscular tube connecting the bladder with the external urethral orifice for excretion. In males and females, urethra has significant anatomic, physiologic, and microscopic differences predisposing to different types of lesions (see Table 4.1; Figs. 4.1a–d, 4.2a–c, and 4.3a, b).

- In men, the urethra is 15–20 cm long and consists of four main anatomic segments: preprostatic (1–1.5 cm intramural within bladder neck), prostatic (3–4 cm), membranous (2 cm, intermediate) and penile (10–15 cm, proximal bulbous, and distal spongy with saccular fossa navicularis).
- In women, the urethra is much shorter (on average 4 cm) and divided into proximal and distal regions corresponding to the prostatic and membranous urethra segments.
- **References**: [1–5].

What Are the Most Common Congenital Abnormalities of Urethra?

Although congenital abnormalities are not commonly encountered in urologic pathology practice, they could be seen on autopsy or enter in the differential diagnosis of the inflammatory or neoplastic lesion. Due to the complex anatomy of male urethra, the majority of developmental abnormalities are seen in boys with a notable exception for urethral diverticulum. (Tables 4.2, 4.3, 4.4, 4.5, and 4.6; Fig. 4.4a, b).
    References: [6–12].

M. Tretiakova (✉)
Department of Pathology, University of Washington, Seattle, WA, USA
e-mail: mariast@uw.edu

Table 4.1 Comparison of the male and female urethra

Feature	Male urethra	Female urethra
Length	15–20 cm	~4 cm
Anatomic segments	Preprostatic, prostatic, membranous, penile	Proximal and distal portions
Orifice	Glans penis	Vaginal vestibule/vulva
Function	Urine excretion and conduit for semen	Urine excretion
Associated periurethral epithelial structures	Prostatic ducts, prostatic utricle, ejaculatory ducts, verumontanum; bulbourethral (Cowper) glands; paraurethral Littre glands (Fig. 4.1a–d)	Paraurethral (Skene) glands
Epithelial lining	Urothelium transitions to pseudostratified columnar epithelium to nonkeratinizing stratified squamous epithelium	Urothelium transitions to nonkeratinizing stratified squamous epithelium or pure squamous
Common congenital lesions	Urethral valves, duplication of urethra, utricle cyst, hypospadias, megalourethra, etc.	Urethral diverticula
Common reactive inflammatory lesions	Fibroepithelial polyps and nephrogenic adenoma (Fig. 4.2a–c)	Most common are squamous metaplasia and caruncle (Fig. 4.3a, b)

What Are the Most Common Reactive/Inflammatory Lesions of Urethra?

Nonneoplastic inflammatory and reactive lesions that typically occur in the bladder could also develop in the urethra. These lesions include, but not limited to, urethritis (nonspecific, polypoid and papillary, glandularis and cystica, radiation induced, HPV-induced with or without Condylomas), malakoplakia, and various types of metaplasia (i.e., squamous, glandular, intestinal, nephrogenic). There are, however, reactive and inflammatory lesions that are specific to

© Springer Nature Switzerland AG 2021
X. J. Yang, M. Zhou (eds.), *Practical Genitourinary Pathology*, Practical Anatomic Pathology,
https://doi.org/10.1007/978-3-030-57141-2_4

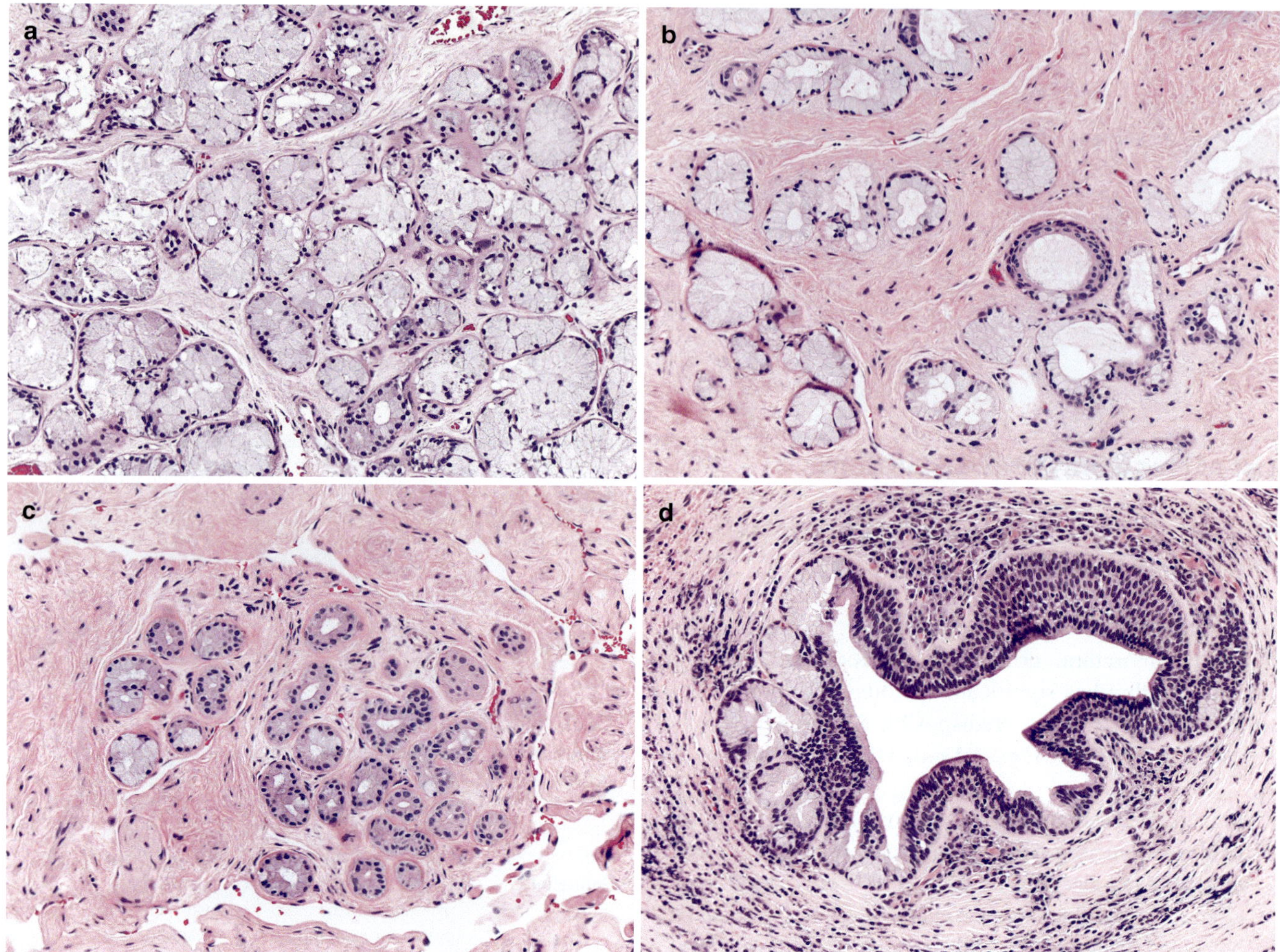

Fig. 4.1 (**a**) Bulbourethral (Cowper) glands have a compact lobular architecture of mucinous acini with small dark nuclei and pale blue foamy cytoplasm. (**b**) Cowper glands can undergo squamous metaplasia and fibrosis, especially in cases of proximal urethral stricture. (**c**) Mucin depletion of Cowper glands with nuclear enlargement and hyperchromasia could be confused with low-grade prostatic adenocarcinoma. (**d**) Periurethral glands of Littre with transitional and mucinous secreting cells embedded into the erectile tissue of corpus spongiosum. Females have morphologically very similar-looking Skene glands

the urethra, which could be divided into solitary polypoid lesions (Table 4.7; Figs. 4.3a, b, 4.5, and 4.6.) and cystic lesions (Table 4.8).

References: [13–18].

Risk Factors and Pathological Diagnoses Associated with Urethral Stricture?

Urethral stricture is a common disease of luminal narrowing and fibrotic scar formation around urethral mucosa. Strictures can occur at any urethral location from the external meatus up to the bladder neck. Every process that causes urethral trauma can finally lead to stricture. It is much often affecting men who can experience obstructive voiding symptoms, urinary retention, and occasionally urinary tract infections including prostatitis and epididymitis.

In the past, urethritis due to sexually transmitted diseases, especially gonorrhea, was the main cause of stricture. As the treatment and prevention of sexually transmitted disease had advanced in the developed world, etiologies have shifted to those that are less well understood and differ by patient age and stricture site. Etiologies of urethral stricture and their relative frequencies are as follows: idiopathic/unknown (~30%), transurethral resection (~20%), pelvic fracture (~12%), urethral catheterization (~11%), hypospadias and other congenital anomalies (~10%), lichen sclerosis (~5%), urethritis (~4%), prostatectomy (~3%), perineal trauma (~2%), cystoscopy (~1%), penile fracture (~1%), and brachytherapy (~1%).

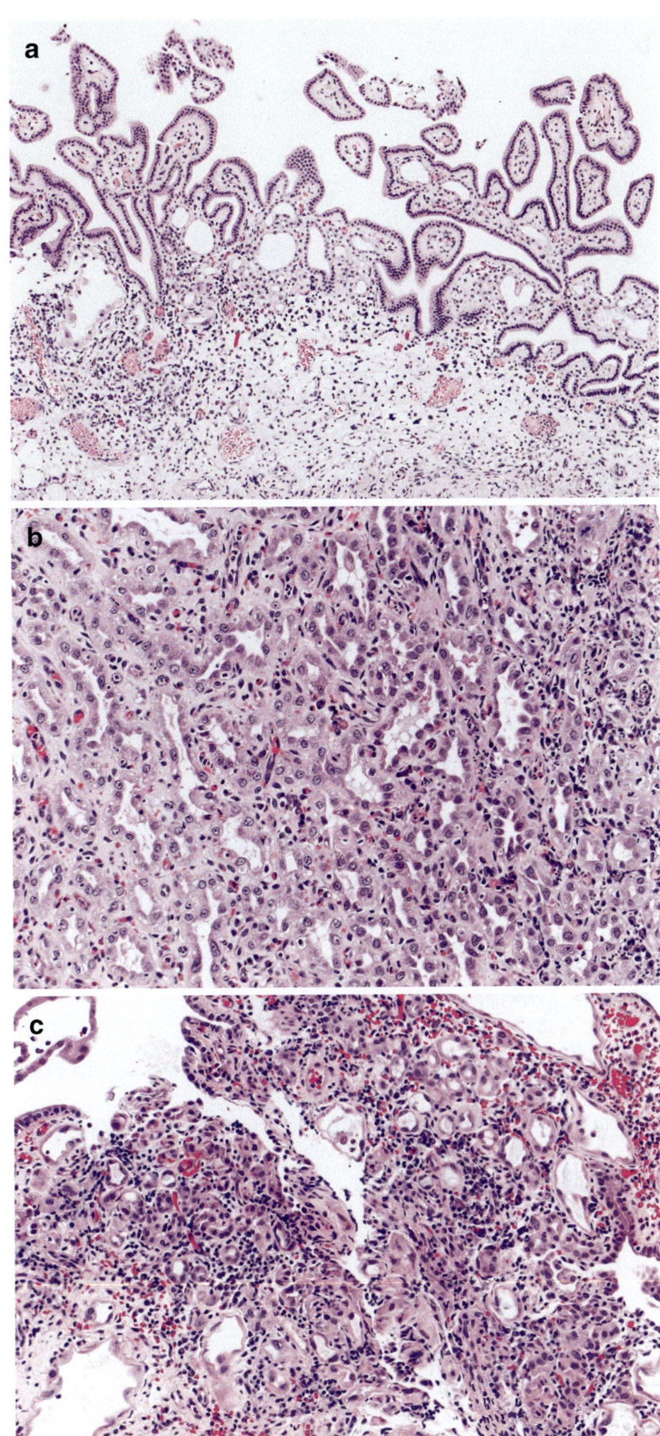

Fig. 4.2 (**a**) Nephrogenic adenoma of the urethra is a common reactive metaplastic process often with papillary structures lined by a single layer of cuboidal epithelium with round hyperchromatic nuclei. (**b**) Deep nephrogenic adenoma of male urethra composed of compact tubules lined by hobnailed and cuboidal cells with round nuclei containing prominent nucleoli, mimicking prostatic adenocarcinoma. (**c**) Nephrogenic adenoma of female urethra could be confused with clear cell adenocarcinoma due to infiltrating features and high-grade nuclei

Male urethral stricture disease can be recurrent and debilitating. Although the rates of urethral stricture have declined in the past decade, costs to the USA health care system are still significant, averaging approximately $6000 per affected insured individual yearly and almost $200 million nationwide. Open reconstruction via anterior urethroplasty is now considered the gold standard treatment for urethral stricture disease. Segments of the strictured urethra and surrounding corpus spongiosum are dissected from surrounding tissues, excised, and if sufficiently short, a primary anastomosis is performed. Complications from stricture treatment include bleeding, infection, incontinence, and impotence and occur in up to 7%.

Below we provide a list of common pathology findings that are frequently encountered in the resection specimens and have been linked to postsurgical complications/recurrence and development of neoplasia.

- *Nonspecific (active) chronic inflammation and fibrosis (most common).*
- Epithelium with squamous metaplasia, sometimes keratinizing and extending to periurethral glands; luminal narrowing, acute and chronic inflammation, subepithelial eccentric or concentric fibrosis involving surrounding erectile tissue (Fig. 4.7a–c).
- *Nephrogenic adenoma/metaplasia*:
- Complex papillary or tubular structures covered by cuboidal hobnailed epithelium with pale to eosinophilic cytoplasm, round nuclei with small nucleoli. The surrounding stroma is often edematous, inflamed, or sclerosed (Fig. 4.7b, c).
- *Lichen sclerosus et atrophicus*:
- Inflammatory phase with squamous metaplasia, atrophy, and band-like chronic inflammation of subepithelial stroma; Sclerosing phase shows basal cell vacuolization and loss overlying thick paucicellular collagenized stroma (Fig. 4.8a–d).
- *Urothelial carcinoma (rare)*:
- Flat or papillary atypical clonal proliferation of urothelium with or without invasion into the underlying tissues.

References: [19–25].

What Are the Most Common Benign Neoplasms of Urethra?

Benign epithelial neoplastic lesions of the urethra are rare and, therefore, could post a significant diagnostic challenge for practicing pathologists. Because of the rarity of these tumors, most cases in the literature represent single case

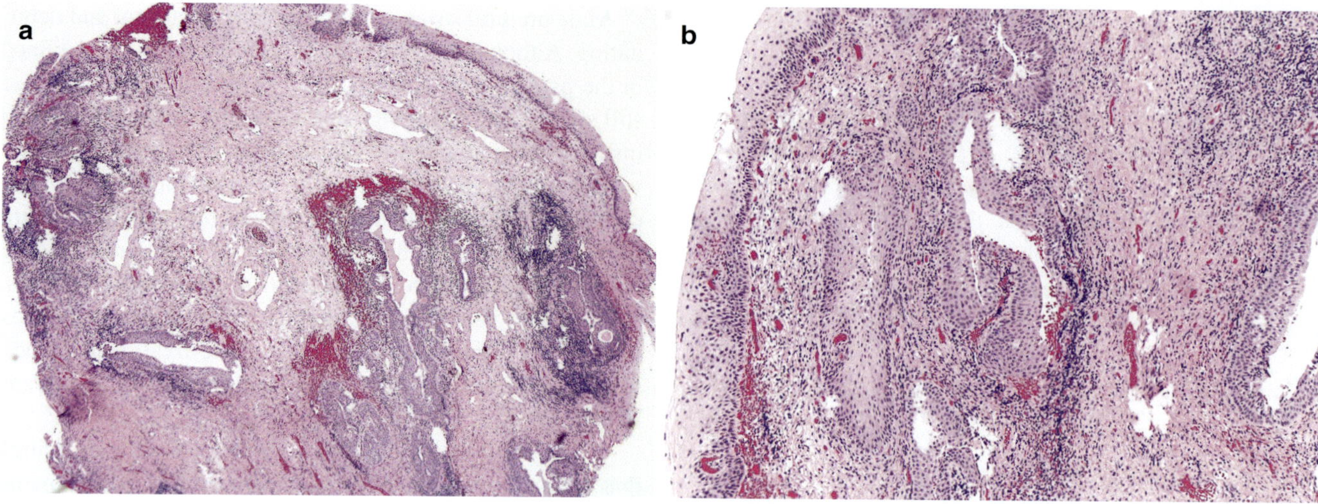

Fig. 4.3 (**a**) Caruncle is a reactive polypoid mass with marked inflammation, abundant vasculature, and hemorrhages. (**b**) Caruncle at higher power shows benign urothelium with invaginations and squamous metaplasia and invariably present dense inflammatory infiltrate

Table 4.2 Urethral duplication

Feature	Description
Definition	Complete (from bladder to meatus) or partial (ending blindly) duplication of urethra; 15% cases connect with the functional urethra
Patients	Males
Symptoms	Asymptomatic (autopsy finding) or present with double stream and incontinence
Histology	Two lumens and walls of urethra with urothelial or squamous lining
Complications	Common: Infection; uncommon: Obstruction due to accumulation of desquamated material and compression of functional urethra

Table 4.3 Urethral valves

Feature	Description
Definition	Posterior or vertical folds, often fused to form a diaphragm or obstructing concentric disk at the level of prostatic (more common) or penile urethra
Patients	Males
Symptoms	Severe cases—Urinary retention with enlarged bladder and hydronephrosis; mild cases—Frequent infections, incontinence, hematuria, weak stream
Histology	Folds with urothelial lining and variable degrees of inflammation
Complications	Hydronephrosis (end-stage kidney), renal insufficiency, sepsis

Table 4.4 Megalouretrha

Feature	Description
Definition	Absence of corpus spongiosum or both corpora spongiosum and cavernosum
Patients	Males
Symptoms	Enlarged deformed penis in neonates
Histology	Lack of erectile tissue around penile urethra
Complications	May be associated with prune belly syndrome or other genitourinary anomalies

Table 4.5 Hypospadias

Feature	Description
Definition	Ectopic urethral opening on the ventral surface of perineum, scrotum or penis
Patients	Males, most common congenital anomaly of urethra (1:125 live male births)
Symptoms	Asymptomatic
Histology	Not required
Complications	May be associated with other penile anomalies and infection

Table 4.6 Urethral diverticulum

Feature	Description
Definition	Outpouching or invagination of urothelial mucosa into the urethral wall
Patients	Females
Symptoms	Asymptomatic, pain, dribbling, and bulging mass
Histology	Invagination of mucosa with squamous metaplasia and chronic inflammation
Complications	Inflammation (diverticulitis), ulceration, fistula, calculi, fibrosis, nephrogenic adenoma, villous adenoma, condyloma; malignant transformation (~5%)

reports or small case series. In Tables 4.9, 4.10, 4.11, and 4.12 we summarized the most important clinicopathologic features of the four main benign urethral tumors. See also Fig. 4.9.

References: [26–31].

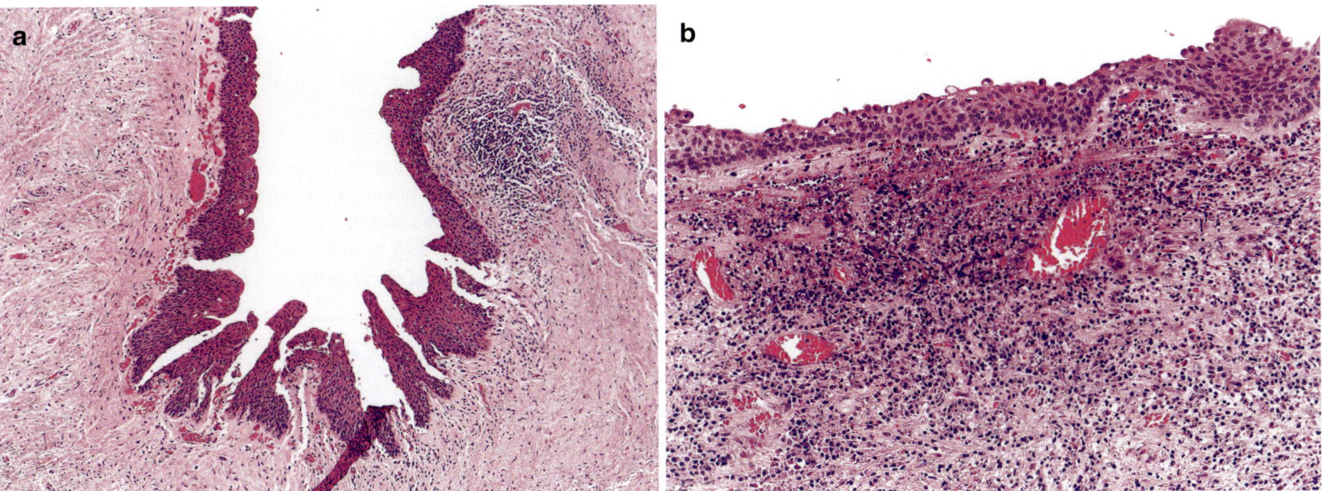

Fig. 4.4 (**a**) Urethral diverticulum is more common in females and represents an invagination of mucosa with squamous metaplasia. (**b**) Diverticulum of the urethra is often associated with active and chronic inflammation and reactive epithelial atypia

Table 4.7 Solitary polypoid lesions of urethra

Entity	Caruncle	Prostatic-type polyp	Fibroepithelial polyp
Patients	Females, postmenopausal	Males, adults	Males, first decade of life
Etiology	Trauma-related or due to mucosal prolapse	Hyperplasia and overgrowth of underlying prostatic epithelium or from ectopic prostatic tissue	Secondary to congenital defect of urethral wall
Location	Distal urethra near meatus	Prostatic urethra or penile urethra	Posterior prostatic urethra adjacent to verumontanum
Symptoms	Asymptomatic could have frequency, bloody spotting, pain, dysuria, or obstruction	Asymptomatic, could have hematuria	Asymptomatic, could have hematuria or obstruction
Gross	Pedunculated or sessile fleshy pink polyp, 1–2 cm	<1 cm	Polypoid mass on narrow stalk, <4 cm
Histology	Invariably inflamed polyp with prominent vasculature, often thrombosed may contain atypical cells (Fig. 4.3a, b)	Irregular papillary fronds covered by prostatic-type epithelium occasionally intermixed with urothelium	Club-like or finger-like projections with urothelial lining and abundant stroma, sometimes atypical (Fig. 4.5)
Immunostains	EMA/ALK negative	PSA/34βE12/p63 positive	PSA negative
Differential	Inflammatory myofibroblastic tumor, urothelial carcinoma	Prostatic adenocarcinoma including ductal; urethritis glandularis, villous adenoma	Polypoid-papillary urethritis (Fig. 4.6) and urothelial papilloma

How to Distinguish Urothelial and Squamous Cell Carcinoma of Urethra?

Primary carcinomas of the urethra are rare accounting for less than 1% of urinary tract malignancies. The histologic type, natural history, treatment, and prognosis of these tumors are largely determined by the segment of the urethra in which they develop (see Table 4.13; Fig. 4.10a, b).

Recently, a new entity of a primary urethral carcinoma showing hybrid features of urothelial and squamous differentiation was proposed by M.D. Anderson Cancer Center urologic pathology group. This carcinoma is distinct from typical urothelial carcinomas developing in the bladder and squamous carcinomas developing in the distal male urethra involving the meatus or glans penis as well as those arising in the vulva of females. Morphologically these tumors are poorly differentiated carcinomas with basaloid features and hybrid squamous as well as urothelial differentiation. They often develop in association with HPV infection and are clinically highly aggressive with frequent regional lymph node and distant organ metastatic spread.

References: [32–38].

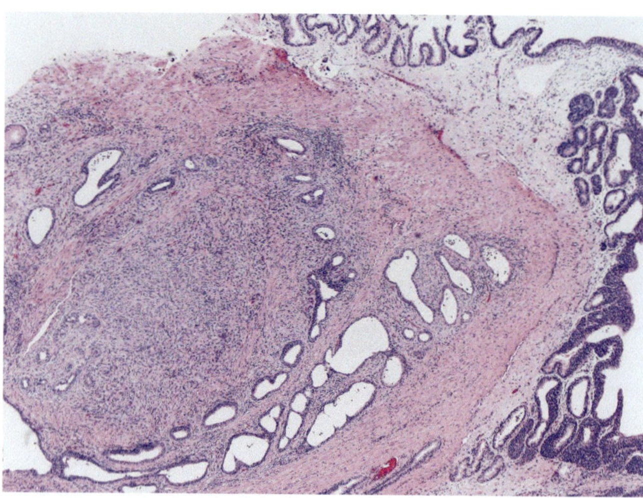

Fig. 4.5 Fibroepithelial polyp of the prostatic urethra is a polypoid mass at the verumontanum area with urothelial lining and abundant underlying stroma

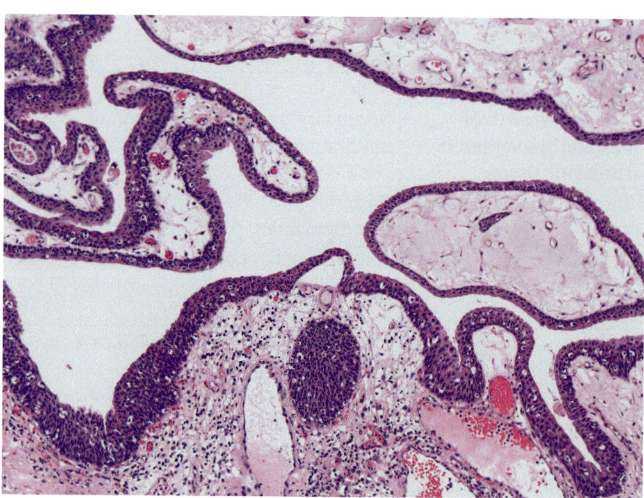

Fig. 4.6 Polypoid urethritis could be an isolated lesion with prominent edematous stroma and dilated vasculature with thickened reactive urothelium and scattered chronic inflammatory cells

What Types of Adenocarcinomas Are Encountered in Male and Female Urethra?

Primary urethral adenocarcinomas are rare tumors accounting for approximately 10% of all urethral cancers. Their incidence is higher in women while the age distribution is similar to other urothelial carcinomas with the peak in the seventh decade.

Three main variants of primary urethral adenocarcinoma are described below and include: (1) Conventional adenocarcinoma (enteric, mucinous, signet-ring, and nonenteric subtypes), (2) Clear cell adenocarcinoma, (3) Adenocarcinoma of accessory glands. Case reports of other primary urethral

Table 4.8 Cystic lesions of urethra

Entity	Skene duct cyst	Cowper gland duct cyst (syringocele)
Patients	Females (from newborn to adult)	Males (wide age range)
Etiology	Obstruction of Skene glands (analog of male prostate gland) secondary to infection	Obstruction of bulbourethral (Cowper) glands with cystic dilatation
Location	Floor of distal urethra	Bulbomembranous urethra
Symptoms	Dysuria and obstruction of voiding	Frequency, urgency, dysuria, postvoid incontinence, hematuria
Gross	Variably sized cystic spaces	Unilocular cystic dilatation
Histology	Cysts with squamous epithelial lining	Syringocele may be denuded with fibrous wall and marked inflammation
Differential	Urethral diverticulum, cystocele, Gartner duct cyst	Congenital urethral lesions: i.e., urethral valves

adenocarcinomas include adenoid cystic carcinoma, adenosquamous carcinoma, and so-called cloacogenic carcinoma.

Secondary urethral adenocarcinomas are more common than primary and their incidence is higher in men because the vast majority of secondary adenocarcinomas are of the prostatic origin. The diagnosis of any primary urethral adenocarcinoma requires ruling out secondary involvement by direct extension or metastatic spread (Tables 4.14, 4.15, and 4.16; Fig. 4.11a–c).

References: [39–46].

Case Presentation

Case 1

Learning Objectives
1. To become familiar with the histologic features of the tumor.
2. To become familiar with the immunohistochemical features of the tumor.
3. To generate the differential diagnosis.

Case History
The 71-year-old healthy male presented with intermittent hematuria.

Gross
Multiple friable pink soft tissue fragments of prostatic urethra measuring 2 × 0.8 × 0.3 cm in aggregate were submitted in total in one cassette.

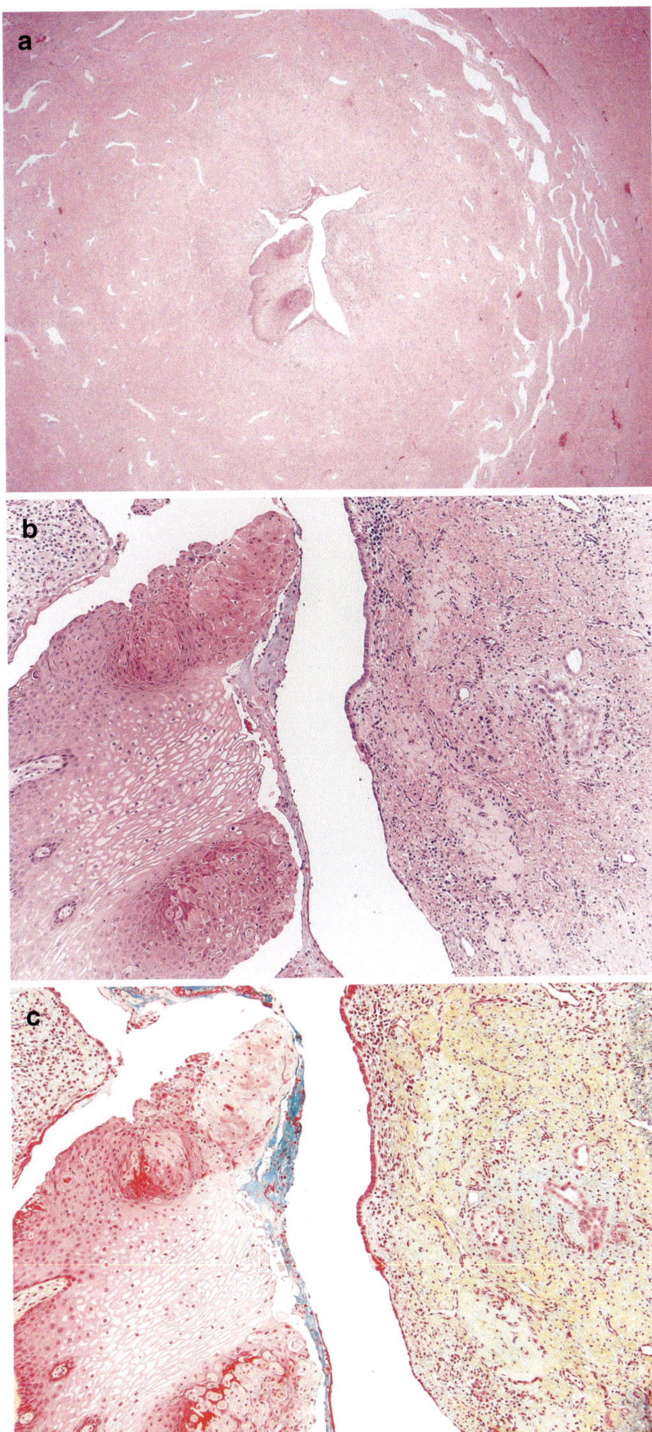

Fig. 4.7 (**a**) Urethral stricture with stellate-shaped luminal narrowing, subepithelial eccentric or concentric fibrosis involving surrounding erectile tissue. (**b**) Urethral stricture shows squamous metaplasia, dyskeratosis, inflammation, and nephrogenic metaplasia with cuboidal lining and small tubules within the fibrotic stroma. (**c**) MOVAT special staining of urethral stricture highlights subepithelial fibrosis (bright yellow stain)

Histologic Findings
- Papillary proliferation with thin fibrovascular cores lined by columnar cells with mild atypia, enlarged nuclei, and focal pseudostratification (Fig. 4.12a).
- Papillary and focally cribriform growth pattern. Elongated crowded tumor cells with hyperchromasia and scattered mitoses (Fig. 4.12b).

Differential Diagnosis
- Prostatic-type urethral polyp.
- Prostatic ductal carcinoma.
- Papillary urothelial carcinoma.

IHC and Other Ancillary Studies
- PSA strongly positive.
- NKX3.1 strongly positive.
- P63 negative.
- GATA3 negative.

Final Diagnosis
Ductal Adenocarcinoma of the Prostate.

Take-Home Messages
1. Prostatic ductal adenocarcinoma can be distinguished from a prostatic urethral polyp by nuclear enlargement and pseudostratification.
2. Prostatic urethral polyps contain two types of cells: basal and luminal, which are not appreciated in this case.
3. Immunohistochemistry with prostate-specific, basal-cell, and urothelial markers are important in making this diagnosis.

References: [47, 48].

Case 2

Learning Objectives
1. To become familiar with gross and histologic features of the lesion.
2. To generate the differential diagnosis.

Case History
A 42-year-old man with history of nephrolithiasis found to have urethral mass during operation.

Gross
Polypoid 1.7 cm fragment of tan-white soft tissue was bisected and submitted in one cassette.

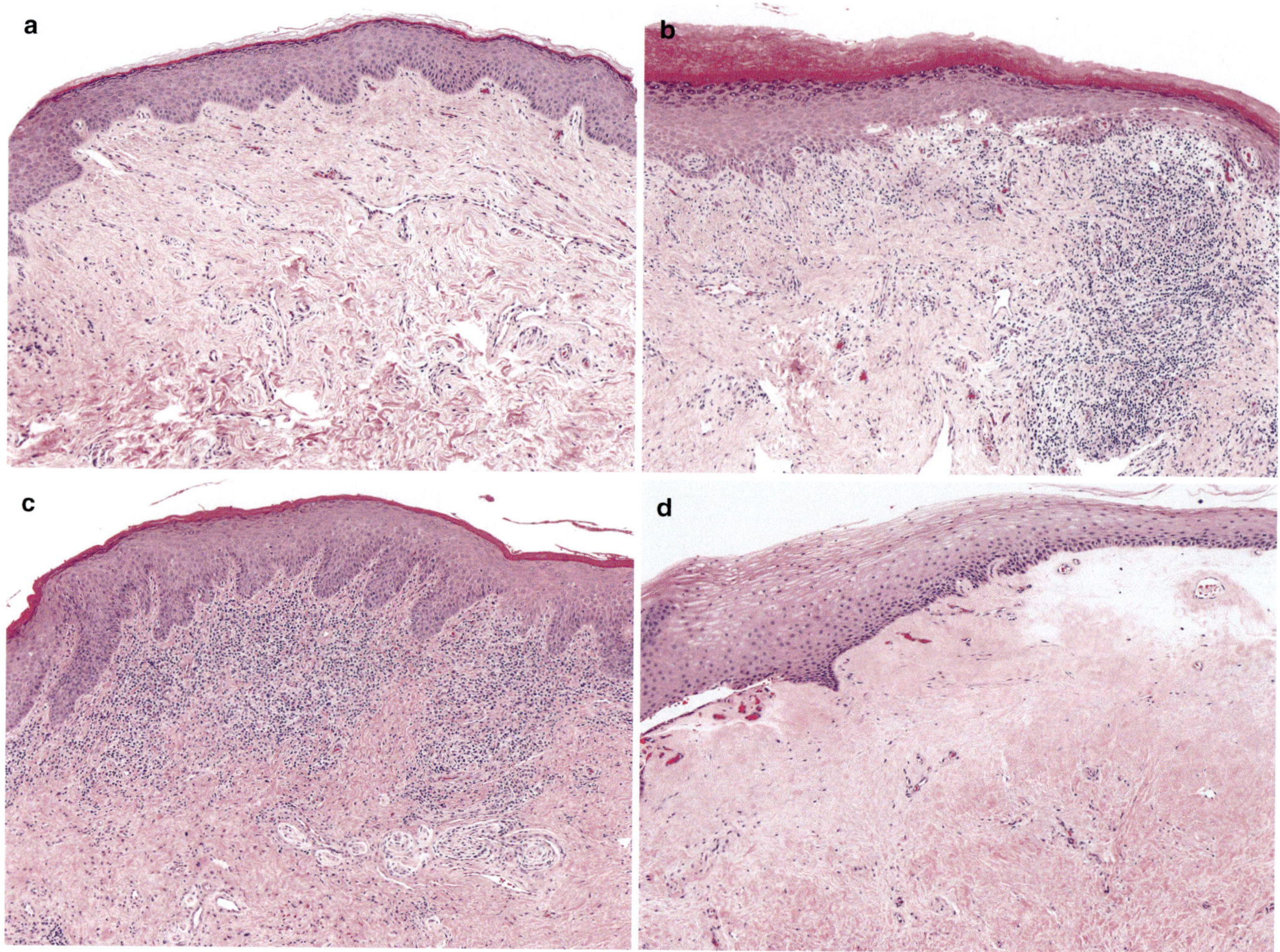

Fig. 4.8 (**a**) Penile urethra with mild keratinizing squamous metaplasia. This photo is taken from the area adjacent to lichen sclerosus for comparison. (**b**) Lichen sclerosus of the penile stricture with increased squamous metaplasia, hyper- and parakeratosis, and nonspecific chronic inflammation. (**c**) Lichen sclerosus at inflammatory phase with band-like chronic inflammation of subepithelial stroma. (**d**) Lichen sclerosus et atrophicus showing basal cell loss, clefting, and underlying paucicellular collagenized and edematous stroma

Histologic Findings

- Low magnification with club-like and finger-like projections of fibrovascular cores lined by benign-appearing urothelium (Fig. 4.13a).
- Unremarkable surface urothelium transitioning into the anastomosing nests with hyperplasia, squamous metaplasia with gland-like and cystic change (Fig. 4.13b).

Differential Diagnosis

- Urothelial papilloma.
- Florid polypoid-papillary urethritis.
- Fibroepithelial polyp.

IHC and Other Ancillary Studies

- Not performed.

Final Diagnosis

Fibroepithelial Polyp Associated with Florid Cystitis Cystica and Glandularis

Take-Home Messages

1. Fibroepithelial polyp is a pseudotumorous condition with marked male predominance and typically occurring in boys under 10 years of age or young adult patients.
2. Fibroepithelial polyps have equally represented fibrous and epithelial components, lack significant stromal edema or inflammation, as well as the history of instrumentation/trauma typical for polypoid-papillary urethritis.
3. In contrast to urothelial papilloma, fibroepithelial polyps do not have true branching of papillary structures, but dis-

Table 4.9 Inverted urothelial papilloma

Feature	Description
Definition	Most common benign proliferative urothelial lesion with endophytic growth
Patients	Males > females
Etiology	Same as in the urinary bladder; controversy about true neoplastic nature
Symptoms	Hematuria, irritative urinary symptoms; rarely asymptomatic
Gross	Polypoid or nodular circumscribed lesion up to 3 cm in size with smooth surface
Histology	Composed of invaginated interconnected cords, anastomosing islands and compressed nests of benign urothelium with endophytic growth and palisading; squamous metaplasia and cyst formation may be seen; cells with nuclear grooving and bland cytology; rare mitoses
Ancillary test	CK20 pattern similar to normal urothelium, low proliferative rare by Ki67
Differential DX	Invasive urothelial carcinoma; florid von Brunn's proliferation
Prognosis	Excellent, rarely recur

Table 4.10 Conventional urothelial papilloma (exophytic)

Feature	Description
Definition	Rare benign proliferative urothelial lesion with exophytic growth
Patients	Males >>> females
Etiology	Same as in the urinary bladder
Symptoms	Hematuria, irritative urinary symptoms; rarely asymptomatic
Gross	Prostatic urethra with exophytic protruding papillary mass
Histology	Discrete papillary projections with thin fibrovascular cores covered by normal-appearing urothelium
Ancillary test	CK20 positive umbrella cells
Differential DX	Low-grade papillary urothelial carcinoma
Prognosis	Excellent, rarely recur

play club-like or finger-like projections of the abundant dense supporting stroma.

References: [49, 50].

Case 3

Learning Objectives
1. To become familiar with the histologic features of the lesion.
2. To become familiar with the immunohistochemical features of the lesion and its mimics.
3. To generate the differential diagnosis.

Table 4.11 Squamous papilloma

Feature	Description
Definition	Very rare benign proliferative squamous lesion
Patients	Females >> males
Etiology	Unknown, but not HPV-related
Symptoms	Asymptomatic or present with irritative urinary symptoms and hematuria
Gross	Small polypoid solitary lesion
Histology	Fibrovascular fronds lined by mature squamous epithelium lacking morphologic features of HPV infection
Ancillary test	Negative for HPV 6/11, 16/18, 31/33; p53 wild-type expression
Differential Dx	Condyloma acuminatum and well-differentiated squamous cell carcinoma
Prognosis	Excellent; no recurrence

Table 4.12 Villous adenoma

Feature	Description
Definition	Benign glandular neoplasm with papillary-villiform growth pattern
Patients	Older patients, males >>> females
Etiology	Uncertain
Symptoms	Hematuria, irritative urinary symptoms; rarely asymptomatic
Gross	Bulbous or prostatic urethra with delicate papillary lesion
Histology	Villiform papillae lined by columnar and goblet cells containing abundant mucin; elongated pseudostratified nuclei with mild to moderate atypia, rare mitoses
Ancillary test	Positive for CK20/CEA; often CK7 positive; negative for CDX2, PSA and PSAP
Differential Dx	Urethritis glandularis, adenocarcinoma (ductal prostatic; primary or secondary)
Prognosis	Excellent prognosis if pure adenoma, but malignant transformation in ~50% cases

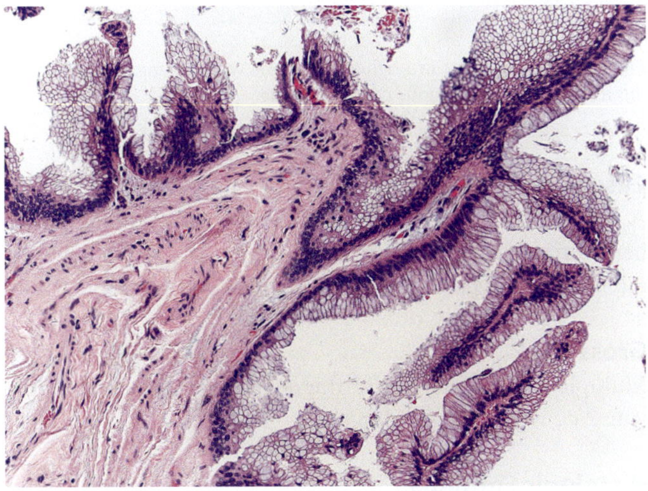

Fig. 4.9 Villous adenoma with papillary formation, columnar, and goblet cells containing abundant mucin, elongated pseudostratified nuclei with mild atypia

Table 4.13 Distinctive clinicopathological characteristics of primary urothelial and squamous cell carcinomas of urethra

Feature	Urothelial carcinoma	Squamous cell carcinoma
Incidence	20% of all urethral cancers	70% of all urethral cancers
Location	Proximal 1/3 of urethra	Distal 2/3 of urethra, meatus
Patients	Mean age 65	Sixth to seventh decade
Associated lesions	Urothelial carcinoma in situ	Urethral stenosis, diverticulum or fistula; squamous metaplasia and CIS
Symptoms	Palpable mass, dysuria, hematuria or obstructive urinary symptoms	Palpable mass, obstructive symptoms; hematuria, infection and irritation signs
Gross	Large endo- or exophytic fleshy hemorrhagic mass	Exophytic cauliflower-like mass could be ulcerated, with cheesy debris or white scaly surface
Histology	Papillary or nonpapillary, majority are high-grade urothelial carcinomas with squamous, glandular or sarcomatoid differentiation (Fig. 4.10a)	Keratinizing or nonkeratinizing with intercellular bridges and keratin pearls; moderately to poorly differentiated with deep invasion (Fig. 4.10b)
Diagnostic criteria	Rule out synchronous or metachronous urothelial carcinoma of the urinary bladder or prostatic ducts	Rule out primary penile or vulvar squamous cell carcinoma
Ancillary studies	Positive for GATA3, CK20, CK7, p63 and Uroplakin; some positive for HPV 6/11	Positive for p53, p63, CK5/6; GATA3, CK7 and Uroplakin negative; >30% positive for HPV 16
Regional spread	Deep pelvic and hypogastric lymph nodes	Inguinal lymph nodes
Prognosis	Stage-related; better than for squamous carcinoma, but worse than primary bladder urothelial carcinoma	Stage-related, but in general poor outcome

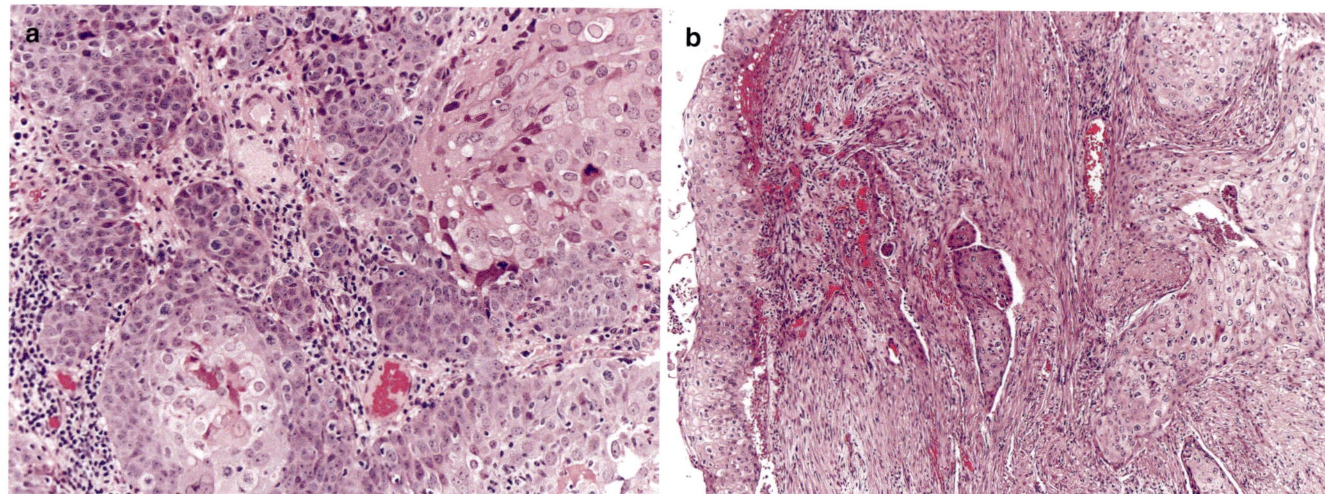

Fig. 4.10 (**a**) Invasive urothelial carcinoma with squamous differentiation. (**b**) Distal segment of urethral with squamous metaplasia and underlying invasive pure squamous cell carcinoma

Case History

A 59-year-old previously healthy woman complained of hematuria and urinary frequency was found to have a polypoid mass in her proximal urethra, which was biopsied.

Gross

Multiple pink hemorrhagic fragments measuring in aggregate 2 cc were submitted in total.

Histologic Findings

– Surface urothelium transitioned to papillary and tubular structures lined by clear to oncocytic cells with hobnailing and slightly enlarged hyperchromatic nuclei (Fig. 4.14a).

– Mixture of superficial papillary architecture and deep compact tubules and glands embedded into edematous stroma with focal hemorrhages (Fig. 4.14b).

– Some glands are cystically dilated and lined by pseudostratified crowded cells with prominent nucleoli but no mitoses; stroma with mucinous change (Fig. 4.14c).

Differential Diagnosis

- Nephrogenic adenoma.
- Reactive proliferation of periurethral Skene glands.
- Clear cell adenocarcinoma.

IHC and Other Ancillary Studies

- CK7/ CK20 positive.

Table 4.14 Conventional adenocarcinoma (~80%)

Feature	Description
Definition	Malignant epithelial neoplasm with pure glandular component
Etiology	Surface urothelium with chronic inflammatory insult or diverticula
Location	Females: Proximal urethra, males: Bulbomembranous urethra
Symptoms	Irritative symptoms, hematuria, recurrent infections, prolapsing mass
Gross	Polypoid-papillary mass with compression or protrusion into the urethra; often with hemorrhage and necrosis
Associated lesions	Diverticula, stricture, fistula, chronic urethritis with glandular, cystic or colonic metaplasia, villous adenoma with dysplasia
Histology	Glandular, papillary and/or cribriform architecture with columnar and goblet cells (enteric type), mucin production (colloid or mucinous type), signet-ring cells or poorly differentiated pleomorphic type (not otherwise specified—NOS)
Ancillary tests	Positive for CEA; could be positive for CK7/CK20/ HMWCK; negative for PSA/PSAP/NKX3.1/ CDX2/β-catenin/GATA3/Uroplakin
Differential DX	Primary urothelial carcinoma with extensive glandular differentiation; secondary involvement by bladder, prostate, or colorectal adenocarcinoma
Prognosis	Similar to urothelial carcinoma (stage dependent)

Table 4.15 Clear cell adenocarcinoma (~15%)

Feature	Description
Definition	Malignant epithelial neoplasm resembling Mullerian clear cell carcinoma (also known as mesonephric or glycogen-rich adenocarcinoma)
Etiology	From metaplastic surface urothelium or periurethral glands
Location	Females >> males: Proximal urethra
Symptoms	Irritative symptoms, gross hematuria, polypoid mass
Gross	Exophytic mass with compression or protrusion into the urethra; hemorrhage and necrosis are common
Associated lesions	Diverticulum and Mullerian-type metaplasia
Histology	Combination of tubulo-papillary, micropapillary, acinar, and solid growth patterns with abundant clear to eosinophilic hobnailed cells containing glycogen (not mucin). Nuclei are large, hyperchromatic and pleomorphic
Ancillary tests	Positive for HNF-β1/CK7/CK20/PAX8/CEA/p53/ P504; negative for PSA/PSAP/NKX3.1/p63/GATA3/ ER/PR
Differential DX	Nephrogenic adenoma; secondary involvement by gynecologic, prostate or renal cell carcinoma
Prognosis	Similar to conventional adenocarcinoma (stage dependent)

- PAX8 positive.
- p53 positive,
- ER/PR negative.

Table 4.16 Adenocarcinoma of accessory glands (~5%)

Feature	Description
Definition	Adenocarcinomas arising from Skene glands in females, Littre or Cowper glands in males
Etiology	Unknown
Location	Females: Distal segment of urethra is most common site; males—Bulbomembranous urethra (Cowper glands) or penile urethra (Littre glands)
Symptoms	Nonspecific: Hematuria, dysuria, progressive urinary obstruction
Gross	Can form a mass or an ulcerated lesion
Associated lesions	Hyperplasia of accessory glands
Histology	Glandular, tubulopapillary, micropapillary architectures with columnar or cuboidal cells with large hyperchromatic nuclei
Ancillary tests	Positive for pan-cytokeratin, CEA and S100 (insufficient studies)
Differential DX	Primary adenocarcinoma, NOS or clear cell adenocarcinoma (both lack involvement of adjacent accessory glands)
Prognosis	Similar to conventional adenocarcinoma (stage dependent)

Final Diagnosis

Clear Cell Adenocarcinoma.

Take-Home Messages

1. Clear cell adenocarcinoma represents 15% of urethral adenocarcinomas with marked female predominance and morphologically are indistinguishable from its Mullerian counterpart.
2. Some cases could have very subtle morphology without frankly malignant features like marked pleomorphism, presence of necrosis, and high mitotic rates, thus closely resembling reactive lesions like nephrogenic adenoma, especially in superficial biopsies.
3. PAX8 is not helpful in the differential diagnosis of primary or metastatic clear cell adenocarcinoma and nephrogenic adenoma, since all these lesions are positive.

References: [51, 52].

Case 4

Learning Objectives

1. To become familiar with the histologic features of the lesion.
2. To become familiar with the immunohistochemical features of the lesion and its mimics.
3. To generate the differential diagnosis.

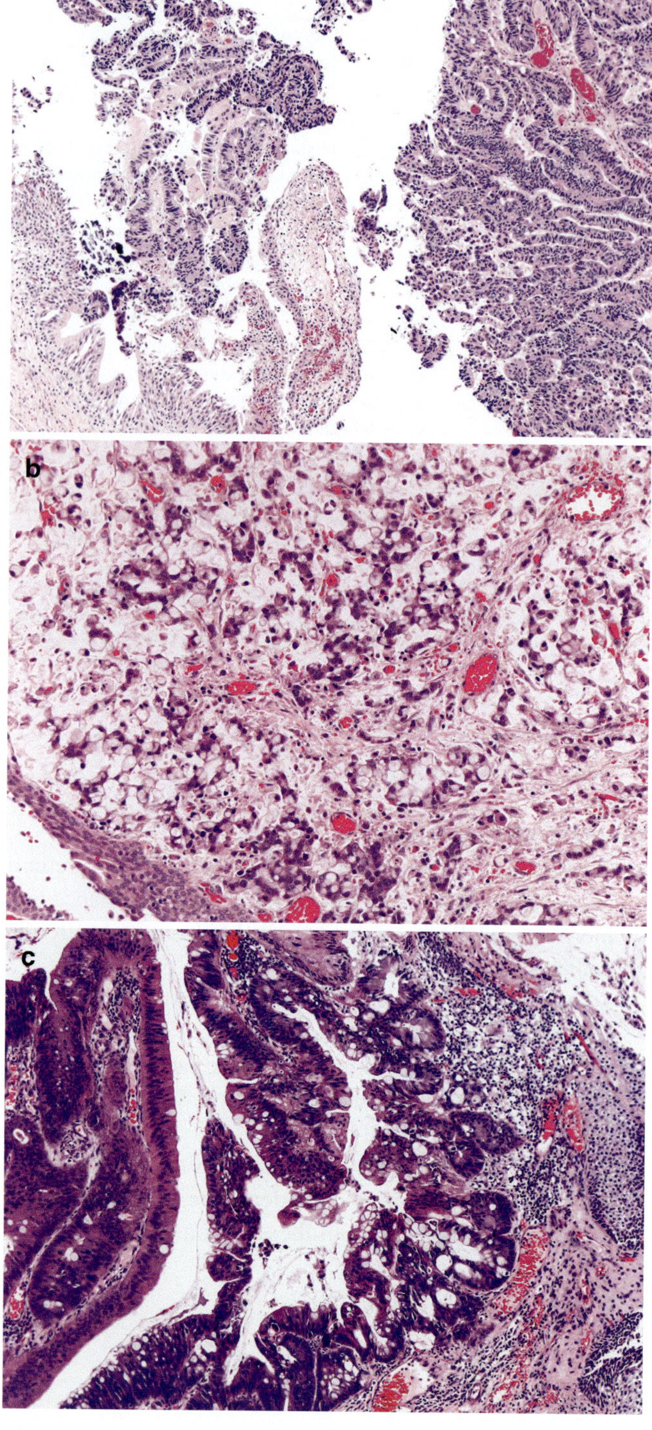

Fig. 4.11 (**a**) Adenocarcinoma of the urethra with glandular and villiform architecture lacking mucin production of intestinal-type differentiation (Adenocarcinoma, NOS). (**b**) Adenocarcinoma with prominent mucin production and signet-ring formation. (**c**) Adenocarcinoma with columnar and goblet cells (enteric type)

Case History

The 69-year-old man has a history of prostate cancer (Gleason $3 + 3 = 6$, clinical T1 prostate cancer), status post prior external beam, external beam radiotherapy and brachytherapy. The patient has recently developed microhematuria in the setting of lower urinary tract symptoms and on cystoscopy he was found to have an obliterative stricture.

Gross

Proximal segment of pink-tan bulbar prostatic urethra resection specimen with a central lumen measuring 0.3–0.5 cm which is serially sectioned and submitted in total.

Histologic Findings

- Ulcerated urethral mucosa associated with marked chronic and active inflammation and near occlusion of the urethral lumen (Fig. 4.15a).
- Focus of infiltrating glandular structures lined by a single layer of atypical flattened to cuboidal epithelium with visible nucleoli (Fig. 4.15b).

Differential Diagnosis

- Prostatic adenocarcinoma.
- Nephrogenic adenoma.
- Inflammation with reactive changes of periurethral glands.

IHC and Other Ancillary Studies

- AMACR (P504) strongly positive.
- P63 negative.
- PAX8 positive (Fig. 4.15c).
- PSA negative.

Final Diagnosis

Nephrogenic Adenoma of the Urethra.

Take-Home Messages

1. Nephrogenic adenoma with pure tubular architecture represent ~15% of all cases in the genitourinary tract and morphologically could mimic prostatic adenocarcinoma.
2. Prostatic adenocarcinoma cannot be distinguished from nephrogenic adenoma by positive AMACR and negative p63 since both lesions show the same staining pattern.
3. Combination of PAX8 and prostate-specific markers are recommended ancillary studies to rule out prostate cancer (PSA/PSAP/NKX3.1 positive) and confirm the diagnosis of nephrogenic adenoma (PAX8 positive as opposed to negative periurethral glands and prostate cancer).

References: [53, 54].

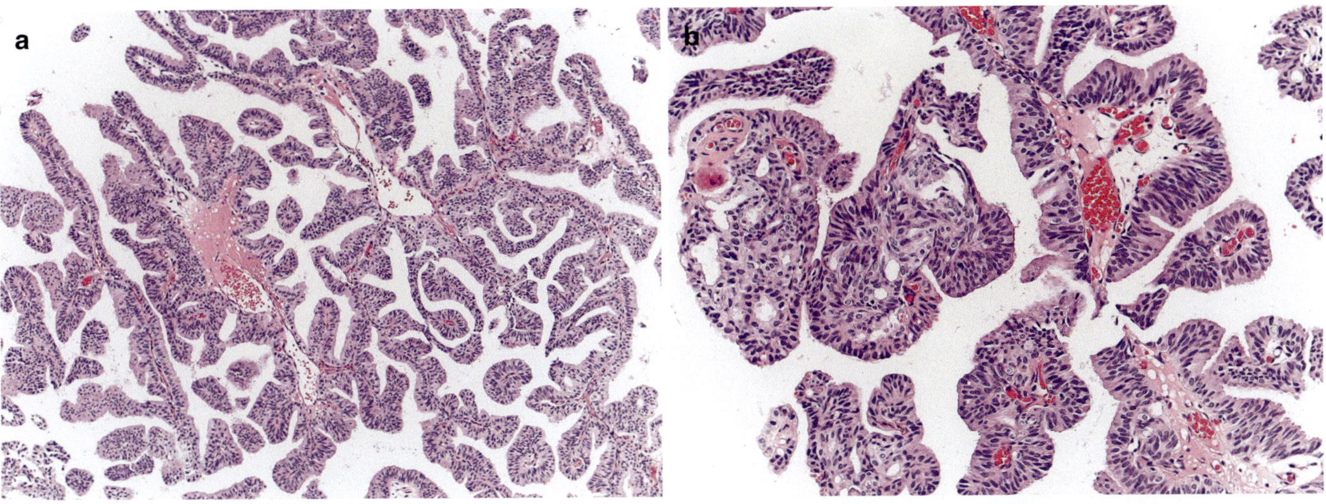

Fig. 4.12 (**a**) Papillary proliferation with thin fibrovascular cores lined by columnar cells with mild atypia, enlarged nuclei, and focal pseudostratification. (**b**) Papillary and focally cribriform growth pattern. Elongated crowded tumor cells with hyperchromasia and scattered mitoses

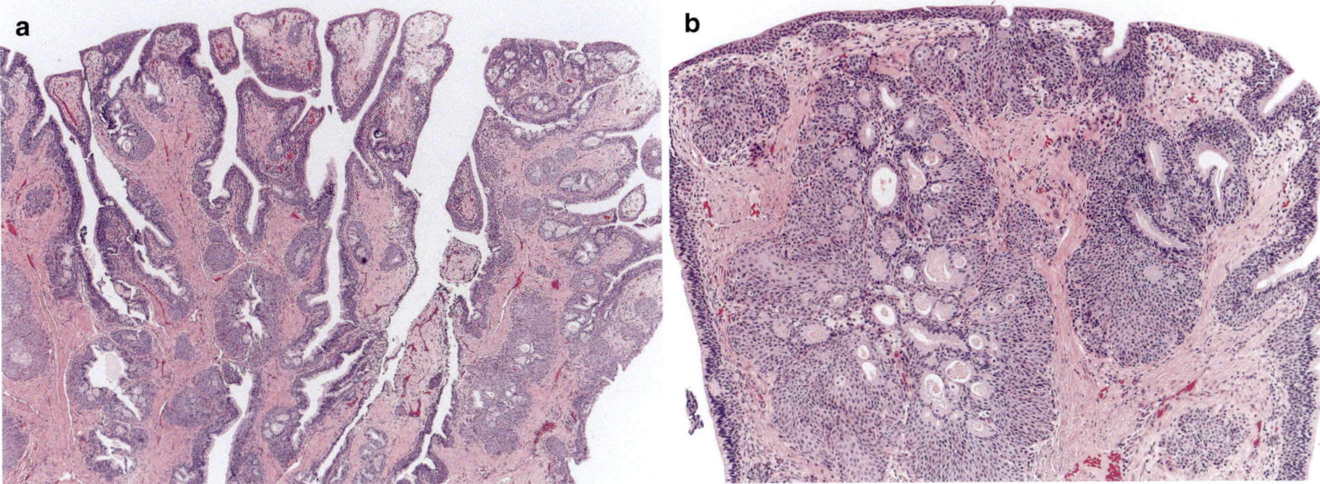

Fig. 4.13 (**a**) Low magnification with club-like and finger-like projections of fibrovascular cores lined by benign-appearing urothelium. (**b**) Unremarkable surface urothelium transitioning into the anastomosing nests with hyperplasia, squamous metaplasia with gland-like and cystic change

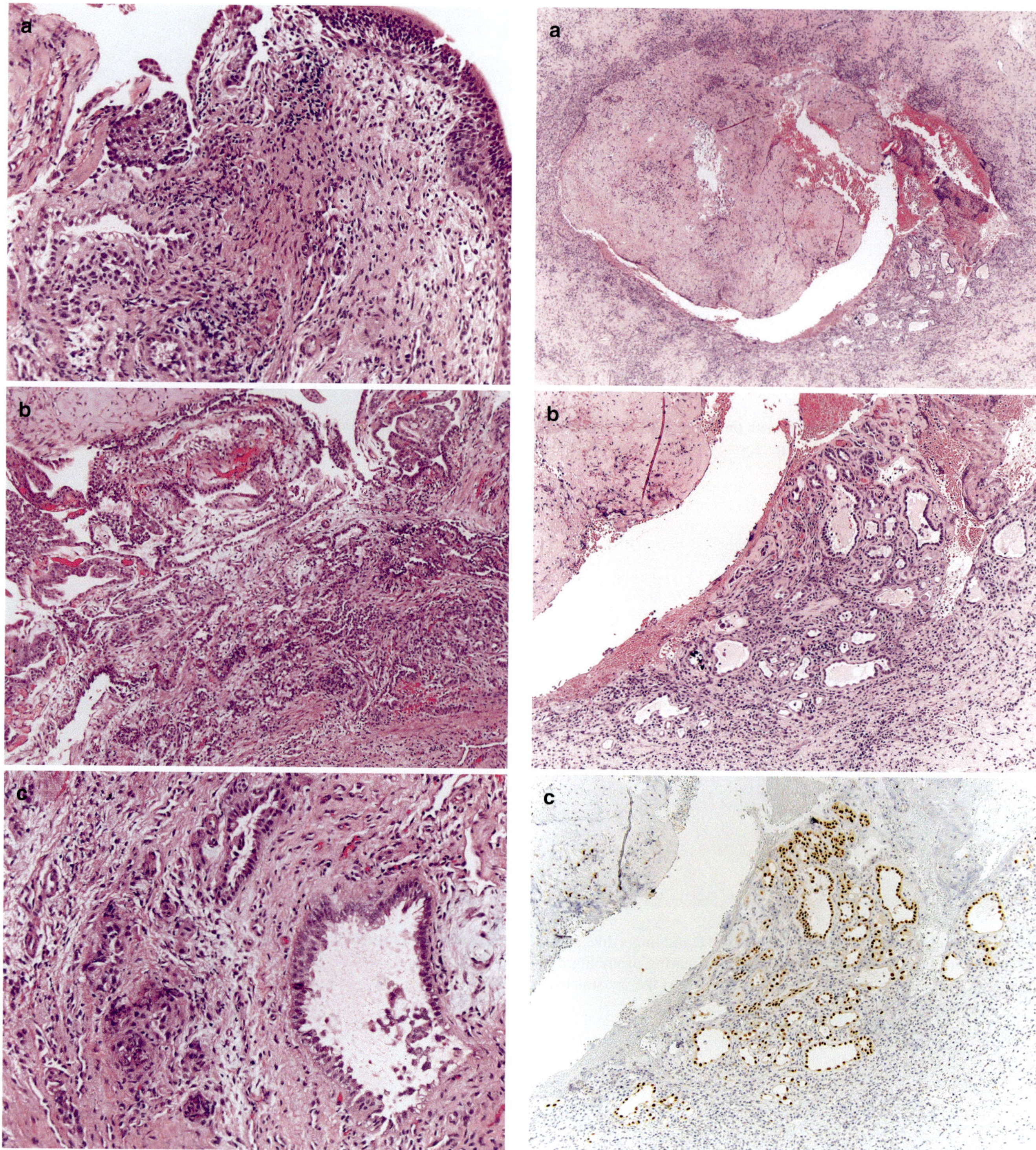

Fig. 4.14 (**a**) Surface urothelium transitioned to papillary and tubular structures lined by clear to oncocytic cells with hobnailing and slightly enlarged hyperchromatic nuclei. (**b**) Mixture of superficial papillary architecture and deep compact tubules and glands embedded into edematous stroma with focal hemorrhages. (**c**) Some glands are cystically dilated and lined by pseudostratified crowded cells with prominent nucleoli but no mitoses; stroma with mucinous change

Fig. 4.15 (**a**) Ulcerated urethral mucosa associated with marked chronic and active inflammation and near occlusion of the urethral lumen. (**b**) Focus of infiltrating glandular structures lined by a single layer of atypical flattened to cuboidal epithelium with visible nucleoli. (**c**) PAX8 positive

References

1. Carroll PR, Dixon CM. Surgical anatomy of the male and female urethra. Urol Clin North Am. 1992;19(2):339–46. Review

2. Krishnan A, de Souza A, Konijeti R, Baskin LS. The anatomy and embryology of posterior urethral valves. J Urol. 2006;175(4):1214–20. Review

3. McNeal JE, Bostwick DG. Anatomy of the prostatic urethra. JAMA. 1984;251(7):890–1.

4. Kurzrock EA, Baskin LS, Cunha GR. Ontogeny of the male urethra: theory of endodermal differentiation. Differentiation. 1999;64(2):115–22.

5. Moore L, Dalley AF, Agur AM. Clinically oriented anatomy, 7th edition, by Keith. Baltimore: Lippincott Williams & Wilkins; 2014.

6. Eckoldt F, Heling KS, Woderich R, Wolke S. Posterior urethral valves: prenatal diagnostic signs and outcome. Urol Int. 2004;73(4):296–301.

7. Dinneen MD, Duffy PG. Posterior urethral valves. Br J Urol. 1996;78(2):275–81.

8. Paulhac P, Fourcade L, Lesaux N, Alain JL, Colombeau P. Anterior urethral valves and diverticula. BJU Int. 2003;92(5):506–9.

9. Prasad N, Vivekanandhan KG, Ilangovan G, Prabakaran S. Duplication of the urethra. Pediatr Surg Int. 1999;15(5–6):419–21.

10. Jones EA, Freedman AL, Ehrlich RM. Megalourethra and urethral diverticula. Urol Clin North Am. 2002;29(2):341–8. vi. Review

11. Wang MH, Baskin LS. Endocrine disruptors, genital development, and hypospadias. J Androl. 2008;29(5):499–505.

12. Thomas AA, Rackley RR, Lee U, Goldman HB, Vasavada SP, Hansel DE. Urethral diverticula in 90 female patients: a study with emphasis on neoplastic alterations. J Urol. 2008;180(6):2463–7.

13. Young RH, Oliva E, Garcia JA, Bhan AK, Clement PB. Urethral caruncle with atypical stromal cells simulating lymphoma or sarcoma--a distinctive pseudoneoplastic lesion of females. A report of six cases. Am J Surg Pathol. 1996;20(10):1190–5.

14. Chan JK, Chow TC, Tsui MS. Prostatic-type polyps of the lower urinary tract: three histogenetic types? Histopathology. 1987;11(8):789–801.

15. Remick DG Jr, Kumar NB. Benign polyps with prostatic-type epithelium of the urethra and the urinary bladder. A suggestion of histogenesis based on histologic and immunohistochemical studies. Am J Surg Pathol. 1984;8(11):833–9.

16. Tsuzuki T, Epstein JI. Fibroepithelial polyp of the lower urinary tract in adults. Am J Surg Pathol. 2005;29(4):460–6.

17. Bevers RF, Abbekerk EM, Boon TA. Cowper's syringocele: symptoms, classification and treatment of an unappreciated problem. J Urol. 2000;163(3):782–4.

18. Miller EV. Skene's duct cyst. J Urol. 1984;131(5):966–7.

19. Singh M, Blandy JP. The pathology of urethral stricture. J Urol. 1976;115(6):673–6.

20. Morgia G, Saita A, Falsaperla M, Spampinato A, Motta M, Cordaro S. Immunohistochemical and molecular analysis in recurrent urethral stricture. Urol Res. 2000;28(5):319–22.

21. Brandes SB. Epidemiology, etiology, histology, classification, and economic impact of urethral stricture disease. In: Current clinical urology: urethral reconstructive surgery: Springer; Humana press, Totowa, NJ. 2008.

22. Santucci RA, Joyce GF, Wise M. Male urethral stricture disease. J Urol. 2007;177(5):1667–74.

23. Cavalcanti AG, Costa WS, Baskin LS, McAninch JA, Sampaio FJ. A morphometric analysis of bulbar urethral strictures. BJU Int. 2007;100(2):397–402.

24. Lumen N, Hoebeke P, Willemsen P, De troyer B, Pieters R, Oosterlinck W. Etiology of urethral stricture disease in the 21st century. J Urol. 2009;182(3):983–7.

25. Voelzke BB. Critical review of existing patient reported outcome measures after male anterior urethroplasty. J Urol. 2013;189(1):182–8.

26. Patel P, Reikie BA, Maxwell JP, Yilmaz A, Gotto GT, Trpkov K. Long-term clinical outcome of inverted urothelial papilloma including cases with focal papillary pattern: is continuous surveillance necessary? Urology. 2013;82(4):857–60.

27. Fine SW, Chan TY, Epstein JI. Inverted papillomas of the prostatic urethra. Am J Surg Pathol. 2006;30(8):975–9.

28. McKenney JK, Amin MB, Young RH. Urothelial (transitional cell) papilloma of the urinary bladder: a clinicopathologic study of 26 cases. Mod Pathol. 2003;16(7):623–9.

29. Gustafson P, Fenster HN, So AI. Urethral squamous cell papilloma: case report and literature review. Can Urol Assoc J. 2014;8(5–6):E364–5.

30. Cheng L, Leibovich BC, Cheville JC, et al. Squamous papilloma of the urinary tract is unrelated to condyloma acuminata. Cancer. 2000;88(7):1679–86.

31. Seibel JL, Prasad S, Weiss RE, Bancila E, Epstein JI. Villous adenoma of the urinary tract: a lesion frequently associated with malignancy. Hum Pathol. 2002;33(2):236–41.

32. Kakizoe T, Tobisu K. Transitional cell carcinoma of the urethra in men and women associated with bladder cancer. Jpn J Clin Oncol. 1998;28(6):357–9. Review

33. Amin MB, Young RH. Primary carcinomas of the urethra. Semin Diagn Pathol. 1997;14(2):147–60. Review

34. Wiener JS, Effert PJ, Humphrey PA, et al. Prevalence of human papillomavirus types 16 and 18 in squamous-cell carcinoma of the penis: a retrospective analysis of primary and metastatic lesions by differential polymerase chain reaction. Int J Cancer. 1992;50(5):694–701.

35. Kim SJ, MacLennan GT. Tumors of the male urethra. J Urol. 2005;174(1):312.

36. Chaux A, Reuter V, Lezcano C, et al. Comparison of morphologic features and outcome of resected recurrent and nonrecurrent squamous cell carcinoma of the penis: a study of 81 cases. Am J Surg Pathol. 2009;33(9):1299–306.

37. Guma S, Maglantay R, Lau R, et al. Papillary urothelial carcinoma with squamous differentiation in association with human papilloma virus: case report and literature review. Am J Clin Exp Urol. 2016;4(1):12–6.

38. Zhang M, Adeniran AJ, Vikram R, et al. Carcinoma of the urethra. Hum Pathol. 2018;72:35–44.

39. Bourque JL, Charghi A, Gauthier GE, et al. Primary carcinoma of Cowper's gland. J Urol. 1970;103(6):758–61.

40. Sacks SA, Waisman J, Apfelbaum HB, et al. Urethral adenocarcinoma (possibly originating in the glands of Littre). J Urol. 1975;113(1):50–5.

41. Meis JM, Ayala AG, Johnson DE. Adenocarcinoma of the urethra in women. A clinicopathologic study. Cancer. 1987;60(5):1038–52.

42. Mostofi FK, Davis CJ Jr, Sesterhenn IA. Carcinoma of the male and female urethra. Urol Clin North Am. 1992;19(2):347–58.

43. Osunkoya AO, Epstein JI. Primary mucin-producing urothelial-type adenocarcinoma of prostate: report of 15 cases. Am J Surg Pathol. 2007;31(9):1323–9.

44. Brimo F, Herawi M, Sharma R, et al. Hepatocyte nuclear factor-1β expression in clear cell adenocarcinomas of the bladder and urethra: diagnostic utility and implications for histogenesis. Hum Pathol. 2011;42(11):1613–9.

45. Alexiev BA, Tavora F. Histology and immunohistochemistry of clear cell adenocarcinoma of the urethra: histogenesis and diagnostic problems. Virchows Arch. 2013;462(2):193–201.

46. Muto M, Inamura K, Ozawa N. Skene's gland adenocarcinoma with intestinal differentiation: a case report and literature review. Pathol Int. 2017;67(11):575–9.

47. Samaratunga H, Letizia B. Prostatic ductal adenocarcinoma presenting as a urethral polyp: a clinicopathological study of eight

cases of a lesion with the potential to be misdiagnosed as a benign prostatic urethral polyp. Pathology. 2007;39(5):476–81.

48. Paner GP, Lopez-Beltran A, So JS, et al. Spectrum of cystic epithelial tumors of the prostate: most cystadenocarcinomas are ductal type with Intracystic papillary pattern. Am J Surg Pathol. 2016;40(7):886–95.

49. Kumar A, Das SK, Trivedi S, et al. Genito-urinary polyps: summary of the 10-year experiences of a single institute. Int Urol Nephrol. 2008;40(4):901–7.

50. Falahatkar S, Neiroomand H, Akbarpour M. Fibroepithelial congenital polyp of prostatic urethra in an adult man. Urol J. 2009;6(4):301–2.

51. Venyo AK. Clear cell adenocarcinoma of the urethra: review of the literature. Int J Surg Oncol. 2015;2015:790235.

52. Rane SR, Ghodke AN, Vishwasrao S. Clear cell adenocarcinoma of female urethra. J Clin Diagn Res. 2017;11(7):ED01–2.

53. López JI, Schiavo-Lena M, Corominas-Cishek A, et al. Nephrogenic adenoma of the urinary tract: clinical, histological, and immunohistochemical characteristics. Virchows Arch. 2013;463(6):819–25.

54. Turcan D, Acikalin MF, Yilmaz E, et al. Nephrogenic adenoma of the urinary tract: a 6-year single center experience. Pathol Res Pract. 2017;213(7):831–5.

Ximing J. Yang and Ming Zhou

Frequently Asked Questions and Answers

What Are the Histologic Features Pathognomonic or Highly Specific for Prostatic Adenocarcinoma?

Three features, namely, mucinous fibroplasia (collagenous micronodules) (Fig. 5.1a), glomerulation (Fig. 5.1b), and perineural invasion (Fig. 5.1c), have not, to date, been reported in benign glands and are considered specific for prostate cancer. A cancer diagnosis can be rendered when one of the three features is present in biopsy, although it is prudent to confirm the cancer diagnosis with basal cell marker immunostains when the focus is small and does not have other cancer-associated features.

References: [1–3]

What Is the Minimal Number of Glands for Diagnosis of Limited Prostatic Adenocarcinoma?

Such a number depends on the degree of architectural and cytological atypia in the glands suspicious for cancer. With significant atypia, fewer glands are required to make a cancer diagnosis. However, most urological pathology experts require at least three or more atypical glands to make a definitive diagnosis if there are no full-blown cancer-associated architectural and cytological features.

References: [3–6]

X. J. Yang (✉)
Department of Pathology, Northwestern Memorial Hospital, Northwestern University Feinberg School of Medicine, Chicago, IL, USA
e-mail: xyang@northwestern.edu

M. Zhou
Department of Pathology and Laboratory Medicine, Tufts Medical Center, Tufts School of Medicine, Boston, MA, USA

What Is the Difference Between Perineural Invasion by Carcinoma and Perineural Indentation by Benign Prostatic Glands?

In perineural invasion, tumor cells either tightly wrap around a nerve or are in direct contact with nerve in perineural space. This represents the "path of least resistance" for the tumor to extend outside the prostate leading to extraprostatic extension. In contrast, benign prostate glands abut and loosely encircle a nerve fiber in perineural indentation.

The differences between perineural invasion and perineural indentation are the following: in perineural invasion, cancer glands usually show features of carcinoma such as prominent nucleoli and lack of basal cells, but benign glands will not have these features

- In perineural invasion, carcinoma cells tend to wrap tightly around a nerve (Fig. 5.2a), while in perineural indentation benign glands may touch the nerve or partially wrap around a nerve, up to 50% of a nerve circumference, but do not circumferentially wrap around a nerve. Rarely could multiple benign glands entirely surround a nerve (Fig. 5.2b, c).
- Basal cells can be identified in benign glands in perineural indentation, but not in malignant glands in perineural invasion. If there is any doubt, basal cell stains will confirm the presence of basal cells in benign glands in perineural indentation and lack of basal cell in carcinoma in perineural invasion.

References: [2, 7]

What Is the Clinical Significance of Perineural Invasion on Biopsy and Prostatectomy?

Perineural invasion identified on needle biopsy correlates with extraprostatic extension in radical prostatectomy. This

© Springer Nature Switzerland AG 2021
X. J. Yang, M. Zhou (eds.), *Practical Genitourinary Pathology*, Practical Anatomic Pathology,
https://doi.org/10.1007/978-3-030-57141-2_5

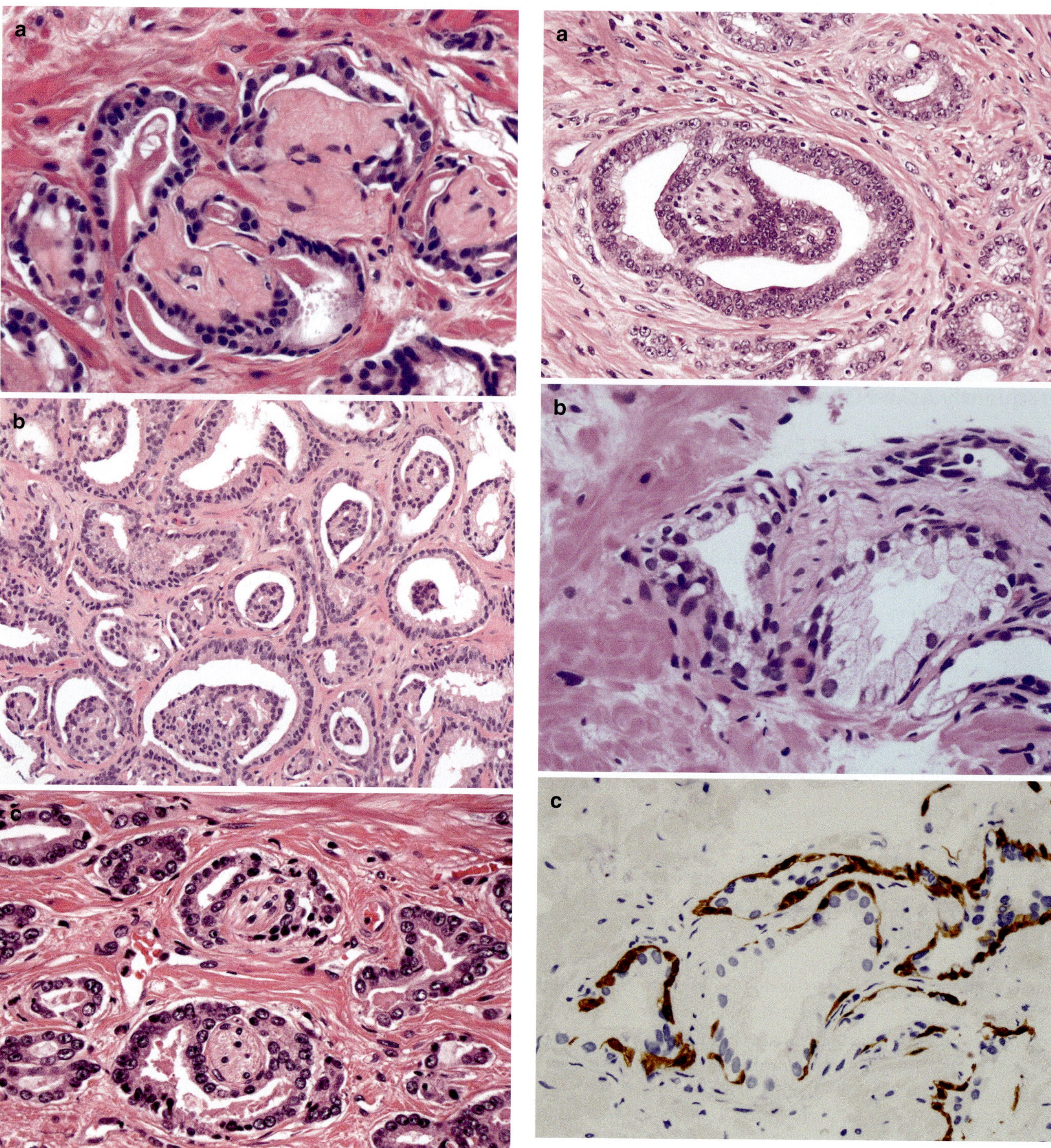

Fig. 5.1 Mucinous fibroplasia (collagenous micronodules) with acellular or hypocellular hyalinized stroma within or outside cancer glands (**a**). Glomeration with balls or tufts of cancer cells within the cancer glands, reminiscent of renal glomeruli (**b**). Perineural invasion with tight, circumferential, or near circumferential encircling of a nerve fiber by cancer glands (**c**)

Fig. 5.2 Perineural invasion by adenocarcinoma. A nerve bundle is wrapped around by a malignant gland (**a**). Perineural indentation by benign glands is characterized by several benign glands surrounding a nerve bundle (**b**). These benign glands do not show cytological atypia and contain basal cells confirmed by positive basal cell immunostaining (p63 + high molecular weight cytokeratin, (**c**)

information may be used by surgeons to plan nerve-sparing surgery. Some radiation oncology studies suggest that it also independently predicts adverse outcomes after radiation therapy. However, it is considered a "category 3" prognostic factor (insufficient data to warrant prognostic utility). It can be reported if found in needle biopsies. Cases that meet biopsy criteria for active surveillance yet have perineural invasion are not significantly different from those without perineural invasion in terms of adverse findings at radical prostatectomy; therefore, perineural invasion in prostate biopsy should not disqualify patients who otherwise meet the inclusion criteria for active surveillance. Perineural invasion is frequently identified in prostatectomy specimens and has not been found to be of prognostic significance for patients after prostatectomy.

References: [8–10]

How to Distinguish Atrophic Carcinoma from Benign Atrophic Glands?

The key for the differential diagnosis is to look for the infiltrating growth pattern and cytological atypia in the suspected atrophic cancer glands.

Despite lacking prominent cytoplasm, atrophic carcinoma still exhibits other architectural and cytological features of prostate cancer. At low magnification (Fig. 5.3), atrophic carcinoma has infiltrative growth and/or crowded glands with scant yet basophilic/amphophilic cytoplasm. Intraluminal secretions including amorphous eosinophilic concretions and blue mucin are often present. The atrophic cancer glands are usually intermixed with nonatrophic conventional acinar adenocarcinoma. Significant nuclear enlargement, hyperchromasia, and prominent nucleoli are usually present and are required for making the diagnosis.

Benign atrophy shows lobulated architecture. It may show mild nuclear atypia. Frank atypia, such as significant nuclear enlargement and prominent nucleoli, is however almost certain indication of atrophic cancer.

In limited sampling such as in needle biopsy with suspcious atrophic glands, it is prudent to apply immunohistochemistry. It is also important to know that atrophic carcinoma may show weaker AMACR reactivity because of scant cytoplasm, but basal cells are absent in atrophic cancer.

References: [2, 11, 12]

What Is Pseudohyperplastic Carcinoma of the Prostate?

Pseudohyperplastic prostate carcinoma is a histological variant of acinar carcinoma that simulates the appearance of nodular prostatic hyperplasia at low magnification due to closely

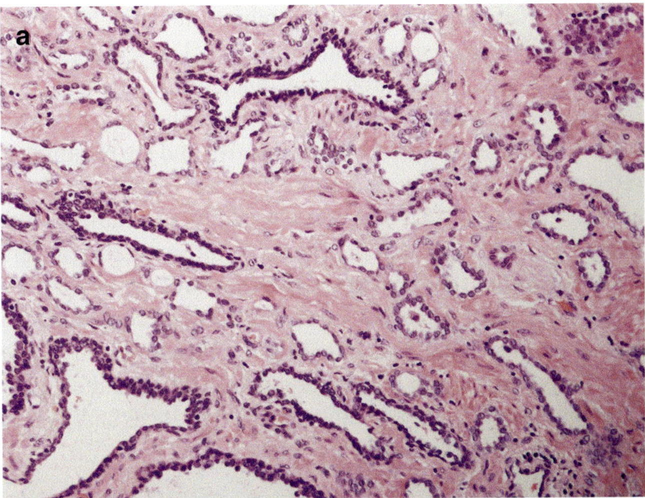

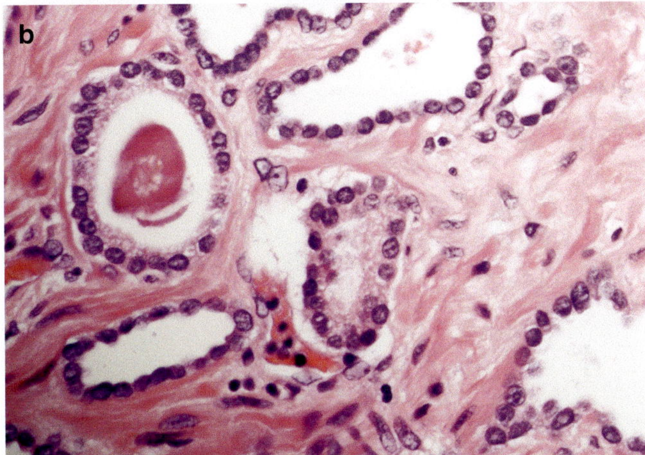

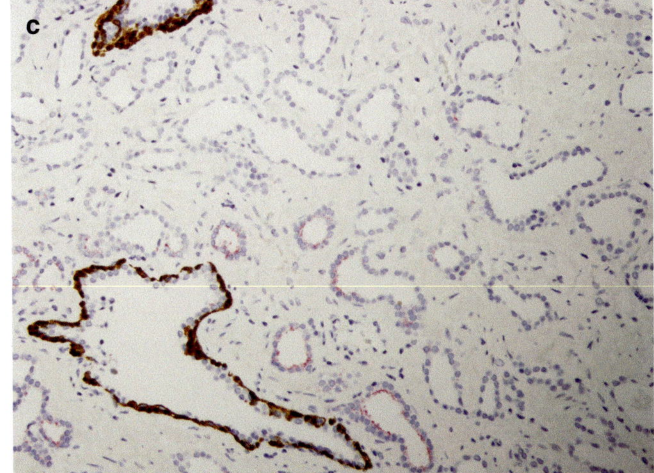

Fig. 5.3 Atrophic prostatic adenocarcinoma. At low magnification, a focus of atrophic carcinoma glands infiltrates between benign glands (**a**). At higher magnification, some cancer glands are not completely atrophic and still display unequivocal malignant histologic features including enlarged nuclei and prominent nucleoli (**b**). Atrophic cancer glands are weakly positive for AMACR and negative for basal cell markers (triple stain, **c**)

packed glands of varying sizes and complex and undulating architecture forming vague nodules. Large glands with undulating architecture are a prominent feature. However, significant nuclear atypia, including nuclear enlargement, hyperchromasia, and prominent nucleoli is present and required for making a cancer diagnosis in needle biopsy (Fig. 5.4). Basal cell markers are negative and are required in most cases. Gleason score for this tumor is usually $3 + 3 = 6$ (grade group 1). The prognosis is likely favorable as the pathological stage is not significantly different for cancers with and without pseudohyperplastic features.

In differential diagnosis, one should always consider nodular hyperplasia and adenosis. While mild nuclear atypia is usually present, frank nuclear atypia should raise the suspicion for cancer. Basal cell staining is often focal and patchy but is nevertheless present.

References: [2, 11, 13]

What Is the Feature of Foamy Gland Carcinoma?

Foamy gland carcinoma is characterized by abundant foamy cytoplasm of the tumor cells that form large (Fig. 5.5a) or small glandular structures. The foamy gland carcinoma cells have deceptively bland cytological features with small and pyknotic nuclei. It is not a stand-alone subtype but a special histologic pattern of prostatic adenocarcinoma. It is almost always associated with adenocarcinoma with typical histological features (Fig. 5.5b). Foamy gland carcinoma is not indicative of an aggressive behavior, so it should be Gleason graded with the same standard as for a typical adenocarcinoma. It important to remember that AMACR immunoreactivity can be weak in some cases of foamy gland carcinoma.

References: [14, 15]

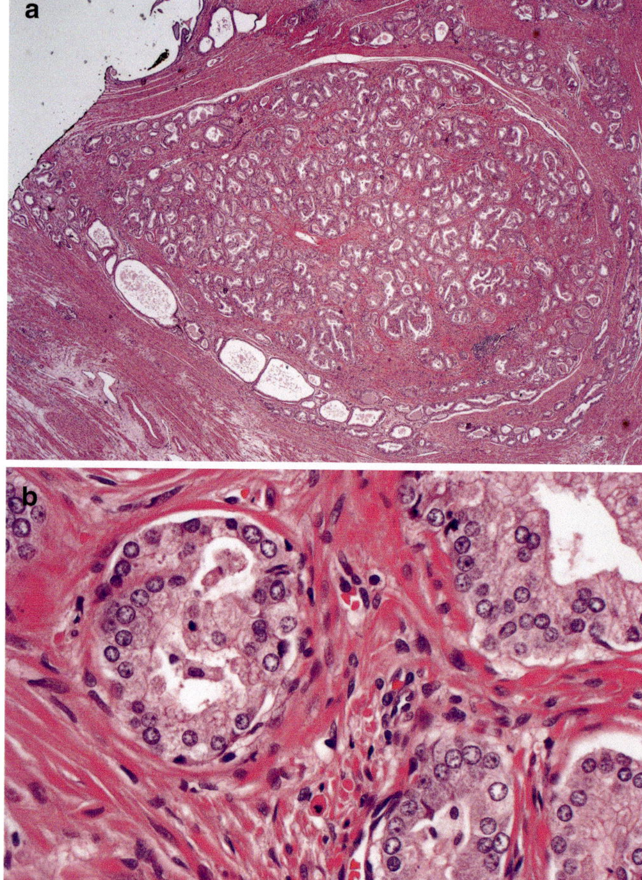

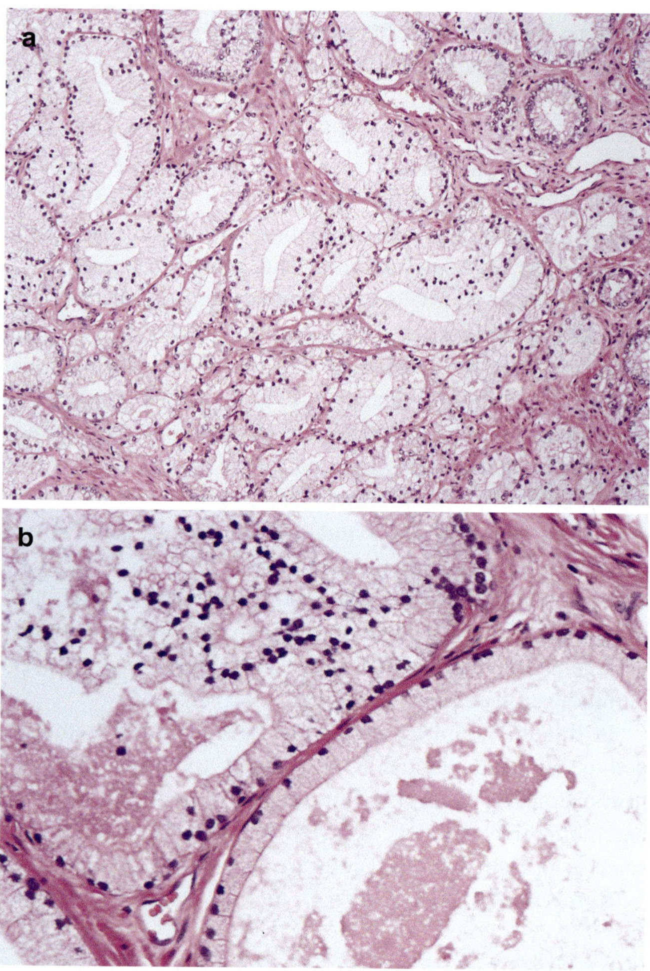

Fig. 5.4 In pseudohyperplastic carcinoma, glands with complex branching demonstrate nodular growth (**a**). At high magnification, cancer glands display cytoplasmic amphophilia and nuclear atypia including nuclear enlargement and prominent nucleoli (**b**)

Fig. 5.5 Foamy gland carcinoma of the prostate (Gleason score 3+4=7, Grade group 2) is composed of cancer glands with abundant foamy cytoplasm and small hyperchromatic nuclei (**a**). Nuclear atypia is not obvious except in a few glands. A few typical cancer glands are usually found (right upper portion). Another case of foamy gland carcinoma composed large foamy glands with a straight luminal border and tumor cells with deceptively bland appearance (**b**)

What Are the Major Diagnostic Criteria for Prostate Cancer?

The histological diagnosis of prostate cancer relies on a combination of architectural and cytological features. Some of these features, however, are more important and more frequently present, and therefore should be weighted heavily for diagnosis and represent major diagnostic criteria. They include infiltrating growth pattern, absence of basal cells, and nuclear atypia.

- The infiltrating growth patterns. The malignant glandular structures often display haphazard infiltrating growth pattern (Fig. 5.6a) instead of the lobular pattern of benign prostatic glands. The rare exceptions are Gleason pattern 2 and rare Gleason pattern 1 that do not demonstrate infiltrating growth pattern.

- Absence of basal cells is the hallmark of prostatic adenocarcinoma (Fig. 5.6b). The absence of basal cell can be confirmed by the negative immunostaining for p63 and high molecular weight cytokeratins (CK5/6, K903, or 34βE12). One caveat is a small subset of p63-positive prostatic adenocarcinoma cells that show diffuse p63 staining. In rare cases, adenocarcinoma may contain patchy basal cells.

- Nuclear atypia is one of the most important features for prostate cancer diagnosis (Fig. 5.6c). It is characterized by the presence of prominent nucleoli, nuclear enlargement, and nuclear hyperchromasia. However, on the needle core biopsy with limited material, up to 20% of prostate cancer cases may not show prominent nucleoli. Furthermore, a number of variants of prostatic adenocarcinoma, such as atrophic carcinoma and foamy gland carcinoma, often do not display prominent nucleoli or other features of atypia. Finally, on rare occasions certain

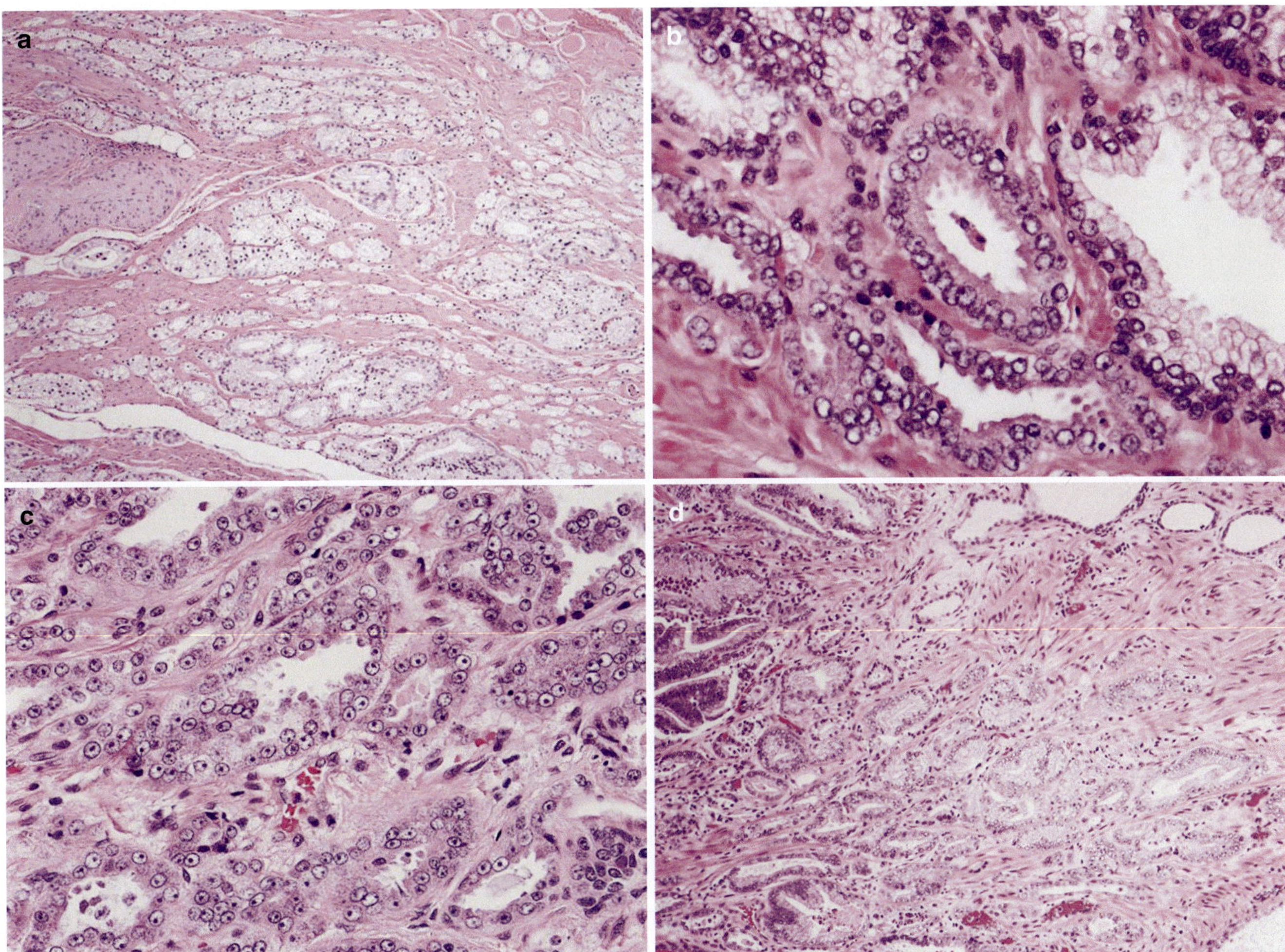

Fig. 5.6 Major diagnostic features of prostatic adenocarcinoma. Prostatic adenocarcinoma exhibits haphazard infiltrating growth pattern with cancer glands extending to the extraprostatic adipose tissue (**a**). Compared to the benign glands with basal cells (**b**), malignant glands (**b**) do not have basal cells. Prostatic adenocarcinoma cells display prominent cytological atypia with prominent nucleoli in most tumor cells (**c**). Typically, prostatic adenocarcinoma shows more than one major diagnostic features. In this case of prostatic adenocarcinoma, infiltrating features, lack of basal cells, and cytological atypia are evident (**d**)

benign conditions such as sclerosing adenosis or reactive atypia may show prominent nucleoli.

In our experience, no single major criterion is sufficient for diagnosis of prostate cancer. In most cases, the diagnosis of prostatic carcinoma will require at least two of the major diagnostic criteria (Fig. 5.6d). It is also important to point out that the application of major criteria should not be rigid; other histological features have to be included in the diagnostic consideration.

References: [2, 5, 16]

What Are Minor Diagnostic Features for Prostate Cancer?

Minor diagnostic features are those histological features that are less strongly associated with cancer, and may also be seen in noncancer lesions. However, they are diagnostically very helpful as the cancer glands with these minor features usually appear significantly different and stand out from the benign glands (Fig. 5.7). These features include the following:

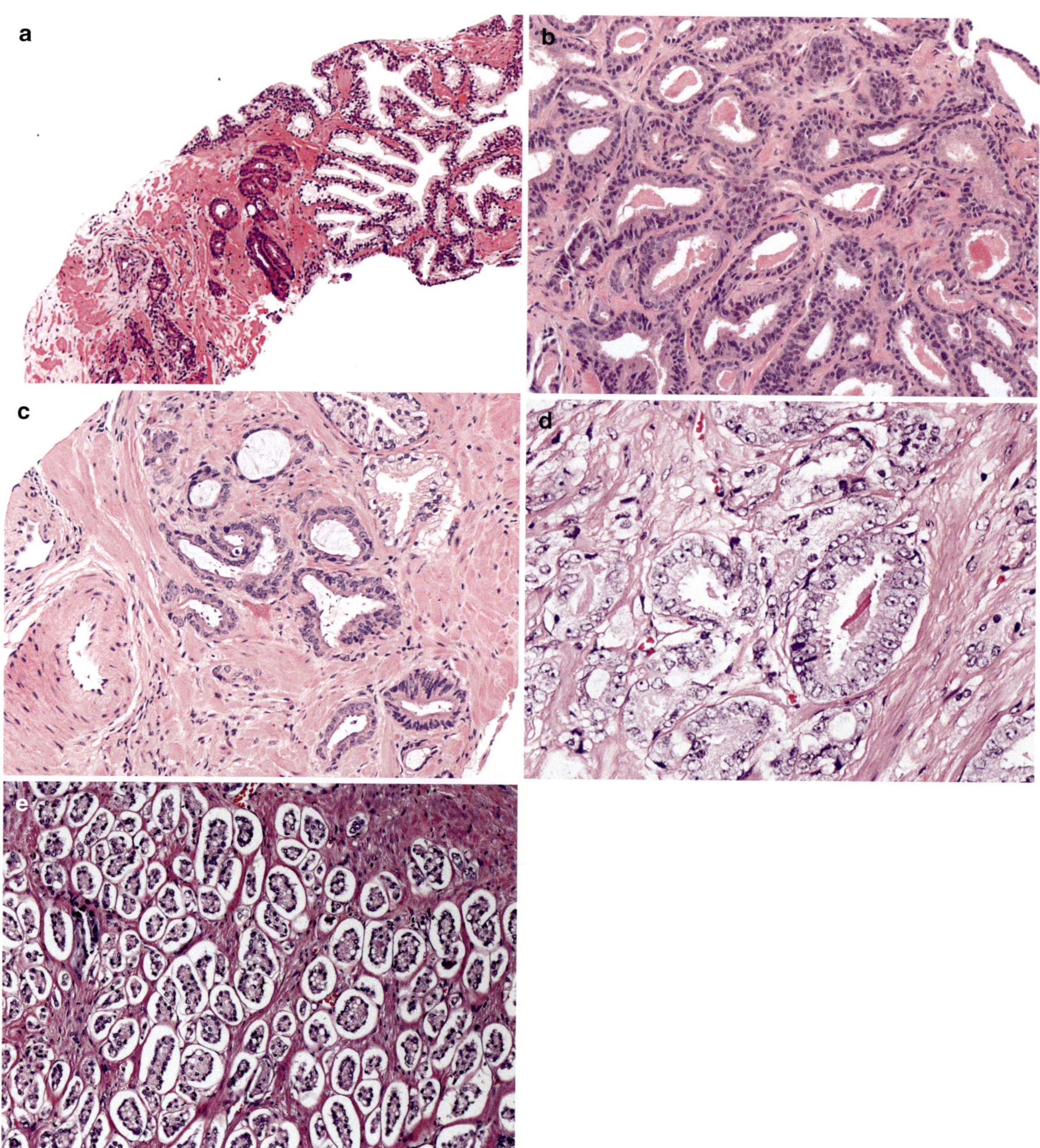

Fig. 5.7 Minor diagnostic features include amphophilic cytoplasm (**a**), amorphous intraluminal secretion (**b**), blue mucin (**c**), crystalloids (**d**), and periacinar retraction clefting (**e**)

- Cytoplasm: cytoplasmic amphophilia (dark cytoplasm) (Fig. 5.7a)
- Intraluminal contents: amorphous secretion, blue mucin, and crystalloids (Fig. 5.7b–d)
- Mitosis and apoptosis
- Periacinar retraction clefting (Fig. 5.7e)
- Adjacent high-grade prostatic intraepithelial neoplasia (HGPIN)

Reference: [2]

How to Make Diagnosis of High-Grade Prostatic Intraepithelial Neoplasia (HGPIN)?

The diagnosis of high-grade PIN is morphological. At low magnification, high-grade PIN glands are dark-appearing with benign architecture. It may partially involve a prostate gland. At high magnification, high-grade PIN glands demonstrate nuclear enlargement, crowding, irregular spacing and stratification with chromatin hyperchromasia, and clumping. The key to the diagnosis is to visualize prominent nucleoli at 20× magnification, or mitosis or pleomorphic nuclei if nucleoli are not prominent (Fig. 5.8). They often have discontinuous basal cell layer marked with HMWCK and p63.

HGPIN should be differentiated from other benign or malignant prostate lesions with "atypical large glandular" pattern, including central zone morphology, reactive atypia to inflammation, infarction or radiation, clear cell cribriform hyperplasia, basal cell hyperplasia, prostate cancer with large glandular pattern, ductal prostate carcinoma, and intraductal carcinoma.

References: [2, 17]

How to Distinguish High-Grade PIN from Prostatic Adenocarcinoma?

HGPIN is defined as neoplastic cell growing within the preexisting ducts or acini of the prostate. Evidence indicates that HGPIN is the precursor of prostate cancer; however, its latency or the time frame of transformation from HGPIN to carcinoma is unknown.

Both HGPIN and adenocarcinoma may display prominent nucleoli and other features of cytologic atypia (Fig. 5.9). However, HGPIN differs from adenocarcinoma by the following features (Table 5.1).

HGPIN glands are usually large with stratified or pseudostratified layers of neoplastic cells, while cancer glands typically contain a single layer of neoplastic cells.

HGPIN is a neoplastic condition confined within preexisting glands. It is not an invasive disease. HGPIN will not

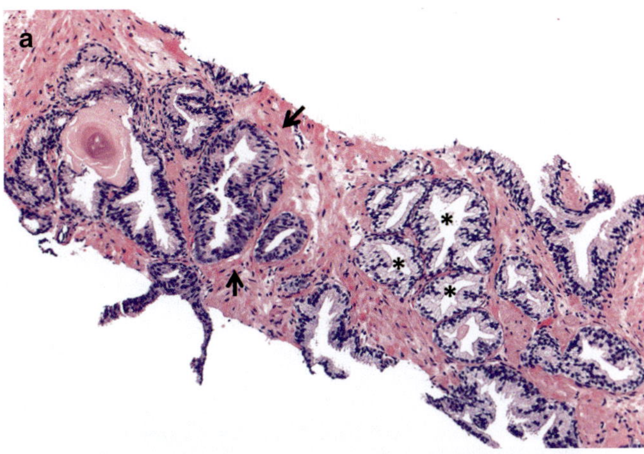

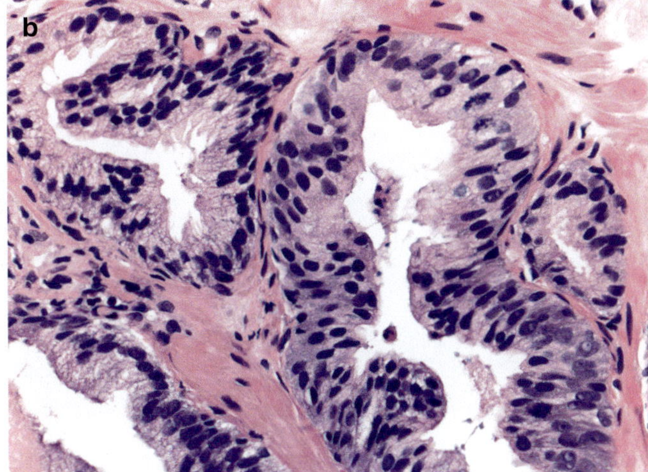

Fig. 5.8 High-grade prostatic intraepithelial neoplasia (HGPIN). At low magnification, HGPIN glands (arrows) are architecturally similar to but appear darker than the adjacent benign glands (asterisks, **a**). At 20× magnification, the secretory cells have crowded, stratified, and enlarged nuclei that have coarse and clumpy chromatin. Importantly, large and conspicuous nucleoli are present in the secretory cells (**b**)

show infiltrative growth, extraprostatic invasion, and perineural invasion, while adenocarcinoma does.

HGPIN retains basal cells, while prostatic adenocarcinoma lacks basal cells. Additionally, AMACR expression is lower in HGPIN than prostatic adenocarcinoma. Cytoplasmic PTEN protein loss is seen in majority of carcinomas and is rarely seen in HGPIN.

References: [18, 19]

What Is the Clinical Significance of High-Grade Prostatic Intraepithelial Neoplasia (HGPIN)?

Although evidence indicates it is a precursor of prostate cancer, the latency of HGPIN to progress to cancer is uncertain. Therefore, HGPIN is currently not an indication for defini-

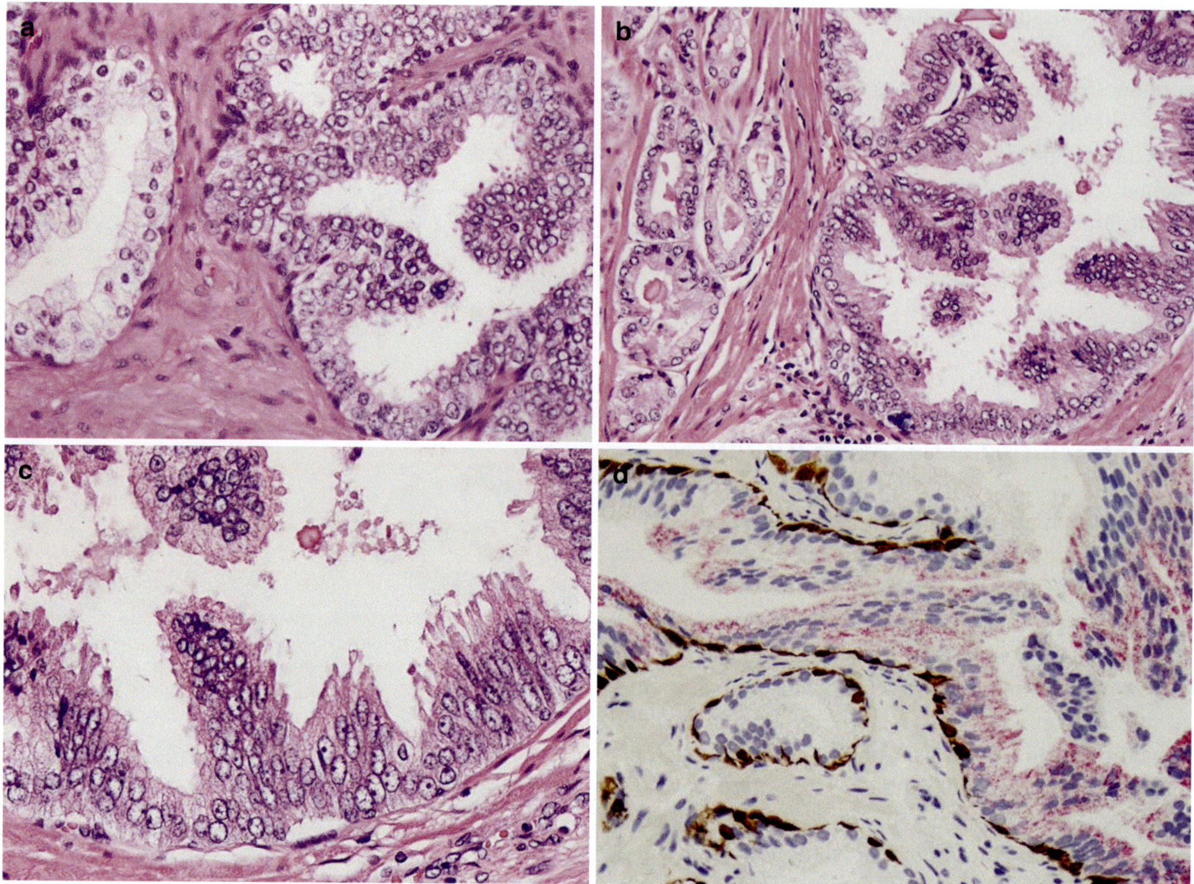

Fig. 5.9 Different from the benign prostatic gland (**a**, arrow), HGPIN gland is expanded and filled with neoplastic cells with cytologic atypia and basal cells can be easily seen (**a**, arrowheads). Compared to carcinoma glands (**b**, arrows), HGPIN gland is larger with papillary infold-ings (**b**, arrowhead). Both show cytologic atypia (**b**). The neoplastic cells in HGPIN show stratified nuclei with prominent nucleoli (**c**). Triple stain demonstrates the presence of basal cells and increased AMACR staining in HGPIN glands (**d**)

Table 5.1 Comparison of high-grade PIN with adenocarcinoma

	High-grade PIN	Adenocarcinoma
Size of the gland	Usually large	Usually small
Layers of proliferating cells	Stratified or pseudostratified	Usually single layer
Crystalloids or blue mucin	Rarely seen	Often seen
Cytological atypia	Present	Present
Infiltrating growth	Absent	Present
Basal cells	Present	Absent
AMACR staining	Only in 50% case Usually weaker	Positive Strong
Ki67 Proliferative activity	Low	Low to high based on the grade
Management option	Follow-up depending on risk for cancer based on serum biomarkers and MRI imaging	Treatment or active surveillance

tive treatments such as surgery, radiation, or hormonal therapy. In the past, isolated HGPIN without concomitant cancer on needle core biopsy would be an indication for a repeat biopsy. However, the current recommendation is that men with HGPIN diagnosed in a single biopsy core do not need a routine repeat biopsy. This is because only a small percentage of these patients will be found to have prostate cancer on repeat biopsy, and the risk is not much higher than a man with a negative prostate biopsy (23% risk for HGPIN vs. 20% risk for benign prostate biopsy). The cancer risk is even lower in the contemporary setting of MRI targeted biopsy, because more prostate cancer cases are detected in the first biopsy. National Comprehensive Cancer Network (NCCN) recommends that men with HGPIN diagnosed in a single biopsy core do not need a routine repeat biopsy. If multiple cores harbor HGPIN, it is recommended additional serum and urine biomarker testing such as free PSA %, prostate health index (PHI) or 4Kscore, and imaging studies to assess the risk of high-grade cancer upon which the decision to perform repeat biopsy may depend.

A clinical trial was previously conducted to prevent prostate cancer with finasteride (an alpha reductase inhibitor) in men with HGPIN. The results from this trial showed slight reduction of prostate cancer incidence in the treated group compared to untreated control group. However, some prostate cancers in the treatment group showed appearance of higher grade prostate cancer. Therefore, finasteride or other medical treatment has not been proven to be beneficial for men with isolated HGPIN.

References: [17, 20–22]

What Is "Atypical Glands Suspicious for Cancer (ATYP)" or "Atypical Small Acinar Proliferation (ASAP)"?

"Atypical glands suspicious for cancer (ATYP)" or "atypical small acinar proliferation (ASAP)" is a diagnostic term used to describe a small focus of prostate glands that exhibits architectural and cytological atypia is suspicious for, yet falls short of, the diagnostic threshold for prostate cancer (Fig. 5.10). It is not a distinct biological entity; rather, it encompasses a range of lesions of varying clinical significance, including under-sampled cancer, high-grade prostatic intraepithelial neoplasia, benign lesions that mimic cancer, and benign prostate glands with reactive atypia.

An ATYP/ASAP diagnosis in prostate needle biopsy is considered a risk factor for finding prostate cancer in subsequent biopsies. Such risk ranges from 27% to 47%, with an average of 42%, in recent studies. National Comprehensive Cancer Network (NCCN) recommends patients with ATYP/ASAP on initial biopsies undergo additional biomarker testing, such as free PSA %, prostate health index (PHI) or 4Kscore, and imaging studies, to assess the risk of high-grade cancer and consider repeated biopsy with relative increased sampling of the site of the atypical diagnosis.

References: [17, 23]

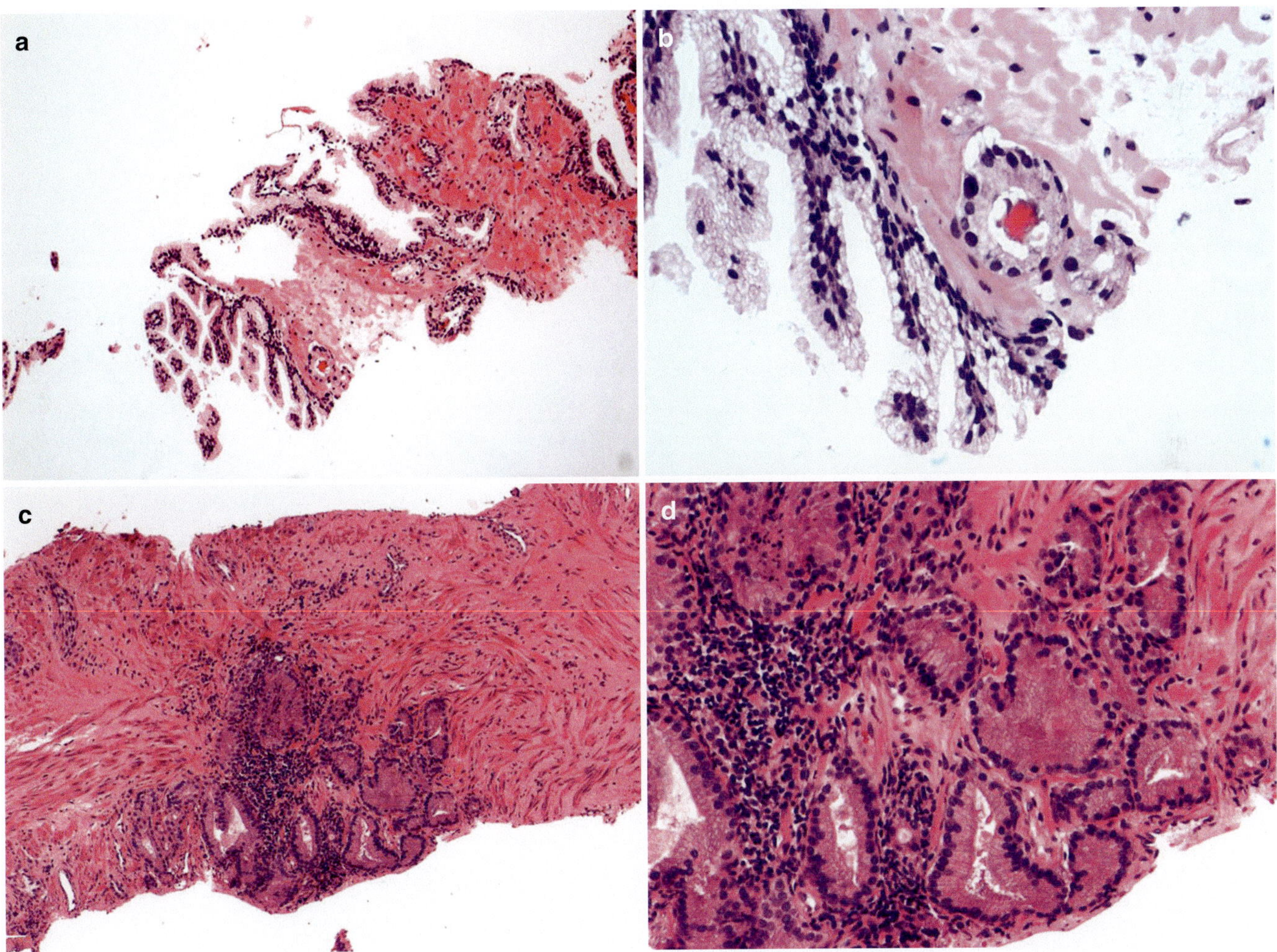

Fig. 5.10 Examples of atypical glands suspicious for but not diagnostic of carcinoma. A small focus of atypical gland can be seen at low magnification because of the presence of crystalloid (**a**, arrow). At higher magnification, there are three glands with nuclear enlargement and hyperchromasia (**b**). However, the focus is too small and cytologi-cal atypia is not conclusive, therefore insufficient for a definitive diagnosis of carcinoma. Another case of atypically glands with background heavy lymphocytic infiltrates at low magnification (**c**). Cytological atypia is not convincing although infiltrating pattern is suspicious (**d**). In this situation, it is also difficult to make a definitive diagnosis of adenocarcinoma

What Are Types of Primary Carcinomas of the Prostate Other Than Adenocarcinomas?

More than 95% of prostatic carcinomas are adenocarcinomas including acinar and ductal types. Other histological types of primary prostatic carcinomas include basal cell carcinoma (Fig. 5.11a), small cell carcinoma (Fig. 5.11b), and large cell (neuroendocrine) carcinoma. The vast majority of urothelial carcinoma of the prostate spreads from the bladder primary tumor. Primary prostatic urothelial carcinoma (Fig. 5.11c) originating from the prostatic urethral urothelium is exceedingly rare. Rarely enteric type adenocarcinoma (Fig. 5.11d) can occur as a primary tumor in the prostate. This type of adenocarcinoma is similar to enteric type adenocarcinoma of the bladder. Carcinosarcoma or sarcomatoid carcinoma may also be seen in the prostate, often following treatment of a high-grade prostate acinar or ductal carcinoma. It is important to make distinction of these tumors because of the therapeutic implications. The key diagnostic features are listed in Table 5.2.

References: [24–26]

How Is Neuroendocrine Differentiation of Prostate Cancer Classified?

Neuroendocrine differentiation in prostate carcinoma has a wide morphological spectrum. Its classification and clinical significance are listed in Table 5.3.

Pure de novo small cell carcinoma of the prostate that likely arises from malignant transformation of preexisting neuroendocrine or neural tissue within the prostate gland is rare (<1% of cases). Great majority of prostate cancers with neuroendocrine differentiation arise from acinar adenocarci-

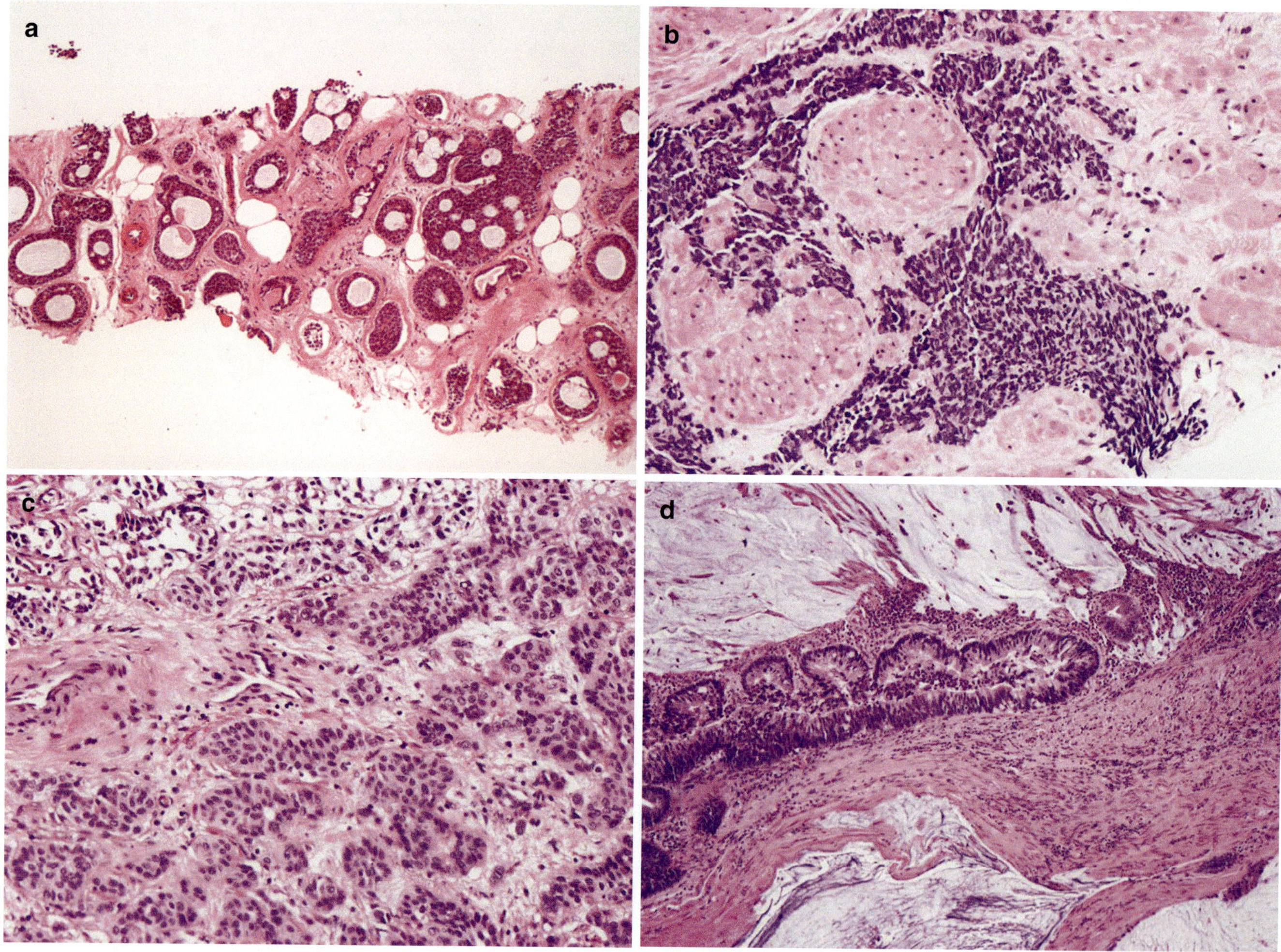

Fig. 5.11 Other histological types of prostate cancer. Basal cell carcinoma of the prostate (**a**), small cell carcinoma of the prostate (**b**), urothelial carcinoma of the prostate (**c**), and enteric adenocarcinoma of the prostate (**d**)

Table 5.2 Comparison of the uncommon types of primary carcinomas of the prostate

	Urothelial carcinoma	Small cell carcinoma	Basal cell carcinoma	Enteric type adenocarcinoma
Key histological features	Nests with more pleomorphic nuclei	Small cells with nuclear molding, salt-pepper chromatin	Nests of infiltrating tumor cells resembling basal cells	Large malignant glands with large amount of mucin and occasional goblet cells
AMACR	Positive	Negative	Negative	Positive
NKX3.1	Negative	Negative or weakly positive	Negative	Negative
PSA	Negative	Negative or weakly positive	Negative	Negative
P63/HMWCK	Positive	Negative	Positive	Negative
GATA3	Positive	Negative	Negative	Negative
CDX2	Negative	Negative	Negative	Positive
Neuroendocrine markers	Negative	Positive	Negative	Negative

Table 5.3 Neuroendocrine differentiation in prostate carcinoma

Type of neuroendocrine (NE) differentiation	Clinical significance
Usual prostate adenocarcinoma with neuroendocrine differentiation	No significance on outcome Should be Gleason graded Paneth cells in nests/cords are not Gleason graded as such
Adenocarcinoma with Paneth cell differentiation (Fig. 5.12)	tumors do not behave like Gleason pattern 5 prostate cancer Routine use of neuroendocrine markers without morphological evidence of neuroendocrine differentiation is not recommended
Well-differentiated neuroendocrine tumor	Protracted prognosis; do not Gleason grade; differentiate from carcinoid-like prostate adenocarcinoma
Small cell carcinoma	Dismal prognosis; any amount of small/large cell neuroendocrine component should be reported; Gleason grade only acinar component
Large cell neuroendocrine carcinoma	
Mixed (small or large cell) neuroendocrine carcinoma—acinar/ductal adenocarcinoma	

noma after treatment and represent emergence of an aggressive terminal phase of the disease.

References: [27, 28]

How to Make Diagnosis of Small Cell Carcinoma of the Prostate?

Small cell carcinoma of the prostate is defined as a primary prostate carcinoma with features of small neuroendocrine cells. Similar to its counterpart of the lung, small cell carcinoma of the prostate is characterized by nuclear molding, high nuclear-to-cytoplasmic (N:C) ratio, fine "salt-and-pepper" chromatin, lack of prominent nucleoli, and no glandular formation, although some rosettes may be seen. Brisk mitotic rate and increased apoptotic bodies are evident (Fig. 5.13) in small cell carcinoma.

Small cell carcinoma is uncommon, accounting for proximately 1% of prostate cancers. It can be found in a pure form but is more often associated with typical prostatic adenocarcinoma (>50% of the cases). The majority cases of prostatic adenocarcinomas associated with small cell carcinoma are high grade (≥ Gleason score 8). In the mixed cases, the adenocarcinomatous component should be graded but not for small cell carcinoma component.

Immunoprofile of small cell carcinoma is different from that of acinar adenocarcinoma. At least one of neuroendocrine markers (chromogranin, synaptophysin, CD56, and neuron-specific enolase) is positive in small cell carcinoma, and TTF1 is positive in 50% of primary small cell carcinoma of the prostate, as opposed to 90% positivity in primary small cell carcinoma of the lung. Prostatic markers such as PSA and NKX3.1 are positive only in a minority of cases, and the expression is typically focal. The expression of P63 or HMWCK is more common in small cell carcinoma than in adenocarcinoma. If all neuroendocrine markers are negative, diagnosis of small cell carcinoma of the prostate should be made with caution, and the histology must be convincing.

Small cell carcinoma of the prostate, similar to its counterpart of the lung, is a very aggressive disease. The diagnosis should be made clear, when it presents with or without adenocarcinoma component. The percentage of small cell component may or may not affect the prognosis, but it will most likely prompt systemic treatment.

Reference: [28]

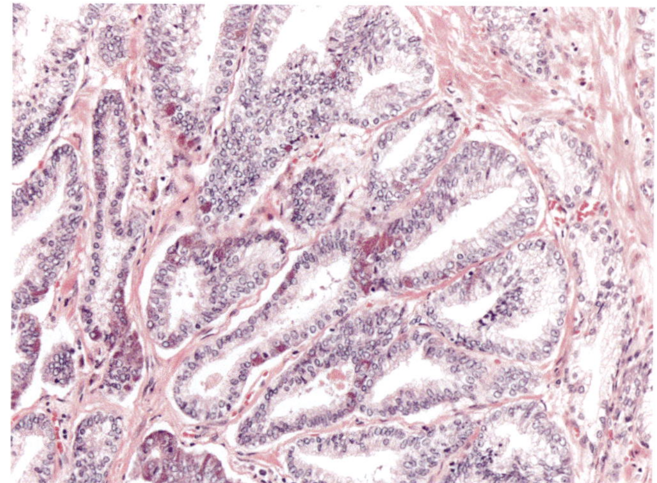

Fig. 5.12 Prostatic acinar adenocarcinoma demonstrates Paneth cell-like neuroendocrine differentiation, characterized by occasional cells with bright eosinophilic cytoplasmic granules resembling Paneth cells in the gastrointestinal tract

What Are Nonprostatic Adenocarcinomas Involving the Prostate?

Secondary adenocarcinomas other than primary prostatic acinar/ductal carcinoma are rare in the prostate. They often are adenocarcinomas of contiguous organs (including the urinary bladder, colon/rectum, or urethra) directly invading the prostate. Distant metastases to the prostate from adenocarcinomas arising in noncontiguous organs (e.g., the lung) are exceptionally rare in clinical specimens. They typically are noted only with disseminated disease at autopsy (5% of cases in some series). Their morphology is similar to the primary tumors. Primary mucin-producing urothelial-type adenocarcinoma of the prostate is a distinct entity that typically arises from the prostatic urethra possibly from urethritis glandularis or glandular metaplasia with malignant transformation, and it is analogous to adenocarcinoma with mucinous differentiation arising from the urinary bladder (Fig. 5.14).

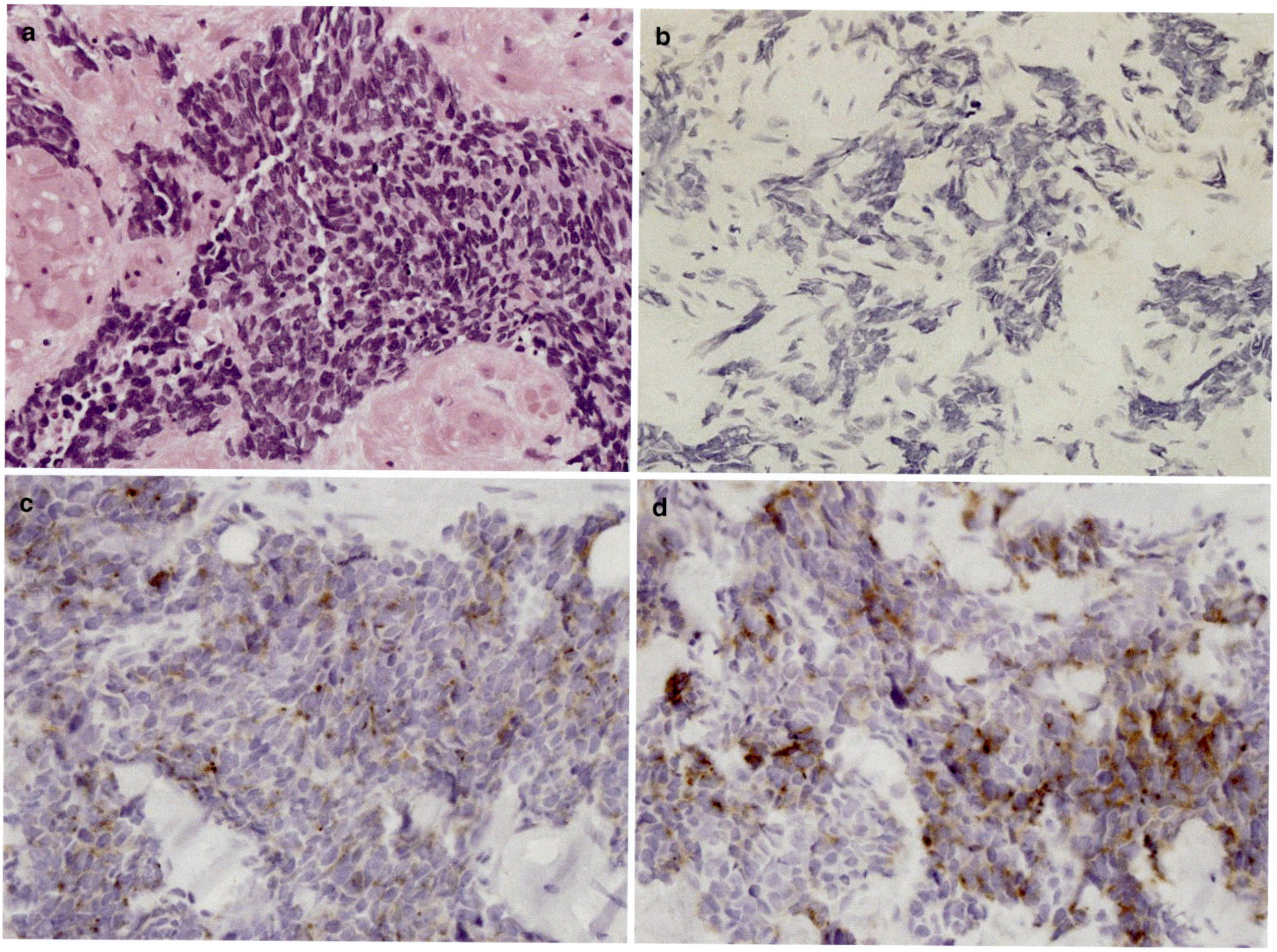

Fig. 5.13 Small cell carcinoma of the prostate is characterized by small tumor cells with scant cytoplasm, nuclear molding, and salt-pepper chromatin without glandular structures (**a**). The tumor cells are typically negative for PSA (**b**), positive for neuroendocrine markers such as neuron-specific enolase (**c**) and synaptophysin (**d**)

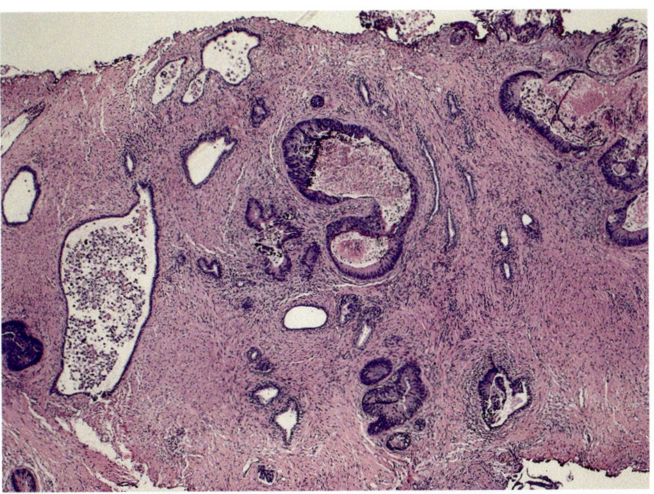

Fig. 5.14 Transurethral resection of the prostate with colonic type adenocarcinoma infiltrating between prostate glands

For the differential diagnosis, one should rule out prostate acinar carcinomas with mucin production, such as "signet ring" cell prostate carcinoma or prostate ductal carcinoma that may have "enteric" morphology. History of primary tumors of other organs should be sought and a battery of immunostains will help establish the correct diagnosis, including prostate specific markers (PSA, PSAP, and NKX3.1) and other lineage specific markers (GATA3 and CDX2).

Reference: [29]

How to Make Diagnosis of Large Cell Neuroendocrine Carcinoma?

Large cell neuroendocrine carcinoma is characterized by high-grade carcinoma with neuroendocrine differentiation that often forms large nests with peripheral palisading and central necrosis. The tumor cells show fine salt-pepper chromatin. The cytology is similar but different from high-grade acinar carcinoma with brisk mitosis and fine chromatin without prominent nucleoli (Fig. 5.15a). This tumor may be present in a pure form or mixed with small cell carcinoma.

This tumor is highly aggressive. Currently, there is no effective treatment for large cell neuroendocrine carcinoma of the prostate. Most of the patients receive chemotherapies designed for small cell carcinoma. It remains to be seen whether these regiments are beneficial or not, due to its rare incidence.

Diagnosis of small cell carcinoma is based primarily on the morphological appearance. However, the diagnosis of large cell neuroendocrine carcinoma requires both morphological features and appropriate immunoprofile (Figs. 5.15b–d) including positive neuroendocrine markers.

References: [28, 30]

How to Determine Whether a Urothelial Carcinoma in the Prostate Is Primary or Secondary?

Secondary urothelial carcinoma involving the prostate can occur in two clinical settings. Most commonly, it represents a bladder urothelial carcinoma involving the prostate, either by so-called transmucosal route (extension of the bladder tumor along the prostatic urethral surface and prostatic ducts with or without stromal invasion) or transmural route (a bladder tumor directly invades through the bladder wall to invade prostatic stroma, seminal vesicles, or other adjacent organs). Rarely, urothelial carcinoma arises within the prostate without concomitant bladder carcinoma. The key to distinguish between these two clinical settings is the clinical history of previous or concurrent bladder cancer diagnosis.

When urothelial carcinoma of the prostate is suspected, it is critical to first rule out prostatic carcinoma because the clinical management is vastly different for urothelial and prostatic carcinomas. Urothelial carcinomas often display significant cytological atypia compared to relatively monotonous cytological atypia in prostate carcinomas. A panel of prostate markers (PSA, NKX3.1, and PSMA) and urothelial /basal cell markers HMWCK K903 and p63, and GATA3 can be used for this differential diagnosis. Urothelial carcinomas are variably positive for urothelial cell markers and GATA3 and negative for prostate-specific markers.

References: [31, 32]

How to Distinguish Basal Cell Carcinoma from Basal Cell Hyperplasia?

Basal cell carcinoma (BCC), also known as basaloid carcinoma, of the prostate is a very rare type of prostate cancer. It is characterized by the proliferation of neoplastic cells with features of prostatic basal cells (Fig. 5.16). Basal cell hyperplasia (BCH) is a common condition often seen as a part of benign prostatic hyperplasia. It is characterized by a lobular proliferation of basal cells confined within the preexisting glands.

The major differences between BCC and BCH are listed in Table 5.4. The key is the infiltrative nature of basal cell carcinoma. The most important features include the following:

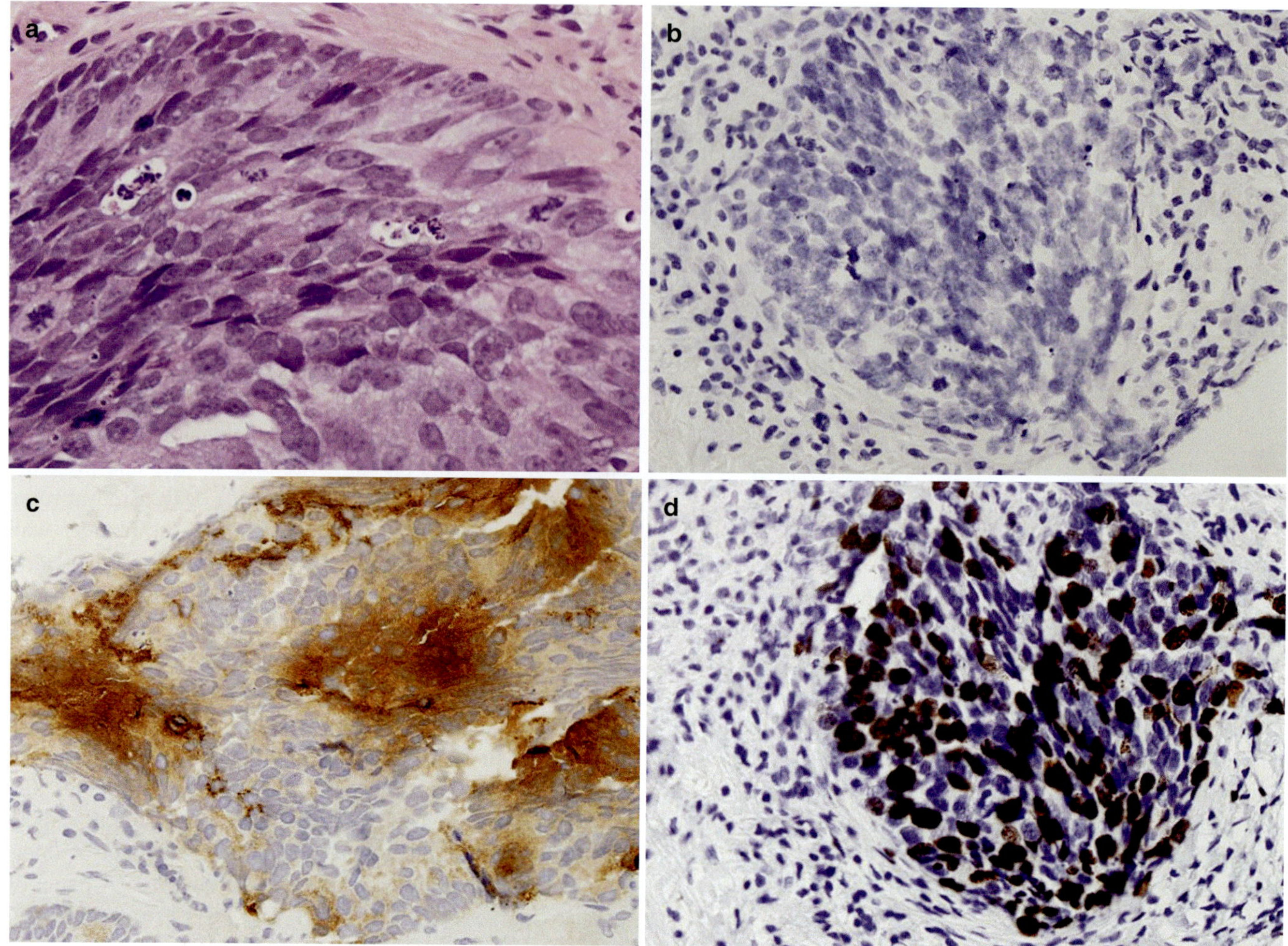

Fig. 5.15 Large cell neuroendocrine carcinoma of the prostate is characterized by large nests of tumor cells with peripheral palisading. The tumor cells are large with fine chromatin and numerous mitoses and apoptotic bodies (**a**). They are negative for PSA (**b**), positive for chromogranin (**c**), and show very high Ki67 proliferative activity (70%) (**d**)

- BCC presents with an invasive pattern while basal cell hyperplasia presents with lobular growth pattern. Perineural invasion or extraprostatic extension by BCC tumor cells can also been seen. Invasive nature is the key for diagnosis. Therefore, the diagnosis of BCC on needle core biopsy should be made with caution.
- The invasive nests of BCC are typically composed of monomorphic neoplastic basal cells without secretory cells, while BCH shows hyperplastic basal cells with secretory cells overlying the surface of proliferating basal cells. Microcalcifications or hyaline globules may be seen in the benign or malignant hyperplastic basal cell nests.

Immunohistochemically, BCC is positive for basal cells markers such as p63 and HMWCK, and be negative for PSA, similar to BCH. However, basal cell carcinoma will have high Ki67 proliferative index, up to 10–30%. BCL2 immunostaining may also be positive in BCC. It is important to note that invasive nature is much more important than the immunoprofile of the lesion for the diagnosis of BCC. The majority of BCC is low grade locally invasive disease, although rare metastasis has been reported. BCC should be distinguished from p63 positive prostatic adenocarcinoma, which have the phenotype of secrotary cells (typical histology of adenocaricnoma).

References: [33, 34]

What Is the Difference Between Intraductal Carcinoma and Invasive Carcinoma of the Prostate?

Intraductal carcinoma of the prostate (IDC-P) refers a unique type of prostatic glandular neoplasia with a propensity to

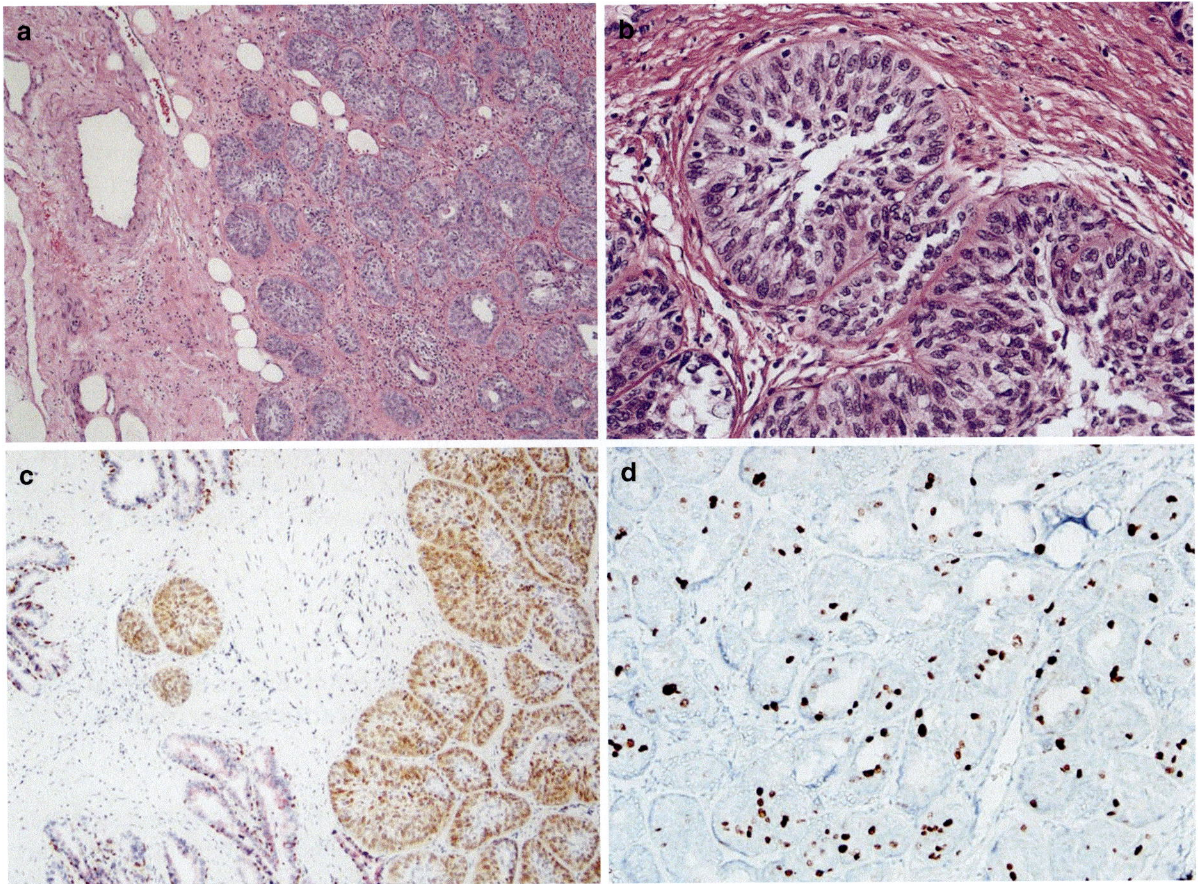

Fig. 5.16 Basal cell carcinoma of the prostate is characterized by cells with features of prostatic basal cells forming solid and cribriform nests invading into extraprostatic adipose tissue (**a**). At higher magnification, the tumor cells are multilayered with mild cytological atypia (**b**). The triple stain shows tumor cells invading seminal vesicle tissue, positive for both p63 and HWMCK and negative for AMACR (**c**). The Ki67 proliferative activity is low to moderate in tumor cells (**d**)

Table 5.4 Comparison of basal cell carcinoma and basal cell hyperplasia of the Prostate

	BCC	BCH
Definition	Malignant neoplasm with basal cell features	Benign basal cell proliferation
Growth pattern	Haphazard invasive growth pattern	Lobular pattern
Association with benign prostatic hyperplasia	No	Yes
Presence of secretory cells in the nests	No or yes	Yes
Perineural invasion	Present	Absent
Extraprostatic extension	Present	Absent
Metastasis	Only occur in a small subset of tumors	No
Ki67	Increased	Not increased
P63 and HMWCK	Positive	Positive
PSA	Negative	Positive in secretory cells
Treatment of choice	Surgery	Similar to BPH

grow within and expand benign prostatic ducts and acini. It retains basal cell layers, at least focally. In contrast, prostate adenocarcinoma (PCa), Gleason pattern 4 or 5 cribriform, and solid pattern, in particular, closely mimic IDC-P, but lack a basal cell lining. Additionally, IDC-P and PCa differ in many other aspects.

- The majority of IDC-P originates from invasive prostate cancer, and in a small subset of cases IDC-P may represent a precursor to invasive PCa, typically more aggressive invasive cancer than seen associated with high-grade PIN.
- IDC-P harbors genetic changes more common in Gleason pattern 4/5 PCa than Gleason pattern 3 PCa.
- IDC-P is almost always associated with aggressive, high-grade and volume PCa and is an independent adverse pathological factor in both radical prostatectomy and needle biopsy specimens and may influence response to current therapeutic regimens for advanced stage PCa.

References: [35, 36]

What Is the Difference Between High-Grade PIN and Intraductal Carcinoma?

High-grade PIN is a precursor lesion of prostate cancer characterized by the presence of neoplastic cells present in preexisting ducts or acini. Intraductal carcinoma of the prostate (IDC-P) is a marker of advanced invasive disease where tumor cells are thought to extend back into the ducts or acini. In practice, it may be difficult to distinguish between the two, as both have retained basal cells.

Several features can be used to separate these two entities (Table 5.5). First, IDC-P has more prominent cell proliferation than high-grade PIN. The neoplastic cells in IDC-P markedly expand the acini or ducts to form large solid or dense cribriform nests (neoplastic cells occupy more than 50% of the lumen) and tend to lose orientation (Fig. 5.17a). Second, intraductal carcinoma has more prominent cytological atypia than high-grade PIN. In IDC-P, nuclei can be six times larger than the nucleus of a normal secretory cell. Third, central necrosis is only seen in IDC-P. Fourth, immunohistochemistry may assist in the differential diagnosis. The IDC-P shows higher AMACR intensity (Fig. 5.17b) and higher Ki67 proliferative index similar to Gleason pattern 4 or 5 tumor, while high-grade PIN (Fig. 5.17c, d) has lower AMACR intensity and low Ki67 proliferative activity, similar to Gleason pattern 3 tumor. PTEN loss and positive ERG protein expression are characteristic of IDC-P. Finally, IDC-P is associated with high-grade invasive prostatic adenocarcinoma in the majority of cases, while high-grade PIN may not be. IDC-P necessitate definitive treatment, even in the absence of invasive carcinoma on prostate biopsies, while isolated high-grade PIN may prompt follow-up.

References: [35, 36]

Table 5.5 Comparison of intraductal carcinoma (IDC) with high-grade PIN

	IDC	High-grade PIN
Definition	Aggressive prostate cancer	Precursor of prostate cancer
	Adenocarcinoma cells invading ducts or acini in a retrograde fashion	Neoplastic cells present in preexisting ducts or acini
Proliferation of neoplastic cells	High Confluent or >75% cribriform lesion	Low
Nuclear atypia	Prominent Greater than 6× of normal nuclei	Present
Mitosis	Frequent, atypical mitosis may be present	Infrequent
Glandular structure	Extended and enlarged, solid and dense cribriform nests	Normal size
Basal cells	Present	Present
AMACR staining	Majority is positive and strong intensity	Only 50% are positive Mild to moderate intensity
Ki67 proliferative index	Increased similar to Gleason pattern 4 tumor	Mildly increased lower than Gleason pattern 3 tumor
Basal cell markers p63 and HMWCK	Positive	Positive
PTEN loss	Present (70%)	No
ERG	Present (70%)	No
Clinical significance when present in biopsy	Associated with high-grade and high volume prostatic adenocarcinoma in >90% cases	Slightly increased risk for detection of prostate cancer on repeat biopsy

What Is the Difference Between Ductal Carcinoma and Intraductal Carcinoma of the Prostate?

A confusing issue is the distinction between "ductal adenocarcinoma" and "intraductal carcinoma." Intraductal carcinoma (IDC-P) refers to the location of neoplastic cells within prostate acini and ducts as the result of retrograde extension of prostate cancer into the preexisting ducts and acini in most cases. Ductal adenocarcinoma is, on the other hand, defined by the cytological features of the tumor with tall pseudostratified columnar epithelium (Fig. 5.18) as opposed to acinar (usual) PCa, which has a simple cuboidal/low columnar lining of epithelium. Ductal adenocarcinoma involves large atypical glands with expansile growth usually with papillary, cribriform, or solid growth patterns with frequent necrosis. The papillae in ductal adenocarcinoma have true fibrovascular cores. The majority of ductal adenocarcinomas are invasive with a lack of basal cells. However, invasive ductal adenocarcinoma is also prone to intraductal spread, mechanistically similar to aggressive acinar PCa. Residual basal cells can be found in ductal adenocarcinoma with intraductal extension into preexisting benign glands (Intraductal ductal adenocarcinoma). In a fashion analogous to the majority of IDC-P cases composed of acinar (usual) PCa, almost all IDC-P cases composed of ductal adenocarcinoma have associated invasive ductal adenocarcinoma. However, just as with IDC-P with acinar cytology, there are rare cases of IDC-P with ductal cytology without concomitant invasive PCa, where the IDC-P is likely a precursor lesion to invasive ductal adenocarcinoma.

References: [2, 36]

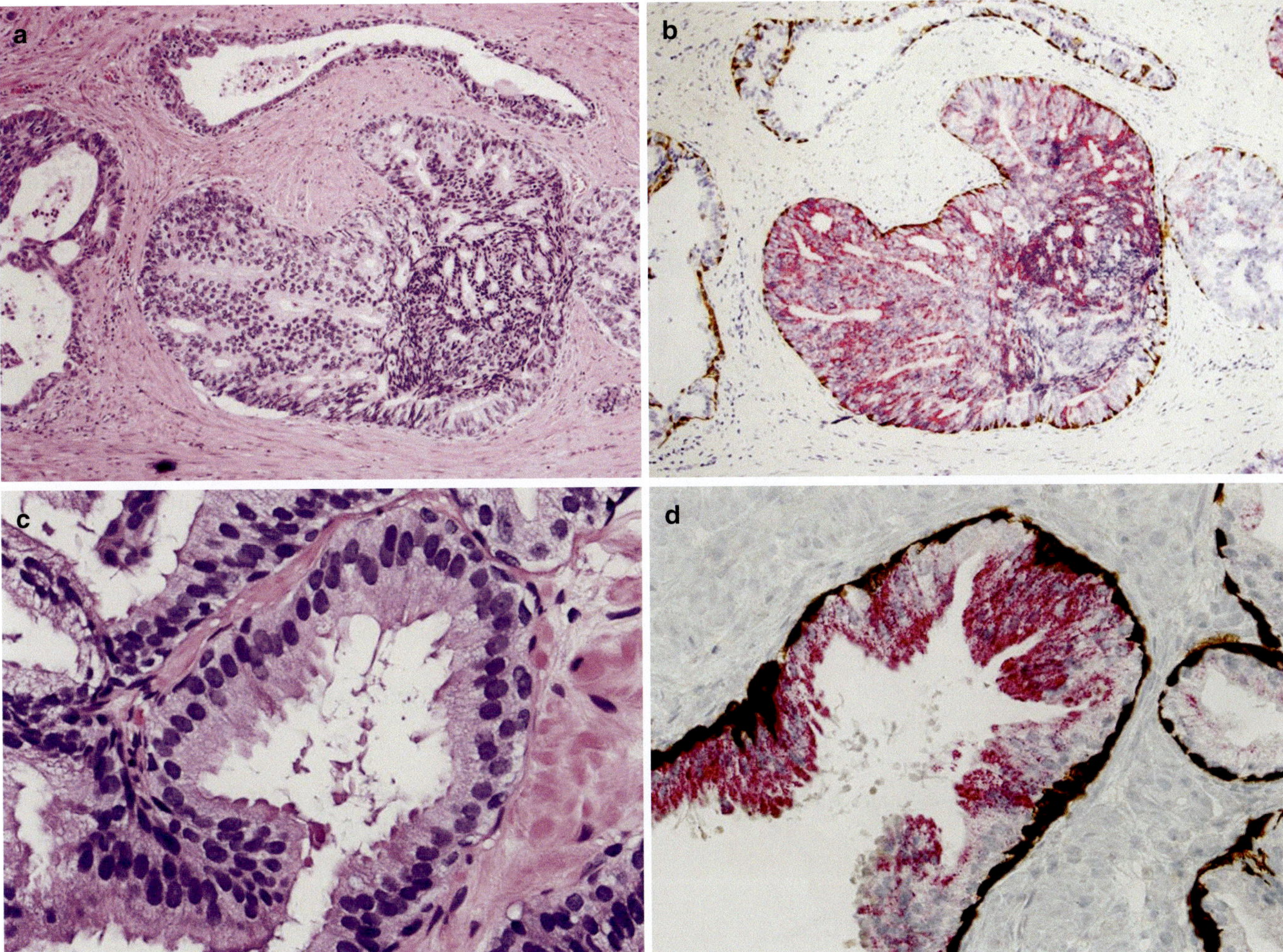

Fig. 5.17 Intraductal carcinoma of the prostate shows a dense cribriform pattern (**a**). It also shows stronger AMACR staining and presence of basal cells (**b**). In contrast, high-grade PIN displays simpler tufted pattern (**c**) and shows focal and moderate AMACR staining with presence of basal cells (**d**)

What Is the Difference Between HGPIN and PIN-like Prostatic Adenocarcinoma?

The majority of prostatic adenocarcinomas are composed of small glands with a single layer of tumor cells. However, some prostatic adenocarcinomas present as larger glands consisting of multiple layers or single layer of tumor cells (Fig. 5.19a, c), similar in appearance to high-grade PIN. In this situation, the PIN-like carcinoma has to be distinguished from high-grade PIN. The key differences are twofold:

- In PIN-like carcinoma, glands are more crowded than in high-grade PIN, and may exhibit confluent growth.
- High-grade PIN retain basal cells while PIN-like adenocarcinoma does not (Fig. 5.19b, d).

Reference: [35]

What Is the Clinical Significance of the "Grade Group" System?

"Grade Group" system is a new patient-centric grade grouping system for prostate cancer. It is still based on Gleason scores but represents a novel way to group Gleason scores. Gleason score 2–6 is Grade Group 1; Gleason score 3 + 4 is Grade Group 2; Gleason score 4 + 3 is Grade Group 3; Gleason score 8 is Grade Group 4; and Gleason score 9–10 is Grade Group 5. Many studies have correlated "Grade Group" with biochemical recurrence, distant metastases, and death following biopsy, radical prostatectomy, and radiation therapy. This new "Grade Group" system more accurately reflects outcomes and prognosis compared to the Gleason scores. It has been accepted as the grading system for prostate cancer by the American Joint Committee on Cancer (AJCC), College of American Pathologists (CAP),

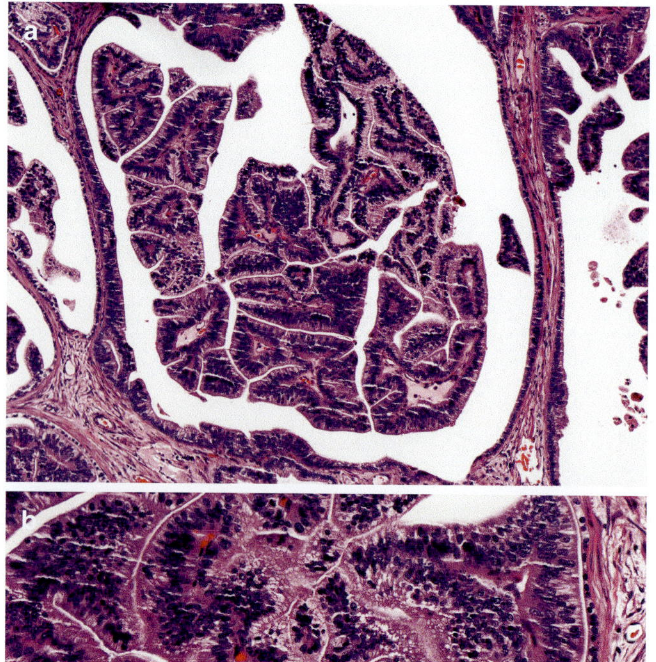

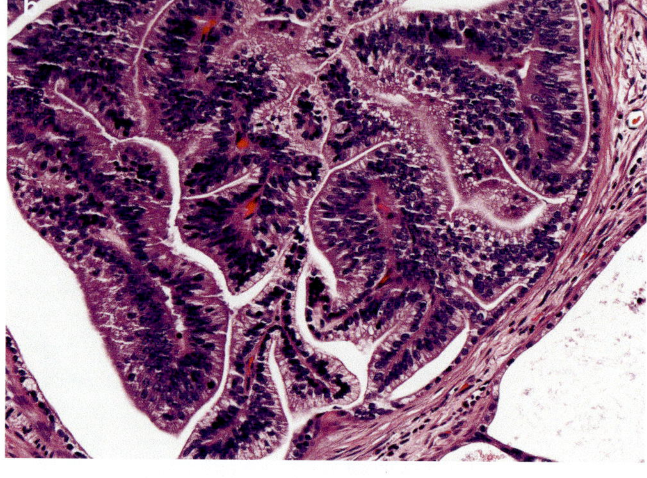

Fig. 5.18 In ductal adenocarcinoma, tumor cells form true papillae (**a**). Glands are lined by tall columnar cells (**b**)

International Society of Urological Pathology (ISUP), World Health Organization (WHO), and other international associations and organizations.

References: [37, 38]

Is It Necessary to Report the Percentage of Gleason 4 Tumor in a Case of Gleason 7 (3 + 4 or 4 + 3) Prostatic Adenocarcinoma?

Yes. The percentage of Gleason pattern 4 tumor in biopsies with Gleason score 3 + 4 = 7 (Grade Group 2) may determine active surveillance eligibility. Studies have demonstrated similar rates of radical prostatectomy adverse pathology for patients with biopsy Grade Group 1 vs. Grade Group 2 with limited Gleason pattern 4. The National Comprehensive Cancer Center Network (NCCN) guidelines now also consider active surveillance for select favorable intermediate risk patients, which includes low-volume Grade Group 2 disease.

Knowing whether the Gleason pattern 4 component of Gleason score 4 + 3 = 7 on biopsy is 60% vs. 90% may be beneficial for patient counseling and treatment decisions. For example, if a biopsy has a Grade Group 3 cancer with 60% Gleason pattern 4, and it is quite likely that the tumor nodule could be Grade Group 2 or Grade Group 3. Such a consideration may affect patient's management decision.

Whether the outcome of patients with Grade Groups 2 and 3 at radical prostatectomy is influenced by the quantity of Gleason pattern 4 is not entirely clear, although demonstrated that increasing percentage of Gleason pattern 4 is associated with decreased rates of biochemical risk-free survival. Currently, pathologists report the percentage of Gleason pattern 4 in both radical prostatectomy and prostate needle core biopsy specimens with Grade Groups 2–3. Although the percentage of Gleason pattern 4 on biopsy is subject of samling eror when the material is limited.

Reference: [39]

How Should Cribriform Prostatic Carcinoma Be Graded?

All cribriform cancer glands, regardless of their size and shape, should be graded as Gleason pattern 4 (Fig. 5.20a, b) or 5, if necrosis is present within the cribriform glands (Fig. 5.20c).

The only caveat is that intraductal carcinoma may show cribriform patterns with comedo necrosis. Therefore, sometimes, it is necessary to distinguish intraductal from invasive carcinoma, because the current recommendation is not to grade intraductal carcinoma (Fig. 5.20d).

Reference: [39]

Should Ductal Carcinoma of the Prostate Be Gleason Graded?

Yes. Ductal carcinoma of the prostate (the old term "endometrioid carcinoma of the prostate" is no longer recommended) should be graded as Gleason pattern 4 or 5 (when solid nests or necrosis is present) because ductal carcinoma behaves like Gleason pattern 4 or 5 tumor and the vast majority of ductal carcinoma cases are associated with Gleason pattern 4 or 5 acinar carcinoma. Furthermore, ductal carcinoma has a high Ki67 proliferative index similar to that of Gleason ≥4 tumor. Therefore, a case of pure ductal carcinoma should be grade as Gleason score 8/9 (Grade group 4 or 5). A case with both ductal and acinar components is graded as Gleason 4 + 3 or 3 + 4 or Gleason 4 + 5 depending on the grade of acinar component.

References: [40, 41]

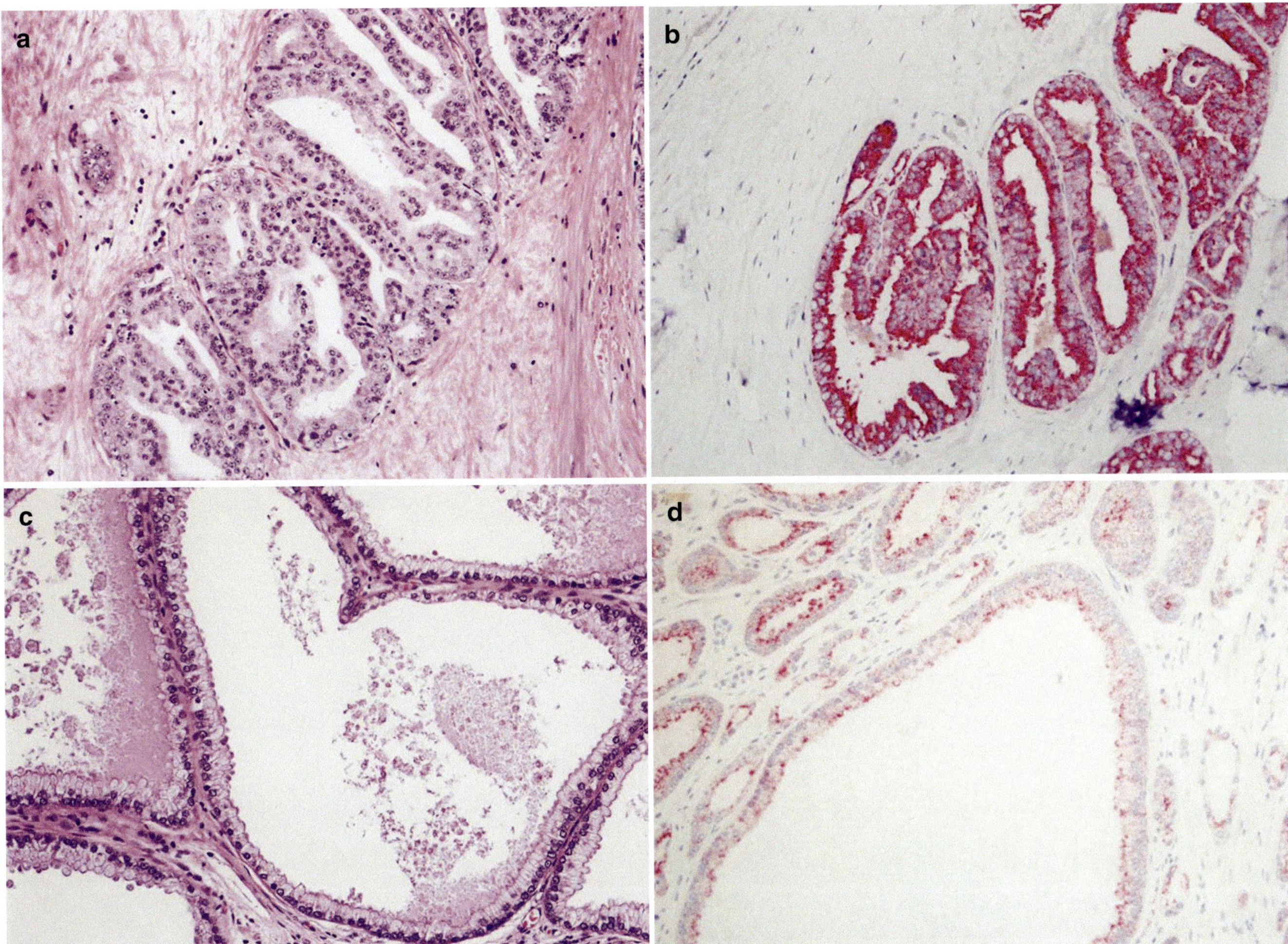

Fig. 5.19 PIN-like prostatic adenocarcinoma mimicking high-grade PIN. A group of large glands with pseudostratified atypical nuclei (**a**). However, no basal cells are present confirmed by the negative immu- nostaining for basal cells and strong AMACR staining (**b**, triple stain). Another case of PIN-like carcinoma composed of large glands with tall columnar cells (**c**). No basal cells are present (**d**, triple stain)

Should Intraductal Carcinoma of the Prostate Be Given a Gleason Grade?

Intraductal carcinoma of the prostate should not be graded when present without invasive prostate cancer. When present with invasive prostate cancer, its presence should not factor in the grade assignment, especially in the setting of low-grade invasive carcinoma.

Reference: [39]

Do Gleason Score 2–5 Tumors Still Exist? Are They Malignant?

Yes. Prostatic adenocarcinomas with Gleason score 2–5 score still exist but are rare. They are malignant based on their biological and histological features. But they are low-grade cancer with a good prognosis falling into Grade Group 1.

Gleason patterns 1 and 2 cancers are characterized by the lobulated pattern composed of back to back, regularly shaped cancer glands. Gleason score 2–3 tumors are rare. Gleason score 4 (Fig. 5.21) or 5 tumors sometimes can be seen on TUR or prostatectomy specimens. However, it is recommended not to report Gleason score 2–5 tumor on needle core biopsy, because it is difficult to appreciate the lobular pattern of Gleason pattern 2 on needle core with limited tissue.

Reference: [42]

Can Gleason Score 6 (Grade Group 1) Tumor Metastasize?

In prostate cancer, regional metastases occur to the pelvic lymph nodes. Ross et al. studied 14,123 radical prostatectomies with Gleason score ≤ 6 and found lymph node metasta-

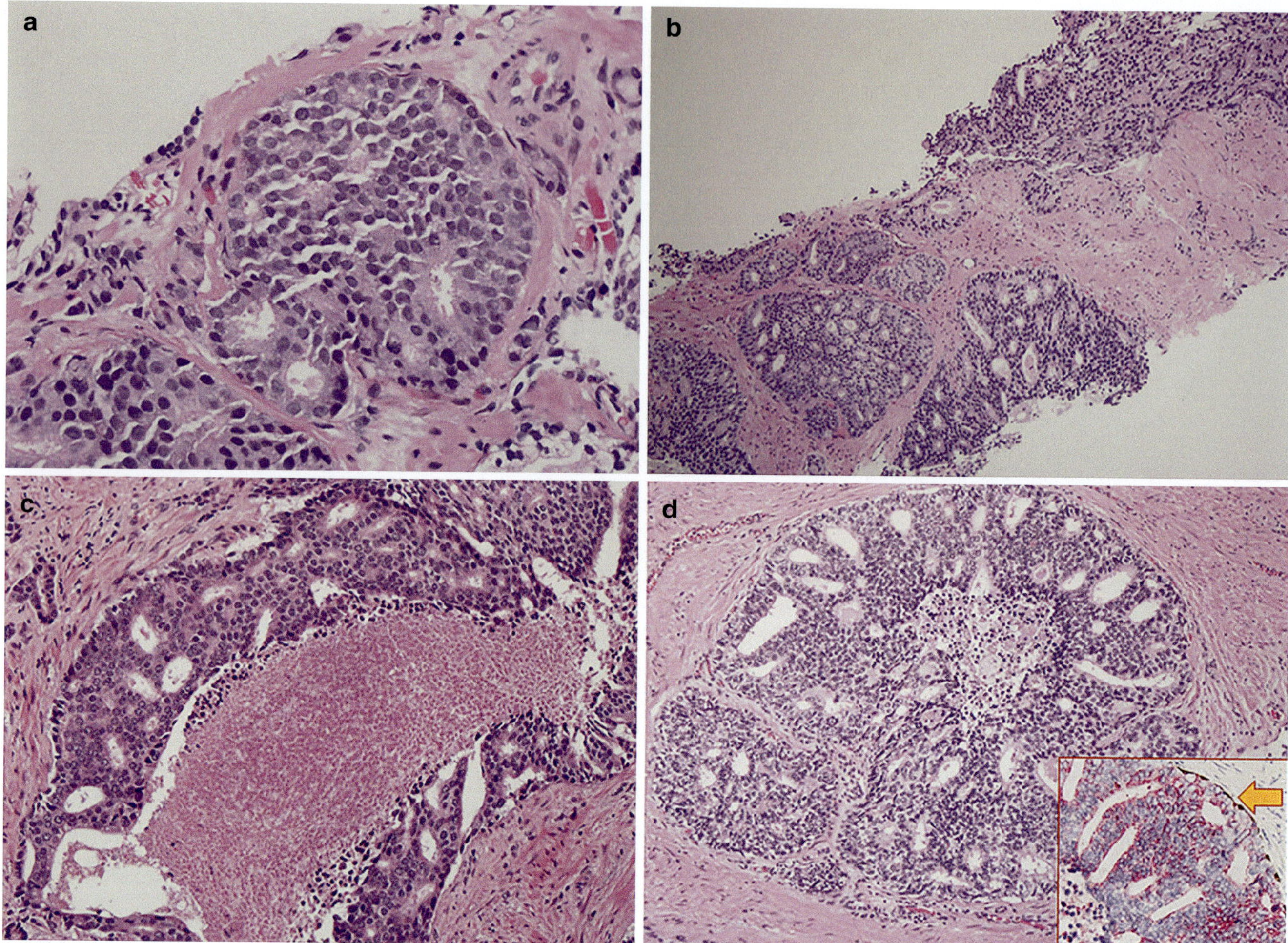

Fig. 5.20 Four examples of cribriform carcinomas with different sizes and contours. In general, they are graded as Gleason pattern 4 (**a**, **b**). The cribriform carcinoma with comedo necrosis is graded as Gleason pattern 5 (**c**). Intraductal carcinoma of the prostate with comedo necrosis should not be assigned a Gleason grade (**d**). Triple immunostaining confirms the presence of basal cells in the intraductal carcinoma (**d**, inset)

ses in 22 patients (0.156%). When these positive cases were reviewed using the contemporary Gleason grading criteria, all showed at least some Gleason pattern 4 components. Therefore, Gleason score 6 (Grade Group 1) prostate cancer, if evaluated in a well sampled prostatectomy specimen with contemporary grading criteria, may not have the potential to metastasize.

However, a Gleason score 6 (Grade Group 1) prostate cancer diagnosed in prostate biopsies cannot be assumed to have indolent biological behavior because of the potential under-grading by prostate biopsies as 20–35% of Gleason score 6 (Grade Group 1) prostate cancer in prostate biopsy are upgraded at radical prostatectomy.

References: [43, 44]

Should a Small Focus of Cancer Be Graded?

Yes. A small focus of prostatic adenocarcinoma on limited tissue such as needle core biopsy should be assigned a Gleason score and not just a Gleason pattern in pathology report: Gleason 3 + 3 = 6, not Gleason 3. For example, a small focus of 3 to 5 well-formed cancer glands (Fig. 5.22) should be graded as Gleason score 3 + 3 = 6 (Grade Group 1). Diagnosis of small focus of high grade (Gleason score 7–10) on needle core biopsy or TUR specimens should be made with caution after excluding possibility of tangential cut or crush artifact.

Grading a small focus of Gleason score 7 tumor can be particularly challenging in deciding whether to assign 3 + 4

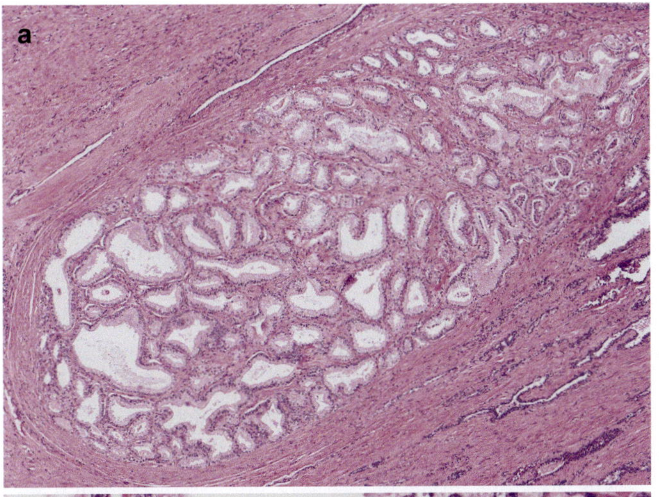

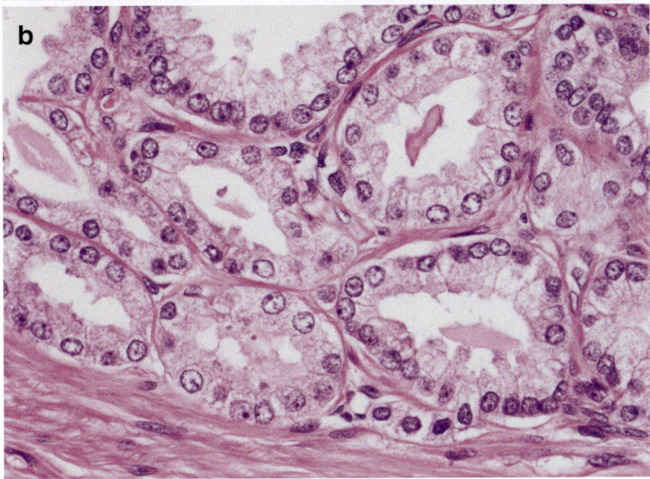

Fig. 5.21 A focus of prostatic adenocarcinoma, Gleason score 2 + 2 = 4 (Grade Group 1). At lower magnification, the focus is arranged in a lobular pattern (**a**), difficult to distinguish from adenosis. However, at higher magnification, the tumor cells exhibit nuclear atypia typical of prostate cancer (**b**)

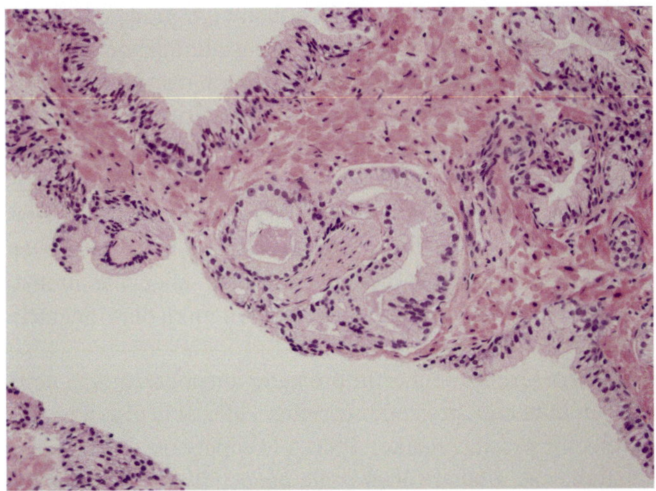

Fig. 5.22 Small focus of prostatic adenocarcinoma composed of three malignant glands with perineural invasion, Gleason score 3 + 3 = 6 (Grade Group 1)

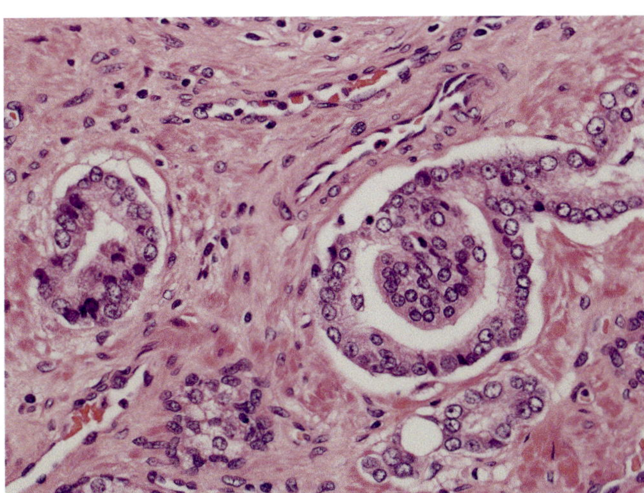

Fig. 5.23 Small focus of prostatic adenocarcinoma, Gleason score 3 + 4 (Grade Group 2). One cancer gland has glomeruloid architecture (Gleason 4 pattern), but the focus is too small to accurately estimate the percentage of Gleason pattern 4 component

(Grade Group 2) or 4 + 3 (Grade Group 3), because of the potential therapeutic implications. In most cases, it is possible to assign Gleason score 3 + 4 or Gleason score 4 + 3 based on the degree of glandular fusion and provide the percentage of Gleason 4 pattern. Occasionally, it is necessary to report Gleason 3 + 4 = 7 (Grade Group 2) without specifying percentage of Gleason pattern 4 component, and with a comment stating that the focus is too small to give an accurate percentage of Gleason pattern 4 component (Fig. 5.23).

Reference: [39]

How to Grade Prostatic Adenocarcinoma with Mucinous Differentiation?

Gleason grading should be based on the architecture of the cancer glands and ignores the mucinous component in the background (Fig. 5.24).

References: [2, 45]

How to Grade Prostatic Adenocarcinoma with Signet Ring Cells?

Signet ring-like cell variant of prostate carcinoma is composed of sheets, cords, and single cells with cytoplasmic vacuoles displacing the nuclei peripherally. At higher magnification, vacuoles are optically clear, and in most cases lack staining for mucin. The signet ring cell carcinoma is graded as Gleason pattern 5 (Fig. 5.25).

Vacuoles may be present in any Gleason pattern cancer and should not be viewed as signet ring cell differentiation,

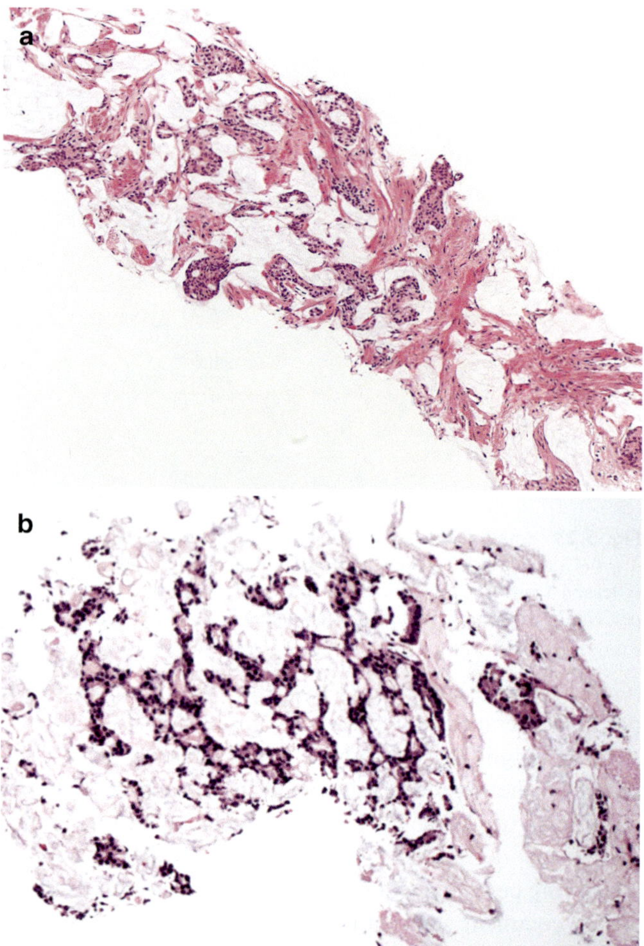

Fig. 5.24 Prostate carcinoma with mucinous features. Cancer glands float within the mucin pool (**a**). Majority of the cancer glands are fused or cribriform with a few well-formed discrete cancer glands. This tumor is graded as 4 + 3 = 7. In another case, interconnecting cancer glands and a few discrete glands float in the extracellular mucin lake and are graded as 4 + 3 = 7 (**b**)

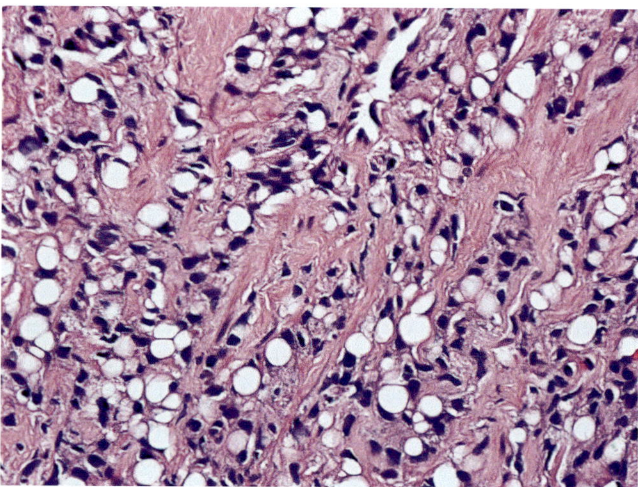

Fig. 5.25 Signet ring-like cell variant of prostate carcinoma comprises cords and single cells with cytoplasmic vacuoles which at higher magnification are optically clear. This tumor is graded as 5 + 5 = 10

and grading in such a setting should be based on underlying architecture of the cancer glands.

Reference: [2]

What Are the Most Specific Immunohistochemical Markers to Determine a Prostatic Origin in a Metastatic Tumor?

Since prostate cancer is one of the most common cancers in men in the United States, pathologists often encounter a situation to determine whether a malignant tumor is a metastatic prostate cancer. Therefore, a panel of prostate specific markers is valuable to help make such a decision.

The first-line prostate markers are NKX3.1, PSA, and PSMA (Fig. 5.26).

- NKX3.1 has the highest sensitivity and highest specificity among all prostate markers. It is present in secretory and basal cells in benign and cancer glands of the prostate. The expression in basal cells of the benign glands is negative or very weakly positive. However, this marker does not distinguish benign from malignant prostate glands. In most cases of prostatic adenocarcinoma with prior therapies, the tumor cells still express NKX3.1, making it a marker to identify prostatic origin in a patient with treated prostate cancer. It is negative in only rare cases of high-grade prostate cancer, particularly small cell carcinoma of the prostate.

- PSA is the most commonly used, highly specific prostatic marker. Only rare cases such as salivary gland carcinoma may express low level PSA. However, the sensitivity of PSA is lower than NKX3.1. It is important to know that benign prostatic glandular cells produce more PSA than adenocarcinoma cells, low-grade prostatic adenocarcinoma cells produce more PSA than high-grade adenocarcinoma cells, and hormone naïve prostatic adenocarcinoma cells produce more PSA than castration resistant prostatic adenocarcinoma cells. Most cases requiring confirmation of metastatic prostatic adenocarcinoma are high grade and often castration resistant tumors; therefore, it is essential to keep in mind that PSA staining in those metastatic prostatic adenocarcinoma cells can be focal or even negative. In the metastatic prostatic adenocarcinoma, negative PSA staining is more common than negative NKX3.1 staining.

- PSMA level is higher in prostatic adenocarcinoma cells than in benign prostatic secretory cells. It is also a highly specific prostate marker. PSMA is widely used in imaging studies as a label for prostate cancer in determining the extent of prostate cancer at primary and metastatic sites.

Second-line prostate markers include Prostein (P501S), AMACR, ERG, and PSAP. These prostate markers have

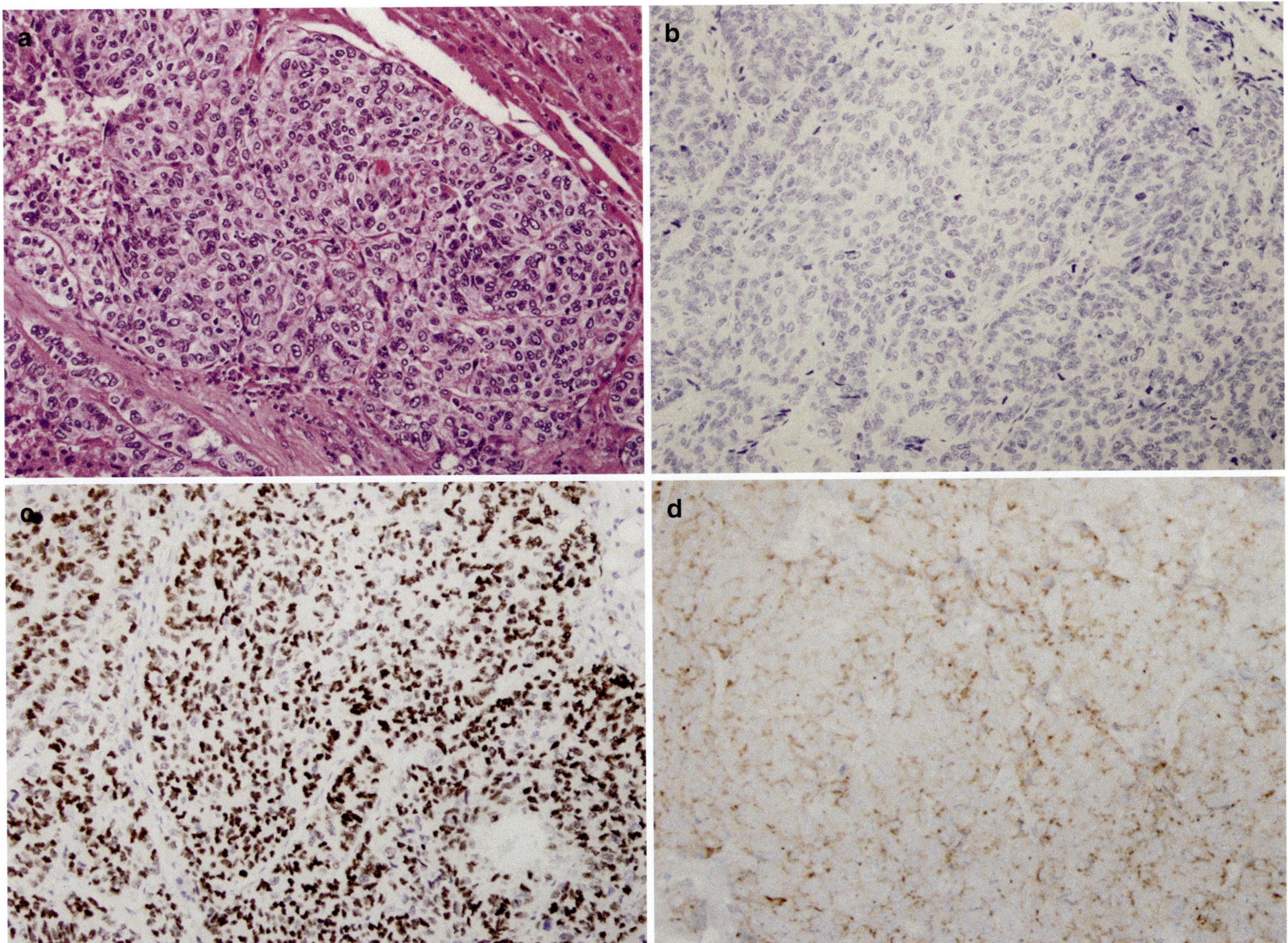

Fig. 5.26 A metastatic prostatic adenocarcinoma in the liver (**a**) shows negative PSA staining (**b**), but strong staining for NKX3.1 (**c**) and weak staining for PSMA (**d**)

a lower specificity or lower sensitivity, which limits their utility as the first-line prostate markers. They may be used when none of the first-line prostate markers works.

Prostein (P501S) is positive in prostate and breast cancer. AMACR (P504S) is the best marker for prostate cancer in prostate tissue, but not at metastatic sites because it is also positive in the majority of colon cancer (90%), papillary renal cell carcinoma (100%), and lower percentages of other tumors. ERG is another useful marker. However, it has low sensitivity as it is positive only in 40–50% of prostate cancer. It is, however, highly specific for prostatic adenocarcinoma with a caveat that it is also positive in endothelium, including angiosarcoma. PSAP tends to have higher background staining and is less specific.

One piece of important information to have when considering prostate as a possible origin of a metastasis is the Gleason score of the primary prostate cancer. Gleason score 6 cancers have virtually no metastatic potential compared with Gleason 7 cancers. The higher the Gleason score, the higher is the probability of developing metastatic disease.

References: [46–51]

What Is the Diagnostic Value of NKX3.1?

NKX3.1 is a highly sensitive and specific immunohistochemical marker to confirm the prostatic origin of a metastatic, poorly or undifferentiated carcinoma, or to distinguish between a high-grade prostatic acinar carcinoma and a metastatic carcinoma to the prostate.

NKX3.1 is an androgen-regulated gene whose expression is predominantly localized to prostate epithelium. It is a nuclear protein positive in the majority of primary prostatic carcinomas (Fig. 5.27). Of clinical importance, NKX3.1 is positive in approximately 92–95% of high-grade (Gleason score 8–10) prostate cancer and 98.6% metastatic prostate

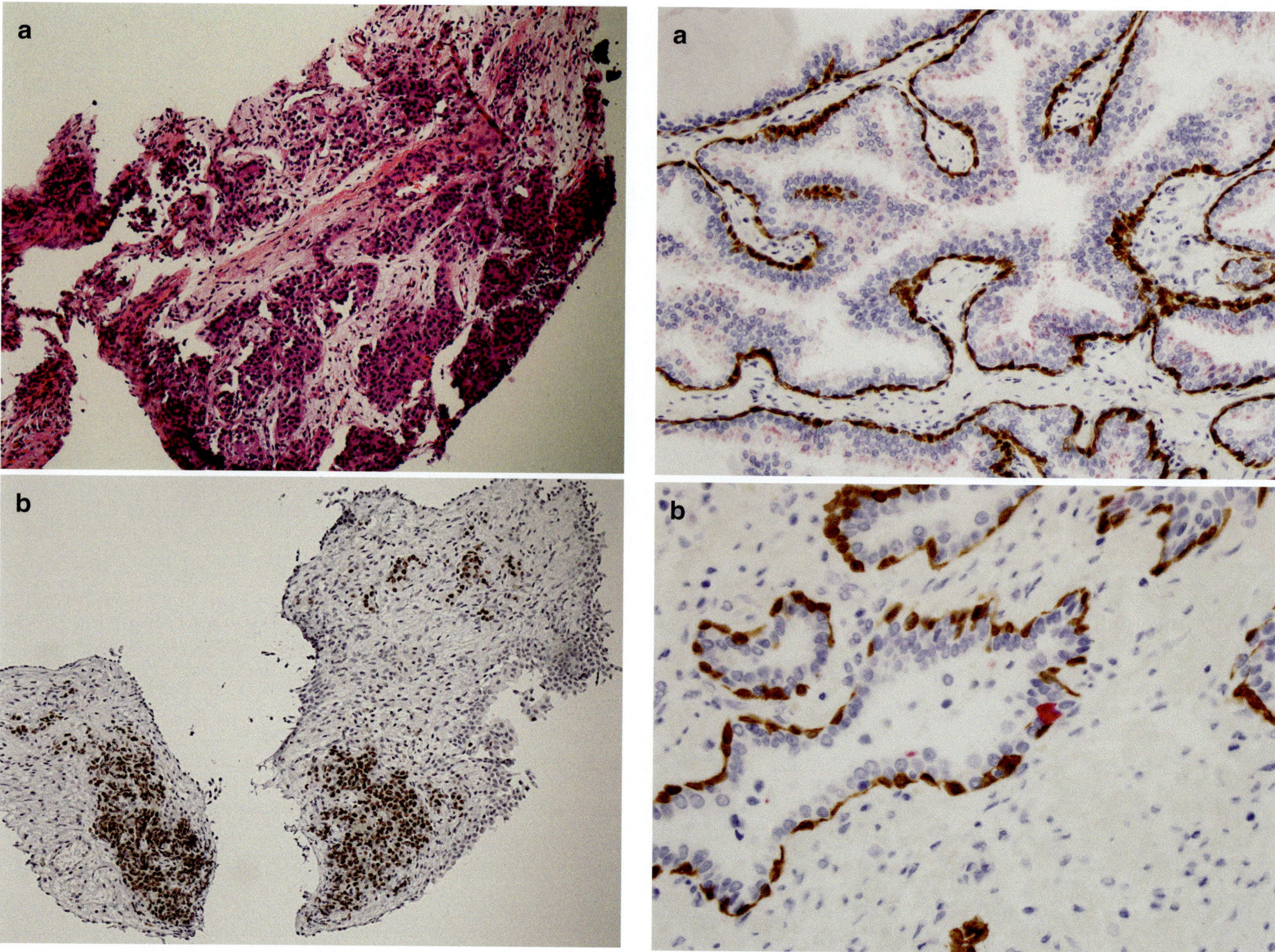

Fig. 5.27 A prostatic adenocarcinoma metastatic to the bladder (**a**) is positive for NKX3.1 (**b**). Note the overlying urothelial cells are negative for NKX3.1

Fig. 5.28 Benign glands have weak but diffuse fine granular staining in the cytoplasm (**a**). Isolated benign prostatic epithelial cells show strong AMACR positivity (**b**)

cancer. The specificity of NKX3.1 was 99.7% (nonprostatic tumor positive for NKX3.1), as its expression is also seen in normal testis, 9% of primary and 5% of metastatic infiltrating ductal breast carcinoma, and 27% of primary and 26% of metastatic infiltrating lobular breast carcinoma.

References: [46, 52]

ules in the cytoplasm of adenocarcinoma cells. Occasionally, benign prostatic glands may contain isolated cells strongly positive for AMACR (Fig. 5.28b), which are believed to be special neuroendocrine cells. A subset of prostatic adenosis and partial atrophy expresses AMACR, usually weak.

References: [26, 53]

Can AMACR Positivity Be Observed in Benign Prostatic Glands?

Yes. The discovery of AMACR as a prostate cancer maker is based on the differential expression of this gene between benign prostatic tissue and prostatic adenocarcinoma, which has a much higher level of expression than benign prostatic glands or stroma. The benign prostatic secretory cells may display a weaker AMACR staining with fine cytoplasmic granules (Fig. 5.28a) compared to the intense coarse gran-

Can Prostatic Adenocarcinoma Show Positivity for P63?

Immunostain for p63, or its isoform p40, is one of the commonly used immunohistochemical markers for working up difficult prostate biopsies, as they are strongly expressed in prostatic basal cells and absent in prostatic acinar carcinomas. However, p63 can rarely be found in prostatic carcinoma cells with uniform and nonbasal cell distribution in so-called p63-positive prostate cancer (Fig. 5.29) that represents a form

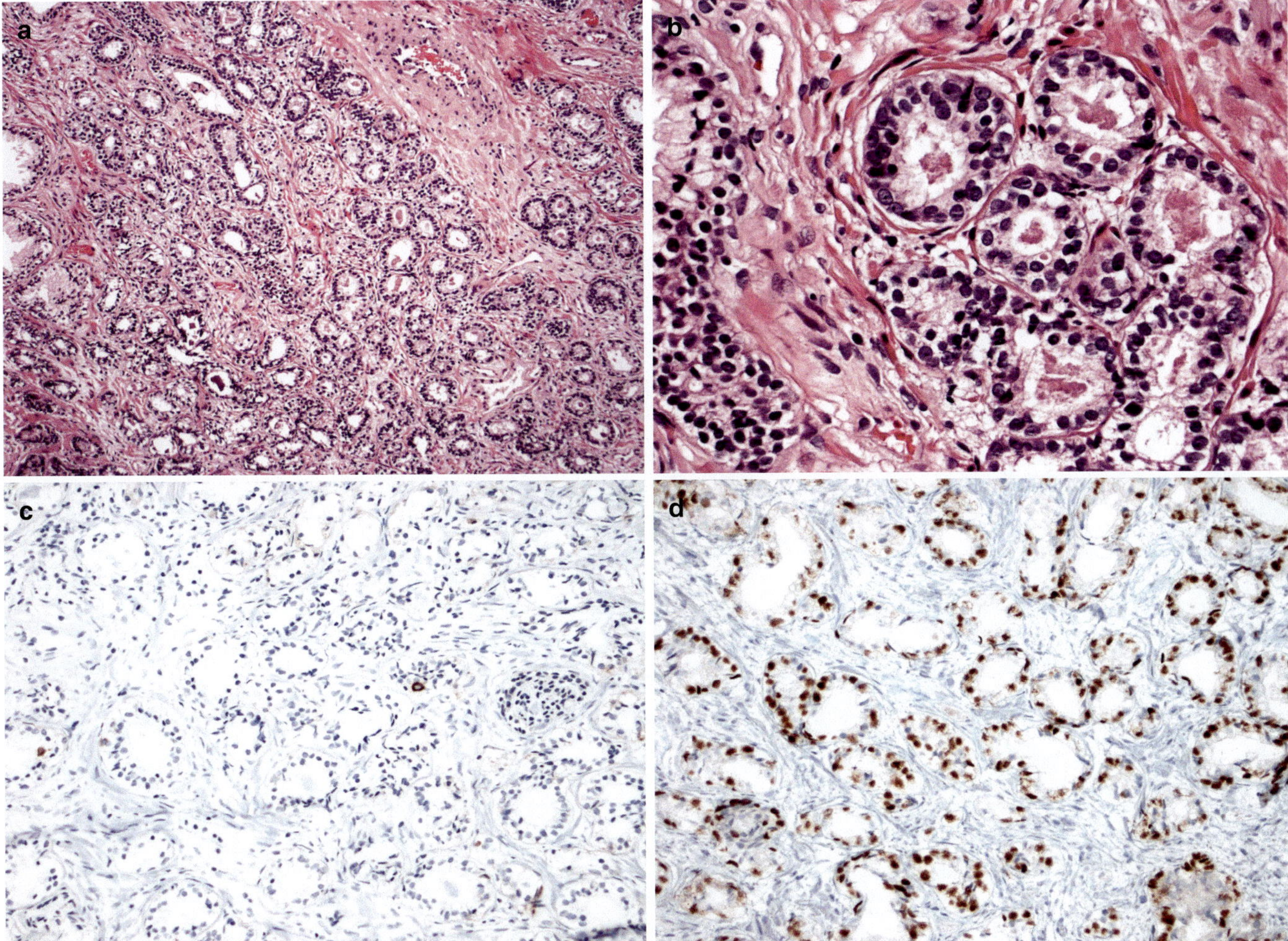

Fig. 5.29 p63-positive prostate cancer. The cancer glands are small and have round rigid lumens (**a**). The nucleoli are prominent (**b**). All the cancer glands are negative for HMWCK (34βE12) (**c**), but uniformly positive for p63 (**d**). Rather than being in basal cell distribution, the staining is found in all cancer cells

of prostate cancer with partial basal-like immunophenotype, molecularly different from the usual acinar cancers.

References: [54, 55]

Can Prostatic Adenocarcinoma Show Positivity for High Molecular Weight Cytokeratin (CK5/CK6, K903)?

Yes. Although lack of basal cells is the hallmark of prostate cancer, exceedingly rare cases of prostatic adenocarcinoma with focal basal cell marker HMWCK positivity have been reported. These cancer glands have typical histological features of invasive prostatic adenocarcinoma, but show focal HMWCK staining. Typically, these tumor cells are present in a small cluster of 5–10 cells, and the positive staining is not in basal cell distribution (Fig. 5.30).

As discussed in the other places in this chapter, intraductal carcinoma also have retained basal cells positive for HMWCK, and basal cell carcinoma of the prostate shows strong staining for HMWCK.

References: [56, 57]

Can any Benign Lesion in the Prostate Display Strong AMACR Positivity But Negative for Basal Cell Markers?

Adenosis, partial atrophy, high-grade prostatic intraepithelial neoplasia (HGPIN) may have discontinuous or even absent basal cell lining, yet are positive, sometimes quite strongly, for AMACR (Fig. 5.31). Nephrogenic adenocarcinoma, which can be found in the prostate, can be strongly positive for AMACR, negative for basal cell markers. Therefore, neg-

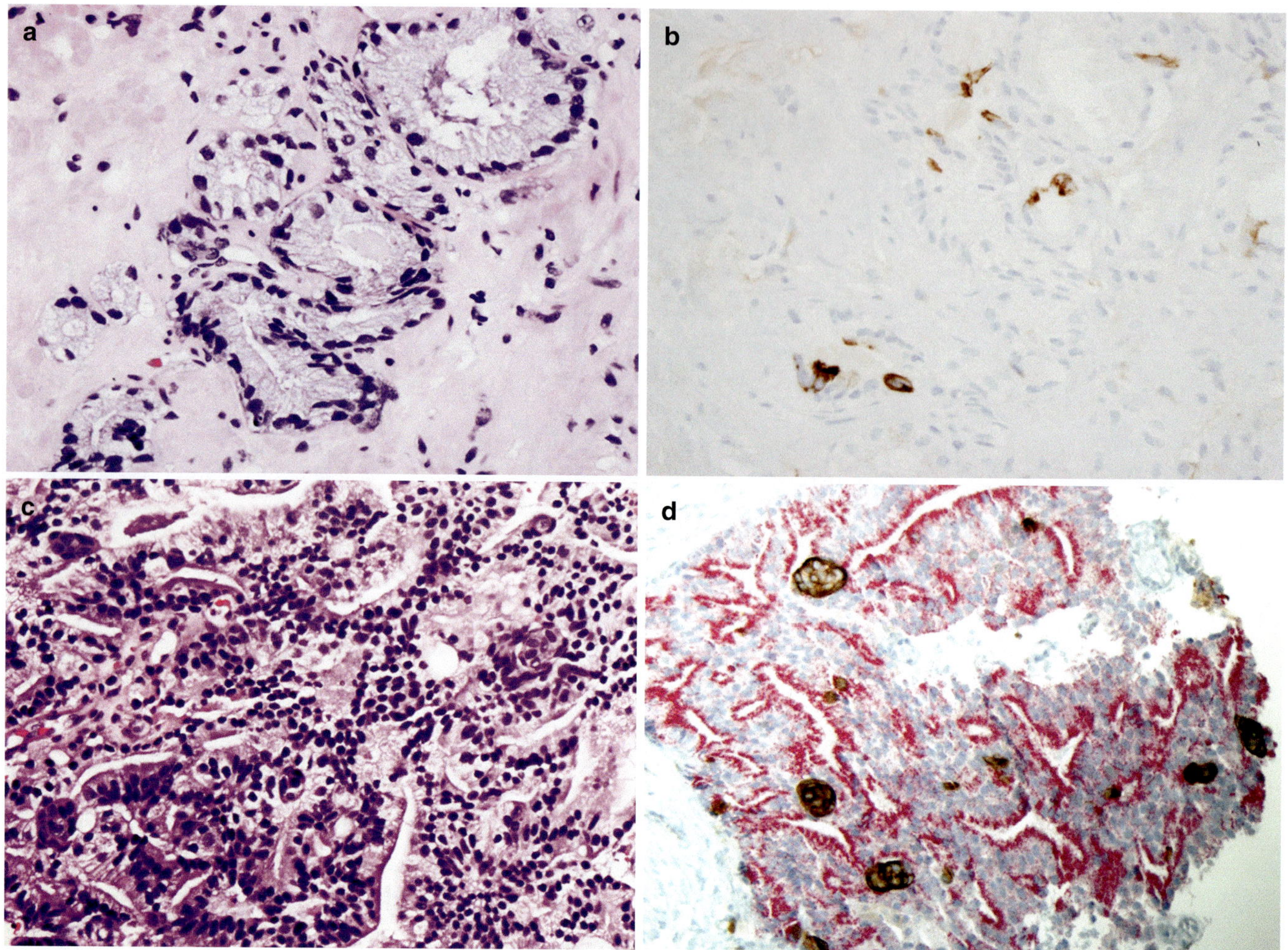

Fig. 5.30 Prostatic adenocarcinoma (**a**) shows focal HMWCK immunoreactivity in scattered tumor cells (**b**). Another case of high-grade prostatic adenocarcinoma (**c**) shows strong AMACR immunoreactivity in the majority of tumor cells, with scattered tumor cells positive for HMWCK (**d**)

ative basal cell marker and positive AMACR staining are by itself not diagnostic of cancer.

References: [53, 58]

What Are the Components of the Triple Stain for the Prostate? When Should We Perform Triple Stains?

Prostate triple stain contains antibodies against AMACR for labeling adenocarcinoma cells, while p63 and high molecular weight cytokeratin (HMWCK) for labeling basal cells. It can be used in the following clinical settings: (1) to ascertain the diagnosis of prostatic adenocarcinoma on needle core biopsy, when the focus has histologic feature of carcinoma but is small (Fig. 5.32); (2) to clarify the nature of a small focus of atypical glands suspicious for adenocarcinoma; (3) to confirm possible benign conditions such as adenosis, partial atrophy, sclerosing adenosis; (4) in evaluation of trans- urethral resection of bladder tumor or prostate to rule out prostate cancer; (5) to distinguish invasive adenocarcinoma from intraductal carcinoma of the prostate; (6) to distinguish PIN-like carcinoma from high-grade PIN; and (7) to confirm recurrent prostate cancer after treatment. Triple stain is particularly useful in the postradiation settings.

The advantage of triple stain is several folds. It is particularly useful on prostate biopsy with limited amount of cancer. It also allows simultaneous evaluation of basal cell marker and AMACR in the same small focus of cancer/atypical glands. Random use of the triple stain for obvious invasive prostatic adenocarcinoma on needle biopsy for financial gain is not recommended and should be strongly discouraged. In a metastatic lesion, the value of the triple stain is also limited because other types of carcinomas often express AMACR. Finally, some benign conditions such as nephrogenic adenoma in the prostate or bladder may show strong AMACR staining without basal cell staining, mimicking prostate cancer.

References: [59, 60]

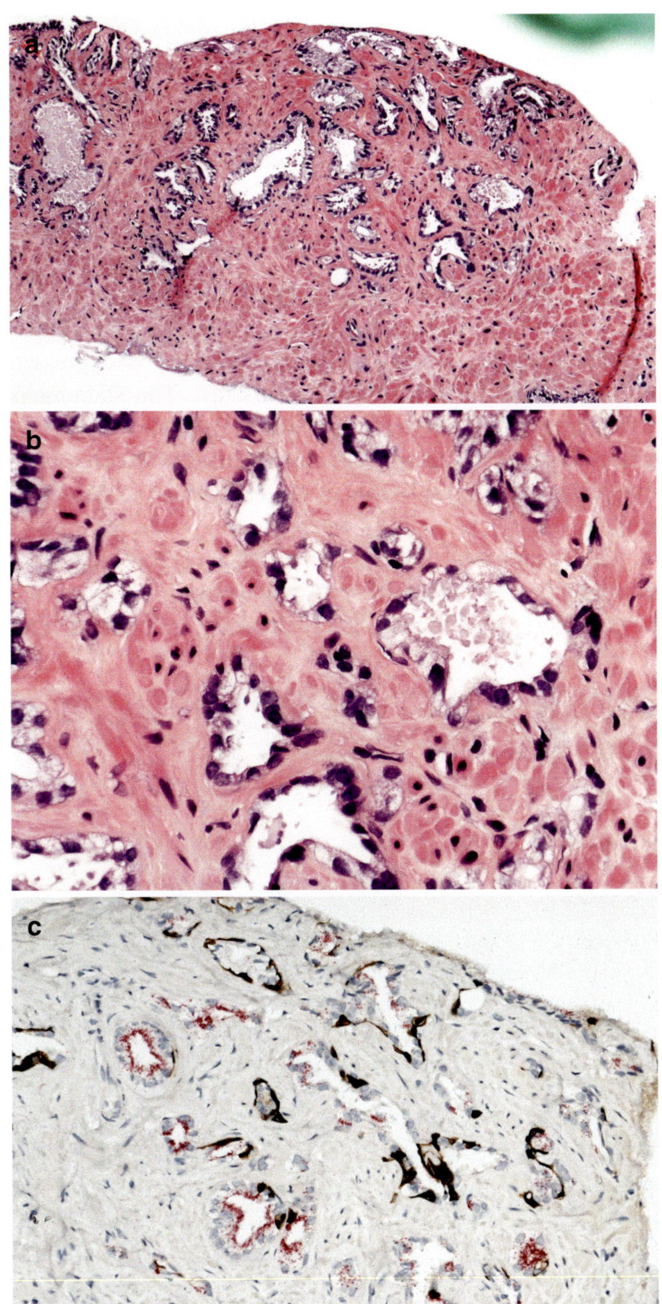

Fig. 5.31 In prostate partial atrophy (**a**, **b**), some glands are focally positive, while other glands are negative, for basal cell markers and strongly positive for AMACR (**c**, triple stain)

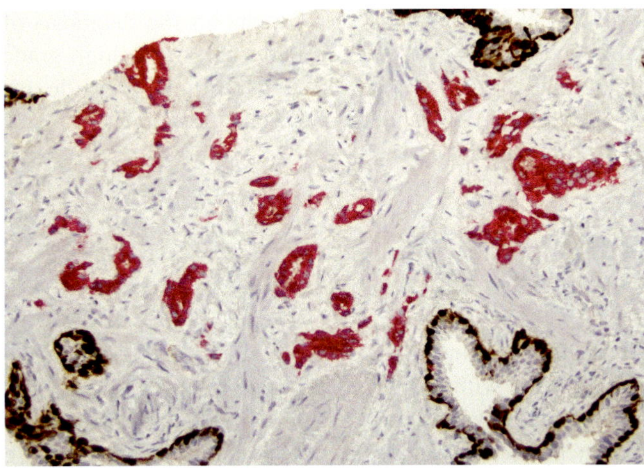

Fig. 5.32 A prostate biopsy with triple staining. The cancer glands are positive for AMACR (red staining) and negative for basal cell markers p63 and HMWCK (brown staining), whereas benign glands are positive for basal cell markers and negative for AMACR

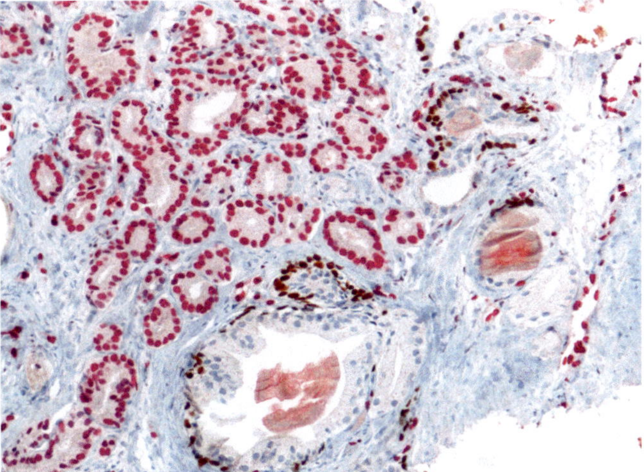

Fig. 5.33 Prostate cancer stained with an antibody cocktail for both basal cell markers p63 (brown nuclear staining) and ERG (red nuclear staining). Cancer glands are positive for ERG and negative for p63, whereas benign glands are positive for p63 and negative for ERG. Endothelial cells serve as internal positive control

What Is the Diagnostic Value of ERG Immunostaining?

ERG is a member of the ETS gene family, which is commonly involved by chromosomal translocation in prostate cancer. ERG immunostaining correlates highly with *ERG* gene alteration. However, ERG is positive in only 40–50% of prostate carcinomas. It is also positive in 20% of HGPIN that intermingles with ERG-positive prostate carcinomas. Positive staining is exceedingly rare in noncancer glands distant from prostate carcinoma. Therefore, ERG has a limited utility in diagnosis of challenging prostate cancer cases in prostate biopsies. A positive ERG staining supports a cancer diagnosis (Fig. 5.33) but lack of staining does not rule out cancer. One scenario in which ERG is helpful is a positive ERG staining in "atypical glands suspicious for cancer," where the diagnosis of high-grade PIN is excluded, supports a cancer diagnosis. Positive ERG staining, coupled with PTEN loss, may be used to support the diagnosis of intraductal carcinoma and distinguish it from high-grade PIN. Finally, ERG, if positive, can confirm the prostatic origin of a poorly differentiated metastatic carcinoma.

References: [50, 61–63]

Is the AMACR Immunostaining in Prostate Cancer Cells Affected by any Treatment?

Generally speaking, the level of AMACR expression does not correlate with the Gleason grade of prostatic adenocarcinoma. However, some therapies, particularly, hormonal treatment such as androgen deprivation therapy (ADT), may reduce the level of AMACR in prostatic adenocarcinoma cells. Furthermore, our studies found that the hormonally treated tumor cells will re-express AMACR when they become castration resistant. Therefore, the diagnosis of hormonal-treated prostate cancer is primarily based on

infiltrative nature of the tumor cells (Fig. 5.34). On the other hand, most recurrent/residual prostatic adenocarcinoma after radiation shows strong AMACR immunoreactivity. Therefore, the triple stain will be very useful in the needle core biopsy interpretation in postradiation cases.

References: [64–66]

What Is the Diagnostic Utility of PSMA?

Prostate-specific membrane antigen (PSMA) is expressed in benign and malignant prostate tissues. The staining is stronger in cancer versus benign and high-grade versus low-grade cancer. The staining patterns in prostate cancer include cytoplasmic and cytoplasmic with membranous accentuation (Fig. 5.35).

PSMA cannot be used to differentiate prostate cancer from its mimickers in the prostate. It may be used to confirm the prostatic origin of a metastatic carcinoma in a patient with

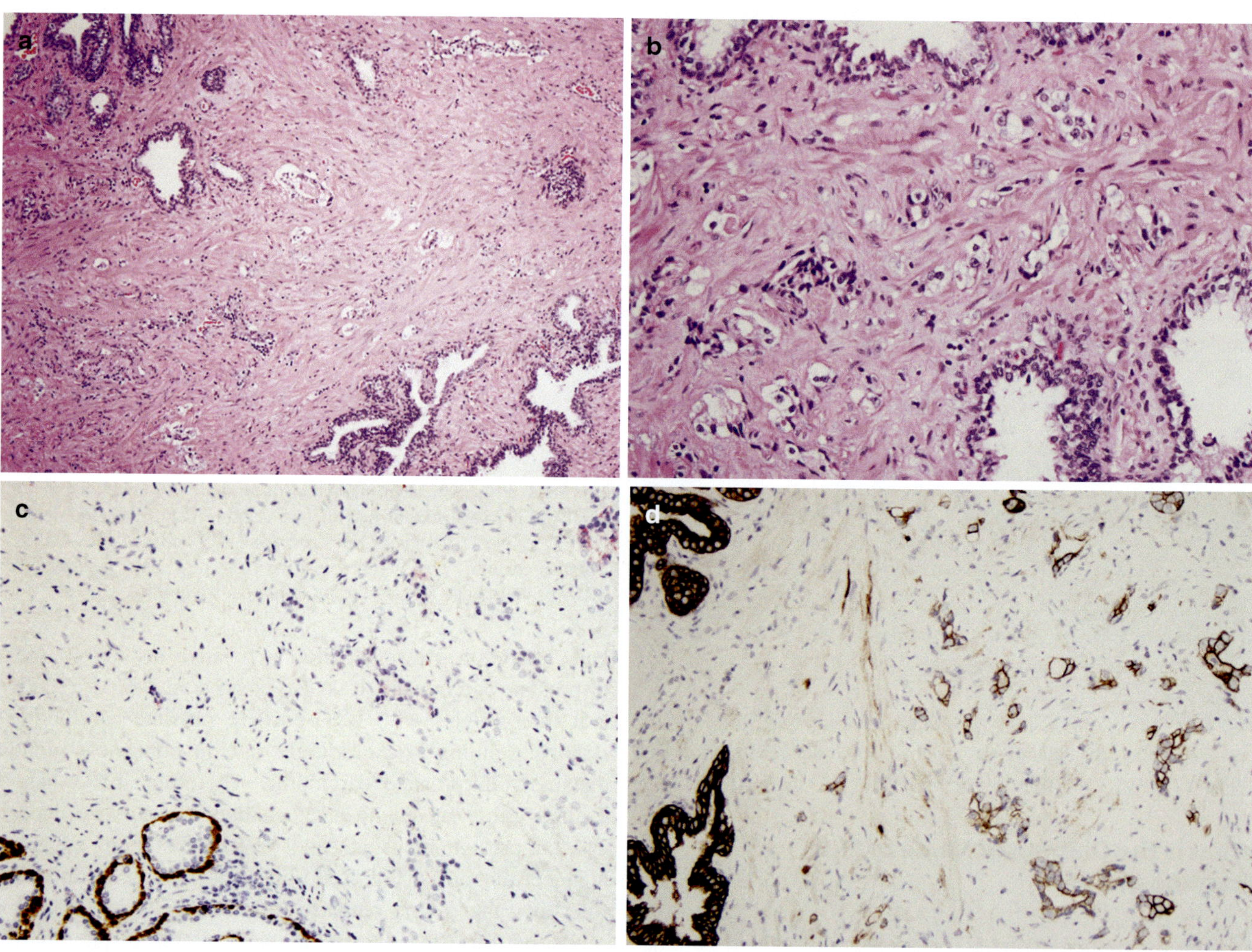

Fig. 5.34 Prostatic adenocarcinoma after androgen deprivation therapy shows marked atrophy (**a**). Occasional cytological atypia can be seen in some tumor cells with prominent nucleoli (**b**). The triple stain shows weak AMACR staining and no basal cell staining in the treated tumor cells (**c**). AE1/AE3 highlights the infiltrating tumor cells (**d**)

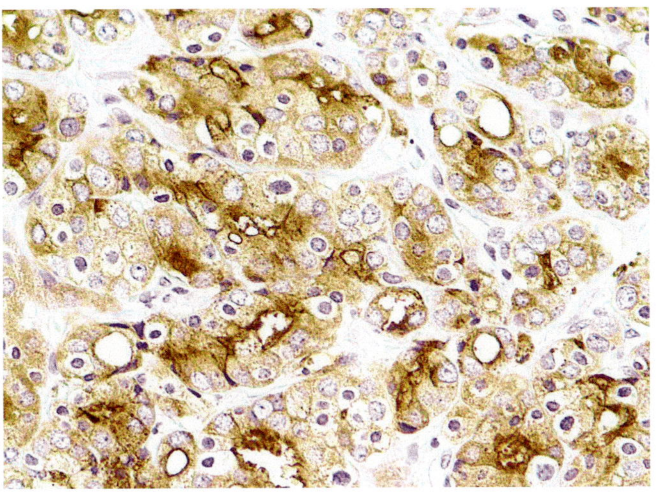

Fig. 5.35 A Gleason score 4 + 4 = 8 prostate cancer is positive for PSMA with mainly cytoplasmic staining and luminal accentuation

known history of prostate cancer. Because it is expressed in other tissues, including kidney, liver, and urinary bladder, and it is associated with tumor neovasculature as well, it cannot be used as the sole marker to confirm the prostatic origin for a metastatic carcinoma of unknown primary.

Studies have also shown that PSMA overexpression correlates with an unfavorable biochemical recurrence-free survival rate. PSMA expression also significantly correlates with Gleason Score in prostate biopsy and prostatectomy specimen, implying a potential prognostic value for PSMA in prostate biopsy as well. However, these findings are preliminary and PSMA as a prognostic marker is not used routinely in clinical settings.

References: [67, 68]

When and How Often Do You See PSA-Negative Prostate Cancer?

The majority of prostatic adenocarcinomas (95–99%) are positive for PSA prior to any treatment. However, a small subset of high-grade prostatic adenocarcinomas may show very low PSA immunoreactivity. Furthermore, treated prostatic adenocarcinoma often shows significantly decreased or negative PSA staining. This is particularly relevant when the biopsy material is limited. With different positive staining thresholds, the PSA positive rate ranges from 30% to 50% in metastatic prostate cancer (Fig. 5.36). It is important to keep

in mind that PSA staining may be very focal (less than 1% tumor cells positive) and may manifest as fine granules in tumor cells only seen at high power magnification.

Significantly reduced or negative PSA staining in treated prostatic adenocarcinoma may lead to diagnostic errors. We have repeatedly seen this mistake in interpreting such weak/focal PSA staining as negative. Therefore, we use a panel of prostate markers including PSA and more sensitive markers, such as NKX3.1 and PSMA, for confirmation of metastatic or advanced prostate cancer.

References: [47, 69, 70]

What Is the Difference Between New and Old Prostate Cancer TNM Staging?

Compared with the previous edition, the 2018 8th edition AJCC TNM staging for prostate cancer includes the following changes:

- Pathologically organ-confined disease is considered pT2 and no longer subclassified by extent of involvement or laterality. T2 is no longer substaged into T2a, b, and c.
- The Gleason score and the Grade Group should both be reported.
- Stage III includes selected organ-confined disease tumors based on prostate-specific antigen (PSA) and Gleason/Grade Group status.

Reference: [31]

What Is Difference Between Focal and Nonfocal Extraprostatic Extension (EPE)?

Focal extraprostatic extension (EPE) is defined as small focus of tumor cells present outside prostate in the extraprostatic tissue (Fig. 5.37a) involving less than one high power (40×) field on one or two slides at most. Multifocal EPE or large focus of EPE (>1 high power field) is considered nonfocal (also known as established or extensive) EPE (Fig. 5.37b, c). Although prostatic adenocarcinoma with focal or nonfocal extraprostatic extension is all staged as pT3a disease, the nonfocal EPE carried a significantly worse prognosis than focal EPE. Extraprostatic extension on biopsy (Fig. 5.37d) can be diagnosed when cancer glands are found in the fat and are typically seen on the tip of a needle core.

Reference: [31]

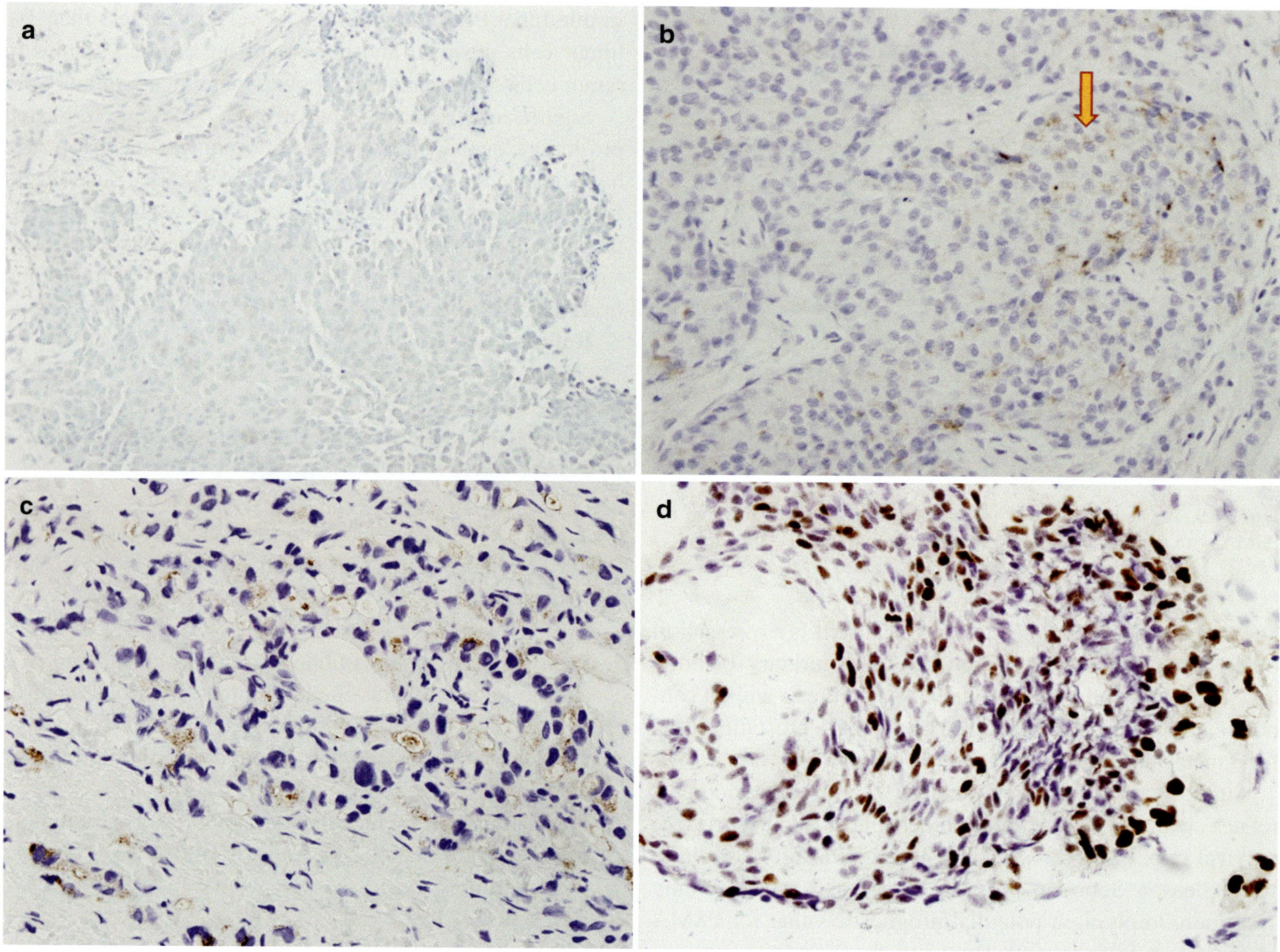

Fig. 5.36 High-grade metastatic prostatic adenocarcinoma negative for PSA (**a**). Another case of metastatic adenocarcinoma shows focal and weak granular PSA staining (**b**, arrow). The same tumor shows focal PSMA staining (**c**) but strong NKX3.1 staining (**d**)

How to Define Seminal Vesicle Invasion by Prostate Cancer?

Seminal vesicle invasion is defined as tumor infiltration of the muscular wall of the seminal vesicle and is staged as pT3b (Fig. 5.38). Only invasion of extraprostatic seminal vesicle invasion is considered as seminal vesicle involvement. Intraprostatic seminal vesicle or ejaculatory duct can be difficult to separate from one another, and involvement of these structures is not considered as pT3b disease. In addition, seminal vesicle invasion should be distinguished from periseminal vesicle soft tissue invasion, which is extraprostatic invasion and staged as pT3a. In prostate biopsies, seminal vesicle may not be reliably distinguished from ejaculatory ducts and hence both are lumped together as "seminal vesicle/ejaculatory duct."

Urologists may perform a biopsy of the seminal vesicle to better stage prostate cancer before prostatectomy. For such biopsies, pathologists should clearly state whether the seminal vesicle tissue is present and whether cancer involves the seminal vesicle tissue.

Reference: [71]

What Is the Difference Between Seminal Vesicle and Ejaculatory Duct?

Seminal vesicles are a pair of tubular structures posterosuperior to the prostate and lateral to the vasa deferentia. Each seminal vesicle and vas deferens join together inside the prostate to form the ejaculatory duct (Fig. 5.39a, b), which then passes through the prostate base and opens into

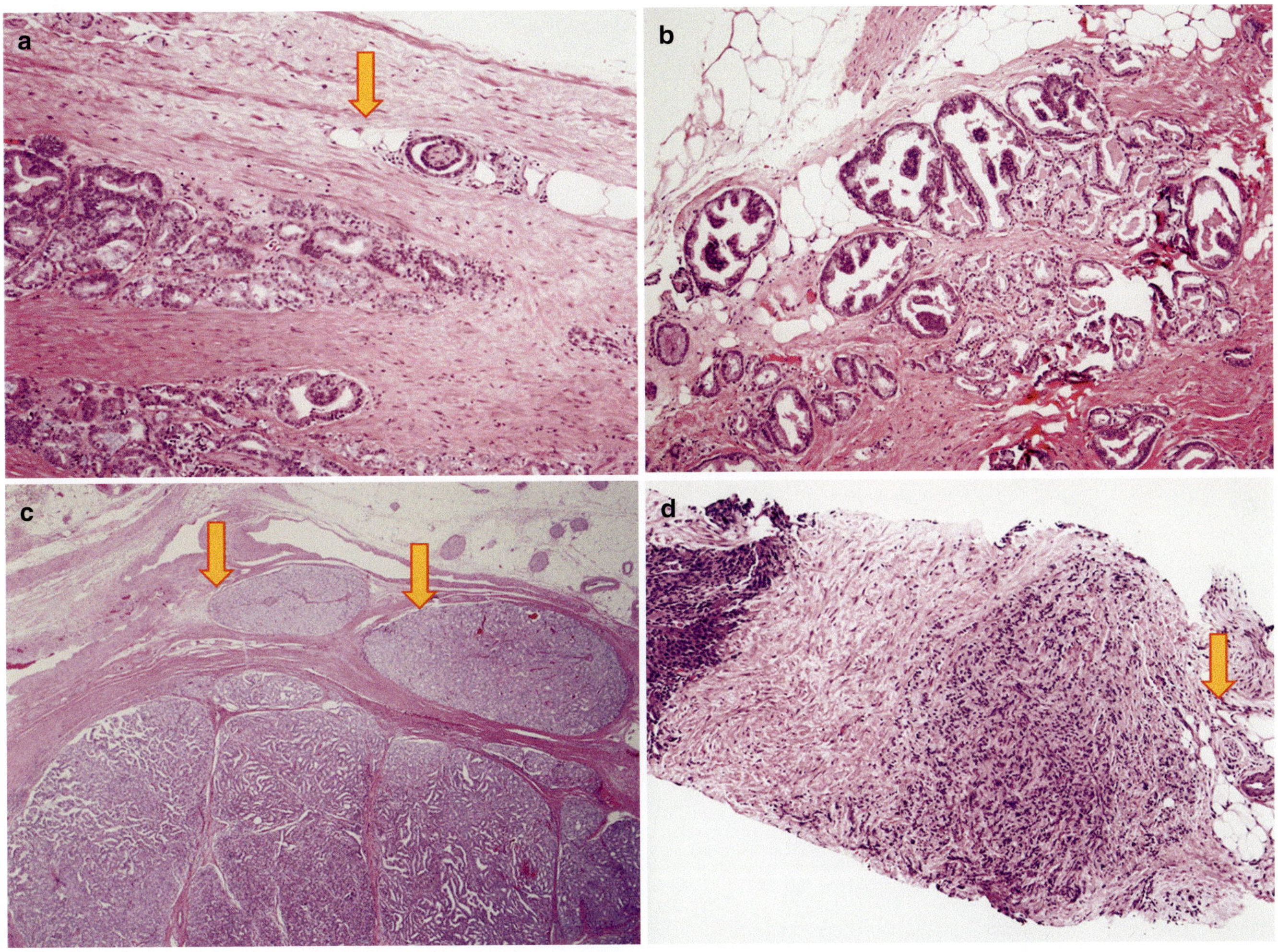

Fig. 5.37 Extraprostatic extension by prostatic adenocarcinoma is categorized as either "focal" when there is only one or a few malignant glands in the adipose tissue (**a**, arrow) or "nonfocal" when there are numerous malignant glands in the adipose tissue (**b**) or large clusters of tumor cells pushing outside into extraprostatic tissue (**c**, arrows). A prostate biopsy core shows high-grade adenocarcinoma cells involving fat, indicative of extraprostatic tissue (**d**, arrow)

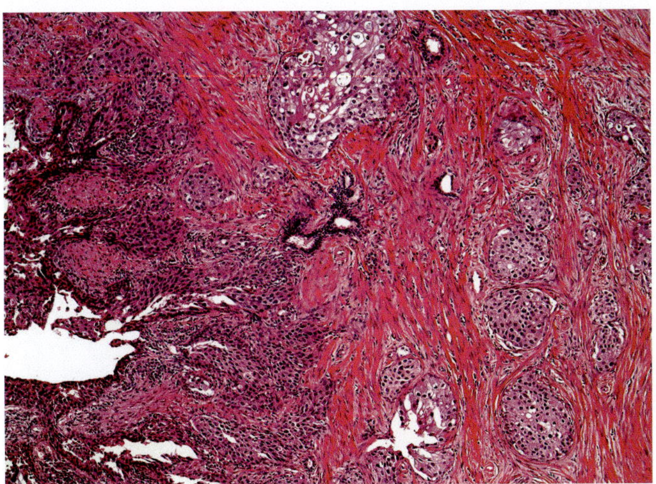

Fig. 5.38 Prostate cancer invading seminal vesicle with cancer glands invading the smooth muscle wall of the seminal vesicle, staged as pT3b

the prostatic urethra at the seminal colliculus adjacent to the verumontanum. Both seminal vesicle and ejaculatory ducts have similar histologic features (Fig. 5.39b) and may be difficult to distinguish from each other in biopsy material. Furthermore, the extraprostatic and intraprostatic seminal vesicles may be even more difficult to distinguish on needle biopsies. However, such distinction is important for staging as prostatic adenocarcinoma involving extraprostatic seminal vesicle is pT3b (Fig. 5.39c), while involvement of intraprostatic seminal vesicle is not considered as pT3b. Therefore, we usually refer these findings as "prostatic adenocarcinoma involving seminal vesicle-type of tissue (Fig. 5.39d), clinical correlation is necessary to determine whether this represents extraprostatic seminal vesicle invasion (pT3b)."

It is important to process the prostatectomy specimen correctly with a cross-section of the base of the seminal vesicles without any prostate tissue, because involvement of the

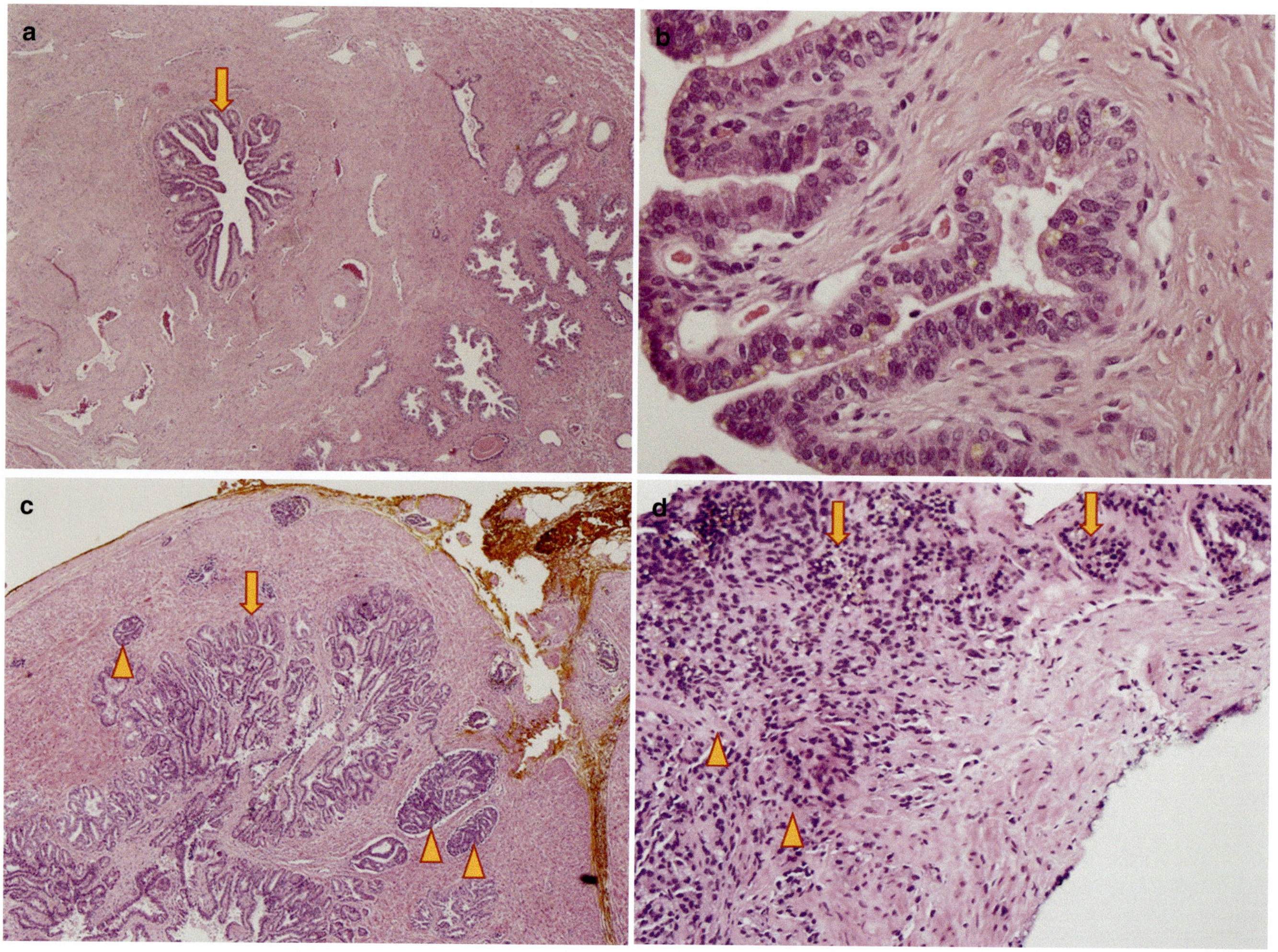

Fig. 5.39 An ejaculatory duct is surrounded by loose fibrovascular tissue and benign prostatic glands (**a**, arrow). The epithelial lining of ejaculatory duct is identical to that of seminal vesicle with cytoplasmic lipofuscin pigment and degenerative cytological atypia (**b**). Seminal vesicle (**c**, arrow) involved by prostatic adenocarcinoma (**c**, arrow heads) in the muscular wall. On biopsy, seminal vesicle tissue (**d**, arrows) is involved by prostatic adenocarcinoma (**d**, arrowheads)

ejaculatory duct surrounded by benign prostatic glands is not considered as stage pT3b disease.

   References: [31, 72]

Can Skeletal Muscle Be Seen inside the Prostate?

Skeletal muscle can be found intraprostatically, usually in the apex and anterior fibromuscular layer. Benign prostate glands can be found within the skeletal muscle fibers (Fig. 5.40). Finding cancer glands within the skeletal muscle fibers therefore does not necessarily indicate extraprostatic extension.

   Reference: [73]

Can Adipocytes Be Seen Within the Prostate?

Yes, but very rarely. Although there are claims of adipocytes in the prostate, it is an exceedingly rare finding. It is

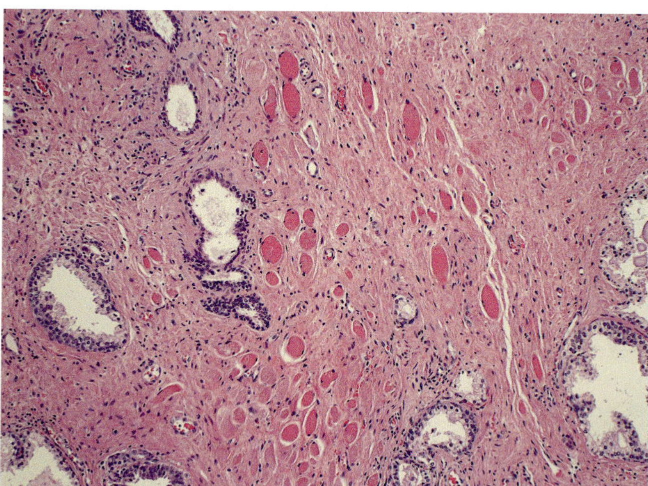

Fig. 5.40 Prostate glands within skeletal muscle fibers in the anterior fibromuscular zone

also rare to see benign glands adjacent to the adipose tissue. In the apex, there is no obvious capsule so adipose tissue intermingles with skeletal and smooth muscle tissue. These adipocytes in the apical region are considered extraprostatic. Therefore, adipocytes involved by adenocarcinoma can be safely interpreted as extraprostatic extension.

References: [74–77]

How to Measure Cancer Extent in Prostate Biopsy?

The tumor extent in prostate biopsy specimens is an important prognostic factor and affects patient management such as active surveillance. The biopsy report should include (1) the number of the biopsy cores involved by cancer and total number of cores and (2) linear length of cancer or percentage of each core involved by cancer. For a specimen with fragmented cores, an overall percentage of cancer over the entire specimen should be estimated. There is no consensus regarding which of these methods is the best one to report the tumor quantity in needle biopsies. If applied consistently, these methods work equally well with a few caveats. Although a high cancer volume in needle biopsy in general correlates with a large-volume cancer in radical prostatectomy, a low volume in biopsy does not necessarily indicate a low-volume cancer in radical prostatectomy.

One issue is how to record discontinuous tumor involvement in which cancer involves a core discontinuous with abundant intervening benign glands. Such a finding may represent a multifocal disease. When estimating the tumor extent in these cases, one could measure from one end of the tumor to the other end without excluding the intervening benign glands. Alternatively, one may report discontinuous involvement by both including and excluding the intervening benign

tissue. Most studies, though, have shown that measuring the cancer length from one end to the other better correlates with radical prostatectomy findings and prognostic outcomes than excluding the intervening benign tissue. Pathologists should communicate with their clinical colleagues regarding the method of tumor volume measurement.

References: [78, 79]

How to Diagnose Bladder Neck Invasion by Prostate Cancer in Radical Prostatectomy Specimens?

Bladder neck, present between distal bladder and prostate base, is composed of large bundles of smooth muscle (Fig. 5.41a) that connect bladder to the urethra. When prostate carcinoma grossly involves the bladder neck and bladder wall, it is staged as T4. These advanced stage tumors are rare, and patients are often not surgical candidates. Microscopic bladder neck involvement requires prostatic adenocarcinoma cells within thick smooth muscle bundles measuring greater than 100–200 nm. These muscle bundles may have scattered adipose tissue, but should not have intermixed benign prostatic glands. However, there is no distinct physical boundary between the bladder neck muscle and surround prostatic stromal tissue. When there is tumor in the adipose tissue present between the thick muscle bundles, it is clearly extraprostatic extension (Fig. 5.41b).

It is still controversial whether the microscopic bladder neck involvement is a significant independent prognostic factor. This is due in part to the poor delineation of the bladder neck region. More studies are necessary to clarify the significance of bladder neck involvement by prostate cancer.

References: [80, 81]

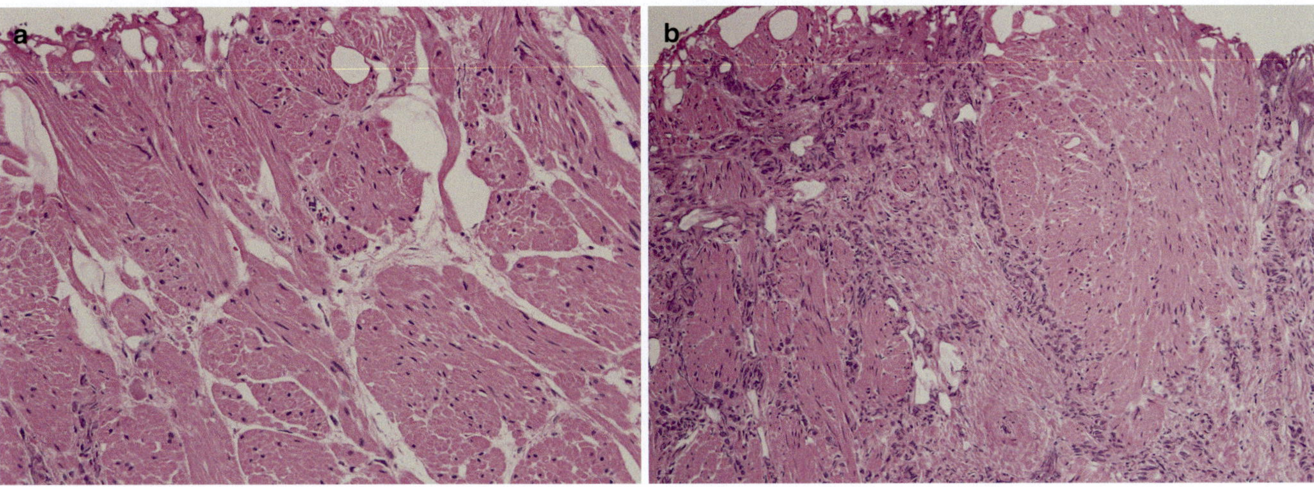

Fig. 5.41 Bladder neck is composed of large smooth muscle bundles with intervening adipocytes (**a**). Prostatic adenocarcinoma involves the bladder neck microscopically (**b**) that is staged as pT3a

How to Grade Multifocal Prostate Cancer in Radical Prostatectomy Specimens?

In a multifocal prostate cancer, the overall Gleason score should be assigned based on the dominant nodule, which is typically the largest in size. The Gleason scores of other foci can be mentioned in the report as well.

However, in 10–20% of multifocal tumors, highest Gleason score, largest tumor size and highest staging parameter do not concur in the same tumor nodules. In such cases, the Gleason scores of individual tumors can be recorded separately. For instance, if there is a large Gleason score 3 + 3 = 6 tumor in the transition zone and a separate smaller Gleason score 4 + 3 = 7 in the peripheral zone, the Gleason scores of both tumor nodules should be reported. The scores should not be averaged to provide an overall score in such cases.

Reference: [82]

How Do You Define Prostate Carcinoma "Dominant Nodule" in Radical Prostatectomy Specimens?

Prostate cancer is often multifocal. Each focus of cancer may have a different Gleason score. A dominant nodule refers as the largest tumor nodule in a multifocal prostate cancer. Typically, the dominant nodule also has the highest Gleason score and staging parameter such as extraprostatic extension (if present). Such a dominant nodule represents the most aggressive disease. We report the size and location of the dominant nodule, which provides important information for clinical, radiographic, and pathological correlation.

However, in a subset (10–20%) of prostate cancer cases, the highest Gleason score and largest size are not present in the same dominant tumor nodule. In such tumors, Gleason scores should be assigned to largest tumor nodule and other significant foci such as those with highest Gleason score and staging parameter. It is controversial to provide an aggregated Gleason score of all tumor foci.

References: [82, 83]

How to Distinguish Adenosis from Prostatic Adenocarcinoma?

Adenosis, also known as atypical adenomatous hyperplasia, is composed of well-circumscribed/lobulated proliferation of large complex glands admixed with small round glands. Mild nuclear atypia including slightly enlarged nuclei and small nucleoli are often seen (Fig. 5.42a–c). Basal cell markers are frequently patchy, or even absent in some small glands. AMACR can be positive, and quite strongly in some cases.

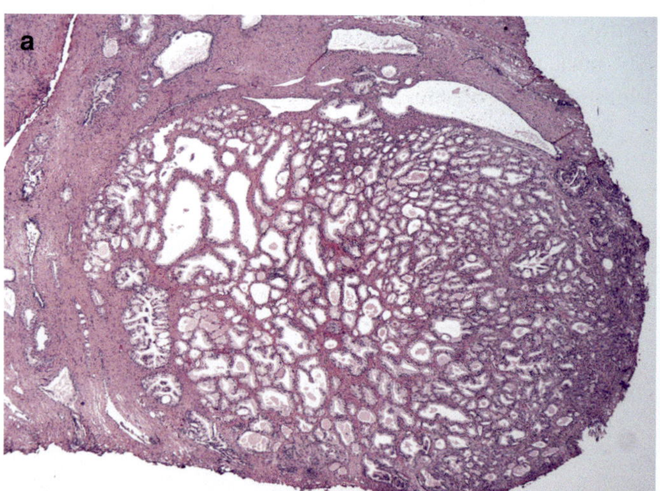

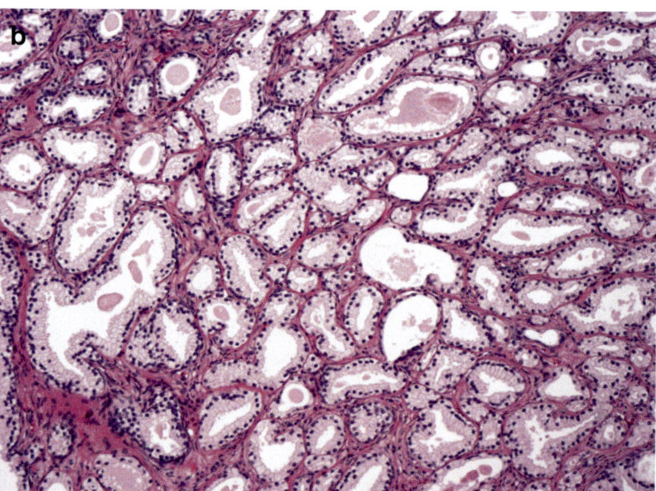

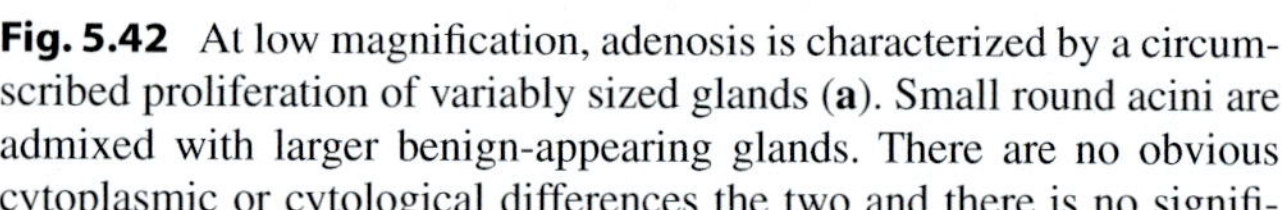

Fig. 5.42 At low magnification, adenosis is characterized by a circumscribed proliferation of variably sized glands (**a**). Small round acini are admixed with larger benign-appearing glands. There are no obvious cytoplasmic or cytological differences the two and there is no significant nuclear atypia (**b**). Basal cell markers demonstrate a patchy-staining pattern (**c**). A pseudohyperplastic carcinoma also has a circumscribed contour (**d**), but cancer glands have significant nuclear atypia (**e**). Basal cell staining is completely negative (**f**)

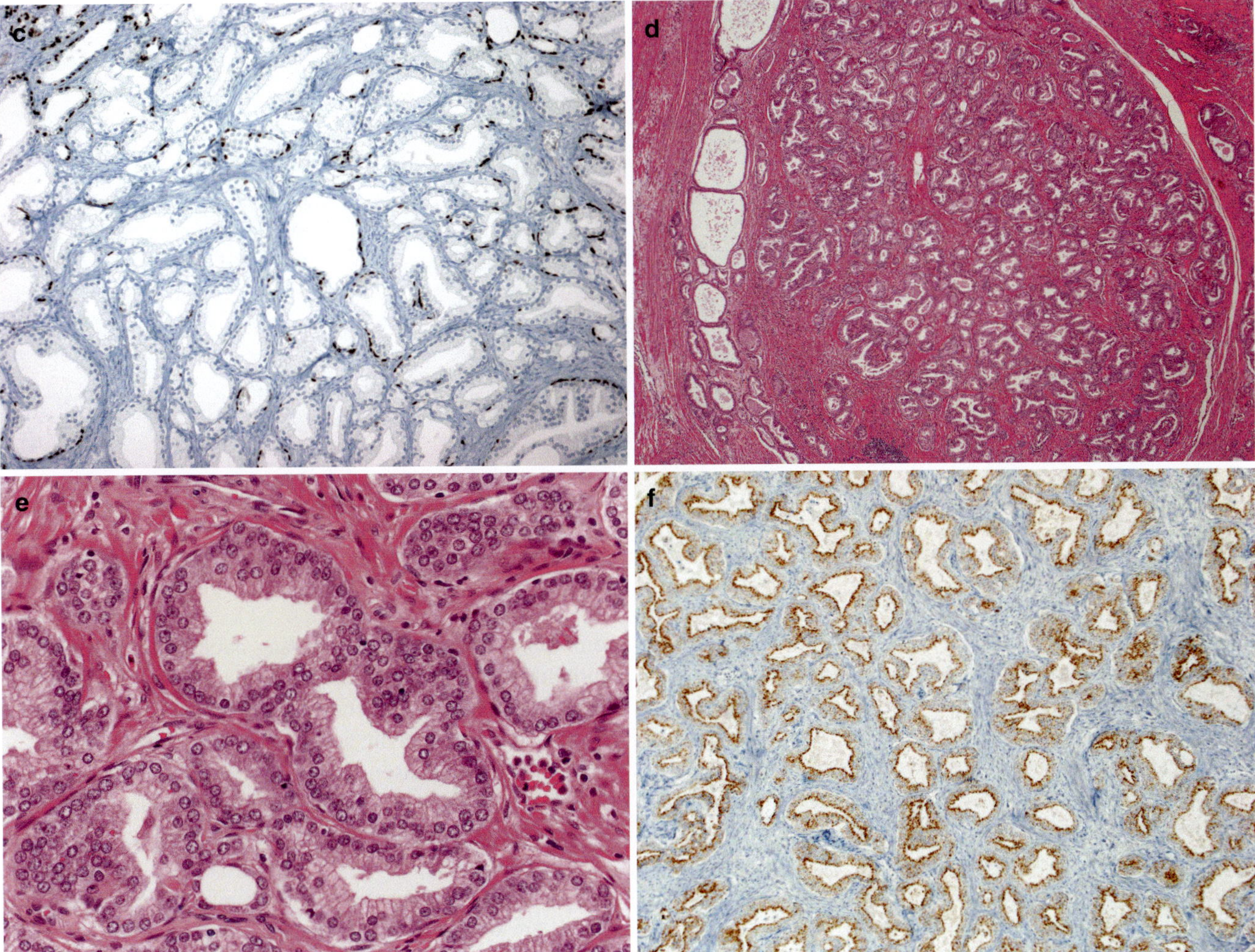

Fig. 5.42 (continued)

When considering a diagnosis of adenosis, one should always consider prostatic adenocarcinoma that also has a circumscribed contour such as pseudohyperplastic variant and those in the anterior/transition zone (Fig. 5.42d, e). In adenosis, small glands are admixed with obvious large hyperplastic benign glands. The cytoplasmic and cytological characteristics of small and large glands appear similar, and the two essentially merge with each other. Cancer glands, in contrast, invariably demonstrate cytoplasmic and cytological features distinct from the adjacent benign glands. Cellular spindly stroma also favors adenosis. Basal cell markers are typically patchy in adenosis but are completely negative in cancer.

Reference: [2]

How to Distinguish Paraganglion Cells from Prostate Cancer?

Paraganglion is a group of neurosecretory cells derived from neural crest (Fig. 5.43). They often are found in close proximity of a nerve or ganglion, and can be seen inside, or more commonly, outside the prostate in the periprostatic tissue.

Paraganglion may be mistaken for high-grade prostate cancer or cancer with treatment effect, but can be distinguished from adenocarcinoma by the following features:

- Paraganglion is a well-circumscribed cluster ranging from a dozen to a few hundreds of cells with a thin cap-

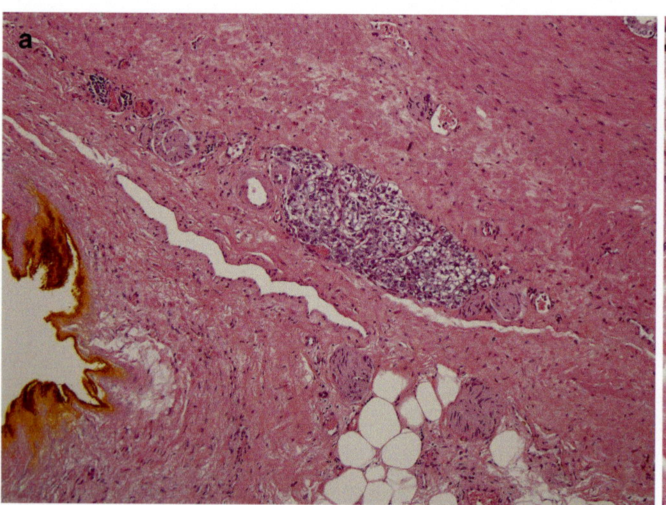

Fig. 5.43 Paraganglion is a well-circumscribed structure within or outside the prostate, often close to a nerve bundle (**a**). It is composed of cluster of solid cells. High magnification shows the epithelioid cells with clear to granular cytoplasm, regular nuclei, and fine chromatin with no prominent nucleoli (**b**)

sule. They are usually well-circumscribed, while cancer cells are more infiltrative without defined borders.

- The nuclei of paraganglion cells are regular and uniform without any cytological atypia.
- Paraganglion nuclei often show salt and pepper chromatin without prominent nucleoli, while adenocarcinoma displays prominent nucleoli.
- Cytoplasm of paraganglion is clear or purplish (amphophilic), while adenocarcinoma cells can have amphophilic cytoplasm but rarely clear cytoplasm.
- Paraganglion cells are negative for basal cell markers (HMWCK or p63), prostate cancer markers (AMACR, NKX3.1 and PSA), but positive for neuroendocrine markers.

References: [84, 85]

How to Recognize Sclerosing Adenosis in the Prostate?

Sclerosing adenosis is largely restricted to the transition zone of the prostate. Therefore, it is extremely rare in prostate needle biopsy and is generally seen as an incidental finding in TURP or radical prostatectomy specimens.

At low magnification, sclerosing adenosis comprises circumscribed proliferation of variably sized and shaped glands and individual cells in a dense spindle cellular stroma (Fig. 5.44a). Glands are usually poorly formed glands with slit-like lumina, cords and single cells with signet ring cell-like features (Fig. 5.44b) are present mimicking high-grade cancer. Stroma surrounding the glands is cellular and hyalinized. Prominent nucleoli, crystalloids, and blue mucin are common. Basal cells in sclerosing adenosis undergo myoepithelial metaplasia and coexpress basal cell markers (high molecular weight cytokeratin and P63) and myoepithelial markers (muscle-specific actin and S-100) (Fig. 5.44c).

High-grade Gleason score 8–10 prostate carcinoma should be considered in the differential diagnosis. The lack of circumscription and negative basal cell markers supports a carcinoma diagnosis.

In summary, when one or more circumscribed cellular lesions are seen in TURP or biopsies from the transition zone of the prostate, the diagnosis of sclerosing adenosis should be ruled out before a high-grade prostate cancer diagnosis is rendered.

Reference: [2]

How to Distinguish Partial Atrophy from Prostate Cancer?

Partial atrophy is one of the most common benign prostate lesions mistaken for prostate cancer.

Partial atrophy is composed of angulated glands with somewhat clear cytoplasm. It can be distinguished from adenocarcinoma by the following features (Fig. 5.45):

- Atrophy retains the lobular pattern, while carcinoma shows haphazard infiltrating pattern.
- On needle core biopsy material, glands in partial atrophy show irregular arrangement with angulated contour and are lined with single layer of cells. However, cells show no significant cytological atypia and prominent nucleoli, which are the features frequently present in prostatic adenocarcinoma.

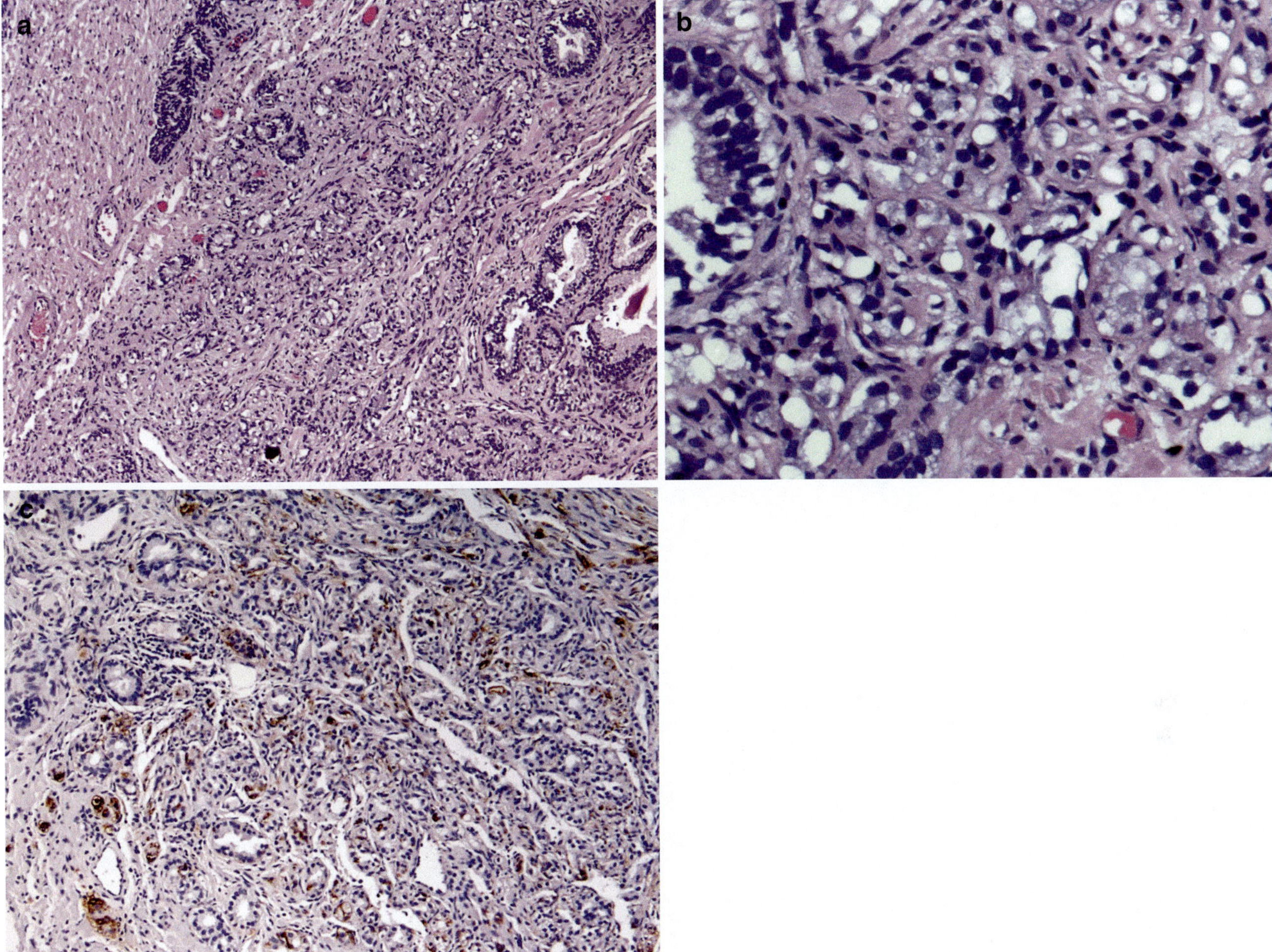

Fig. 5.44 Sclerosing adenosis comprises circumscribed proliferation of poorly formed and complex glands. Stroma between glands is cellular (**a**). At high magnification, glands are ill-formed and fused. Single cells with signet ring features are also present (**b**). Basal cells are positive for basal cell markers (not shown) and S-100 (**c**)

- Basal cells in partial atrophy are flat and inconspicuous but can be identified. Prostatic adenocarcinoma does not have basal cells.
- By immunohistochemistry, partial atrophy will show patchy or scattered basal cells and weak or moderately AMACR staining, in contrast to the strong AMACR immunoreactivity and negative basal staining in prostatic adenocarcinoma.

References: [26, 86, 87]

- Central zone glands (Fig. 5.46a)
- Clear cell cribriform hyperplasia (Fig. 5.46b)
- Reactive atypia
- Basal cell hyperplasia

In addition, cribriform architecture may be seen in high-grade PIN, intraductal carcinoma, invasive cancer, and ductal prostate carcinoma.

Reference: [2]

Can You See Benign Cribriform Lesions in the Prostate?

Cribriform lesions refer to proliferation of prostate glandular epithelial cells to form lumen-spanning mass with distinctive "spaces" or "holes" in between cells, imparting a "Swiss cheese" appearance. The cribriform architecture can be seen in a number of benign lesions, including:

Can Any Benign Prostatic Lesion Be Associated with Elevated Serum PSA?

PSA is produced by prostatic secretory cells and prostatic adenocarcinoma cells that have the phenotype of secretory cells. Serum PSA is a screening test rather than a diagnostic one. Several benign conditions can cause significant elevation of serum PSA. Benign conditions associated with tissue

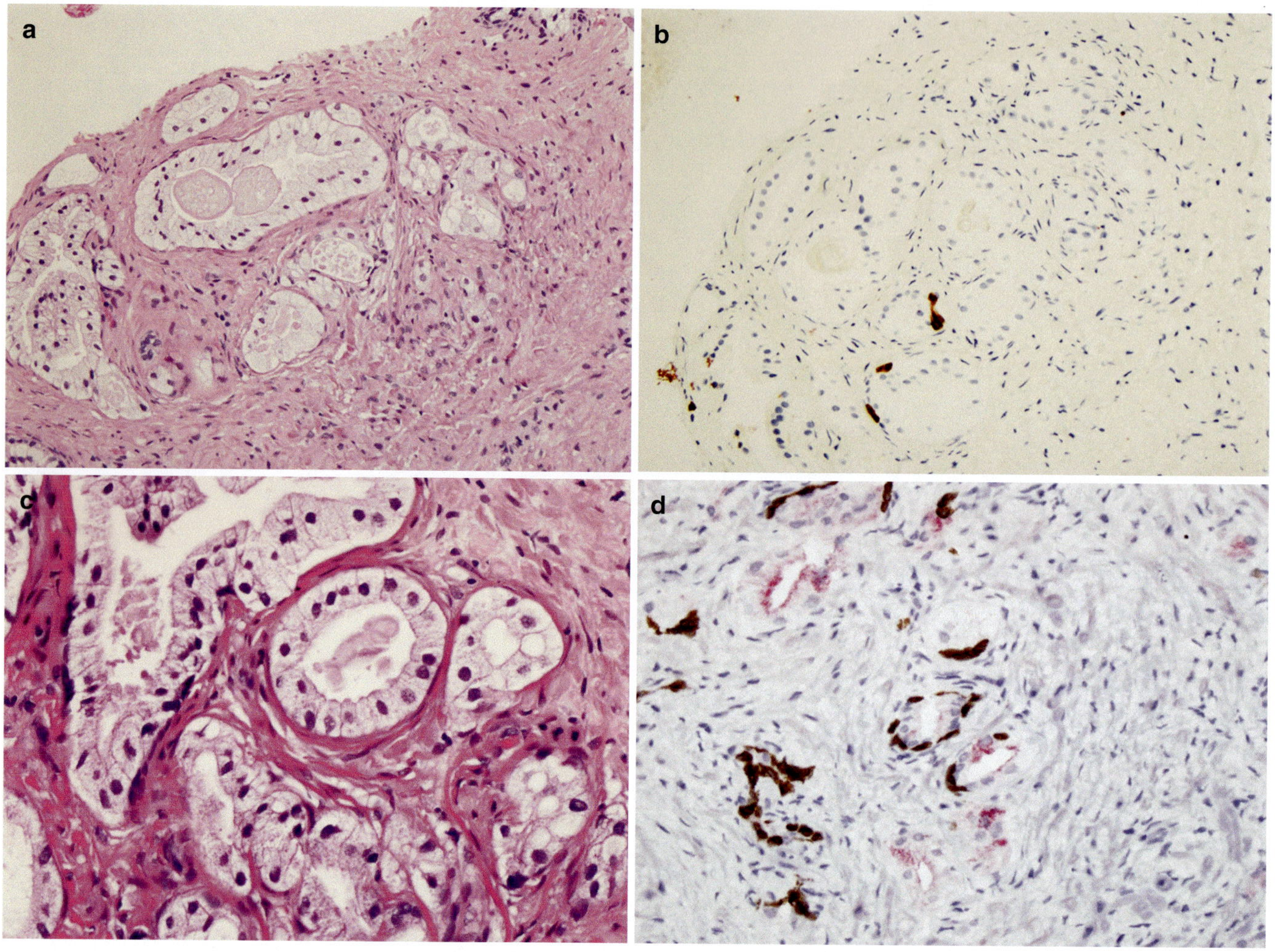

Fig. 5.45 Partial atrophy has a lobular pattern characterized by pale glandular cells that appear to be a single-layered but without significant cytological atypia (**a**). Triple staining shows patchy basal cells and no AMACR staining (**b**). Another case of partial atrophy showing no significant cytologic atypia (**c**) with patchy basal cells and moderate AMACR staining (**d**)

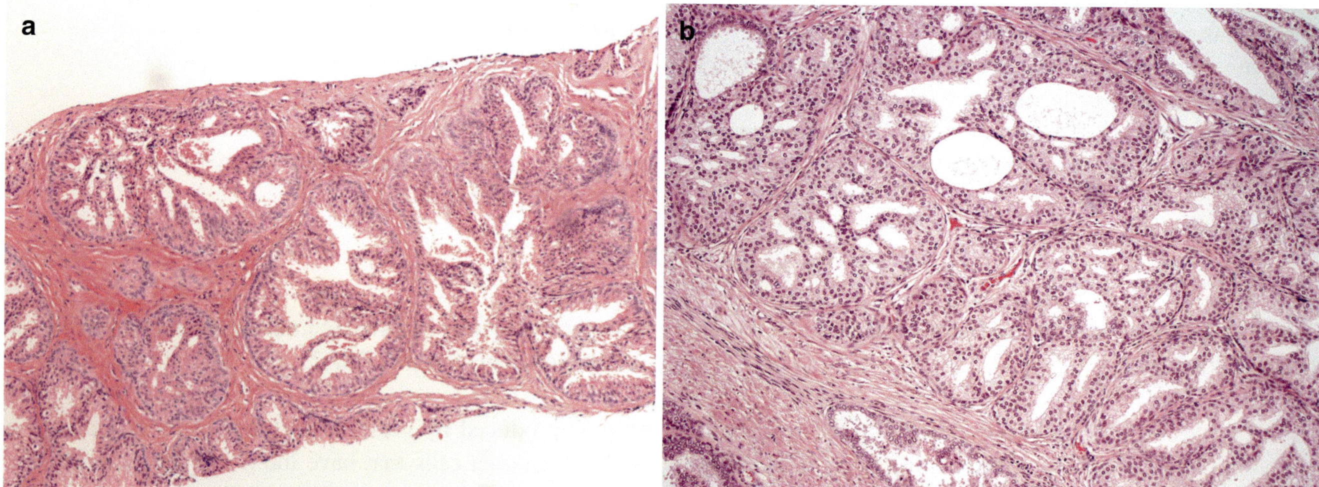

Fig. 5.46 Prostate glands in central zone show loose cribriform architecture (**a**). In clear cell cribriform hyperplasia, there is a nodular proliferation of nonconfluent cribriform glands with clear-to-eosinophilic cytoplasm (**b**). No nuclear atypia is found in benign cribriform lesions

injury may also lead to elevated serum PSA. While elevated serum PSA may prompt prostate biopsy to look for cancer, it should never be factored in the diagnosis on needle core biopsy.

Several benign conditions that are known to cause elevation of serum PSA include the following:

- *Infarct or necrosis of the prostate.* The tissue necrosis in this condition will lead to release a large amount PSA from damaged secretory cells. We have seen serum PSA over 100 ng/mL in a patient with prostate infarct.
- *Inflammation of the prostate.* Acute inflammation, extensive chronic inflammation, and nonspecific granulomatous prostatitis can all lead to destruction of secretory cells and release of PSA into circulation. These benign conditions should be included in the pathology report.
- *Benign prostatic hyperplasia (BPH).* In BPH, the glandular epithelial cell proliferation is prominent, which can cause increased production of PSA. Furthermore, BPH is often associated with urinary obstruction and secondary infection, which further contribute to the elevation of serum PSA. Generally, BPH should not be diagnosed in needle core biopsy, but should be considered in TUR specimens.

References: [88–90]

Should Treated Prostate Cancer Be Graded?

Prostate cancer with treatment effect should not be Gleason-graded as therapy-induced architectural changes, upon which Gleason grading is based, are not indicative of its biological behavior. However, cancer should be graded if there are no significant therapy-related changes.

Reference: [91]

What Is the Cytological Effect of Androgen Deprivation (ADT) on Prostate Cancer?

Androgen deprivation, either by surgical or chemical castration, produces similar histologic changes in the prostate. The treatment affects both benign secretory epithelial cells and adenocarcinoma cells. Typically, the tumor cells show atrophic and degenerative changes, including pyknotic nuclei, clear or vacuolated cytoplasm, and irregularity of glandular structures (Fig. 5.47), which may simulate the appearance of higher grade carcinoma. Nuclear enlargement and prominent nucleoli in carcinoma cells are diminished or absent, although the infiltrating patterns of the tumor cells are retained.

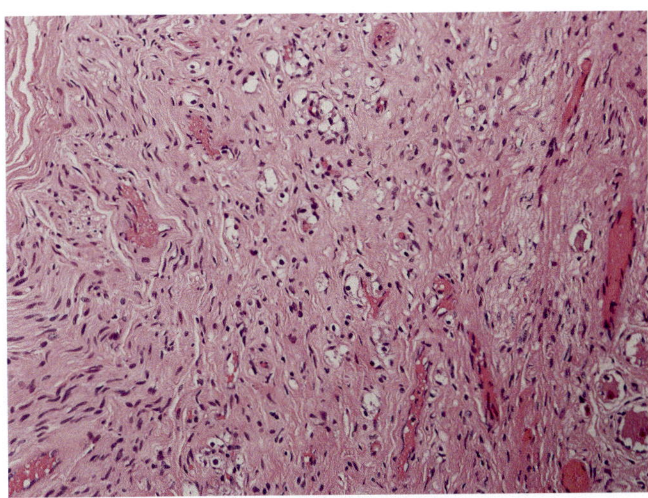

Fig. 5.47 Prostatic adenocarcinoma after androgen deprivation therapy shows prominent atrophic changes, vacuolated cytoplasm, and loss of lumina

As the result, androgen deprivation prior to biopsy or prostatectomy may cause difficulties in diagnosis or staging. Furthermore, because of the severe histologic changes in tumor cells caused by hormonal therapy, assignment of a Gleason score may be unreliable in this situation and should not be done.

However, if there is no obvious treatment effect in the tumor cells, a Gleason score should be assigned, because the tumors that escaped the treatment often have an aggressive behavior. Whether prostatic adenocarcinomas with prominent treatment effects should be graded may warrant further studies.

References: [92, 93]

What Are the Cytological Effects of Radiation on Prostate Tissue?

Radiation produces significant histological changes in both benign and malignant prostate tissues. Benign prostate tissue demonstrates marked glandular atrophy with stromal predominance (Fig. 5.48). Atrophic glands still maintain their lobular architecture. Glands have highly irregular contour and are lined with multiple layers of cells that predominantly display basal cell immunophenotype. Their cytoplasm is eosinophilic. The nuclei are piled up with degenerative appearance and there are scattered enlarged and hyperchromatic nuclei. Radiation-induced vascular changes, including intimal thickening with atheroma-like changes and medial fibrosis, can be seen. The degree of radiation-induced changes varies with the dose and duration and the interval between treatments.

Following radiation, cancer glands exhibit atrophic changes with atrophic cytoplasm and pyknotic nuclei and

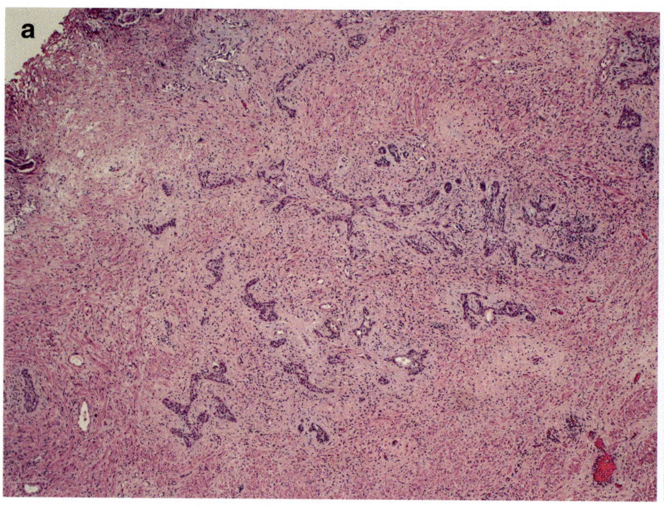
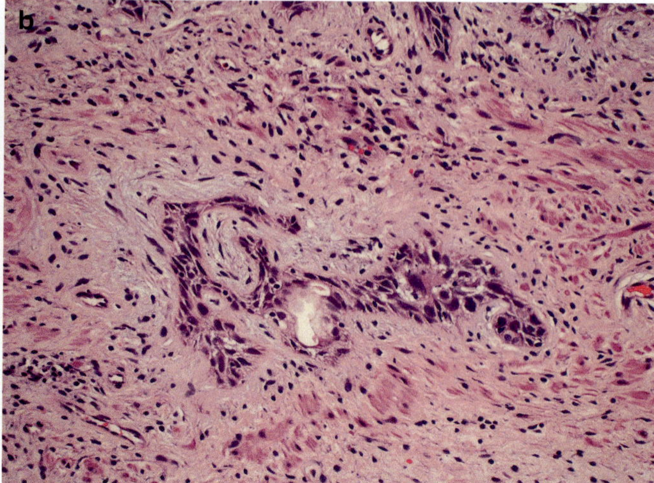

Fig. 5.48 Benign prostatic tissue showing radiation atypia. The glands maintain their lobular architecture (**a**). They have an irregular contour and are lined with multiple layers of cells. The cytoplasm is eosino-philic. The nuclei are piled up with degenerative appearance. There are scattered, enlarged, and hyperchromatic nuclei (**b**)

may be indistinguishable from benign atrophy (Fig. 5.49). But they still exhibit characteristic infiltrative growth pattern. Cancer glands may disintegrate into poorly formed, small clusters or single cells that have abundant vacuolated, clear or foamy cytoplasm and small pyknotic nuclei and may resemble histiocytes. The cancer glands are negative for basal cell markers and may have reduced prostate markers such as PSA but PSMA expression is reported unchanged.

Reference: [91]

Does Finasteride Have Any Effect on the Histological Appearance of Prostate Cancer Cells?

Finasteride and dutasteride are 5-alpha reductase inhibitors that inhibit the conversion of testosterone to more potent dihydrotestosterone (DHT). They are widely used at low doses for treatment of benign prostatic hyperplasia (BPH) leading to reduced hyperplastic cells (Fig. 5.50a) in BPH. Both finasteride and dutasteride appear to have a minimum to mild effect on morphology of prostatic adenocarcinomas in biopsy specimens (Fig. 5.50b) in contrast to other antiandrogen agents. The affected glands have slightly disorganized architecture, atrophic cytoplasm, and small and dark nuclei without prominent nucleoli. Therefore, the histologic diagnosis of prostate cancer on biopsy specimens from men receiving finasteride or dutasteride is not more difficult. However, grading these finasteride-treated prostate cancers may be difficult and unreliable if the morphological changes due to treatment is significant (Fig. 5.50c, d), which may appear of higher grade.

References: [94, 95]

What Histologic Changes Do You See in Alternative Treatments of Prostate Cancer Such as High Intensity Focused Ultrasound (HIFU), Cryoablation, or Microwave?

Cryoablation utilizes multiple cryoprobes filled with circulating liquid nitrogen to freeze and destroy prostate tissue. Hyperthermia uses high temperature generated by various sources (high-intensity focused ultrasound [HIFU], microwave, and laser) to destroy prostate tissue. Prostate tissue sampling is rarely done during acute phase following treatment. At later stage, prostate tissue shows features of tissue damage and repair, including marked reduction of glandular tissue and prominent stroma with myxoid degeneration, hemorrhage and hemosiderin deposition, fibrosis, and chronic inflammation. Residual viable glands show regenerative changes (Fig. 5.51), basal cell hyperplasia, and squamous cell metaplasia. Residual prostate cancer may show architectural distortion due to tissue injury and should not be Gleason graded.

References: [96–98]

How to Recognize Lymphoma in the Prostate?

Lymphoma can involve any organs in the genitourinary tract including the prostate. However, lymphomas are more commonly seen in pelvic lymph nodes and the testis than in the prostate. The most common type of lymphoma involving the prostate is non-Hodgkin lymphoma, particularly small lymphocytic lymphoma/chronic lymphocytic leukemia. Prostatic lymphoma is mostly the secondary involvement of

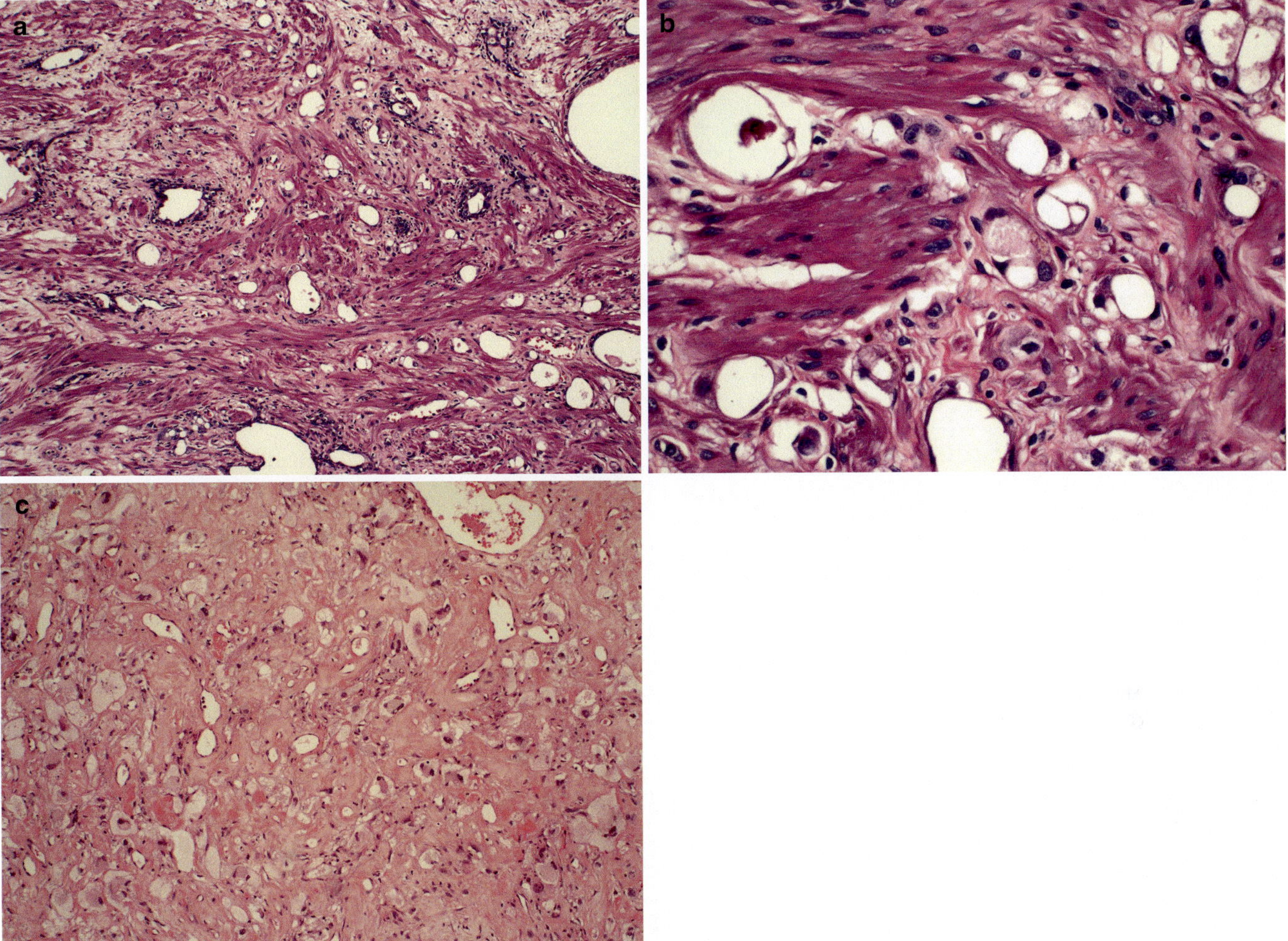

Fig. 5.49 Prostate cancer glands with radiation effect. The cancer glands infiltrate between benign glands (**a**) and have atrophic cytoplasm and pyknotic nuclei (**b**). Cancer demonstrates single and cords of cells with voluminous foamy cytoplasm and pyknotic nuclei (**c**)

the prostate rather than a primary lesion. Therefore, when a lymphoma is identified in the prostate, it is important to determine the extent of the systemic disease.

Prostatic lymphoma is characterized by the heavy lymphocytic infiltrates (Fig. 5.52a). The neoplastic lymphocytes are monotonous and have no other inflammatory cells such as neutrophils, eosinophils, or plasma cells (Fig. 5.52b). The diffuse large B-cell lymphoma may display significant cytological atypia mimicking high-grade prostatic adenocarcinoma.

It is usually difficult to diagnose lymphoma on prostate needle core biopsies. But one should suspect lymphoma when lymphocytic infiltrates are diffuse and involve the prostate stroma away from prostate glands. A panel of lymphoma markers (Fig. 5.52c, d) helps establish the diagnosis.

References: [99–101]

How to Distinguish Sarcomatoid Carcinoma from a True Sarcoma?

The majority of the sarcomas in the prostate are sarcomatoid carcinomas that are biphasic malignant tumors displaying both epithelial and mesenchymal differentiation (Fig. 5.53). Patients often have a precedent history of acinar adenocarcinoma treated with radiation or hormonal ablation. Virtually all tumors have a concurrent high-grade acinar adenocarcinoma or unusual variant of prostate cancer, even in minute amount that requires extensive sampling to identify. Sarcomatoid component may consist of undifferentiated spindled cells. Heterologous elements such as osteosarcoma, chondrosarcoma, and rhabdomyosarcoma may be present. The sarcomatous component may be positive for cytokeratins or prostate markers such as PSA.

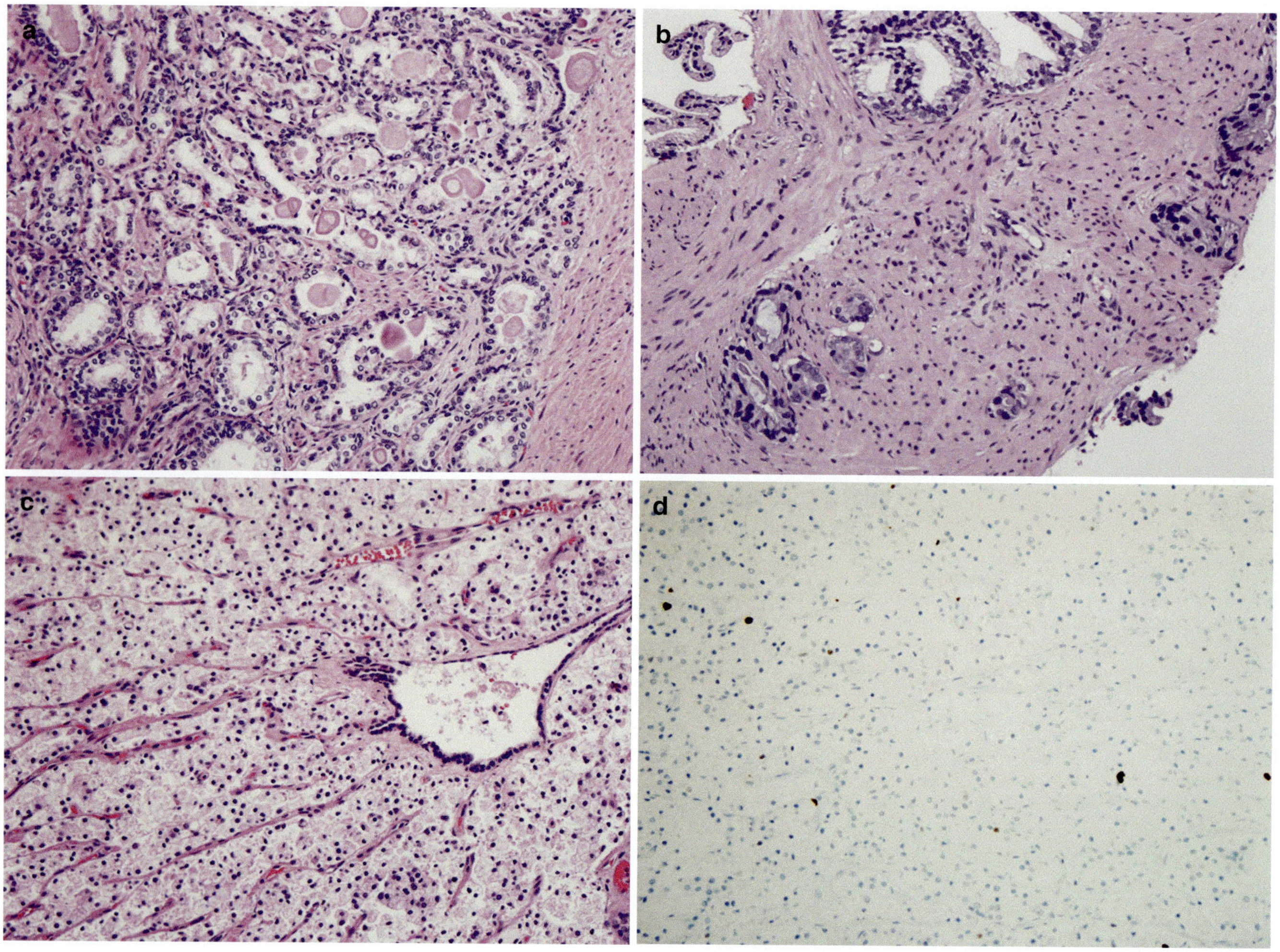

Fig. 5.50 Benign prostatic hyperplasia shows atrophic changes after finasteride treatment (**a**). Prostatic adenocarcinoma in a patient who previously received finasteride retains the typical histological features such as prominent nucleoli, infiltrating growth pattern, and lack of basal cells (**b**). However, in another finasteride-treated case, cancer glands are fused and lack well-formed lumen, which could be interpreted as Gleason score 4 + 5 (Grade Group 5) (**c**). However, the Ki67 proliferative activity in this case is very low (**d**), lower than the typical Gleason score 4 + 5 cancer

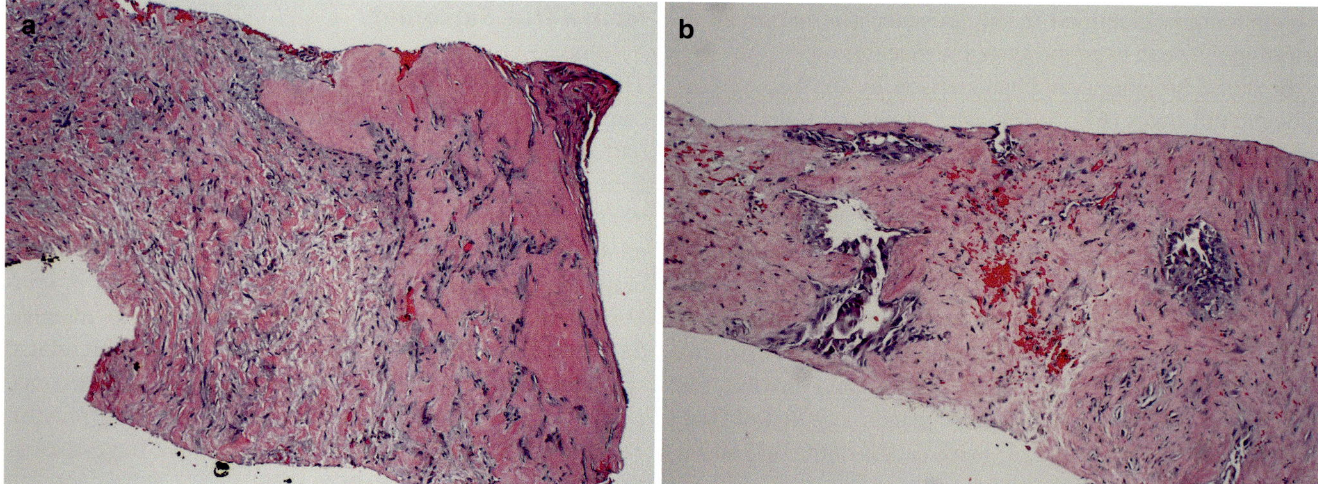

Fig. 5.51 Following cryoablation, affected prostate tissue shows marked reduction of glandular tissue and prominent stroma fibrosis and myxoid degeneration (**a**). Residual benign glands show regenerative changes (**b**)

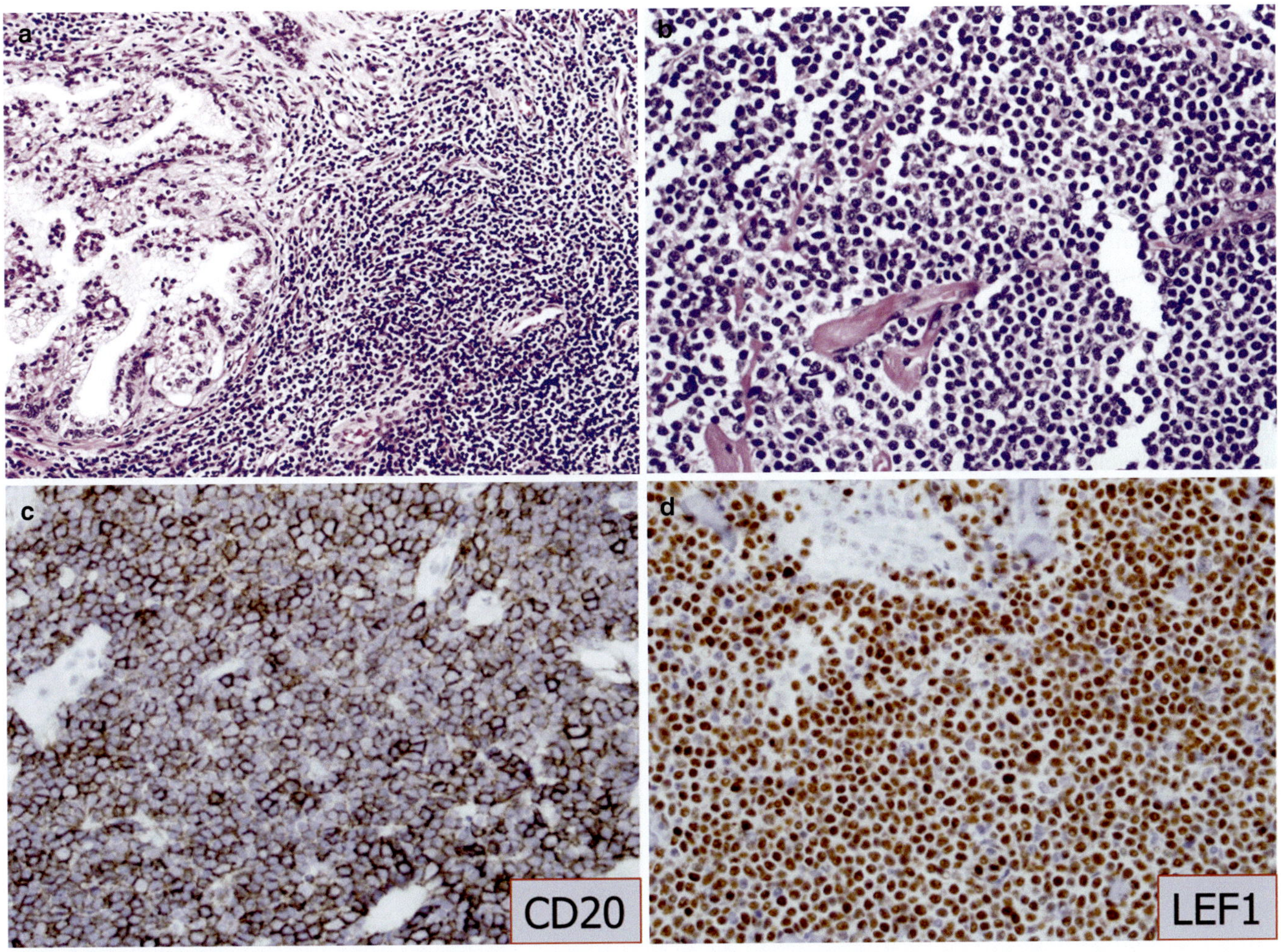

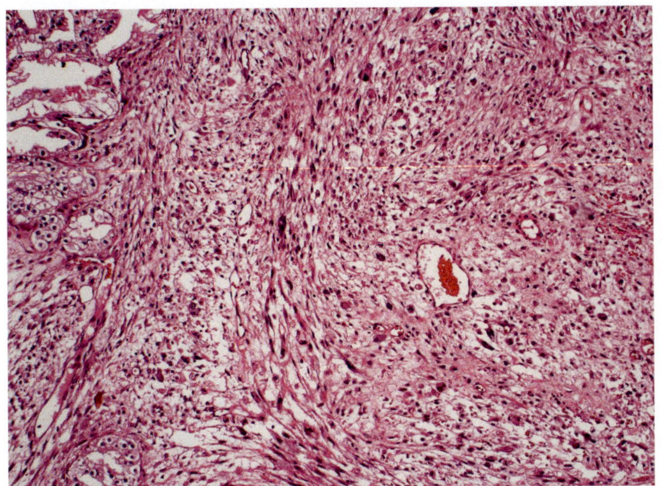

Fig. 5.52 Small lymphocytic lymphoma involving prostate showing infiltrating pattern (**a**). The neoplastic lymphocytes are monotonous without other inflammatory cells (**b**). They are positive for CD20 (**c**) and LEF1 (**d**) confirming the diagnosis

Fig. 5.53 Prostate sarcomatoid carcinoma has both acinar component (left of the image) and high-grade undifferentiated spindle cell component

Rarely a prostate sarcoma represents a primary sarcoma, such as prostatic stromal sarcoma, leiomyosarcoma, rhabdomyosarcoma, and malignant solitary fibrous tumor. Patients do not have a history of prostate acinar carcinoma. There is no concomitant epithelial component after extensive tissue sampling. The stains for cytokeratins and prostate markers are negative.

References: [102, 103]

How to Distinguish Florid Benign Prostatic Hyperplasia (BPH) from Prostate Stroma Tumor of Uncertain Malignant Potential (STUMP)?

Benign prostatic hyperplasia (BPH) is characterized by nodular proliferation of prostatic stromal and glandular epithelial cells. The ratio of stromal and glandular components is variable in each BPH nodule. Sometimes, there is predominantly stromal proliferation with minimal or no glandular component. However, BPH exhibits nodular pattern without infiltrative features (Fig. 5.54a). Multinodularity, prominent blood vessels with some degree of hyalinization, and presence of chronic inflammatory cells are often seen. Stromal cells in BPH do not show cytological atypia although they can have a relative high cellularity (Fig. 5.54b).

Prostatic stromal tumor of uncertain malignant potential (STUMP) is a neoplastic proliferation of specialized stromal cells of the prostate, and was previously called phyllodes tumor or atypical smooth muscle hyperplasia that are no longer recommended. This neoplasm often diffusely involves the prostate without nodular pattern. On needle biopsies, multiple cores are usually involved (Fig. 5.54c). Several histological patterns are described. Most commonly, hypercellular stroma with scattered atypical degenerative cells admixed with benign prostate glands (Fig. 5.54d).

References: [104, 105]

How to Differentiate Nonspecific Granulomatous Prostatitis from Other Types of Granulomatous Prostatitis?

Nonspecific granulomatous prostatitis (NSGP), a granulomatous inflammation of the prostate without a specific causative agent, is a relatively common condition. It is most likely an inflammatory reaction to ruptured ducts or acini. Clinically, digital rectal examination often reveals firm indurated prostate worrisome for a high-grade prostate cancer. Serum PSA is increased, typically 5–10 ng/mL. Transrectal ultrasound may show a hypoechoic region, also suggestive of carcinoma.

Histologically, NSGP is characterized by heavy mixed inflammation composed of lymphoplasmacytic infiltrate and scattered neutrophils and eosinophils (Fig. 5.55a). Well-formed granulomas are not a typical histologic feature. Instead, poorly formed granulomas composed of epithelioid histocytes are present. The granulomatous inflammation

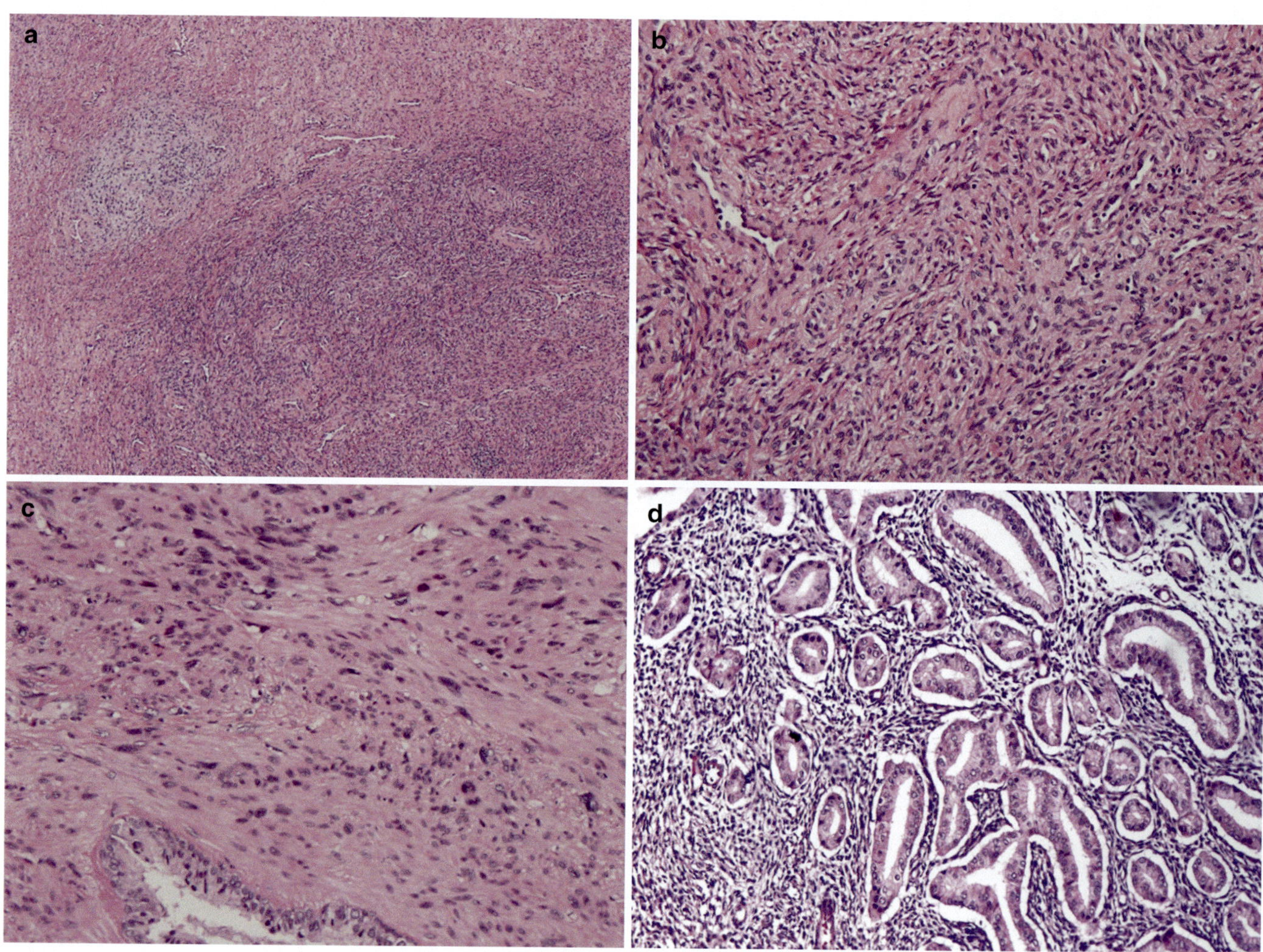

Fig. 5.54 A stroma predominant BPH nodule has a nodular appearance. Small- to medium-sized vessels with hyalinized walls are evident (**a**). Although there is high cellularity, no cytological atypia is observed (**b**). STUMP shows hypercellular stromal cells with marked cytological atypia admixed with benign prostate glands (**c**). Another case of STUMP shows neoplastic stromal cells infiltrating between benign glands (**d**)

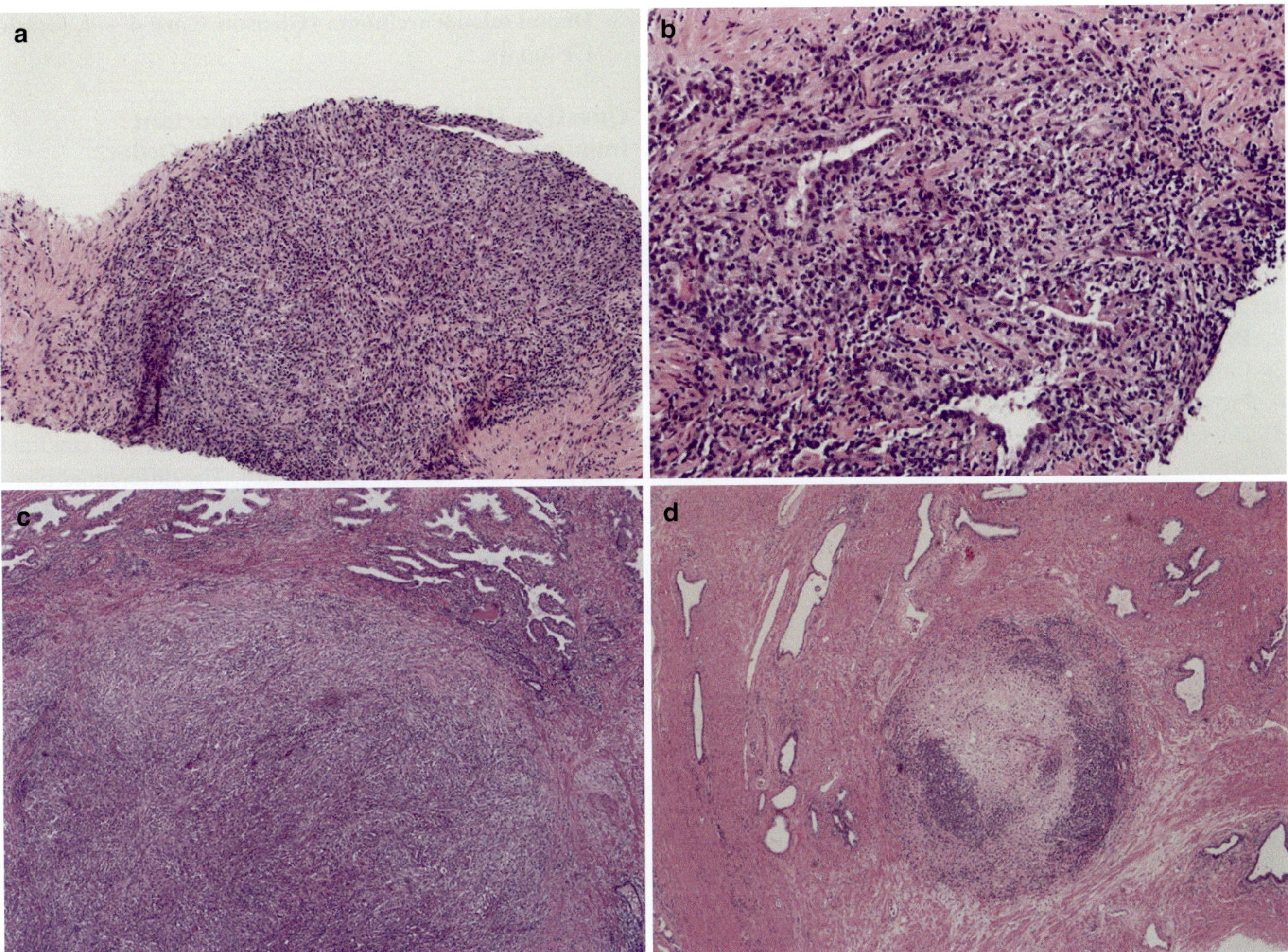

Fig. 5.55 Nonspecific granulomatous prostatitis is characterized by granulomatous inflammation composed of mixed lymphocytes and histiocytes (**a**). The granulomas are poorly formed and around ruptured glands (**b**). BCG granuloma is more defined, predominantly with epithelioid histiocytes and occasional multinuclear giant cells (**c**). Post-biopsy granulomas along the needle track are small with well-defined borders (**d**)

usually surrounds ruptured glandular structures (Fig. 5.55b), sometimes with foamy macrophages and multinuclear giant cells. Caseating necrosis is rarely seen. Special stains for microorganisms are negative.

The prostatic epithelial cells may display reactive and regenerative changes, mimicking prostatic adenocarcinoma. When granulomatous and chronic inflammation is florid and diffuse, prostate ducts may be obliterated, raising suspicion for a high-grade, Gleason pattern 5 carcinoma. We have seen several cases of NSGP misdiagnosed as high-grade prostatic adenocarcinoma. It is also important to know that occasionally small foci of prostatic adenocarcinoma may be obscured by the granulomatous inflammation on needle core biopsy. Careful examination is the key to rule out prostatic carcinoma. If necessary, triple stain and other prostatic markers may help identify coexisting carcinoma.

Several other types of granulomatous inflammation can be seen in the prostate. The two most common ones to be distinguished from NSGP is mycobacteria (BCG) induced granulomas and post-biopsy/post-TUR granulomas. BCG, used for treatment of superficial bladder cancer, may elicit granulomatous inflammation involving the prostate, so clinical history is important. BCG granulomas, sometimes with caseating necrosis in the center (Fig. 5.55c), histologically are different from NSGP granulomas. Post biopsy/TUR granulomas typically exhibit fibroid central necrosis of "geographic shape." Foreign body giant cells are commonly seen. In practice, we rarely perform GMS/AFB stains for prostatic granulomas since a treatment history can be solicited in most cases. Needle track is a single, small, well-defined granuloma without background chronic inflammation in surrounding prostatic tissue (Fig. 5.55d).

References: [106, 107]

Case Discussion

Case 1: Ductal Adenocarcinoma

A 65-year-old man with prostate needle core biopsy, which is showed in Fig. 5.56a, b:

Question 1A: Which of the Following Is the LEAST LIKELY Diagnosis based on H& E stain?

1. Aggressive carcinoma
2. **Prostatic adenocarcinoma, Gleason score 3 + 3**
3. Intraductal carcinoma
4. Prostatic adenocarcinoma, Gleason score 4 + 4
5. Ductal carcinoma

Question 1B: What Is the Most Likely Diagnosis?

1. High-grade PIN
2. Prostatic adenocarcinoma, Gleason score 3 + 3
3. Prostatic adenocarcinoma, Gleason score 5 + 5
4. Urothelial carcinoma

5. **Ductal adenocarcinoma (Gleason score 4 + 4, Grade Group 4)**

Question 1C: What Is the Most Important Immunostain That You Would Like to Order?

1. **Triple stain**
2. PSA
3. NKX3.1
4. Ki67
5. GATA3

Discussion

The lesion is composed of tall columnar cells forming large glands (Fig. 5.56a). The nuclei are elongated and stratified with prominent nucleoli (Fig. 5.56b). The differential diagnosis should include high-grade PIN (but too much cytological atypia), intraductal carcinoma (if there are basal cells), and ductal adenocarcinoma (if there are no basal cells). Ductal carcinoma should be graded as Gleason pattern 4 or 5, if necrosis is present. Prostatic adenocarcinoma should be

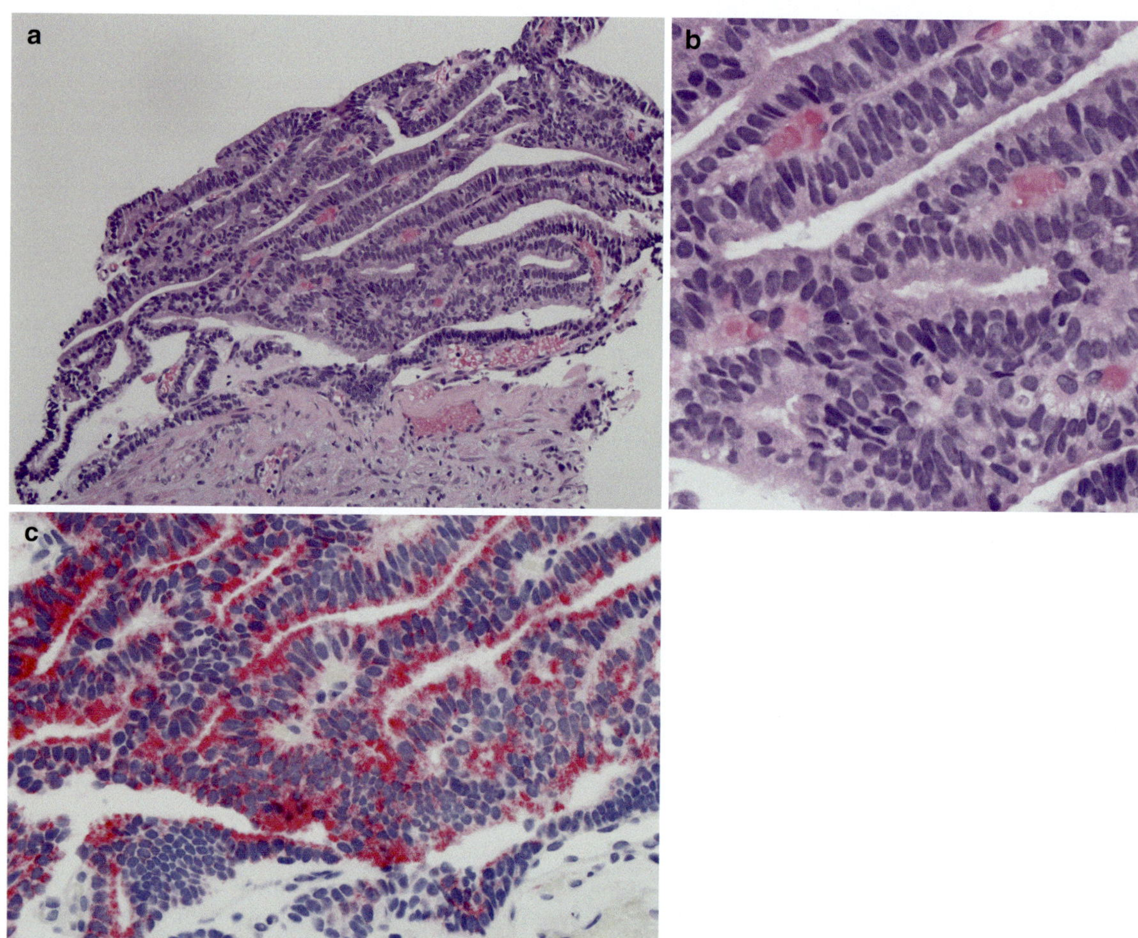

Fig. 5.56 Case discussion 1. Ductal carcinoma of the prostate (H&E stain **a** and **b**, Triple immunostain **c**)

considered, more likely to be Gleason 4 + 4, but not Gleason 3 + 3.

The two most likely diagnoses are ductal adenocarcinoma and intraductal carcinoma. The basal cell markers in triple stain are the most important stains to distinguish invasive ductal from intraductal carcinoma. Triple staining shows lack of basal cells and positive AMACR expression (Fig. 5.56c).

Case 2: Partial Atrophy

A 65-year-old man with prostate needle core biopsy, which is shown in Fig. 5.57.

Question 2A. What Is the Most Likely Diagnosis based on the H&E stain?

1. Adenocarcinoma
2. Sclerosing Adenosis
3. **Partial atrophy**
4. Atrophic hyperplasia
5. Basal cell hyperplasia

Question 2B. What Is the Most Important Feature for Diagnosis?

1. Lack of basal cells
2. AMACR immunoreactivity
3. PSA immunoreactivity
4. **H&E histological features**
5. Infiltrating pattern

Discussion

Partial atrophy is one of the most common benign mimickers of adenocarcinoma. Features of this condition include (1) vague lobular pattern (Fig. 5.57a); (2) angulated glands that appear infiltrative (Fig. 5.57b); (3) single cells may be present due to tangential cut of angulated glands (Fig. 5.57c); (4) minimal cytological atypia without prominent nucleoli (Fig. 5.57b, c) and (5) very patchy basal cells and weak or negative AMACR staining (Fig. 5.57d). The diagnosis is based mostly on the histological features. Incomplete or focal loss of basal cells on immunostaining should not be mistaken for cancer.

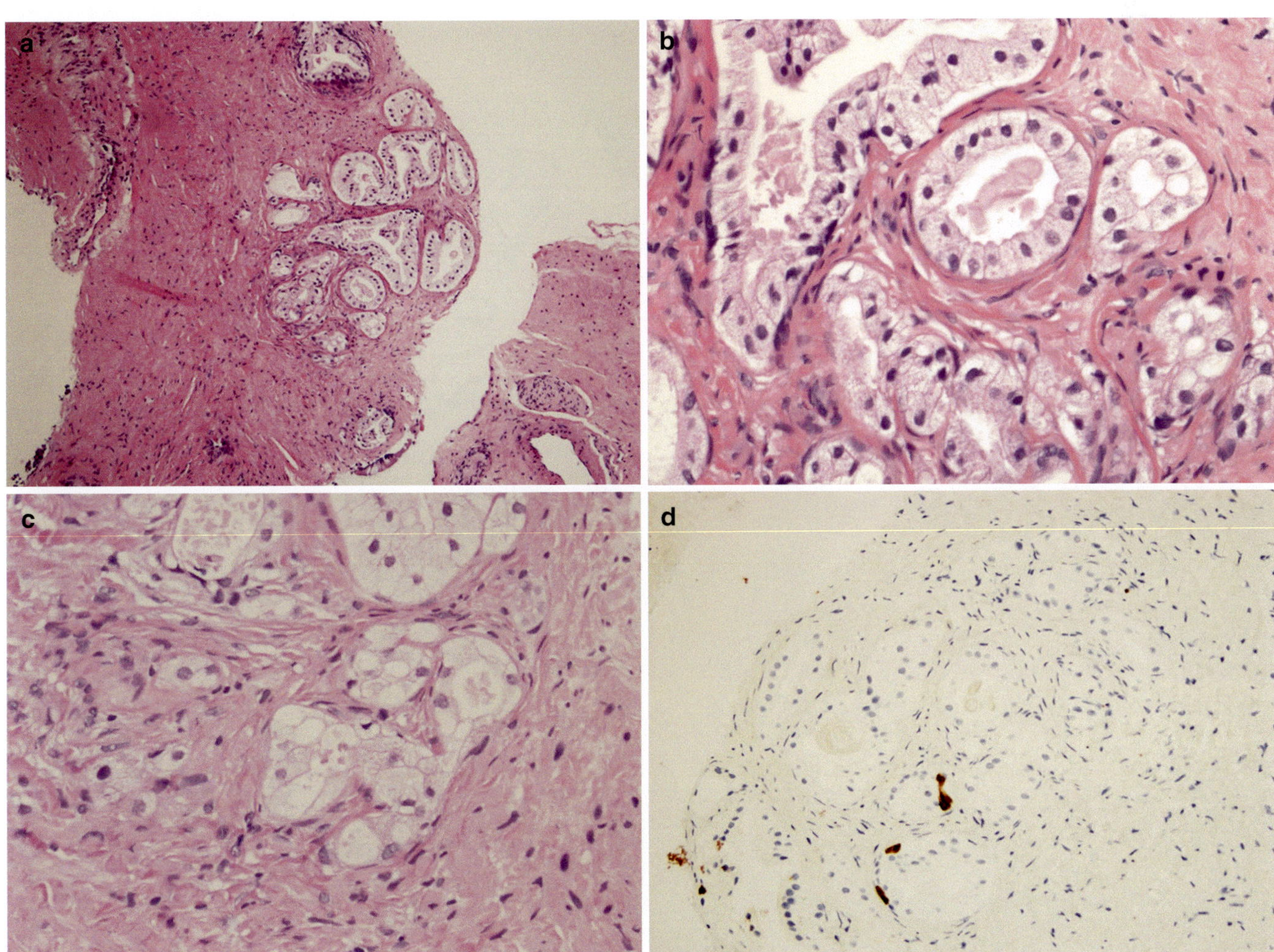

Fig. 5.57 Case discussion 2. Partial atrophy (H &E stains **a** and **c**, triple immunostains **b** and **d**)

Case 3: Benign Atrophy of the Prostate

A 72-year-old man with prostate needle core biopsy as shown in Fig. 5.58a.

Question 3. Which of the Following Statements Is INCORRECT?

1. Atrophy can be confused with prostatic adenocarcinoma.
2. **Atrophy is a not proliferative process.**
3. Atrophy retains a lobular pattern.
4. Atrophy shows no cytological atypia.

Discussion

Benign atrophy is a very common finding in prostate needle core biopsy. It is characterized by atrophic prostate glands in lobular patterns and no significant cytological atypia in the atrophic cells. In Fig. 5.58a, a focus of atrophic glands with scant cytoplasm is present the upper portion of the image. Immunostaining confirms the presence of basal cells (Fig. 5.58b). In another case of atrophy, also known as sclerosing atrophy, the atrophic glands are embedded in fibrotic stroma (Fig. 5.58c). There are often marked glandular distortions. Immunostaining confirms the presence of patchy basal cells in the focus (Fig. 5.58d).

Case 4: Post Radiation Change in Benign and Prostate Cancer Cells

A 70-year-old man with history of prostate cancer status post radiation, now with elevated PSA, undergoes prostate needle core biopsy, which is shown in Fig. 5.59a.

Question 4. What Is NOT True About Postradiation Change?

1. Benign epithelial cells show cytological atypia.
2. Adenocarcinoma cells may show atrophic changes.
3. Adenocarcinoma cells still display infiltrating patterns.

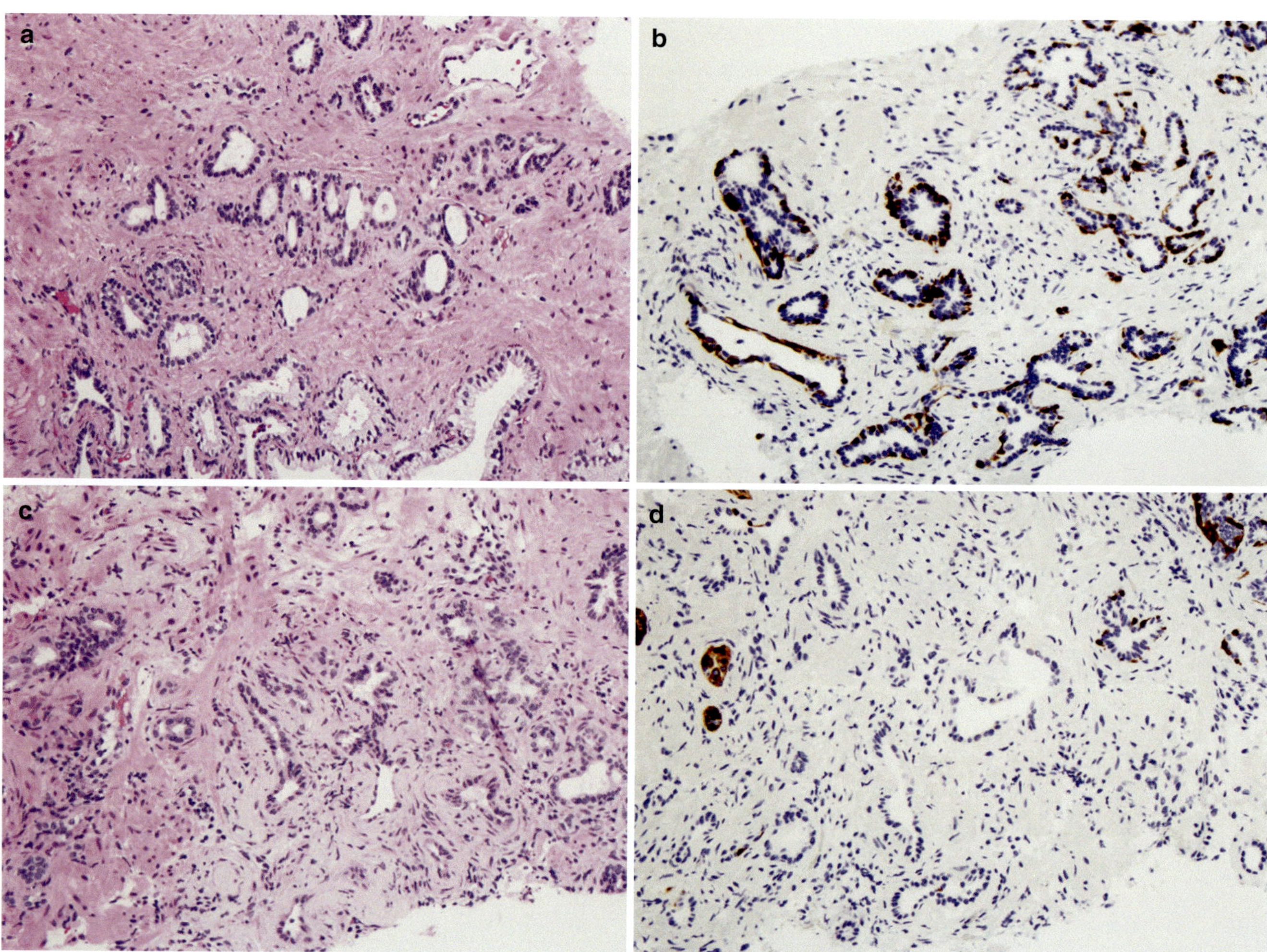

Fig. 5.58 Case discussion 3. Atrophy. Benign atrophic glands (H &E stains **a** and **c**, triple immunostains **b** and **d**)

4. **AMACR will be positive in benign irradiated glandular cells.**
5. AMACR will be positive in prostatic adenocarcinoma cells.

Discussion

After radiation, benign glands may show marked degenerative cytological atypia with cytoplasmic vacuoles (Fig. 5.59a). However, the majority of the cells are basal cells that express basal cell markers p63 and HMWCK (Fig. 5.59b, triple stain). On the other hand, adenocarcinoma cells exhibit atrophic changes with bland nuclei and pale cytoplasm (Fig. 5.59c, arrows), but they are still strongly positive for AMACR and negative for basal cell markers (Fig. 5.59d, triple stain).

Case 5: Foamy Gland Carcinoma of the Prostate

A 72-year-old man with prostate needle core biopsy as shown in Fig. 5.60a.

Question 5. What Should You Not Do as the Next Step When Encountering a Prostate Needle Biopsy with Such a Morphology based on the H&E stain ?

1. Order deeper levels
2. Order triple stain
3. **Make a diagnosis of benign glands because there are no nucleoli**
4. Make a diagnosis of atypical glands suspicious for carcinoma and send out for consultation

Discussion

Foamy gland carcinoma of the prostate is characterized by the presence of deceptively benign appearance with foamy cytoplasm and bland cytological features in the tumor cells (Fig. 5.60a, arrow). You may have difficulty finding prominent nucleoli even at higher magnification (Fig. 5.60b). However, the infiltrating pattern is present and nuclear atypia can be observed in this focus (Fig. 5.60a, arrow) and at higher magnification (Fig. 5.60c). The presence of adenocarcinoma

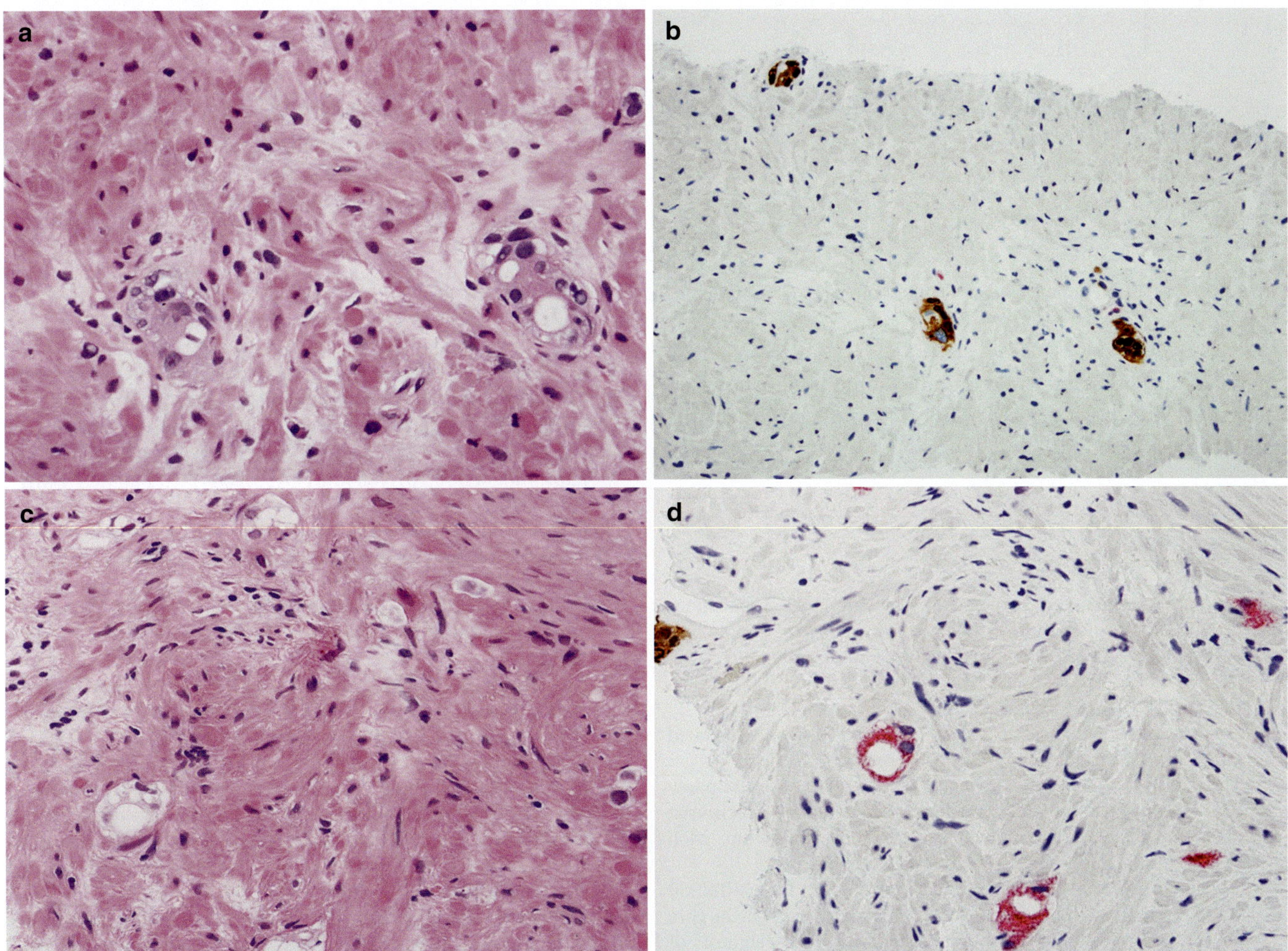

Fig. 5.59 Case discussion 4. Post radiation changes of benign prostate (**a**, **b**) and adenocarcinoma (**c**, **d**). Triple immunostains (**b**, **d**)

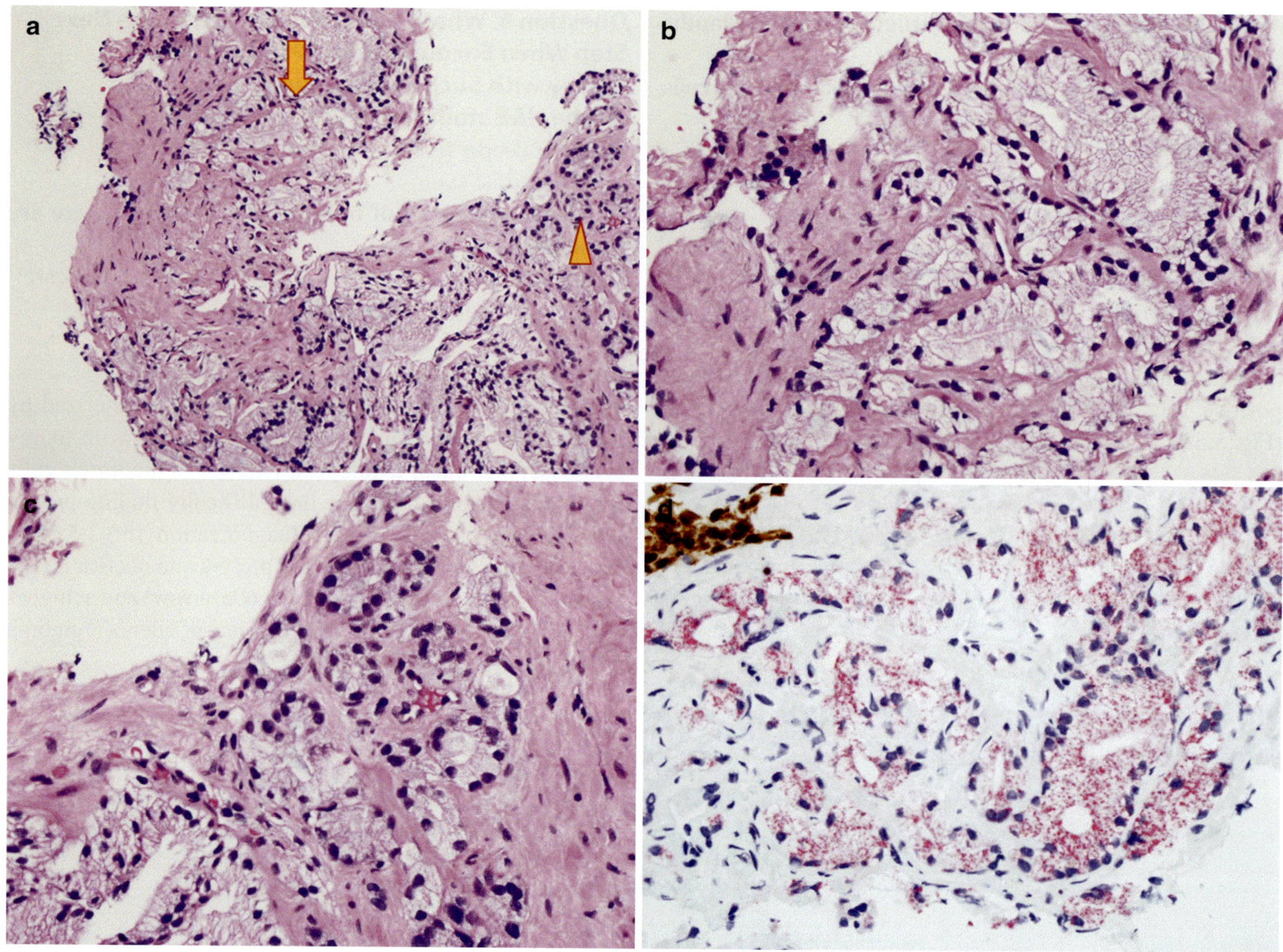

Fig. 5.60 Case discussion 5. Foamy gland adenocarcinoma of the prostate (H &E stains **a–c**, triple immunostain **d**)

can be confirmed using triple immunostaining that shows no basal cells and positive AMACR immunoreactivity in the tumor cells (Fig. 5.60d).

References

1. Baisden BL, Kahane H, Epstein JI. Perineural invasion, mucinous fibroplasia, and glomerulations: diagnostic features of limited cancer on prostate needle biopsy. Am J Surg Pathol. 1999;23(8):918–24. https://doi.org/10.1097/00000478-199908000-00009. PubMed PMID: 10435561.
2. Shah R, Zhou M. Prostate biopsy interpretation: an illustrated guide. 2nd ed. Berlin Heidelberg: Springer-Verlag; 2019.
3. Thorson P, Vollmer RT, Arcangeli C, Keetch DW, Humphrey PA. Minimal carcinoma in prostate needle biopsy specimens: diagnostic features and radical prostatectomy follow-up. Mod Pathol. 1998;11(6):543–51. PubMed PMID: 9647592.
4. Algaba F, Epstein JI, Aldape HC, Farrow GM, Lopez-Beltran A, Maksem J, et al. Assessment of prostate carcinoma in core needle biopsy--definition of minimal criteria for the diagnosis of cancer in biopsy material. Cancer. 1996;78(2):376–81. https://doi.org/10.1002/(SICI)1097-0142(19960715)78:2<376::AID-CNCR32>3.0.CO;2-R. PubMed PMID: 8674022.
5. Epstein JI. Diagnostic criteria of limited adenocarcinoma of the prostate on needle biopsy. Hum Pathol. 1995;26(2):223–9. https://doi.org/10.1016/0046-8177(95)90041-1. PubMed PMID: 7860053.
6. Iczkowski KA, Bostwick DG. Criteria for biopsy diagnosis of minimal volume prostatic adenocarcinoma: analytic comparison with nondiagnostic but suspicious atypical small acinar proliferation. Arch Pathol Lab Med. 2000;124(1):98–107. https://doi.org/10.1043/0003-9985(2000)1242.0.CO;2. PubMed PMID: 10629139.
7. Ali TZ, Epstein JI. Perineural involvement by benign prostatic glands on needle biopsy. Am J Surg Pathol. 2005;29(9):1159–63. https://doi.org/10.1097/01.pas.0000160980.62586.05. PubMed PMID: 16096404.
8. Harnden P, Shelley MD, Clements H, Coles B, Tyndale-Biscoe RS, Naylor B, et al. The prognostic significance of perineural invasion in prostatic cancer biopsies: a systematic review. Cancer. 2007;109(1):13–24. https://doi.org/10.1002/cncr.22388. PubMed PMID: 17123267.
9. Truong M, Rais-Bahrami S, Nix JW, Messing EM, Miyamoto H, Gordetsky JB. Perineural invasion by prostate cancer on MR/US fusion targeted biopsy is associated with extraprostatic exten-

sion and early biochemical recurrence after radical prostatectomy. Hum Pathol. 2017;66:206–11. Epub 2017/07/11. PubMed PMID: 28705708. https://doi.org/10.1016/j.humpath.2017.06.017.

10. Al-Hussain T, Carter HB, Epstein JI. Significance of prostate adenocarcinoma perineural invasion on biopsy in patients who are otherwise candidates for active surveillance. J Urol. 2011;186(2):470–3. Epub 2011/06/15. PubMed PMID: 21679997. https://doi.org/10.1016/j.juro.2011.03.119.

11. Humphrey PA. Variants of acinar adenocarcinoma of the prostate mimicking benign conditions. Mod Pathol. 2018;31(S1):S64–70. https://doi.org/10.1038/modpathol.2017.137. PubMed PMID: 29297496.

12. Farinola MA, Epstein JI. Utility of immunohistochemistry for alpha-methylacyl-CoA racemase in distinguishing atrophic prostate cancer from benign atrophy. Hum Pathol. 2004;35(10):1272–8. https://doi.org/10.1016/j.humpath.2004.06.015. PubMed PMID: 15492996.

13. Levi AW, Epstein JI. Pseudohyperplastic prostatic adenocarcinoma on needle biopsy and simple prostatectomy. Am J Surg Pathol. 2000;24(8):1039–46. https://doi.org/10.1097/00000478-200008000-00001. PubMed PMID: 10935644.

14. Tran TT, Sengupta E, Yang XJ. Prostatic foamy gland carcinoma with aggressive behavior: clinicopathologic, immunohistochemical, and ultrastructural analysis. Am J Surg Pathol. 2001;25(5):618–23. https://doi.org/10.1097/00000478-200105000-00008. PubMed PMID: 11342773.

15. Hudson J, Cao D, Vollmer R, Kibel AS, Grewal S, Humphrey PA. Foamy gland adenocarcinoma of the prostate: incidence, Gleason grade, and early clinical outcome. Hum Pathol. 2012;43(7):974–9. Epub 2012/01/04. PubMed PMID: 22221706. https://doi.org/10.1016/j.humpath.2011.09.009.

16. Epstein JI. Diagnosis and reporting of limited adenocarcinoma of the prostate on needle biopsy. Mod Pathol. 2004;17(3):307–15. https://doi.org/10.1038/modpathol.3800050. PubMed PMID: 14739905

17. Tosoian JJ, Alam R, Ball MW, Carter HB, Epstein JI. Managing high-grade prostatic intraepithelial neoplasia (HGPIN) and atypical glands on prostate biopsy. Nat Rev Urol. 2018;15(1):55–66. Epub 2017/08/31. PubMed PMID: 28858331. https://doi.org/10.1038/nrurol.2017.134.

18. Iczkowski KA. Current prostate biopsy interpretation: criteria for cancer, atypical small acinar proliferation, high-grade prostatic intraepithelial neoplasia, and use of immunostains. Arch Pathol Lab Med. 2006;130(6):835–43. https://doi.org/10.1043/1543-2165(2006)130[835:CPBICF]2.0.CO;2. PubMed PMID: 16740037

19. Lotan TL, Gumuskaya B, Rahimi H, Hicks JL, Iwata T, Robinson BD, et al. Cytoplasmic PTEN protein loss distinguishes intraductal carcinoma of the prostate from high-grade prostatic intraepithelial neoplasia. Mod Pathol. 2013;26(4):587–603. Epub 2012/12/07. https://doi.org/10.1038/modpathol.2012.201. PubMed PMID: 23222491; PubMed Central PMCID: PMCPMC3610824.

20. Patel P, Nayak JG, Biljetina Z, Donnelly B, Trpkov K. Prostate cancer after initial high-grade prostatic intraepithelial neoplasia and benign prostate biopsy. Can J Urol. 2015;22(6):8056–62. PubMed PMID: 26688133.

21. D'Amico AV, Barry MJ. Prostate cancer prevention and finasteride. J Urol. 2006;176(5):2010–2; discussion 2-3. https://doi.org/10.1016/j.juro.2006.07.045. PubMed PMID: 17070238.

22. Thompson IM, Lucia MS, Redman MW, Darke A, La Rosa FG, Parnes HL, et al. Finasteride decreases the risk of prostatic intraepithelial neoplasia. J Urol. 2007;178(1):107–9; discussion 10. Epub 2007/05/11. PubMed PMID: 17499284. https://doi.org/10.1016/j.juro.2007.03.012.

23. Zhou M, Magi-Galluzzi C. Clinicopathological features of prostate cancers detected after an initial diagnosis of 'atypical glands suspicious for cancer'. Pathology. 2010;42(4):334–8. https://doi.org/10.3109/00313021003767280. PubMed PMID: 20438405

24. Ali TZ, Epstein JI. Basal cell carcinoma of the prostate: a clinicopathologic study of 29 cases. Am J Surg Pathol. 2007;31(5):697–705. https://doi.org/10.1097/01.pas.0000213395.42075.86. PubMed PMID: 17460452.

25. Simper NB, Jones CL, MacLennan GT, Montironi R, Williamson SR, Osunkoya AO, et al. Basal cell carcinoma of the prostate is an aggressive tumor with frequent loss of PTEN expression and overexpression of EGFR. Hum Pathol. 2015;46(6):805–12. Epub 2015/02/26. https://doi.org/10.1016/j.humpath.2015.02.004. PubMed PMID: 25870120

26. Adley BP, Maxwell K, Dalton DP, Yang XJ. Urothelial-type adenocarcinoma of the prostate mimicking metastatic colorectal adenocarcinoma. Int Braz J Urol. 2006;32(6):681–7; discussion 7-8. https://doi.org/10.1590/s1677-55382006000600009. PubMed PMID: 17201946

27. Moch HHP, Ulbright TM, Reuter VE. WHO classification of tumours of the urinary system and male genital organs. Lyon: International Agency for Research on Cancer; 2016.

28. Epstein JI, Amin MB, Beltran H, Lotan TL, Mosquera JM, Reuter VE, et al. Proposed morphologic classification of prostate cancer with neuroendocrine differentiation. Am J Surg Pathol. 2014;38(6):756–67. https://doi.org/10.1097/PAS.0000000000000208. PubMed PMID: 24705311; PubMed Central PMCID: PMCPMC4112087.

29. Osunkoya AO. Mucinous and secondary tumors of the prostate. Mod Pathol. 2018;31(S1):S80–95. https://doi.org/10.1038/modpathol.2017.132. PubMed PMID: 29297488.

30. Evans AJ, Humphrey PA, Belani J, van der Kwast TH, Srigley JR. Large cell neuroendocrine carcinoma of prostate: a clinicopathologic summary of 7 cases of a rare manifestation of advanced prostate cancer. Am J Surg Pathol. 2006;30(6):684–93. https://doi.org/10.1097/00000478-200606000-00003. PubMed PMID: 16723845.

31. Amin MBES, Greene FL, et al. AJCC Cancer staging manual. 8th ed. New York: Springer; 2017.

32. Patel AR, Cohn JA, Abd El Latif A, Miocinovic R, Steinberg GD, Paner GP, et al. Validation of new AJCC exclusion criteria for subepithelial prostatic stromal invasion from pT4a bladder urothelial carcinoma. J Urol. 2013;189(1):53–8. Epub 2012/11/16. https://doi.org/10.1016/j.juro.2012.09.006. PubMed PMID: 23164389.

33. Thorson P, Swanson PE, Vollmer RT, Humphrey PA. Basal cell hyperplasia in the peripheral zone of the prostate. Mod Pathol. 2003;16(6):598–606. https://doi.org/10.1097/01.MP.0000073526.59270.6E. PubMed PMID: 12808066.

34. Yang XJ, Tretiakova MS, Sengupta E, Gong C, Jiang Z. Florid basal cell hyperplasia of the prostate: a histological, ultrastructural, and immunohistochemical analysis. Hum Pathol. 2003;34(5):462–70. https://doi.org/10.1016/s0046-8177(03)00121-7. PubMed PMID: 12792920.

35. Zhou M. High-grade prostatic intraepithelial neoplasia, PIN-like carcinoma, ductal carcinoma, and intraductal carcinoma of the prostate. Mod Pathol. 2018;31(S1):S71–9. https://doi.org/10.1038/modpathol.2017.138. PubMed PMID: 29297491.

36. Montironi R, Zhou M, Magi-Galluzzi C, Epstein JI. Features and prognostic significance of intraductal carcinoma of the prostate. Eur Urol Oncol. 2018;1(1):21–8. Epub 2018/05/15. https://doi.org/10.1016/j.euo.2018.03.013. PubMed PMID: 31100224.

37. Epstein JI, Zelefsky MJ, Sjoberg DD, Nelson JB, Egevad L, Magi-Galluzzi C, et al. A contemporary prostate cancer grading system: a validated alternative to the Gleason score. Eur Urol. 2016;69(3):428–35. Epub 2015/07/10. https://doi.org/10.1016/j.eururo.2015.06.046. PubMed PMID: 26166626; PubMed Central PMCID: PMCPMC5002992.

38. Epstein JI. Prostate cancer grading: a decade after the 2005 modified system. Mod Pathol. 2018;31(S1):S47–63. https://doi.org/10.1038/modpathol.2017.133. PubMed PMID: 29297487.

39. Epstein JI, Amin MB, Reuter VE, Humphrey PA. Contemporary Gleason grading of prostatic carcinoma: an update with discussion on practical issues to implement the 2014 International Society of Urological Pathology (ISUP) consensus conference on Gleason grading of prostatic carcinoma. Am J Surg Pathol. 2017;41(4):e1–7. https://doi.org/10.1097/PAS.0000000000000820. PubMed PMID: 28177964.

40. Aydin H, Zhang J, Samaratunga H, Tan N, Magi-Galluzzi C, Klein E, et al. Ductal adenocarcinoma of the prostate diagnosed on transurethral biopsy or resection is not always indicative of aggressive disease: implications for clinical management. BJU Int. 2010;105(4):476–80. Epub 2009/08/25. https://doi.org/10.1111/j.1464-410X.2009.08812.x. PubMed PMID: 19709071.

41. Liu T, Wang Y, Zhou R, Li H, Cheng H, Zhang J. The update of prostatic ductal adenocarcinoma. Chin J Cancer Res. 2016;28(1):50–7. https://doi.org/10.3978/j.issn.1000-9604.2016.02.02. PubMed PMID: 27041926; PubMed Central PMCID: PMCPMC4779765.

42. Gansler T, Fedewa SA, Lin CC, Amin MB, Jemal A, Ward EM. Trends in diagnosis of Gleason score 2 through 4 prostate cancer in the National Cancer Database, 1990-2013. Arch Pathol Lab Med. 2017;141(12):1686–96. Epub 2017/05/30. https://doi.org/10.5858/arpa.2016-0611-OA. PubMed PMID: 28557615.

43. Ross HM, Kryvenko ON, Cowan JE, Simko JP, Wheeler TM, Epstein JI. Do adenocarcinomas of the prostate with Gleason score (GS) ≤6 have the potential to metastasize to lymph nodes? Am J Surg Pathol. 2012;36(9):1346–52. https://doi.org/10.1097/PAS.0b013e3182556dcd. PubMed PMID: 22531173; PubMed Central PMCID: PMCPMC3421030.

44. Epstein JI, Feng Z, Trock BJ, Pierorazio PM. Upgrading and downgrading of prostate cancer from biopsy to radical prostatectomy: incidence and predictive factors using the modified Gleason grading system and factoring in tertiary grades. Eur Urol. 2012;61(5):1019–24. Epub 2012/02/08. https://doi.org/10.1016/j.eururo.2012.01.050. PubMed PMID: 22336380; PubMed Central PMCID: PMCPMC4659370.

45. Lane BR, Magi-Galluzzi C, Reuther AM, Levin HS, Zhou M, Klein EA. Mucinous adenocarcinoma of the prostate does not confer poor prognosis. Urology. 2006;68(4):825–30. https://doi.org/10.1016/j.urology.2006.04.028. PubMed PMID: 17070361.

46. Gurel B, Ali TZ, Montgomery EA, Begum S, Hicks J, Goggins M, et al. NKX3.1 as a marker of prostatic origin in metastatic tumors. Am J Surg Pathol. 2010;34(8):1097–105. https://doi.org/10.1097/PAS.0b013e3181e6cbf3. PubMed PMID: 20588175; PubMed Central PMCID: PMCPMC3072223.

47. Sheridan T, Herawi M, Epstein JI, Illei PB. The role of P501S and PSA in the diagnosis of metastatic adenocarcinoma of the prostate. Am J Surg Pathol. 2007;31(9):1351–5. https://doi.org/10.1097/PAS.0b013e3180536678. PubMed PMID: 17721190.

48. Huang H, Guma SR, Melamed J, Zhou M, Lee P, Deng FM. NKX3.1 and PSMA are sensitive diagnostic markers for prostatic carcinoma in bone metastasis after decalcification of specimens. Am J Clin Exp Urol. 2018;6(5):182–8. Epub 2018/10/20. PubMed PMID: 30510970; PubMed Central PMCID: PMCPMC6261873.

49. Zhou M, Chinnaiyan AM, Kleer CG, Lucas PC, Rubin MA. Alpha-Methylacyl-CoA racemase: a novel tumor marker over-expressed in several human cancers and their precursor lesions. Am J Surg Pathol. 2002;26(7):926–31. https://doi.org/10.1097/00000478-200207000-00012. PubMed PMID: 12131161.

50. Yaskiv O, Zhang X, Simmerman K, Daly T, He H, Falzarano S, et al. The utility of ERG/P63 double immunohistochemical staining in the diagnosis of limited cancer in prostate needle biopsies. Am J Surg Pathol. 2011;35(7):1062–8. https://doi.org/10.1097/PAS.0b013e318215cc03. PubMed PMID: 21623182.

51. Hassan O, Han M, Zhou A, Paulk A, Sun Y, Al-Harbi A, et al. Incidence of Extraprostatic extension at radical prostatectomy with pure Gleason score 3 + 3 = 6 (grade group 1) cancer: implications for whether Gleason score 6 prostate cancer should be renamed "not cancer" and for selection criteria for active surveillance. J Urol. 2018;199(6):1482–7. Epub 2017/11/15. https://doi.org/10.1016/j.juro.2017.11.067. PubMed PMID: 29154905

52. Gelmann EP, Bowen C, Bubendorf L. Expression of NKX3.1 in normal and malignant tissues. Prostate. 2003;55(2):111–7. https://doi.org/10.1002/pros.10210. PubMed PMID: 12661036.

53. Yang XJ, Wu CL, Woda BA, Dresser K, Tretiakova M, Fanger GR, et al. Expression of alpha-Methylacyl-CoA racemase (P504S) in atypical adenomatous hyperplasia of the prostate. Am J Surg Pathol. 2002;26(7):921–5. https://doi.org/10.1097/00000478-200207000-00011. PubMed PMID: 12131160.

54. Osunkoya AO, Hansel DE, Sun X, Netto GJ, Epstein JI. Aberrant diffuse expression of p63 in adenocarcinoma of the prostate on needle biopsy and radical prostatectomy: report of 21 cases. Am J Surg Pathol. 2008;32(3):461–7. https://doi.org/10.1097/PAS.0b013e318157020e. PubMed PMID: 18300803.

55. Tan HL, Haffner MC, Esopi DM, Vaghasia AM, Giannico GA, Ross HM, et al. Prostate adenocarcinomas aberrantly expressing p63 are molecularly distinct from usual-type prostatic adenocarcinomas. Mod Pathol. 2015;28(3):446–56. Epub 2014/09/12. https://doi.org/10.1038/modpathol.2014.115. PubMed PMID: 25216229; PubMed Central PMCID: PMCPMC4344845.

56. Giannico GA, Ross HM, Lotan T, Epstein JI. Aberrant expression of p63 in adenocarcinoma of the prostate: a radical prostatectomy study. Am J Surg Pathol. 2013;37(9):1401–6. https://doi.org/10.1097/PAS.0b013e31828d5c32. PubMed PMID: 23774168.

57. Yang XJ, Lecksell K, Gaudin P, Epstein JI. Rare expression of high-molecular-weight cytokeratin in adenocarcinoma of the prostate gland: a study of 100 cases of metastatic and locally advanced prostate cancer. Am J Surg Pathol. 1999;23(2):147–52. https://doi.org/10.1097/00000478-199902000-00002. PubMed PMID: 9989840.

58. Wu CL, Yang XJ, Tretiakova M, Patton KT, Halpern EF, Woda BA, et al. Analysis of alpha-methylacyl-CoA racemase (P504S) expression in high-grade prostatic intraepithelial neoplasia. Hum Pathol. 2004;35(8):1008–13. https://doi.org/10.1016/j.humpath.2004.03.019. PubMed PMID: 15297968.

59. Daoud NA, Li G, Evans AJ, van der Kwast TH. The value of triple antibody (34βE12 + p63 + AMACR) cocktail stain in radical prostatectomy specimens with crushed surgical margins. J Clin Pathol. 2012;65(5):437–40. Epub 2012/01/31. https://doi.org/10.1136/jclinpath-2011-200533. PubMed PMID: 22294716.

60. Epstein JI, Egevad L, Humphrey PA, Montironi R. Group MotIIiDUP. Best practices recommendations in the application of immunohistochemistry in the prostate: report from the International Society of Urologic Pathology consensus conference. Am J Surg Pathol. 2014;38(8):e6–e19. https://doi.org/10.1097/PAS.0000000000000238. PubMed PMID: 25029122.

61. Park K, Tomlins SA, Mudaliar KM, Chiu YL, Esgueva R, Mehra R, et al. Antibody-based detection of ERG rearrangement-positive prostate cancer. Neoplasia. 2010;12(7):590–8. https://doi.org/10.1593/neo.10726. PubMed PMID: 20651988; PubMed Central PMCID: PMCPMC2907585.

62. Yaskiv O, Rubin BP, He H, Falzarano S, Magi-Galluzzi C, Zhou M. ERG protein expression in human tumors detected with a rabbit monoclonal antibody. Am J Clin Pathol. 2012;138(6):803–10. https://doi.org/10.1309/AJCP3K5VUFALZTKC. PubMed PMID: 23161713.

63. Shah RB, Tadros Y, Brummell B, Zhou M. The diagnostic use of ERG in resolving an "atypical glands suspicious for cancer" diagnosis in prostate biopsies beyond that provided by basal cell and α-methylacyl-CoA-racemase markers. Hum Pathol. 2013;44(5):786–94. Epub 2012/11/14. https://doi.org/10.1016/j.humpath.2012.06.024. PubMed PMID: 23158212.

64. Sung MT, Jiang Z, Montironi R, MacLennan GT, Mazzucchelli R, Cheng L. Alpha-methylacyl-CoA racemase (P504S)/34betaE12/p63 triple cocktail stain in prostatic adenocarcinoma after hormonal therapy. Hum Pathol. 2007;38(2):332–41. Epub 2006/11/28. https://doi.org/10.1016/j.humpath.2006.08.016. PubMed PMID: 17134736.

65. Suzue K, Montag AG, Tretiakova M, Yang XJ, Sahoo S. Altered expression of alpha-methylacyl-coenzyme A racemase in prostatic adenocarcinoma following hormone therapy. Am J Clin Pathol. 2005;123(4):553–61. https://doi.org/10.1309/H4JX-0XEH-DAC8-YL3P. PubMed PMID: 15743746.

66. Yang XJ, Laven B, Tretiakova M, Blute RD, Woda BA, Steinberg GD, et al. Detection of alpha-methylacyl-coenzyme A racemase in postradiation prostatic adenocarcinoma. Urology. 2003;62(2):282–6. https://doi.org/10.1016/s0090-4295(03)00259-0. PubMed PMID: 12893336.

67. Queisser A, Hagedorn SA, Braun M, Vogel W, Duensing S, Perner S. Comparison of different prostatic markers in lymph node and distant metastases of prostate cancer. Mod Pathol. 2015;28(1):138–45. Epub 2014/06/13. https://doi.org/10.1038/modpathol.2014.77. PubMed PMID: 24925052.

68. Kinoshita Y, Kuratsukuri K, Landas S, Imaida K, Rovito PM, Wang CY, et al. Expression of prostate-specific membrane antigen in normal and malignant human tissues. World J Surg. 2006;30(4):628–36. https://doi.org/10.1007/s00268-005-0544-5. PubMed PMID: 16555021.

69. Bernacki KD, Fields KL, Roh MH. The utility of PSMA and PSA immunohistochemistry in the cytologic diagnosis of metastatic prostate carcinoma. Diagn Cytopathol. 2014;42(7):570–5. Epub 2013/11/22. https://doi.org/10.1002/dc.23075. PubMed PMID: 24273068.

70. Jia L, Jiang Y, Michael CW. Performance of different prostate specific antibodies in the cytological diagnosis of metastatic prostate adenocarcinoma. Diagn Cytopathol. 2017;45(11):998–1004. Epub 2017/09/09. https://doi.org/10.1002/dc.23809. PubMed PMID: 28888085.

71. Berney DM, Wheeler TM, Grignon DJ, Epstein JI, Griffiths DF, Humphrey PA, et al. International Society of Urological Pathology (ISUP) consensus conference on handling and staging of radical prostatectomy specimens. Working group 4: seminal vesicles and lymph nodes. Mod Pathol. 2011;24(1):39–47. Epub 2010/09/03. https://doi.org/10.1038/modpathol.2010.160. PubMed PMID: 20818343.

72. Meeks JJ, Walker M, Bernstein M, Eastham JA. Seminal vesicle involvement at salvage radical prostatectomy. BJU Int. 2013;111(8):E342–7. Epub 2013/03/15. https://doi.org/10.1111/bju.12034. PubMed PMID: 23495695.

73. Fine SW, Al-Ahmadie HA, Gopalan A, Tickoo SK, Scardino PT, Reuter VE. Anatomy of the anterior prostate and extraprostatic space: a contemporary surgical pathology analysis. Adv Anat Pathol. 2007;14(6):401–7. https://doi.org/10.1097/PAP.0b013e3181597a9c. PubMed PMID: 18049129.

74. Billis A. Intraprostatic fat: does it exist? Hum Pathol. 2004;35(4):525. https://doi.org/10.1016/j.humpath.2003.12.003. PubMed PMID: 15116338.

75. Joshi A, Shah V, Varma M. Intraprostatic fat in a prostatic needle biopsy: a case report and review of the literature. Histopathology. 2009;54(7):912–3. Epub 2009/05/11. https://doi.org/10.1111/j.1365-2559.2009.03299.x. PubMed PMID: 19469911.

76. Nazeer T, Kee KH, Ro JY, Jennings TA, Ross J, Mian BM, et al. Intraprostatic adipose tissue: a study of 427 whole mount radical prostatectomy specimens. Hum Pathol. 2009;40(4):538–41. Epub 2009/01/03. https://doi.org/10.1016/j.humpath.2008.10.004. PubMed PMID: 19121845

77. Sung MT, Eble JN, Cheng L. Invasion of fat justifies assignment of stage pT3a in prostatic adenocarcinoma. Pathology. 2006;38(4):309–11. https://doi.org/10.1080/00313020600820914. PubMed PMID: 16916718

78. Karram S, Trock BJ, Netto GJ, Epstein JI. Should intervening benign tissue be included in the measurement of discontinuous foci of cancer on prostate needle biopsy? Correlation with radical prostatectomy findings. Am J Surg Pathol. 2011;35(9):1351–5. https://doi.org/10.1097/PAS.0b013e3182217b79. PubMed PMID: 21836493.

79. Fontugne J, Davis K, Palanisamy N, Udager A, Mehra R, McDaniel AS, et al. Clonal evaluation of prostate cancer foci in biopsies with discontinuous tumor involvement by dual ERG/SPINK1 immunohistochemistry. Mod Pathol. 2016;29(2):157–65. Epub 2016/01/08. https://doi.org/10.1038/modpathol.2015.148. PubMed PMID: 26743468; PubMed Central PMCID: PMCPMC4732921.

80. Dash A, Sanda MG, Yu M, Taylor JM, Fecko A, Rubin MA. Prostate cancer involving the bladder neck: recurrence-free survival and implications for AJCC staging modification. American Joint Committee on Cancer. Urology. 2002;60(2):276–80. https://doi.org/10.1016/s0090-4295(02)01727-2. PubMed PMID: 12137826.

81. Zhou M, Reuther AM, Levin HS, Falzarano SM, Kodjoe E, Myles J, et al. Microscopic bladder neck involvement by prostate carcinoma in radical prostatectomy specimens is not a significant independent prognostic factor. Mod Pathol. 2009;22(3):385–92. Epub 2008/11/28. https://doi.org/10.1038/modpathol.2008.190. PubMed PMID: 19043400.

82. Huang CC, Deng FM, Kong MX, Ren Q, Melamed J, Zhou M. Re-evaluating the concept of "dominant/index tumor nodule" in multifocal prostate cancer. Virchows Arch. 2014;464(5):589–94. Epub 2014/03/12. https://doi.org/10.1007/s00428-014-1557-y. PubMed PMID: 24619626.

83. Billis A, Freitas LLL, Costa LBE, Angelis CM, Carvalho KR, Magna LA, et al. Does index tumor predominant location influence prognostic factors in radical prostatectomies?. Int Braz J Urol. 2017;43(4):686–97. https://doi.org/10.1590/S1677-5538.IBJU.2016.0335. PubMed PMID: 28379672; PubMed Central PMCID: PMCPMC5557445.

84. Howarth SM, Griffiths DF, Varma M. Paraganglion of the prostate gland: an uncommon mimic of prostate cancer in needle biopsies. Histopathology. 2005;47(1):114–5. https://doi.org/10.1111/j.1365-2559.2005.02043.x. PubMed PMID: 15982332.

85. Maniar KP, Unger PD, Samadi DB, Xiao GQ. Incidental prostatic paraganglia in radical prostatectomy specimens: a diagnostic pitfall. Int J Surg Pathol. 2011;19(6):772–4. Epub 2011/07/26. https://doi.org/10.1177/1066896911414567. PubMed PMID: 21791487.

86. Oppenheimer JR, Wills ML, Epstein JI. Partial atrophy in prostate needle cores: another diagnostic pitfall for the surgical pathologist. Am J Surg Pathol. 1998;22(4):440–5. https://doi.org/10.1097/00000478-199804000-00008. PubMed PMID: 9537471.

87. Przybycin CG, Kunju LP, Wu AJ, Shah RB. Partial atrophy in prostate needle biopsies: a detailed analysis of its morphology, immunophenotype, and cellular kinetics. Am J Surg Pathol. 2008;32(1):58–64. https://doi.org/10.1097/PAS.0b013e318093e3f6. PubMed PMID: 18162771.

88. Rowe EW, Laniado ME, Walker MM, Anup P. Incidental acute prostatic inflammation is associated with a lower percentage of free prostate-specific antigen than other benign conditions of the prostate: a prospective screening study. BJU Int. 2006;97(5):1039–

42. https://doi.org/10.1111/j.1464-410X.2006.06132.x. PubMed PMID: 16643488.

89. Umbehr MH, Gurel B, Murtola TJ, Sutcliffe S, Peskoe SB, Tangen CM, et al. Intraprostatic inflammation is positively associated with serum PSA in men with PSA <4 ng ml(−1), normal DRE and negative for prostate cancer. Prostate Cancer Prostatic Dis. 2015;18(3):264–9. Epub 2015/05/05. https://doi.org/10.1038/pcan.2015.19. PubMed PMID: 25939516; PubMed Central PMCID: PMCPMC4537352.

90. Lloyd SN, Collins GN, McKelvie GB, Hehir M, Rogers AC. Predicted and actual change in serum PSA following prostatectomy for BPH. Urology. 1994;43(4):472–9. https://doi.org/10.1016/0090-4295(94)90234-8. PubMed PMID: 7512298.

91. Evans AJ. Treatment effects in prostate cancer. Mod Pathol. 2018;31(S1):S110–21. https://doi.org/10.1038/modpathol.2017.158. PubMed PMID: 29297495.

92. Têtu B. Morphological changes induced by androgen blockade in normal prostate and prostatic carcinoma. Best Pract Res Clin Endocrinol Metab. 2008;22(2):271–83. https://doi.org/10.1016/j.beem.2008.01.005. PubMed PMID: 18471785.

93. Vailancourt L, Ttu B, Fradet Y, Dupont A, Gomez J, Cusan L, et al. Effect of neoadjuvant endocrine therapy (combined androgen blockade) on normal prostate and prostatic carcinoma. A randomized study. Am J Surg Pathol. 1996;20(1):86–93. https://doi.org/10.1097/00000478-199601000-00010. PubMed PMID: 8540613.

94. Carver BS, Kattan MW, Scardino PT, Eastham JA. Gleason grade remains an important prognostic predictor in men diagnosed with prostate cancer while on finasteride therapy. BJU Int. 2005;95(4):509–12. https://doi.org/10.1111/j.1464-410X.2005.05375.x. PubMed PMID: 15705069; PubMed Central PMCID: PMCPMC1939940.

95. Yang XJ, Lecksell K, Short K, Gottesman J, Peterson L, Bannow J, et al. Does long-term finasteride therapy affect the histologic features of benign prostatic tissue and prostate cancer on needle biopsy? PLESS Study Group. Proscar Long-Term Efficacy and Safety Study. Urology. 1999;53(4):696–700. https://doi.org/10.1016/s0090-4295(98)00579-2. PubMed PMID: 10197843.

96. Borkowski P, Robinson MJ, Poppiti RJ, Nash SC. Histologic findings in postcryosurgical prostatic biopsies. Mod Pathol. 1996;9(8):807–11. PubMed PMID: 8871920.

97. Biermann K, Montironi R, Lopez-Beltran A, Zhang S, Cheng L. Histopathological findings after treatment of prostate cancer using high-intensity focused ultrasound (HIFU). Prostate. 2010;70(11):1196–200. https://doi.org/10.1002/pros.21154. PubMed PMID: 20564422.

98. Van Leenders GJ, Beerlage HP, Ruijter ET, de la Rosette JJ, van de Kaa CA. Histopathological changes associated with high intensity focused ultrasound (HIFU) treatment for localised adenocarcinoma of the prostate. J Clin Pathol. 2000;53(5):391–4. https://doi.org/10.1136/jcp.53.5.391. PubMed PMID: 10889823; PubMed Central PMCID: PMCPMC1731195.

99. Görgel SN, Şefik E, Olğunelma V, Şahin E, Balcı U, Çallı AO. Primary non-Hodgkin follicular lymphoma of the prostate: a case report. Turk J Urol. 2014;40(1):57–8. https://doi.org/10.5152/tud.2014.68466. PubMed PMID: 26328148; PubMed Central PMCID: PMCPMC4548646.

100. Petrakis G, Koletsa T, Karavasilis V, Rallis G, Bobos M, Karkavelas G, et al. Primary prostatic lymphoma with components of both diffuse large B-cell lymphoma (DLBCL) and MALT lymphoma. Hippokratia. 2012;16(1):86–9. PubMed PMID: 23930067; PubMed Central PMCID: PMCPMC3738403.

101. Rao RN, Bansal M, Raghuvanshi S, Ansari MS, Neyaz Z. Diffuse large B-cell non-Hodgkin lymphoma of the prostate presenting with urinary outlet obstruction: a case report. Urol Ann. 2015;7(1):100–3. https://doi.org/10.4103/0974-7796.148637. PubMed PMID: 25657557; PubMed Central PMCID: PMCPMC4310096.

102. Hansel DE, Herawi M, Montgomery E, Epstein JI. Spindle cell lesions of the adult prostate. Mod Pathol. 2007;20(1):148–58. https://doi.org/10.1038/modpathol.3800676. PubMed PMID: 17170745.

103. McKenney JK. Mesenchymal tumors of the prostate. Mod Pathol. 2018;31(S1):S133–42. https://doi.org/10.1038/modpathol.2017.155. PubMed PMID: 29297486.

104. Herawi M, Epstein JI. Specialized stromal tumors of the prostate: a clinicopathologic study of 50 cases. Am J Surg Pathol. 2006;30(6):694–704. https://doi.org/10.1097/00000478-200606000-00004. PubMed PMID: 16723846.

105. Murer LM, Talmon GA. Stromal tumor of uncertain malignant potential of the prostate. Arch Pathol Lab Med. 2014;138(11):1542–5. https://doi.org/10.5858/arpa.2013-0212-RS. PubMed PMID: 25357117.

106. Oppenheimer JR, Kahane H, Epstein JI. Granulomatous prostatitis on needle biopsy. Arch Pathol Lab Med. 1997;121(7):724–9. PubMed PMID: 9240909.

107. Wilkinson C, Chowdhury F, Scarsbrook A, Smith J. BCG-induced granulomatous prostatitis--an incidental finding on FDG PET-CT. Clin Imaging. 2012;36(4):413–5. Epub 2012/06/08. https://doi.org/10.1016/j.clinimag.2011.09.004. PubMed PMID: 22726988.

Debra L. Zynger and Charles C. Guo

List of Frequently Asked Questions

What Is the Difference Between Prepubertal and Postpubertal Testicular Germ Cell Tumors?

There are critical differences between prepubertal and postpubertal testicular germ cell tumors.

- Postpubertal testicular germ cell neoplasms have as their precursor germ cell neoplasia in situ (GCNIS). These tumors characteristically demonstrate 12p abnormalities (isochromosome formation, increase in copy number) and have an increased risk with cryptorchidism.
- GCNIS is not a precursor for prepubertal tumors.
- Prepubertal germ cell tumors are composed of pure teratoma, pure yolk sac tumor, or very rarely a mixture of teratoma and yolk sac tumor. Pure teratoma in the prepubertal population is an indolent lesion with teratoma composed of neuroendocrine tumor with atypical features such as necrosis and mitoses being the possible exception.
- Teratoma in the postpubertal population is malignant.
- Epidermoid cysts (squamous lined cysts filled with keratin debris) and dermoid cysts (squamous lining with dermal structures such as adnexa) are lesions that are not associated with GCNIS and are cured with complete excision.
- It is imperative to carefully evaluate the surrounding testicular parenchyma for GCNIS or scarring that could indicate a regression of other germ cell tumor components in a postpubertal patient before rendering a diagnosis of an epidermoid cyst.

The remainder of the text describing germ cell tumors will refer to the postpubertal population unless otherwise indicated.

What Is the Most Common Type of Germ Cell Tumor? What Are Other Components of Germ Cell Tumors?

A germ cell tumor can be comprised of one ("pure") or multiple subtypes (Table 6.1). Pure seminoma is more common than mixed germ cell tumor. A tumor with multiple components is called a mixed germ cell tumor. Common subtypes found within mixed germ cell tumors are seminoma, embryonal carcinoma, teratoma, yolk sac tumor, and choriocarcinoma. Rare types include teratoma with somatic-type malignancy and the nonchoriocarcinomatous placental tumors placental site trophoblastic tumor, epithelioid trophoblastic tumor, and cystic trophoblastic tumor.

- Pure seminoma accounts for approximately 60% of testicular germ cell tumors.
- Within mixed germ cell tumor, embryonal carcinoma is the most frequent tumor type followed by teratoma, yolk sac tumor, seminoma, and least frequently choriocarcinoma.

Reference: [1]

Table 6.1 Invasive testicular germ cell tumor components

Seminoma
Embryonal carcinoma
Yolk sac tumor
Teratoma
Teratoma with somatic-type malignancy
Choriocarcinoma
Placental site trophoblastic tumor
Epithelioid trophoblastic tumor
Cystic trophoblastic tumor

D. L. Zynger (✉)
Department of Pathology, The Ohio State University Medical Center, Columbus, OH, USA
e-mail: debra.zynger@osumc.edu

C. C. Guo
Department of Pathology, The University of Texas MD Anderson Cancer Center, Houston, TX, USA

© Springer Nature Switzerland AG 2021
X. J. Yang, M. Zhou (eds.), *Practical Genitourinary Pathology*, Practical Anatomic Pathology,
https://doi.org/10.1007/978-3-030-57141-2_6

What Is the Significance of Different Germ Cell Tumor Types? In which Specimens Is It Required to List Each Germ Cell Tumor Type and Providing Percentages of Each? How Can the Estimation Percentage of Each Tumor Type Be Performed?

Diagnosing a tumor as pure seminoma impacts pT categorization and treatment. Amounts of embryonal carcinoma, choriocarcinoma, yolk sac tumor, and teratoma have been correlated with other adverse pathological features and outcome. Histologic features can be used to estimate percentages. Immunohistochemistry can be used as an aid to corroborate the histologic impression of tumor type. Tumor percentages should be documented for all germ cell tumor specimens including orchiectomy, retroperitoneal lymph node dissection, and distant metastasis.

- Size is a prognostic parameter of pure seminoma that is reflected in the subclassification of pT1a ($\leq$3 cm) and pT1b (>3 cm), although 4 cm is a more cited and studied size threshold.
- Lymphovascular invasion is the most robust prognostic indicator in nonseminomatous tumors and in these patients retroperitoneal lymph node dissection or adjuvant chemotherapy can be considered. In patients with nonseminomatous tumors undergoing active surveillance, relapse occurred in 44% of those with lymphovascular invasion compared to 14% without.
- Presence of teratoma within a primary tumor increases the likelihood of residual teratoma in a postchemotherapy retroperitoneal mass.
- Presence of teratoma in a retroperitoneal metastasis suggests consideration of resection of all lung metastases as histologic concordance of retroperitoneal and lung metastases is high (75%).
- It is recommended that all residual retroperitoneal masses >1 cm be resected unless the primary tumor was pure seminoma.
- Predominance or pure choriocarcinoma portends aggressive behavior.
- Higher amounts of embryonal carcinoma and lower amounts of teratoma and yolk sac tumor are associated with worse pathologic features.

- The presence of teratoma with somatic-type malignancy, particularly in a metastasis, is correlated with a worse outcome.

References: [2–24]

What Is the Clinical Presentation of Seminoma Compared to a Nonseminomatous Germ Cell Tumor?

Seminoma presents at a mean age of 35–37 years with 72–80% clinical stage I. Serum lactate dehydrogenase is often elevated with normal to modestly increased serum human chorionic gonadotropin and normal alpha fetal protein levels. Mean tumor size is 3.9–4.3 cm. In patients diagnosed over 60 years of age, most germ cell tumors (82%) are seminoma.

Patients with nonseminoma have a mean age of 28–31 years and more frequently present at higher stage (60% clinical stage I). Serum levels of human chorionic gonadotropin and alpha fetal protein can be markedly elevated depending upon presence and amount of choriocarcinoma and yolk sac tumor, respectively. Mean tumor size is 4.1–4.7 cm. Within clinical stage I, relapse is more common in nonseminomatous germ cell tumors (19%) compared to seminoma (13%).

References: [1, 10, 13, 15, 25–28]

What Are the Key Histologic Clues to Diagnose GCNIS? What Is the Expression Profile of GCNIS?

GCNIS is the precursor lesion of postpubertal germ cell tumors. Within seminiferous tubules, seminoma-like cells are seen.

- The key histologic feature is the location of these cells in that they are found against the basement membrane (within the spermatogonial niche) rather than dispersed throughout the tubule (Table 6.2; Fig. 6.1a).
- Other important histologic features include vacuolated cytoplasm, nucleomegaly, and hyperchromatic nuclei with occasional prominent nucleoli.

Table 6.2 Features and differential diagnosis of germ cell neoplasia in situ (GCNIS)

	Location in seminiferous tubule	Tubule appears filled with cells/necrosis	Cells within tubule are homogenous	OCT3/4
GCNIS	Against basement membrane	No	No	+
Intratubular seminoma/embryonal carcinoma	Dispersed	Yes	Variable	+
Germ cells with delayed maturation	Dispersed	Yes	No	+
Sertoli-only tubules	Against basement membrane	No	Yes	−

- Tubules with GCNIS typically lack spermatic maturation and thus the tubules appear predominately empty or have lumens with mostly flocculent pink cytoplasm rather than nucleated cells.

Immunohistochemical stains can corroborate the diagnosis of GCNIS:

- Positive: SALL4, PLAP, CD117/c-kit, D2-40/podoplanin, and OCT3/4 (Fig. 6.1b, c).
- Negative: CD30, WT1, inhibin.

References: [29–32]

What Is Intratubular Tumor and How Is It Different Than GCNIS? What Are Other Mimickers of GCNIS?

Other types of intratubular neoplasia such as intratubular seminoma, intratubular embryonal carcinoma, and intratubular teratoma are much less common than GCNIS.

- These lesions can be differentiated from GCNIS as these lesions fill the lumen of the seminiferous tubule with tumor cells or necrosis rather than exist only against the basement membrane (Table 6.2).
- Intratubular seminoma will have an identical immunophenotype as GCNIS.
- Intratubular embryonal carcinoma will have weaker expression of PLAP, minimal expression of CD117/c-kit, and D2-40/podoplanin and will be positive using CD30.
- Germ cells with delayed maturation as can be seen in cryptorchid testes mimic GCNIS.

- These cells are also OCT3/4 positive but occur sprinkled throughout the seminiferous tubule.
- Tubules containing only Sertoli cells can mimic GCNIS.
- A tubule with GCNIS usually contains cells that appear less homogenous than a Sertoli-only tubule.
- Sertoli cells will show positivity for inhibin and WT1 and negativity for SALL4 and OCT3/4.

References: [29–32]

What Are the Histologic Features and Immunohistochemical Expression Pattern of Seminoma?

Seminoma is unencapsulated with a border that sometimes shows growth between tubules (Fig. 6.2a). The tumor can look nodular at low power with expansile sheets of cells separated by fibrous bands containing lymphocytes (Fig. 6.2b; Table 6.3). Cells are monotonous with cleared out to pale, eosinophilic cytoplasm (Fig. 6.2c). The cleared-out cytoplasm, attributable to glycogen, with the remaining nuclei gives rise to a "fried egg" appearance. Nonoverlapping cells and the empty cytoplasm yield a fine, sharp cell membrane, and a polygonal shape to cells. Nuclei have clumped chromatin and prominent nucleoli. Mitotic figures are frequent.

The immunoprofile of seminoma is (Table 6.4):

- Positive: SALL4, PLAP, CD117/c-kit, D2-40/podoplanin, and OCT3/4.
- Negative: AE1/3, CD30, glypican 3, AFP, GATA3, CK7, HCG, inhibin.
- Seminoma can mimic other germ cell tumor types and other lesions.

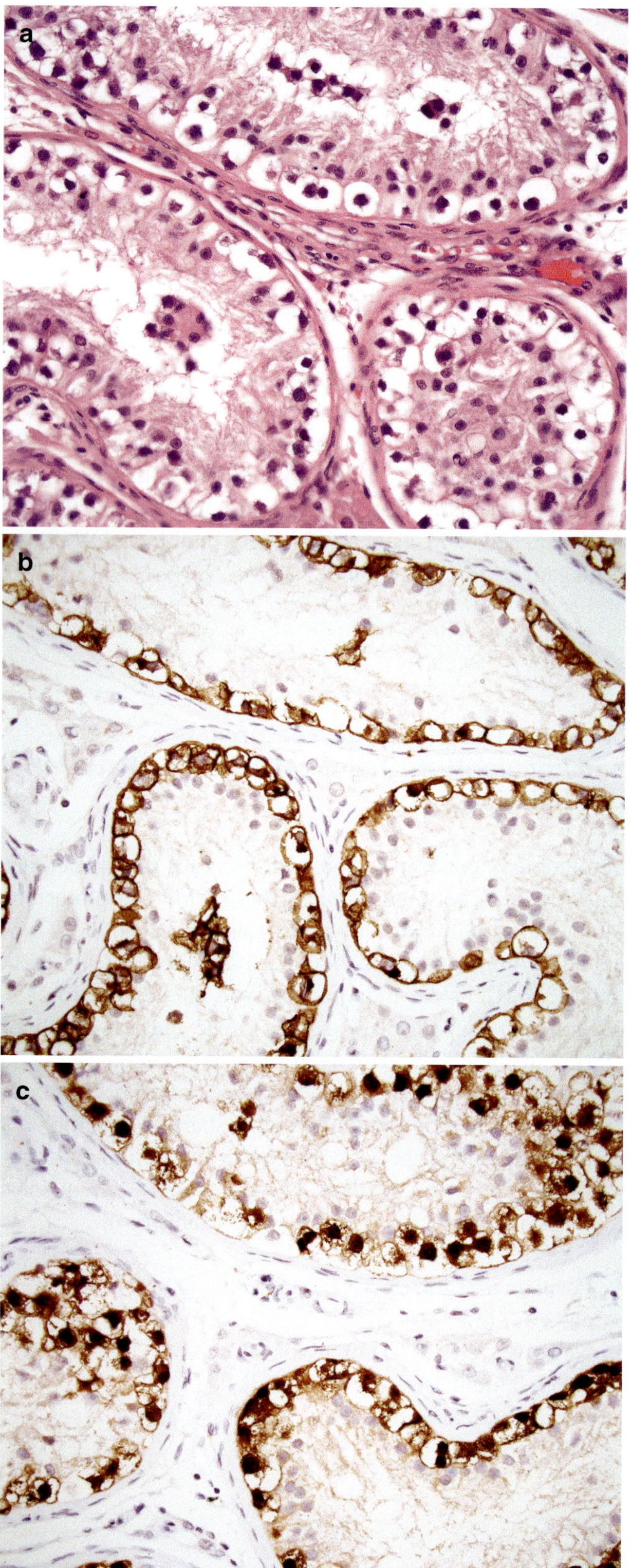

Fig. 6.1 GCNIS. (**a**) GCNIS displays atypical, vacuolated cells lined up against the basement membrane of the seminiferous tubule. (**b**) GCNIS expresses CD117/c-kit in a predominately membranous pattern. (**c**) GCNIS expresses strong, diffuse nuclear OCT3/4

- Pseudoglandular growth or poorly fixed specimens can mimic embryonal carcinoma.
- A microcystic growth patterns resembles yolk sac tumor (Fig. 6.2d).
- Seminoma can have abundant granulomatous inflammation, masking tumor cells, mimicking granulomatous orchitis.
- Nongerm cell tumors to be considered include diffuse large B-cell lymphoma (positive CD20/negative OCT3/4), particularly in an older man, and Sertoli cell tumor (positive inhibin/negative OCT3/4), both of which are readily differentiated from seminoma using immunohistochemistry.

References: [33–36]

What Are Syncytiotrophoblastic Cells in Seminoma and What Is the Clinical Significance of Their Presence?

Syncytiotrophoblastic cells are present in approximately 15% of seminomas. These are typically are seen in scattered clusters near capillaries. The cells are large, have multiple nuclei, and vary from ample cytoplasm to more abundant nuclei ("mulberry" type cells) (Fig. 6.3). These cells usually express HCG and keratin and the presence of these cells has been correlated with detectable increases in serum HCG.

If identified, these tumors can be diagnosed as "seminoma with syncytiotrophoblast cells" and should not be diagnosed as a choriocarcinoma component. Admixture with cytotrophoblasts required for a diagnosis of choriocarcinoma in contrast to seminoma with syncytiotrophoblast cells in which the cells are encountered intermixed with seminoma cells. Their presence does not change clinical management. There is minimal published on this phenomenon in the literature from the past 30 years. Other multinucleate cells, such as Langerhans type giant cells with peripheral nuclei and no expression of HCG or keratin, may be seen.

References: [35–38]

What Is the Significance of a High Mitotic Rate in Seminoma?

Seminoma with high mitotic rate (so called "anaplastic seminoma") has no known prognostic significance and does not impact management. It has been recommended that these diagnostic modifiers not be used to avoid confusion and inappropriate treatment.

References: [31, 39–41]

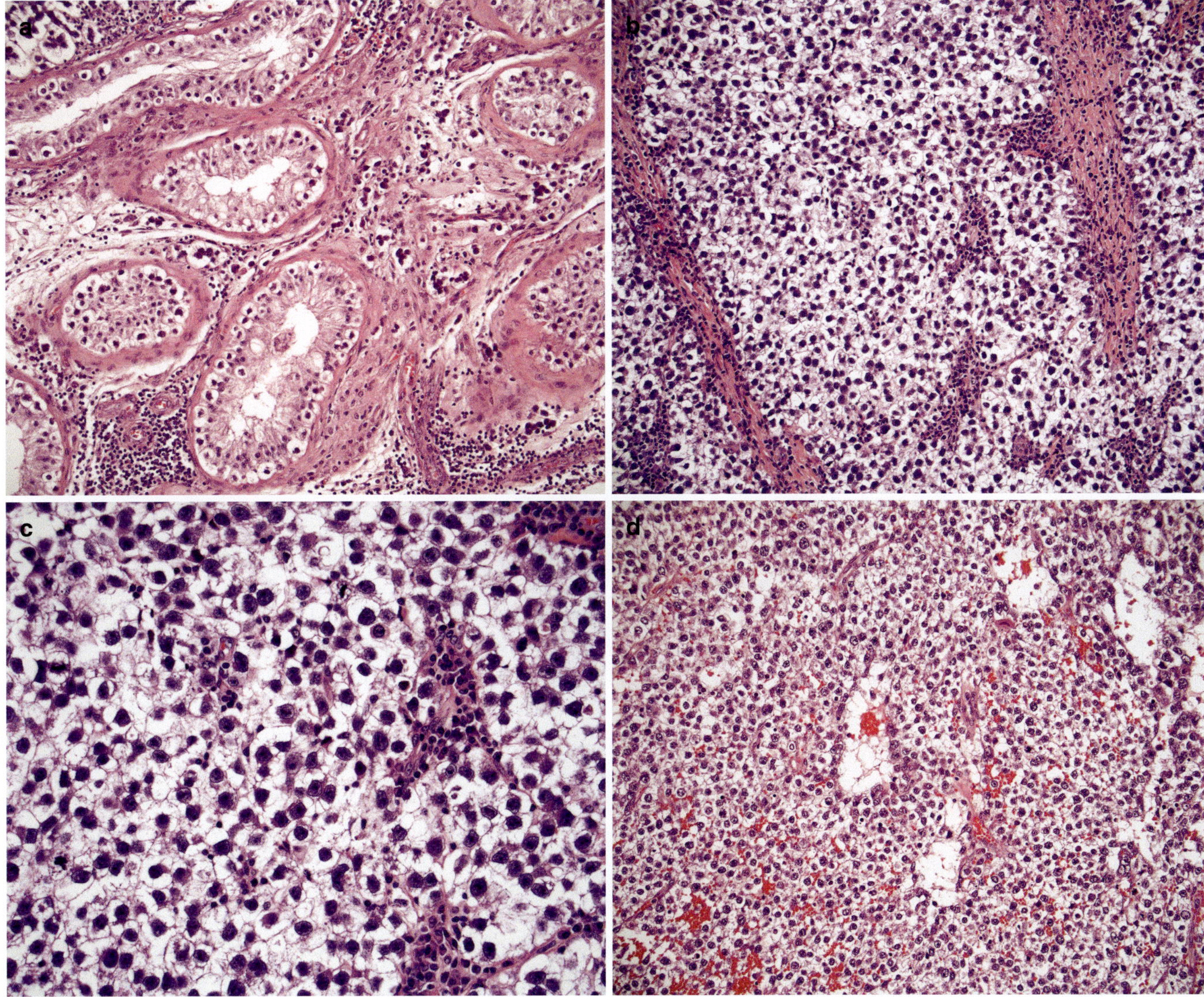

Fig. 6.2 Seminoma. (**a**) Seminoma with tumor infiltrating between tubules at the periphery of the tumor (intertubular growth). (**b**) Fibrous bands containing lymphocytes are characteristic of seminoma. (**c**) Seminoma is composed of sheets of distinctive, monotonous cells with prominent cell membranes and cleared-out cytoplasm. (**d**) Microcystic growth in seminoma can mimic yolk sac tumor

Table 6.3 Histologic features of germ cell tumor subtypes

	Architecture	Distinct cell borders/no cellular overlap	Cytology	Most important germ cells tumor mimics
Seminoma	Expansile nodules separated by fibrous bands containing lymphocytes	Yes	Monotonous cells with pale to cleared-out cytoplasm	Embryonal carcinoma, yolk sac tumor
Embryonal carcinoma	Sheet-like, glandular and papillary growth predominate	No	Pleomorphic, high-grade cells	Seminoma, yolk sac tumor
Yolk sac tumor	Microcystic/reticular pattern most common	No		Seminoma, embryonal carcinoma
Teratoma	Variable	Variable	Variable	Yolk sac tumor
Choriocarcinoma		No-syncytial cells Yes-mononucleate cells		Embryonal carcinoma

Table 6.4 Immunohistochemical expression of common germ cell tumor types

	Seminoma	Embryonal carcinoma	Yolk sac tumor	Choriocarcinoma	Teratoma
SALL4 (nuclear)	+	+	+	+	Variable
PLAP	+	+/weak	−	−	−
CD117/c-kit	+	−/weak	−	−	−
D2-40/podoplanin	+	−/weak	−	−	Variable
OCT3/4 (nuclear)	+	+	−	−	−
CD30	−	+	−	−	−
AE1/3	−/weak	+/weak	+	+	Variable
Glypican 3	−	−	+	+	Variable
AFP	−	−	+	+	Variable
GATA3 (nuclear)	−	−	+	+	Variable
CK7	−	−	−/focal	+	Variable
HCG	−	−	−	+	−
Inhibin	−	−	−	+ (syncytial cells)	−
WT1 (nuclear)	−	−	−	−	−
Calretinin	−	−	−	−	−

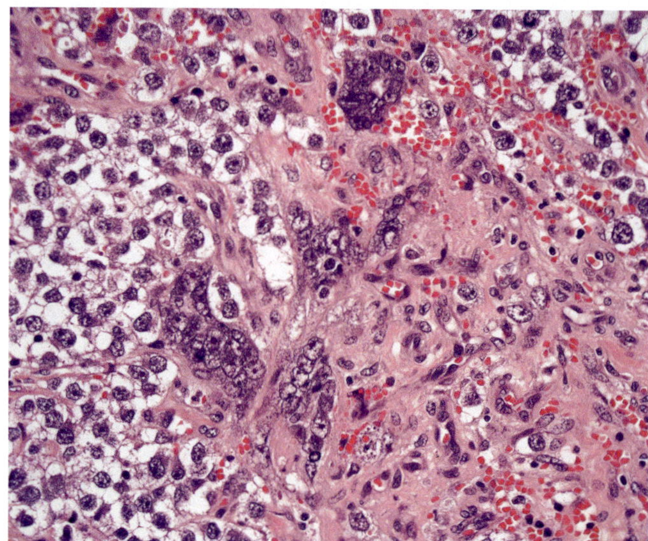

Fig. 6.3 Seminoma with syncytiotrophoblast cells. Multinucleated cells are clustered together

The immunoprofile of embryonal carcinoma is (Table 6.4):

- Positive: SALL4, OCT3/4, CD30.
- Positive/weak: PLAP, AE1/3.
- Negative/weak: CD117/c-kit, D2-40/podoplanin.
- Negative: glypican 3, AFP, GATA3, CK7, HCG, inhibin.
- Embryonal carcinoma can mimic other germ cell tumor types and other lesions.
- Diffuse growth mimics poorly fixed seminoma, especially if admixed with lymphocytes (Fig. 6.4d).
- Degenerative areas and areas with hemorrhage mimics choriocarcinoma.
- Papillary and glandular patterns mimic yolk sac tumor and teratoma (Fig. 6.4b, c).
- In the metastatic setting, embryonal carcinoma is a mimicker of poorly differentiated carcinoma.

References: [33–36, 38, 42, 43]

What Are the Histologic Features and Immunohistochemical Expression Pattern of Embryonal Carcinoma?

Embryonal carcinoma is a primitive, high-grade tumor. The most common growth pattern is diffuse, sheets of cells (55%), but numerus other growth patterns can be seen, and glandular (175) and papillary (11%) patterns are frequent (Fig. 6.4a–c; Table 6.3). Cells are large and overlapping with indistinct cell borders. There is a moderate amount of amphophilic cytoplasm. Nuclei are pleomorphic with prominent nucleoli and frequent mitotic figures present. Necrosis and hemorrhage are frequent. Lymphovascular invasion is often present.

What Are the Histologic Features and Immunohistochemical Expression Pattern of Yolk Sac Tumor?

Yolk sac tumor has a vast array of growth patterns in which multiple can coexist in the same tumor (Table 6.5).

The most common is microvesicular/reticular in which haphazard, varying-sized, anastomosing small cysts are present (Fig. 6.5a, b). The cysts are lined by cuboidal to flattened cells, which can appear lipoblast-like or signet ring. Hyaline globules and wispy myxoid material can be seen in the cyst spaces. Cells are blander than other types of germ cell tumors and mitotic figures, while present, are more difficult to appreciate.

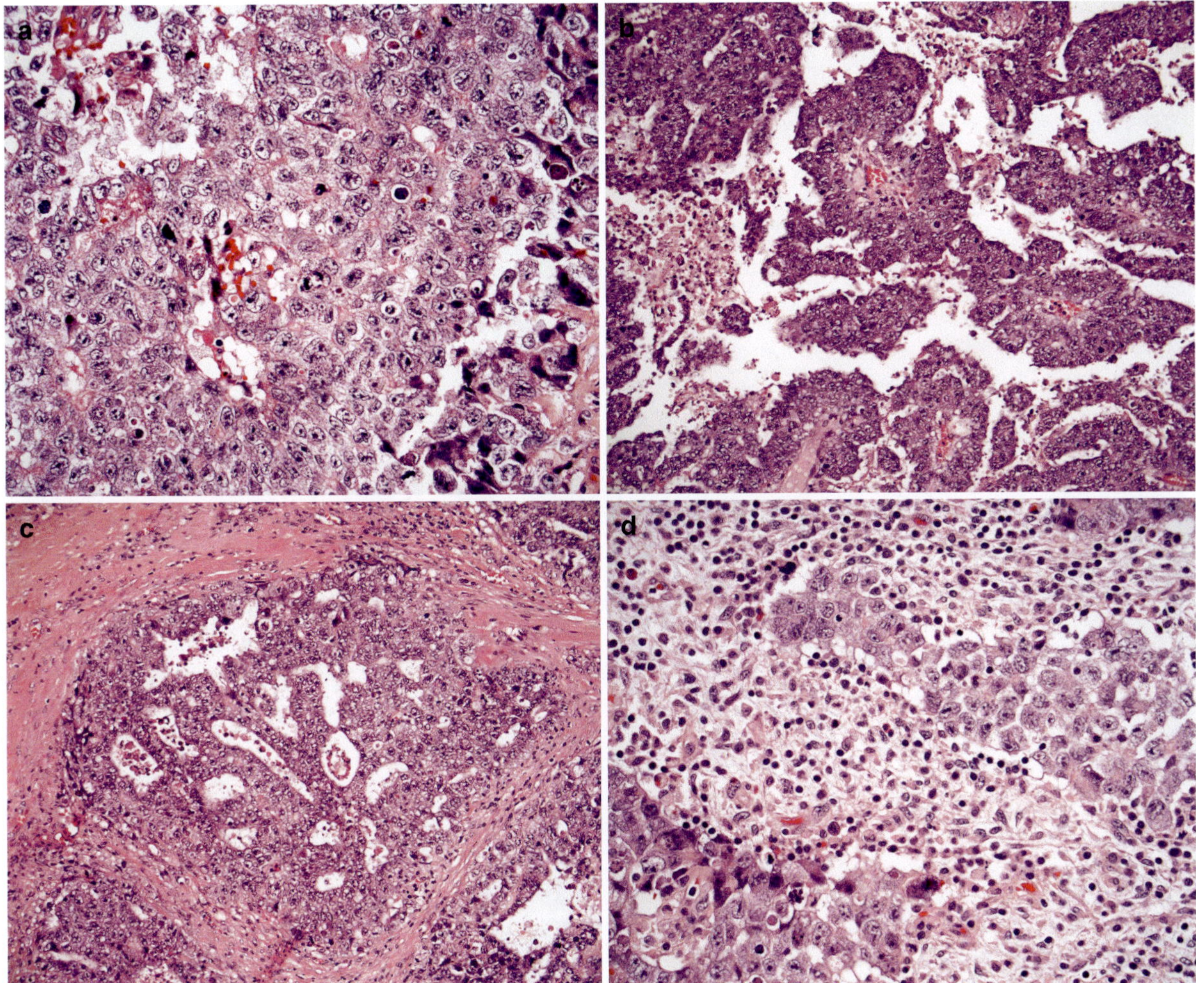

Fig. 6.4 Embryonal carcinoma. (**a**) Embryonal carcinoma usually has a sheet-like growth. Cells are crowded with amphophilic cytoplasm, macronucleoli, and frequent mitotic figures. (**b**) Papillary growth can minim yolk sac tumor. (**c**) Pseudoglandular or cystic growth can mimic yolk sac tumor. (**d**) Embryonal carcinoma admixed with lymphocytes mimics seminoma

Table 6.5 Growth patterns of yolk sac tumor

Yolk sac tumor growth patterns	Features
Microcystic/ reticular	Most common
Myxomatous	Myxoid background
Macrocystic	Large cysts
Solid	Sheets of larger cells, mimicker of seminoma
Glandular/alveolar	Simple, complex, or secretory endometrial appearing; mimics adenocarcinoma and teratoma
Endodermal sinus/ perivascular	Shiller-Duval bodies
Hepatoid	Recapitulates liver, including expression
Papillary	Thin fibrovascular cores or micropapillary clusters
Sarcomatoid/ spindle cell	Mimics sarcoma or teratoma with somatic-type malignancy
Parietal	Intervening eosinophilic basement membrane
Polyvesicular vitelline	Prominent microcysts, classically pear shaped

The myxomatous pattern has similar morphology with more abundant myxoid stroma and cords or strands of cells throughout (Fig. 6.5c). Larger cysts are seen in the macrocystic pattern. The solid pattern has sheets of cells that are monotonous, have well-delineated cell membranes and a moderate amount of pale to cleared-out cytoplasm (Fig. 6.5d). Simple or anastomosing gland like structures can be seen in the glandular/alveolar pattern as can glands resembling secretory endometrium with supra- and subnuclear vacuolization (Fig. 6.5e). The endodermal sinus patter is uncommon and displays a central papillary core surrounded by cuboidal tumor cells (Shiller-Duval bodies) within a background of microcysts (Fig. 6.5f). The cells in the hepatoid pattern grow in nests and cords, have abundant eosinophilic cytoplasm, and express liver markers (Fig. 6.5g). Papillary pattern has thin fibrovascular cores or clumps of micropapillary tumor clusters lacking fibrovascular cores (Fig. 6.5h). Sarcomatoid or spindle cell growth has diffuse growth of somewhat bland, stellate cells. Recent research has shown that some high-

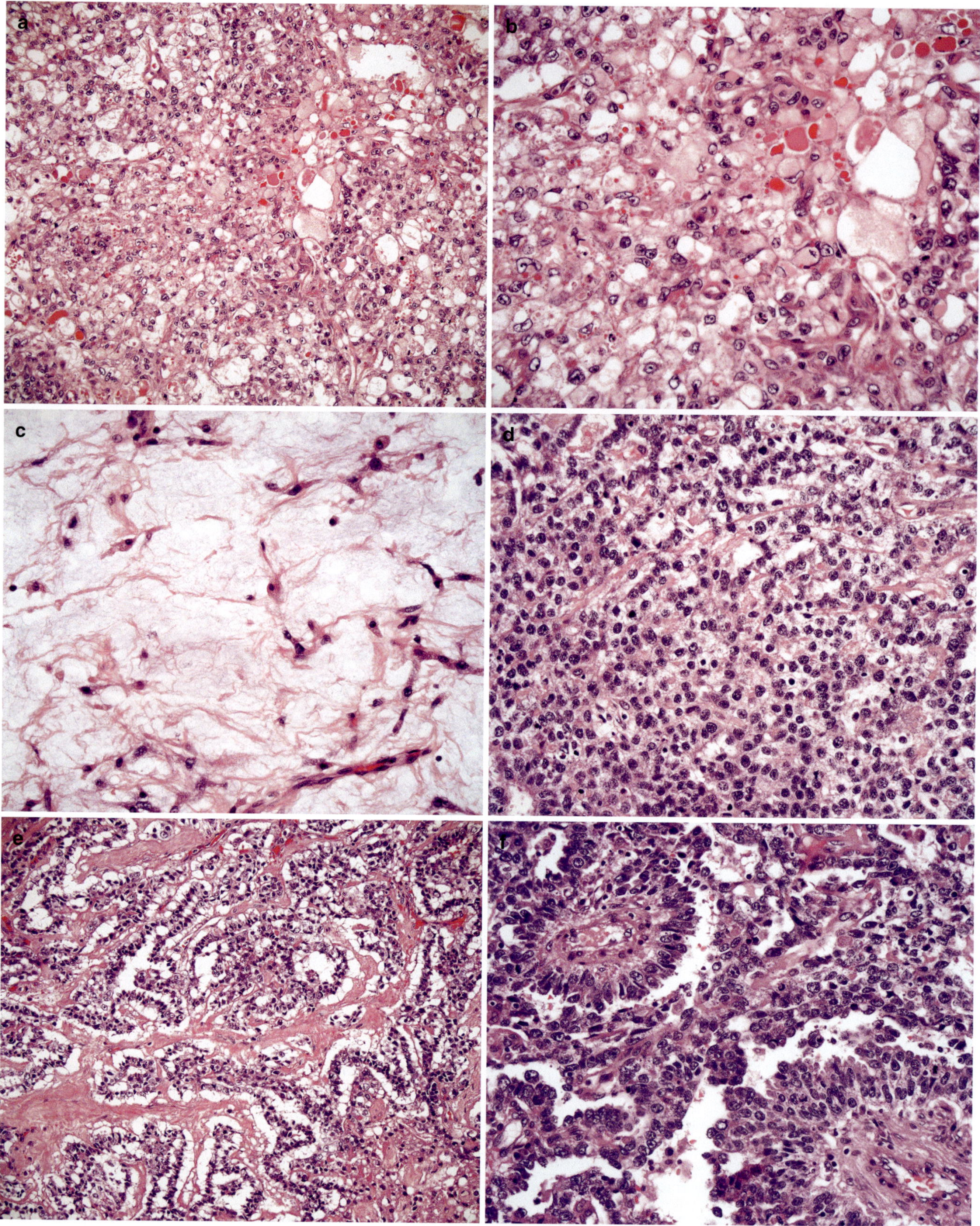

Fig. 6.5 Yolk sac tumor. (**a**) The microcystic/reticular pattern is most common. (**b**) Cells appear flattened and bland. Hyaline globules are seen. (**c**) The myomatous pattern is easily overlooked. (**d**) Solid growth mimics seminoma. (**e**) Glandular/alveolar has an appearance of adeno-carcinoma. (**f**) The endodermal sinus pattern has Shiller-Duval bodies (upper left and lower right). (**g**) Hepatoid pattern. (**h**) Papillary pattern

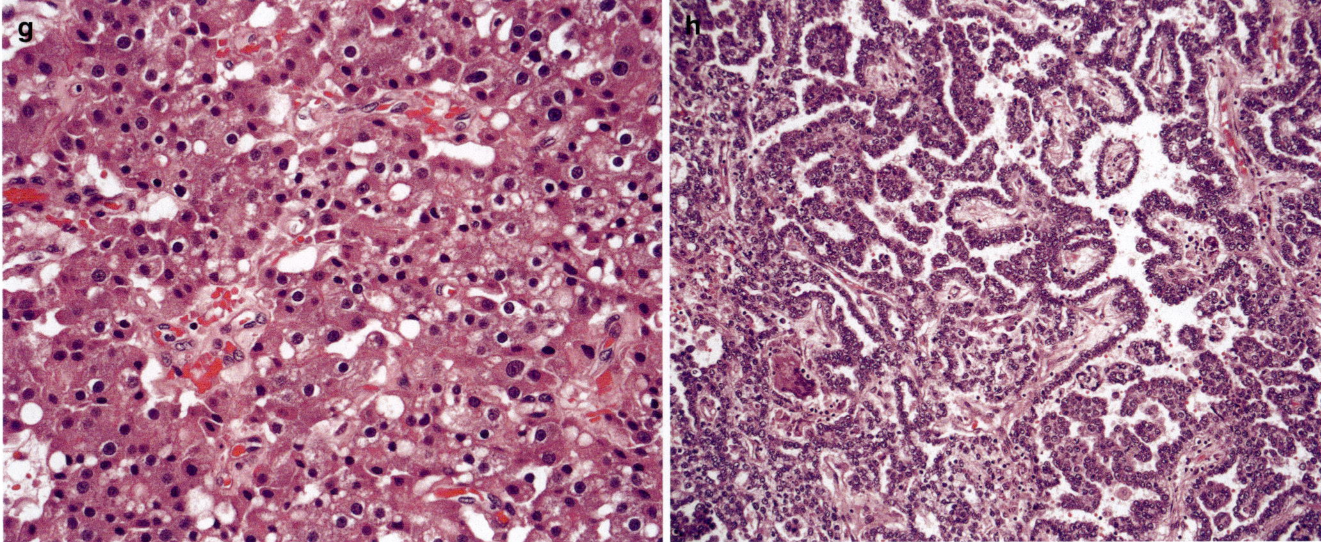

Fig. 6.5 (continued)

grade sarcomatoid tumor that were previously thought to be teratoma with somatic-type malignancy, especially in post-chemotherapy metastases, are actually high-grade sarcomatoid yolk sac tumor. The parietal pattern refers to tumor with eosinophilic clumps or bands of basement membrane material typically between areas with microvesicular/reticular growth. Polyvesicular vitelline pattern has microcysts lined by cuboidal to flattened cells in a hypocellular, edematous to densely cellular background. The microcysts range from pear shaped to irregular and anastomosing.

The immunoprofile of yolk sac tumor is as follows (Table 6.4):

- Positive: SALL4, AE1/3, glypican 3, AFP, GATA3.
- Focal/negative: CK7.
- Negative: PLAP, CD117/c-kit, D2-40/podoplanin, OCT3/4, CD30, HCG, inhibin.
- Yolk sac tumor can mimic other germ cell tumor types and other lesions (Table 6.3).
- Solid yolk sac tumor mimics seminoma (Fig. 6.5d).
- Sarcomatoid yolk sac mimics primary sarcoma and teratoma with somatic-type transformation.
- Glandular yolk sac tumor mimics adenocarcinoma and teratoma (Fig. 6.5e).

References: [17, 33–35, 42–45]

What Is Polyembryoma and How Should It Be Diagnosed in a Pathology Report?

Polyembryoma is the intimate co-mingling of embryonal carcinoma and yolk sac tumor to form structures that resemble the early presomite embryo (embryoid-bodies) (Fig. 6.6a, b).

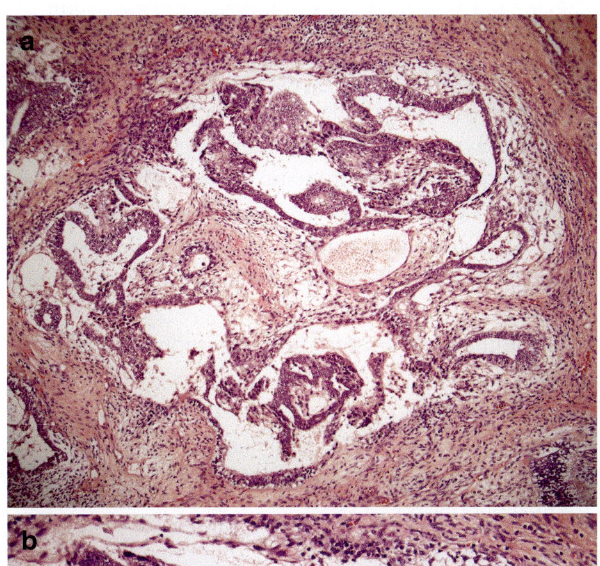

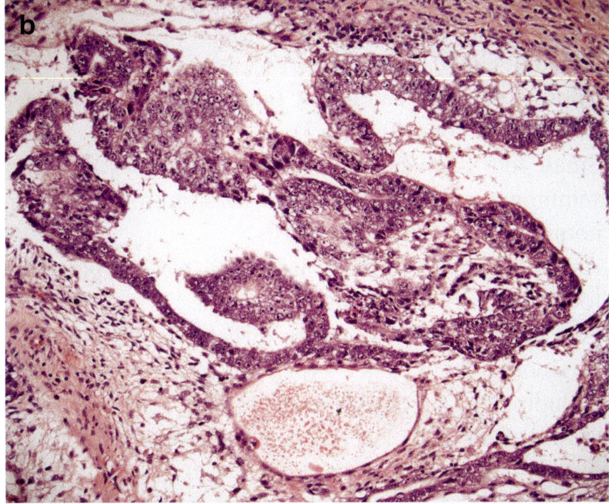

Fig. 6.6 Polyembryoma. (**a**) Numerous embryoid bodies. (**b**) Embryoid body. Basophilic cells are embryonal carcinoma and wispy cells are yolk sac tumor

- A cuplike shape is seen lined by cuboidal to columnar embryonal carcinoma cells.
- Cells within and around the cup lining are made of yolk sac tumor with reticular or myxomatous growth.
- Polyembryoma exists alongside other germ cell tumor types and therefore is a part of a mixed germ cell tumor.
- It is not necessary to mention polyembryoma growth in a pathology report but rather to recognize the structures in order to correctly identify and quantify each germ cell tumor type that is present.

References: [42, 46]

What Are the Histologic Features and Immunohistochemical Expression Pattern of Choriocarcinoma?

Choriocarcinoma is composed of syncytial cells, called syncytiotrophoblasts, and mononucleated trophoblasts (cytotrophoblasts and intermediate trophoblasts). These cells grow admixed and are usually associated with adjacent hemorrhage (Fig. 6.7a). Classically, the syncytiotrophoblasts grow as a cap overlying the mononucleated trophoblasts (Fig. 6.7b). Syncytiotrophoblasts are large cells with multiple pleomorphic, hyperchromatic nuclei. They have abundant, dense, eosinophilic cytoplasm and indistinct cell borders. Mononucleated trophoblasts are medium sized with pale eosinophilic cytoplasm with distinct cell borders (Fig. 6.7c).

The immunoprofile of choriocarcinoma is shown in Table 6.4.

- Positive: SALL4, AE1/3, glypican 3, AFP, GATA3, CK7, HCG, inhibin (syncytiotrophoblasts), p63 (cytotrophoblasts).
- Negative: PLAP, CD117/c-kit, D2-40/podoplanin, OCT3/4, CD30.
- Choriocarcinoma can mimic other germ cell tumor types and other lesions (Table 6.3).
- Small foci admixed with other tumor types can mimic seminoma with syncytiotrophoblasts or embryonal carcinoma with syncytiotrophoblasts.
- As the syncytial cells are large and pleomorphic, small foci can mimic embryonal carcinoma.
- Post chemotherapy, it can be difficult to discern choriocarcinoma from other types of trophoblastic tumors including cystic trophoblastic tumor, epithelial trophoblastic tumor and placental site trophoblastic tumor.

References: [4, 22, 46, 47]

What Are the Histologic Features and Immunohistochemical Expression Pattern of Teratoma?

Teratoma can form any mature or fetal cell type. Common tissue types include spindled mesenchymal stroma, squamous epithelium, respiratory epithelium, intestinal epithelium, cartilage (often with cytologic atypia), and immature neural elements (Fig. 6.8a, b). Spindled smooth muscle or fibroblastic areas of teratoma are easily overlooked but should be included in the diagnosis and quantification of teratoma.

The diagnosis of teratoma is almost always made by recognition of multiple tissue types and the expression pattern is highly variable, depending on the tissue that is recapitulated. SALL4 expression is inconsistent and cannot be relied upon to rule out the presence of teratoma in limited biopsy specimens.

The immunoprofile of choriocarcinoma is as follows (Table 6.4):

- Variable: SALL4, AE1/3, glypican 3, AFP, GATA3, CK7, D2-40/podoplanin.
- Negative: PLAP, CD117/c-kit, OCT3/4, CD30, HCG.

Reference: [33]

Does Immature Teratoma Need to Be Diagnosed Separately from Mature Teratoma?

Both immature and mature teratoma elements are malignant in a postpubertal tumor (Fig. 6.8b). There is no clinical relevance to the presence of immature teratoma in a postpubertal tumor, and therefore only the presence and amount of teratoma, inclusive of mature and immature teratoma, need to be included in a pathology report.

Reference: [33]

How Is Teratoma with Somatic-Type Malignancy Diagnosed?

Teratoma with somatic-type malignancy is defined as overgrowth of one teratoma element occupying a 4×-magnification field or 0.5 cm. It is most frequent in metastases and has a corresponding poor prognosis as the patients usually have a relapse. Presence in a primary tumor may not yield a worse prognosis. Teratoma with somatic malignancy must be differentiated from sarcomatoid yolk sac tumor or glandular

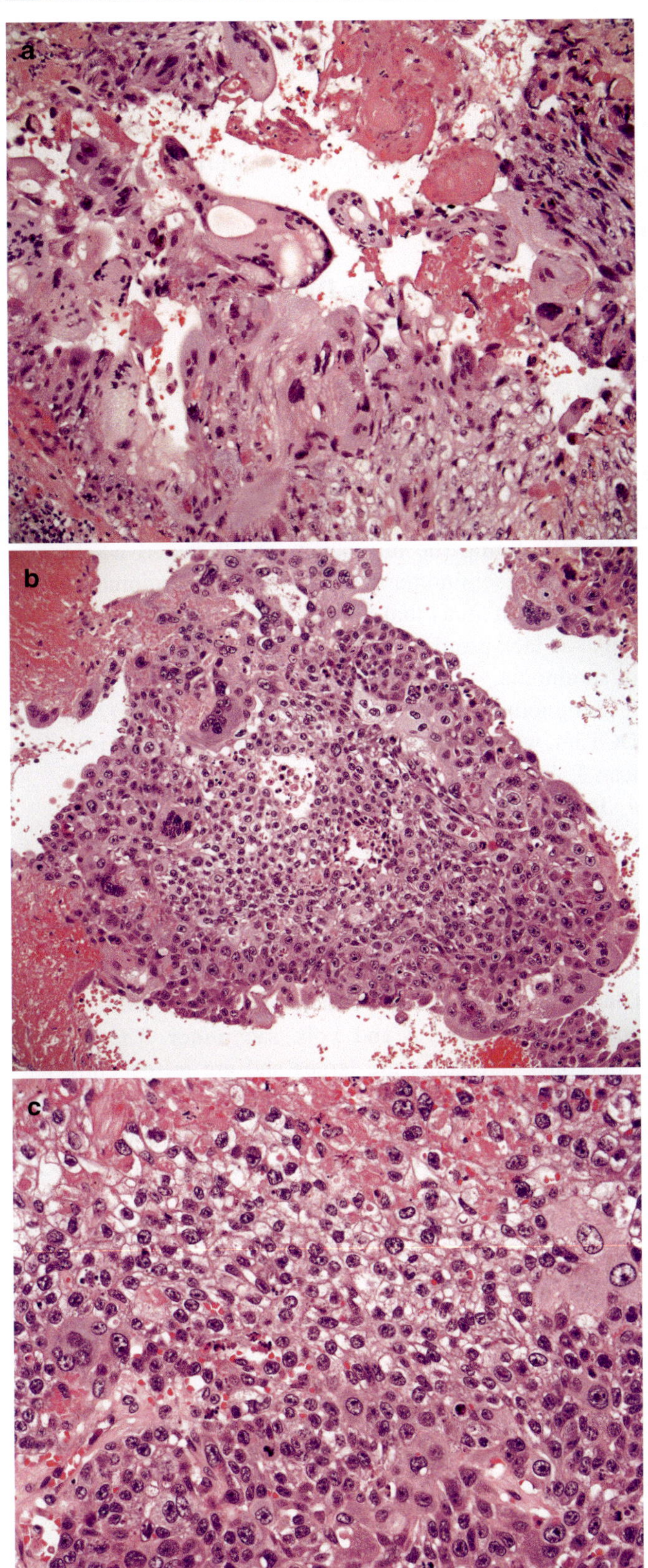

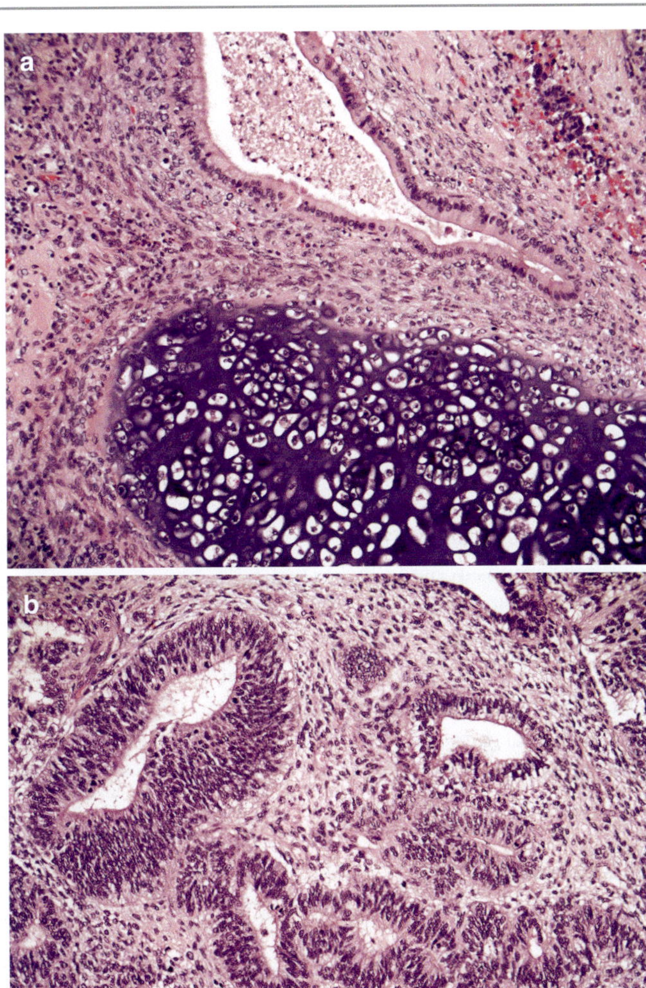

Fig. 6.8 Teratoma. (**a**) Cartilage, glandular epithelium and spindled mesenchymals cells. Spindled cells are easily overlooked but should be included in the diagnosis and quantification of teratoma. (**b**) Immature neural elements. This is included in teratoma as there is no distinction between immature and mature teratoma made in postpubertal testicular germ cell tumors

yolk sac tumor, frequent mimickers in postchemotherapy metastases.

Teratoma with somatic-type malignancy can mimic other germ cell tumor types and other lesions.

- Teratoma with somatic sarcoma can mimic sarcomatoid yolk sac tumor.
- Teratoma with somatic adenocarcinoma can mimic glandular yolk sac tumor.
- Teratoma with somatic squamous cell carcinoma can mimic choriocarcinoma and other nonchoriocarcinomatous germ cell tumor types.

Fig. 6.7 Choriocarcinoma. (**a**) Syncytiotrophoblasts predominate with associated hemorrhage and peripheral mononucleated trophoblasts. (**b**) Characteristic capping of the syncytiotrophoblasts over the trophoblasts is more apparent in areas with greater numbers of mononucleated cells. (**c**) The solid growth of mononucleated trophoblasts mimics seminoma and embryonal carcinoma

- Metastasis from nongerm cell tumor such as primary sarcoma, adenocarcinoma, and squamous cell carcinoma must be excluded in metastases.

References: [17, 45, 48–50]

What Are the Most Common Forms of Teratoma with Somatic-Type Malignancy?

Types of somatic type malignancy vary in prevalence (Table 6.6). The majority are sarcoma (63%). The presence of sarcoma may indicate a worse prognosis than other types.

The most common types in order of decreasing frequency are as follows:

- Rhabdomyosarcoma (35%) (Fig. 6.9a, b)
- Sarcoma, not otherwise specified (24%) (Fig. 6.9c)
- Adenocarcinoma
- Primitive neuroectodermal tumor (lacks t(11;22) translocation, medulloepithelioma appearance) (Fig. 6.9d)
- Neuroglial tumor (lacks consistent results with *ATRX*, *IDH*, *BRAF*) (Fig. 6.9e)
- Squamous cell carcinoma

References: [48–53]

How Can Seminoma Be Differentiated from Embryonal Carcinoma?

Both seminoma and embryonal carcinoma can have solid growth. Seminoma has fibrous septae admixed with lymphocytes that is not present in embryonal carcinoma. Seminoma is composed of uniform cells while embryonal carcinoma is more pleomorphic. Seminoma cells are not overlapping while cells are more crowded and cell borders are less distinct in embryonal carcinoma. The cytoplasm in seminoma is usually much paler than is seen in embryonal carcinoma.

Table 6.6 Most common types of teratoma with somatic-type malignancy

Somatic type	Features
Rhabdomyosarcoma (35%)	
Sarcoma, not otherwise specified (24%)	Must exclude sarcomatoid yolk sac tumor
Adenocarcinoma	Must exclude glandular yolk sac tumor
Primitive neuroectodermal tumor	Lacks t(11;22) translocation, medulloepithelioma appearance
Neuroglial tumor	Lacks consistent results with *ATRX*, *IDH*, *BRAF*
Squamous cell carcinoma	Must exclude cystic trophoblastic tumor

Seminoma expresses CD117/c-kit and D2-40 while embryonal carcinoma is positive for CD30 (Fig. 6.10a, b). Both can express PLAP, but reactivity is stronger in seminoma. Adjacent GCNIS can serve as an excellent internal control for staining that is consistent with seminoma.

References: [34, 35]

How Can Seminoma Be Differentiated from Yolk Sac Tumor?

Both seminoma and yolk sac tumor can have solid or microcystic growth. Yolk sac tumor lacks fibrous septae containing lymphocytes as is seen in seminoma. Seminoma nuclei are larger and more uniform. Microcysts in yolk sac tumor have well-defined lumens dispersed haphazardly. The cells lining the microcysts are flattened whereas in microcystic seminoma the cells remain polygonal and the cysts form in areas that appear discohesive. Cells in solid yolk sac lack prominent cell borders that are characteristic of seminoma.

Seminoma expresses PLAP, CD117/c-kit, D2-40 and OCT3/4, while yolk sac tumor is positive using AE1/3, glypican 3, AFP, and GATA3.

References: [34, 35]

How Can Embryonal Carcinoma Be Differentiated from Yolk Sac Tumor?

Glandular and papillary structures can be seen in both embryonal carcinoma and yolk sac tumor. The cells of embryonal carcinoma are larger and are infrequently flattened compared to yolk sac tumor. The cytoplasm of embryonal carcinoma is denser and more basophilic and the nuclei are larger and have increased pleomorphism. Mitoses are easier to identify in embryonal carcinoma.

Embryonal carcinoma expresses OCT3/4 and CD30 while yolk sac tumor is positive using glypican 3 and AFP (Fig. 6.11a–c).

References: [34, 35]

How Can Choriocarcinoma Be Differentiated from Other Common Types of Germ Cell Tumor?

Choriocarcinoma is easily overlooked as it grows in conjunction with other tumor types often as minute foci and is further obscured by the association with hemorrhage (Fig. 6.12a–e). A key finding in addition to hemorrhage is the large syncytiotrophoblast with indistinct cell borders capping mononucleated cytotrophoblasts. Mononucleated

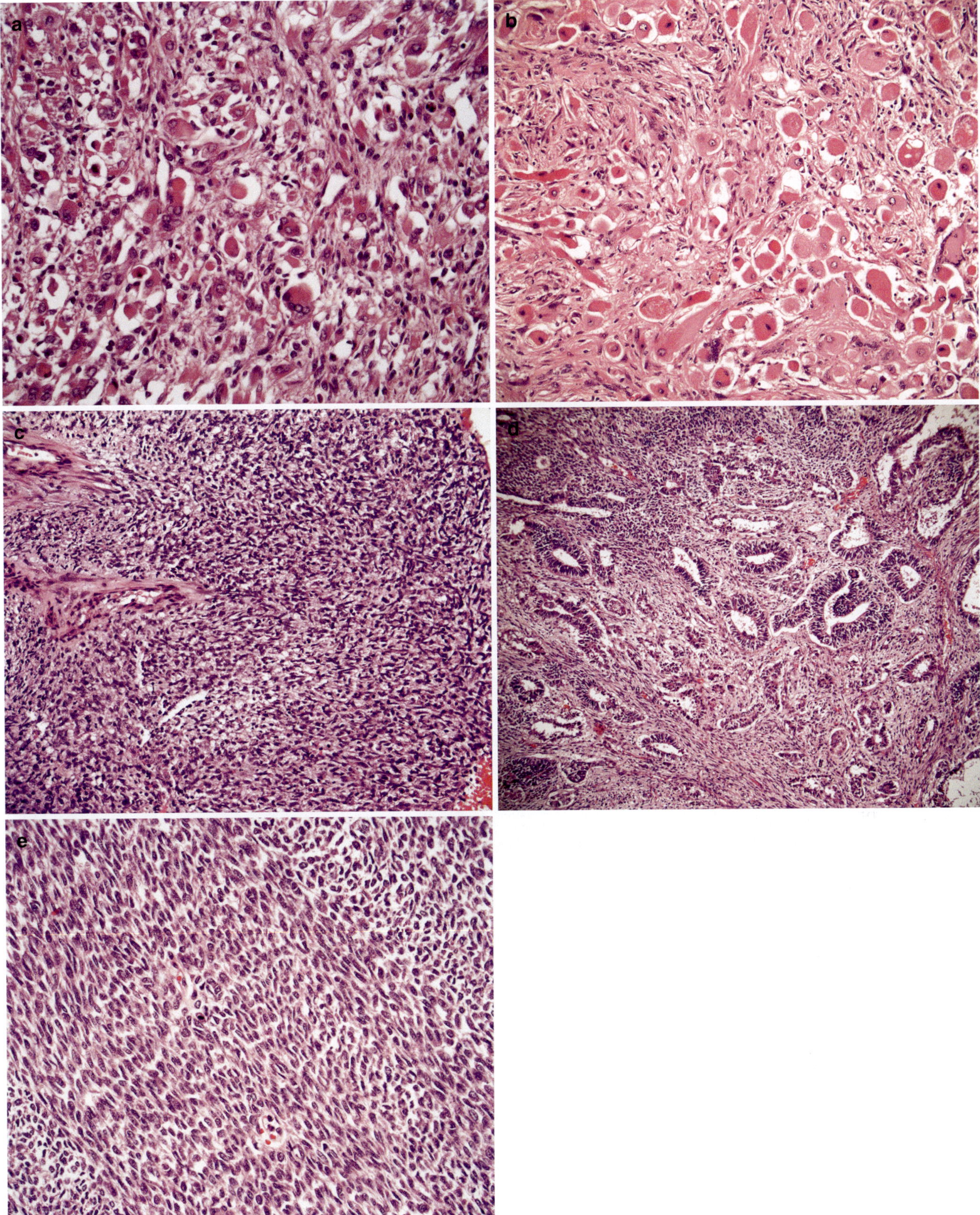

Fig. 6.9 Teratoma with somatic-type malignancy. (**a**) Rhabdomyosarcoma within a testicle. This is the most common somatic-type malignancy. (**b**) Rhabdomyosarcoma in a lung metastasis. Somatic-type malignancy is more frequent in metastases than primary tumors. (**c**) Sarcoma not otherwise specified in a mediastinal metastasis. (**d**) Primitive neuroectodermal tumor within a testicle. Primitive neural elements occupied over 2 cm. (**e**) Spindle cell malignancy with neural differentiation (NGFR positive) in a retroperitoneal metastasis

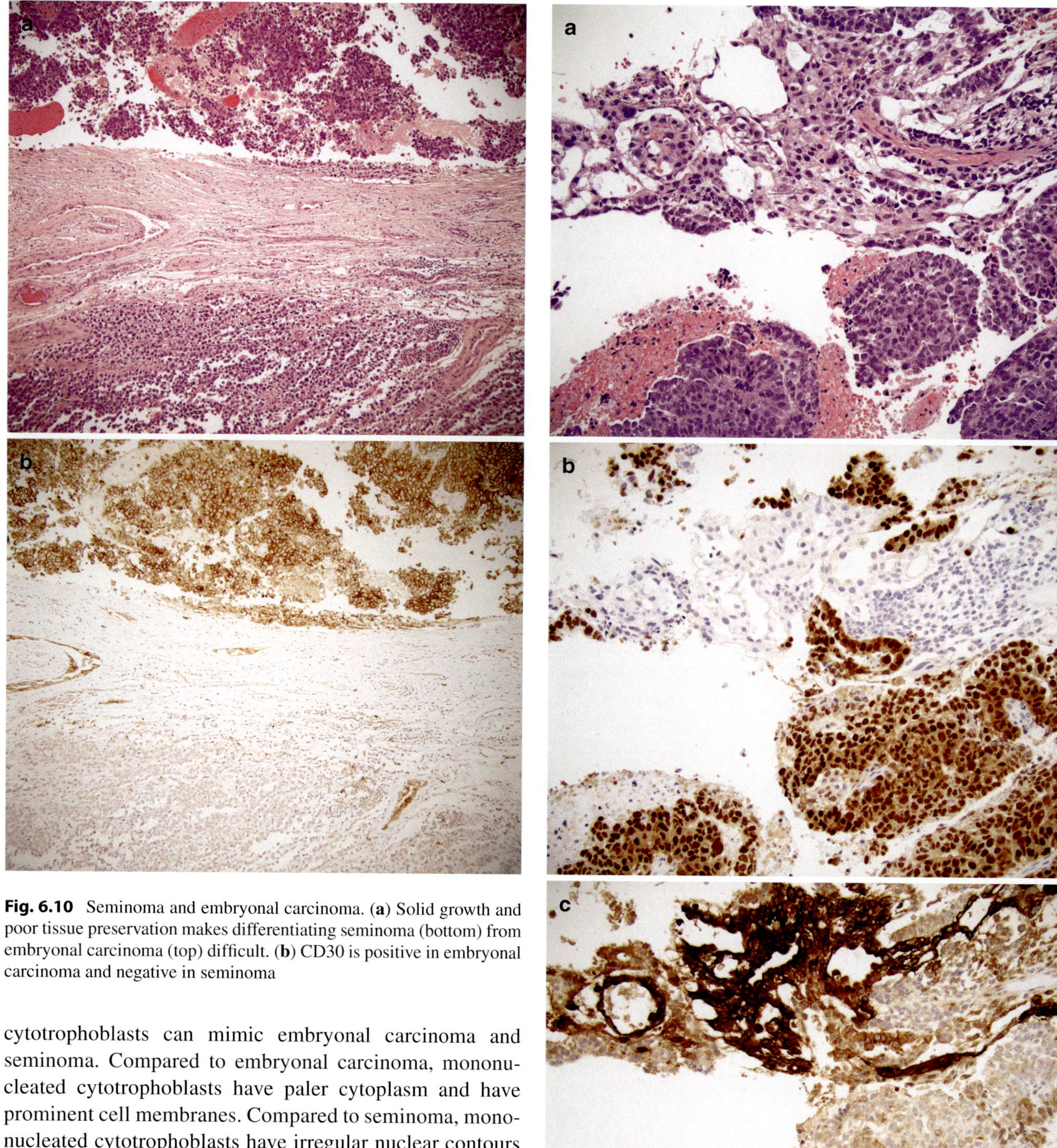

Fig. 6.10 Seminoma and embryonal carcinoma. (**a**) Solid growth and poor tissue preservation makes differentiating seminoma (bottom) from embryonal carcinoma (top) difficult. (**b**) CD30 is positive in embryonal carcinoma and negative in seminoma

cytotrophoblasts can mimic embryonal carcinoma and seminoma. Compared to embryonal carcinoma, mononucleated cytotrophoblasts have paler cytoplasm and have prominent cell membranes. Compared to seminoma, mononucleated cytotrophoblasts have irregular nuclear contours while seminoma nuclear contours are smooth.

Choriocarcinoma expresses GATA3, CK7, HCG, inhibin (syncytiotrophoblasts) and p63 (cytotrophoblasts) while seminoma expresses PLAP, CD117/c-kit, D2-40/podoplanin, and OCT3/4 and embryonal carcinoma has robust reactivity for as OCT3/4 and CD30 (Fig. 6.12a–e).

References: [34, 35]

Fig. 6.11 Embryonal carcinoma and yolk sac tumor. (**a**) In this brain metastasis minute amounts of fragmented tumor make diagnosing the embryonal carcinoma (bottom) and yolk sac tumor (top) difficult. (**b**) OCT3/4 is positive in embryonal carcinoma and negative in yolk sac tumor. (**c**) Glypican 3 is positive yolk sac tumor and weak in embryonal carcinoma

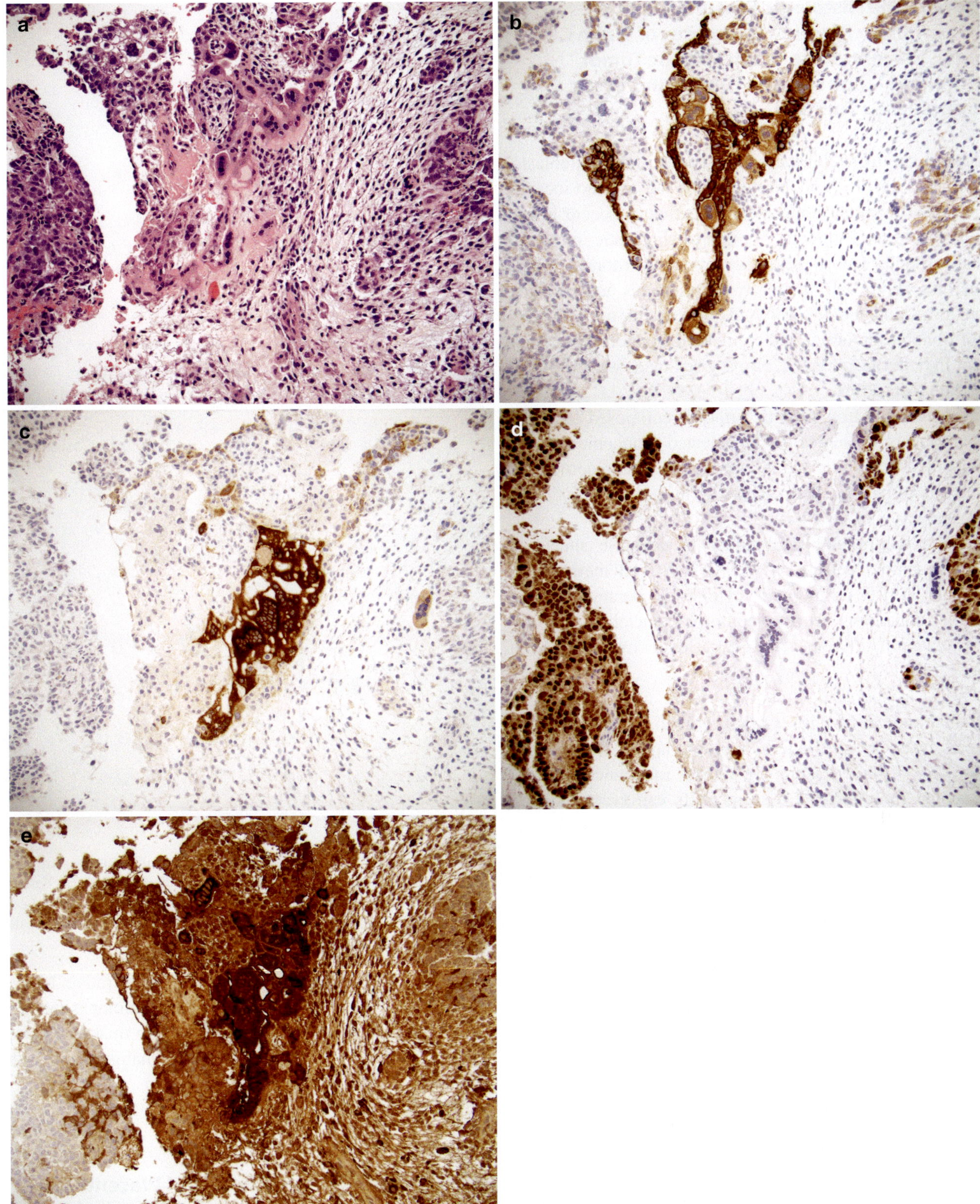

Fig. 6.12 Choriocarcinoma admixed with embryonal carcinoma and teratoma. (**a**) Minute amounts pf choriocarcinoma (center, predominately syncytiotrophoblasts), in a background of teratoma (spindle cells) and embryonal carcinoma (left and far right). (**b**) CK7 os positive in choriocarcinoma and weak to negative in embryonal carcinoma and the spindle cell component of teratoma. (**c**) Inhibin is positive in syncytiotrophoblasts of choriocarcinoma and is negative in embryonal carcinoma and the spindle cell component of teratoma. (**d**) OCT3/4 is positive in embryonal carcinoma and negative in choriocarcinoma and teratoma. (**e**) HCG is positive in choriocarcinoma but due to bleed artifact is a subpar marker

What Are the Histologic Features of Uncommon Placental Subtypes of Germ Cell Tumor, Placental Site Trophoblastic Tumor, Epithelioid Trophoblastic Tumor, and Cystic Trophoblastic Tumor?

Placental site trophoblastic tumor, epithelioid trophoblastic tumor, and cystic trophoblastic tumor are nonchoriocarcinoma gestational trophoblastic tumors that can occur in testicular germ cell tumors. Cystic trophoblastic tumor is usually found in post-chemotherapy retroperitoneal lymph node dissections and has the same prognosis and management as residual tumor composed only of teratoma. Placental site trophoblastic tumor and epithelioid trophoblastic tumor occur in both the untreated, primary setting as well as in distant, late metastases.

Placental site trophoblastic tumor is composed of discohesive sheets of large, mononucleated trophoblasts with abundant eosinophilic cytoplasm, very large pleomorphic nuclei, prominent nucleoli, numerous mitoses, apoptotic figures, and vascular invasion.

Epithelioid trophoblastic tumor of cohesive sheets of large, squamoid cells with well-defined cell membranes, abundant, dense, eosinophilic cytoplasm, intracytoplasmic vacuoles containing debris, pleomorphic nuclei with prominent nucleoli, mitoses, and occasional multinucleation (Fig. 6.13).

Cystic trophoblastic tumor grows in conjunction with teratoma and always has a cystic growth. Large irregular-shaped cysts are lined one to multiple layers of squamoid cells (Fig. 6.14a, b). Cells are mostly mononucleate with occasional multinucleation seen. Cells can be vacuolated with eosinophilic debris in the vacuoles. Nuclei are hyper-

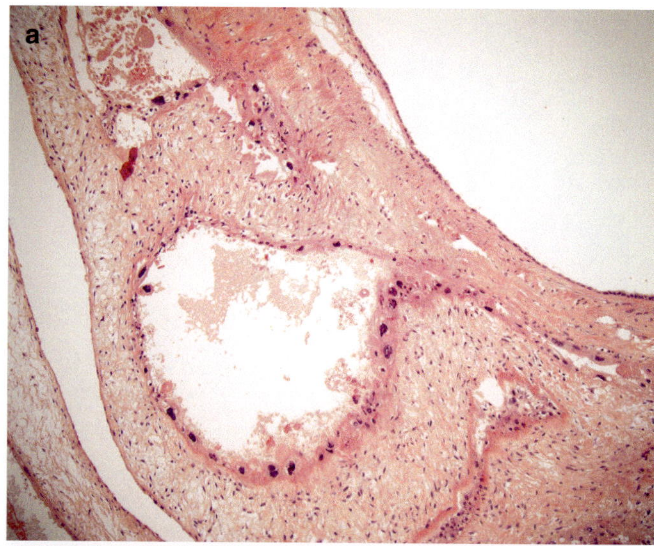

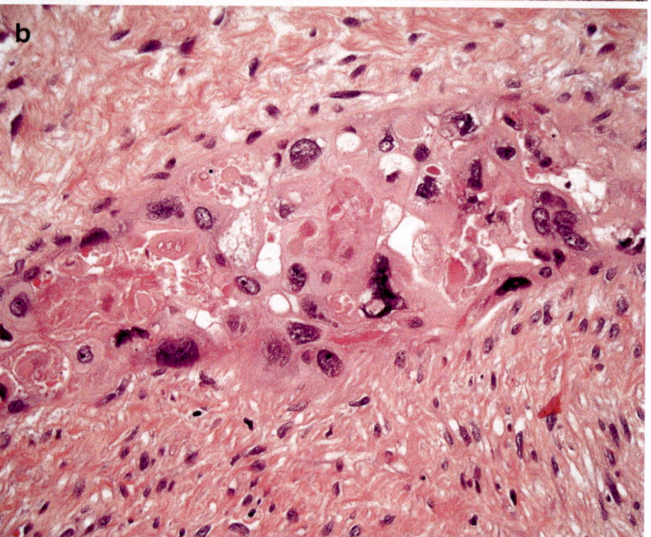

Fig. 6.14 Cystic trophoblastic tumor (postchemotherapy retroperitoneal lymph node mass in which teratoma was also present). (**a**) Variable-sized cysts are present lined by hobnailed to flattened squamoid cells. (**b**) Nuclei are smudgy, degenerative, and occasionally multinucleated

chromic and often appear smudged or degenerative. Mitoses are not identified. As cystic trophoblastic tumor is managed similar to teratoma, it is imperative not to mistaken it for a squamous cell carcinoma somatic malignancy within teratoma.

References: [30, 31, 53–55]

What Is the Expression Profile of Placental Site Trophoblastic Tumor, Epithelioid Trophoblastic Tumor and Cystic Trophoblastic Tumor?

The immunoprofile of testicular nonchoriocarcinoma gestational trophoblastic tumors is not well studied and shows expression overlap.

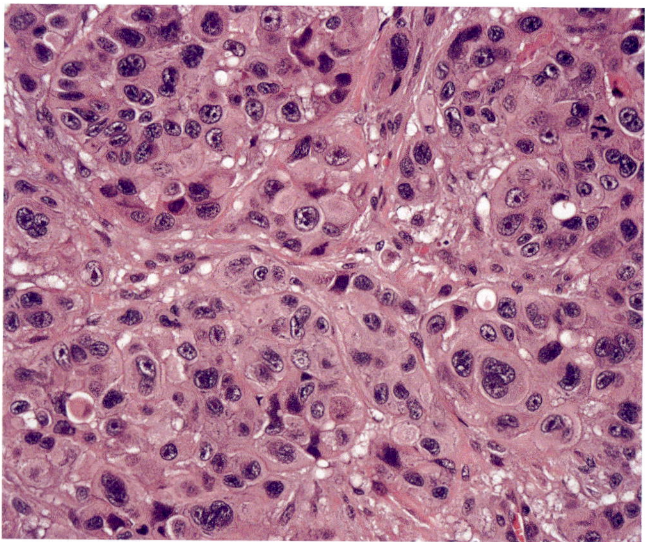

Fig. 6.13 Epithelioid trophoblastic tumor (chest metastasis). Sheets of squamoid cells are seen

Placental site trophoblastic tumor expresses the following:

- Positive: HCG, GATA3, human placental lactogen (HPL).
- Negative: PLAP, p63.

Epithelioid trophoblastic tumor expresses the following:

- Positive: PLAP, CK7, inhibin, GATA3, p63.
- Variable HCG.
- Negative: HPL.

Cystic trophoblastic tumor expresses the following:

- Positive: glypican 3, GATA3, inhibin (focal).
- Variable: HCG, p63.
- Negative: HPL.

References: [30, 47, 53, 54]

What Is a Regressed Germ Cell Tumor and What Are the Characteristic Findings?

Testicular germ cell tumors can present with spontaneous complete or partial regression of the primary tumor. Patients most commonly present with a retroperitoneal metastasis. There is no apparent difference in prognosis between complete and partial regression. Currently, there is no data comparing the prognosis of regressed versus nonregressed testicular germ cell tumors.

Within the testicle, a grossly identifiable scar is seen (Fig. 6.15a). Adjacent to a fibrotic scar with admixed lymphoplasmacytic inflammation, seminiferous tubules are atrophic and have peritubular fibrosis (Fig. 6.15b, c). Half of cases contain GCNIS (Fig. 6.15d). Large coarse calcifications are less common but if an intratubular pattern is seen, this is consistent with tumoral regression. Pure seminoma (40%) is the most common tumor type identified within the testicle in tumors with incomplete regression.

References: [56, 57]

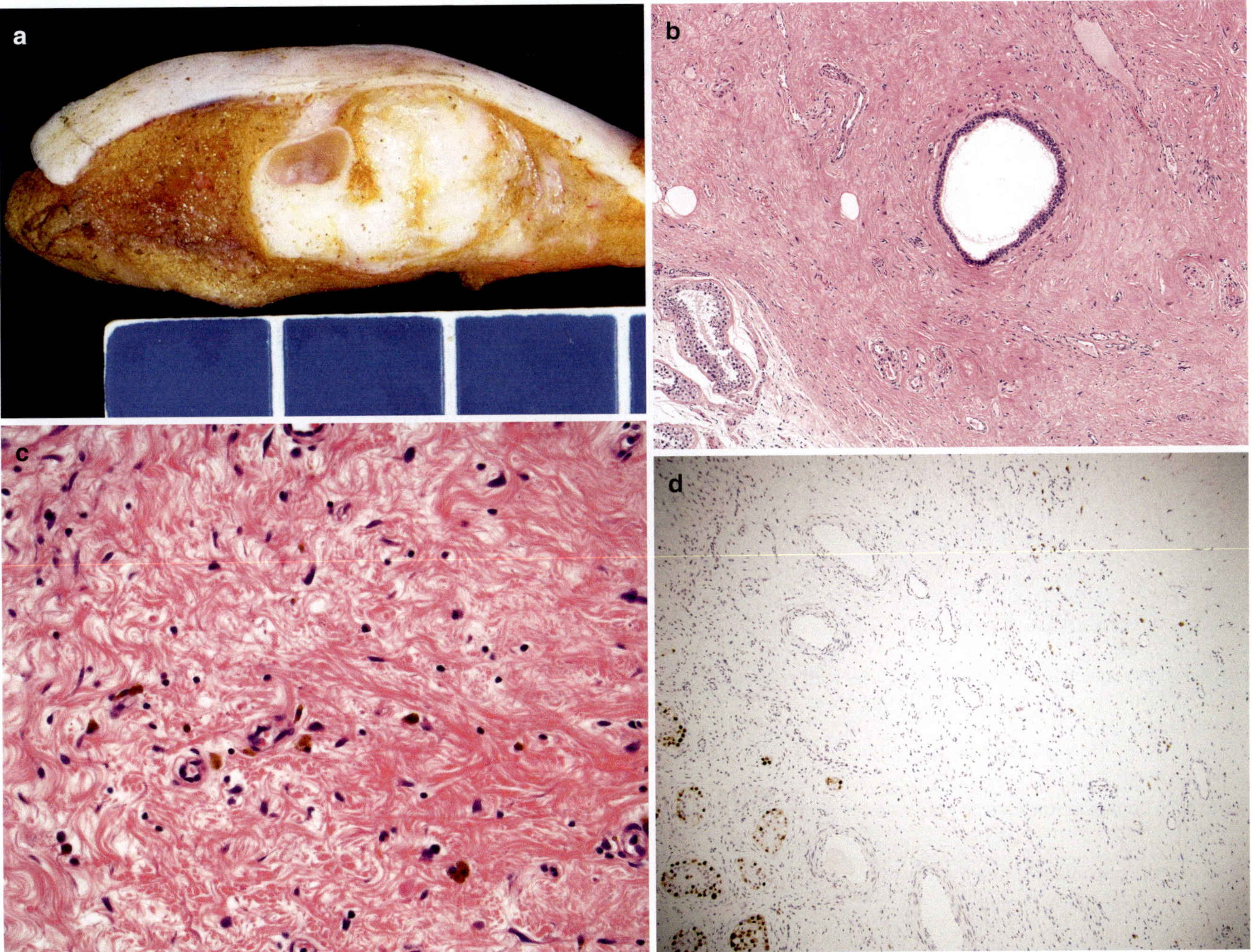

Fig. 6.15 Regressed germ cell tumor with minimal viable teratoma. (**a**) Grossly, a white scar is seen. (**b**) Teratoma (cyst) is seen within a well-demarcated scar. (**c**) Most of the lesion is fibrotic, paucicellular, with hemosiderin, small vessels, and scattered lymphocytes. (**d**) OCT3/4 highlights GCNIS in the tubules adjacent to the scar

What Are Post-chemotherapy Findings of a Germ Cell Tumor and how Is This Different Than a Regressed Germ Cell Tumor?

Chemotherapeutic changes are seen most frequently in retroperitoneal lymph node dissections or in other distant metastases but can be given neoadjuvantly prior to orchiectomy. Pseudocysts filled with necrosis and histiocytic inflammation are the most common findings, which are not seen in regressed tumors (Fig. 6.16). Ghosts of tumor cells can often be seen. Fibrotic scars are not present. Residual teratoma can display an increased degree of atypia and this does not have prognostic significance.

References: [43, 58]

What Are the Most Common Histologic Mimics Misdiagnosed as Testicular Germ Cell Tumors?

The following are critical nongerm cell lesions that mimic germ cell tumors (Table 6.7).

Sertoli cell tumor versus seminoma:

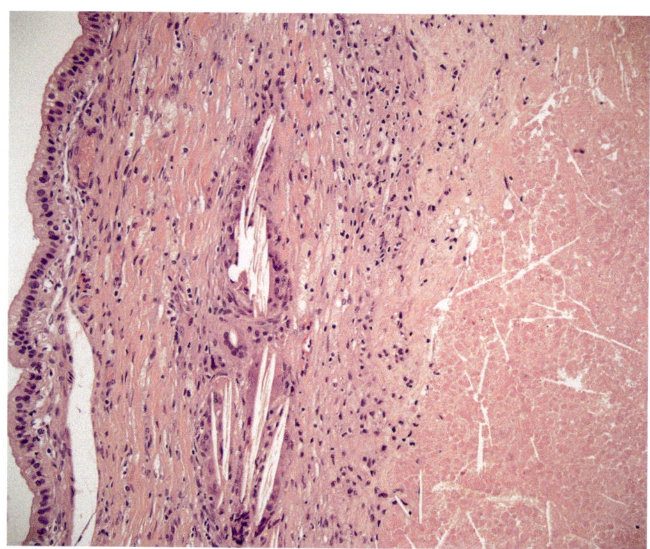

Fig. 6.16 Post-chemotherapy lung metastasis with residual teratoma (far left), histocytes, and necrosis containing ghost cells of nonviable tumor (right)

- Both have sheet-like growth and can have pale cytoplasm.
- The nuclei of Sertoli tumor are blander and mitotic rate is much lower and GCNIS will not be present.
- Sertoli cell tumor is negative for PLAP and OCT 3/4 and is usually positive for inhibin.

Granulomatous orchitis versus seminoma:

- Both can have granulomatous inflammation.
- GCNIS will not be present in granulomatous orchitis.
- OCT3/4 is negative in granulomatous orchitis.

Spermatocytic tumor versus seminoma:

- Both have sheet-like growth.
- Spermatocytic tumor lacks fibrous septae with lymphocytes, lacks GCNIS, have variable cell size, and patients are a mean age of 55, older that seminoma.
- Spermatocytic tumor is negative for PLAP and OCT3/4.

Lymphoma versus embryonal carcinoma or seminoma:

- All can have sheet-like growth of aggressive appearing cells.
- Lymphoma has rounded, more uniform nuclei and more dispersed chromatin and lacks GCNIS. Patients are also typically older.
- Lymphoma is usually positive for CD45 and negative for SALL4 and OCT3/4.

Dermoid cyst versus teratoma:

- Both have squamous cysts.
- Dermoid cysts have adjacent lipogranulomatous reaction and retained spermatogenesis but lack cytologic atypia or GCNIS.

Scar versus regressed germ cell tumor:

- Most importantly, a scar not derived from a regressed germ cell tumor will not have evidence of metastases.
- Additionally, there will not be residual viable tumor identified and GCNIS will be absent.

Table 6.7 Immunohistochemical expression of nonchoriocarcinoma gestational trophoblastic tumors

	PLAP	Glypican 3	CK7	HCG	GATA3	inhibin	p63	HPL
Placental site trophoblastic tumor	−			+	+		−	+
Epithelioid trophoblastic tumor	+		+	Variable	+	+	+	−
Cystic trophoblastic tumor		+		Variable	+	+ (focal)	Variable	−

Table 6.8 Common mimics of testicular germ cell tumors

Nongerm cell tumor mimicked	Germ cell tumor mimicked
Sertoli cell tumor	Seminoma
Granulomatous orchitis	Seminoma
Spermatocytic tumor	Seminoma
Lymphoma	Embryonal carcinoma or seminoma
Dermoid cyst	Teratoma
Carcinoma	Embryonal carcinoma or choriocarcinoma

Carcinoma of nongerm cell origin versus embryonal carcinoma or choriocarcinoma:

- Outside of the testicle, carcinoma is a critical consideration, especially years after treatment of a germ cell tumor.
- Carcinoma will be negative for SALL4, OCT3/4, and HCG and will express site specific markers (Table 6.8).

References: [34, 35, 46]

Which Immunostains Can Help Identify a Testicular Germ Cell Tumor in the Metastatic Setting?

SALL4 has reliable nuclear expression in all germ cell tumor types with the exception of variable reactivity in teratoma (Fig. 6.17a, b). It is thus an ideal marker in the metastatic setting. The inclusion of OCT3/4 adds a marker with strong nuclear expression of seminoma and embryonal carcinoma. Further immunostains can be used based on the histologic impression.

Reference: [59]

Which Florescent In Situ Hybridization (FISH) Test Can Help Identify a Testicular Germ Cell Tumor in the Metastatic Setting?

Testicular germ cell tumor has a high frequency of chromosomal 12p abnormalities including i(12p) and copy number increase of 12p. FISH testing for 12p can identify these aberrations corroborating the diagnosis of a germ cell tumor. Specifically, in the metastatic setting it sometimes difficult to determine if a tumor is a de novo sarcoma or a somatic-type malignancy derived from teratoma. Somatic-type malignancies demonstrated abnormalities for 12p in 78% of cases that were tested.

References: [60, 61]

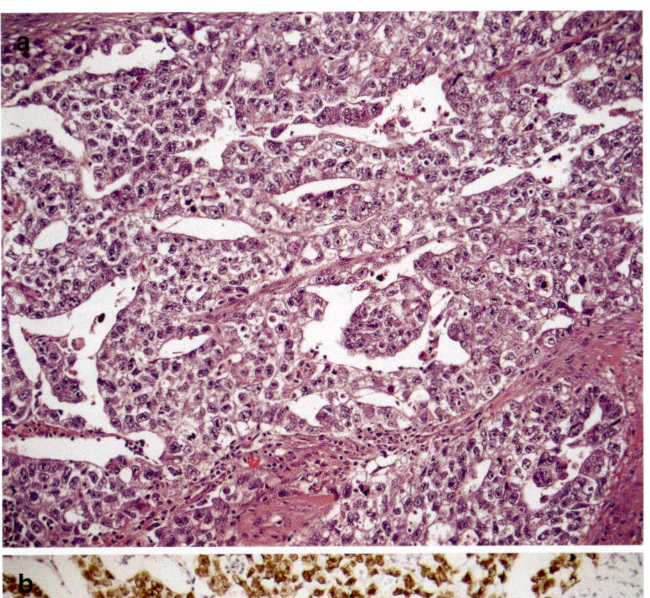

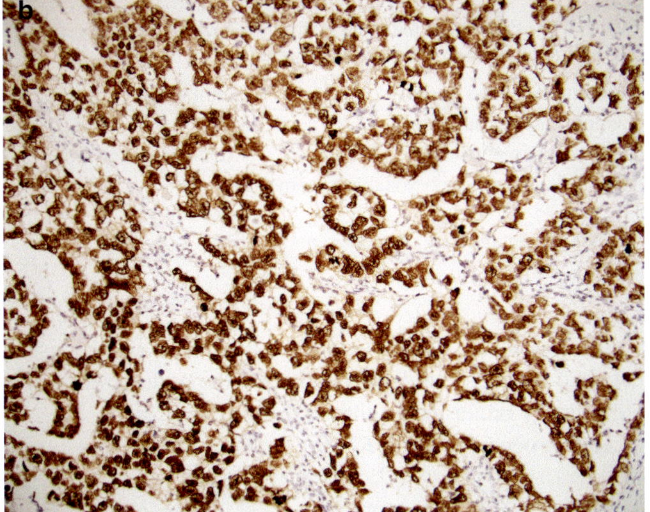

Fig. 6.17 Embryonal carcinoma with SAPPl4 expression. (**a**) Embryonal carcinoma with pseudoglandular spaces. (**b**) SALL4, with strong nuclear expression confirms a germ cell origin of the tumor and can be helpful in the metastatic setting

How Is the PT Classification for Seminoma Different Than a Mixed Germ Cell Tumor?

For tumors confined to the testis and that lack lymphovascular invasion, seminoma has a dichotomized pT1 category based on size (pT1a <3 cm, pT1b ≥3 cm) based on the AJCC Cancer Staging Manual eighth edition, while mixed germ cell tumors are not dichotomized (pT1) (Table 6.9). The rationale for this split is that size is a prognostic parameter of pure seminoma (Table 6.10). Because size is a prognostic parameter, it is imperative that multinodular tumors be measured in largest aggregate single dimension and that this is used for the pT category rather than listing the sizes of indi-

Table 6.9 pT category based on AJCC Cancer Staging Manual 8th edition

Primary tumor (pT)	
pTX	Cannot be assessed
pT0	No evidence of primary tumor
pTis	Germ cell neoplasia in situ
pT1	Germ cell tumor other than pure seminoma confined to testis/tunica albuginea/rete and no lymphovascular invasion
pT1a	Seminoma <3 cm confined to testis/tunica albuginea/rete and no lymphovascular invasion
pT1b	Seminoma ≥3 cm confined to testis/tunica albuginea/rete and no lymphovascular invasion
pT2	Lymphovascular, hilar fat, epididymal or tunica vaginalis invasion
pT3	Direct spermatic cord soft tissue invasion
pT4	Direct scrotum invasion

Table 6.10 Pathologic parameters predictive of aggressive germ cell tumor clinical course on multivariable analysis

Nonseminomatous tumor	Seminoma
Lymphovascular invasion	Size
Hilar soft tissue invasion	Rete testis invasion
Higher percentage embryonal carcinoma	Lymphovascular invasion
Higher percentage/pure choriocarcinoma	Pathologic stage

vidual adjacent nodules. Sectioning intervening tissue between nodules can demonstrate that the nodules are a single primary rather than multiple primary tumors.

References: [2, 7, 13, 62]

What Is the Relevance of Rete Testis Stromal Invasion and Is There Any Clinical Relevance of Pagetoid Extension of Germ Cell Tumor into the Rete Testis?

Rete testis stromal invasion is defined as tumor in the stroma on both sides of a rete testis duct (Fig. 6.18a). This contrasts pagetoid spread of tumor within the confined of the rete testis ducts (Fig. 6.18b).

Within nonseminomatous tumors:

- Rete testis stromal invasion is present in 25% of cases and there have been conflicting results regarding association with metastasis at initial diagnosis and relapse.
- Pagetoid extension is described in 17% of cases but is not associated with higher clinical stage or relapse.

Within pure seminoma tumors:

- Rete testis stromal invasion is seen in 47–58% of cases and pagetoid extension in 19%.

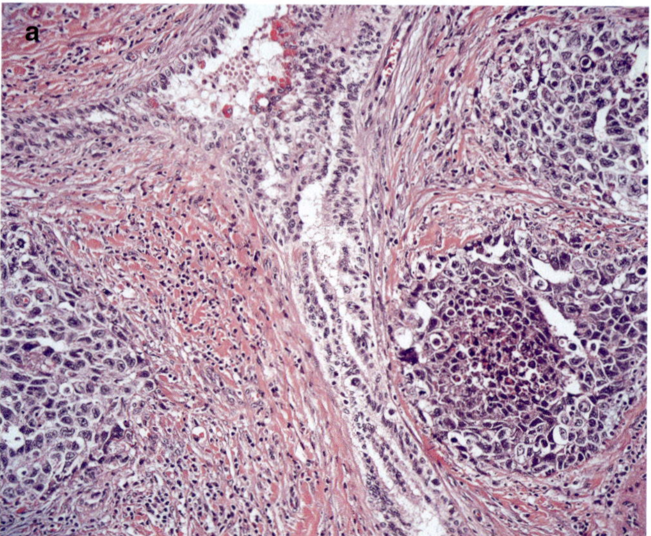
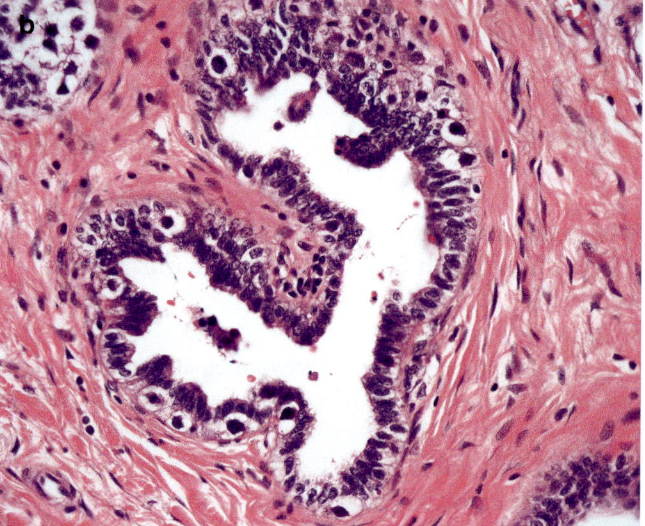

Fig. 6.18 Rete testis involvement. (**a**) Rete testis stromal invasion by embryonal carcinoma. Tumor is on either side of the rete testis duct (center). (**b**) Pagetoid involvement of the rete testis by GCNIS with enlarged atypica cells along the basement membrane of the rete duct. This currently does not need to be reported

- Recent data suggests that neither pattern of rete testis involvement is associated with advanced stage at presentation or of future relapse.
- However, these findings are controversial and a recent study has utilized the presence of rete testis invasion as the sole factor to stratify patients for adjuvant chemotherapy.

Rete testis stromal invasion should be documented in a pathology report while it is optional to report pagetoid extension. Neither impact pT category. If rete testis involvement by pagetoid extension is reported, it is important that the mode of extension be explicitly stated due to the lack of clinical significance.

References: [25, 27, 36, 63–66]

How Does Lymphovascular Invasion Impact PT Category for Germ Cell Tumors?

Testicular germ cell tumors with lymphovascular invasion are categorized as pT2 (Fig. 6.19; Table 6.9).

Within nonseminomatous tumors:

- Lymphovascular invasion is present in 41–43% of cases and is significantly associated with metastasis at initial diagnosis on multivariable analysis (Table 6.10).

Within pure seminoma tumors:

- Lymphovascular invasion is present in 15–18% of cases and was significantly associated metastasis at initial diagnosis in a recent, rigorous analysis. However, older literature has not identified this association.

Lymphovascular invasion should be documented in a pathology report. Lymphovascular invasion is a relative contraindication to surveillance in nonseminomatous tumors and patients are offered adjuvant chemotherapy. Lymphovascular invasion typically does not impact therapy of pure seminoma.

References: [2, 10, 25–27]

Which Histologic Findings Support the Diagnosis of Lymphovascular Invasion Over Pseudoinvasion in Germ Cell Tumor?

The following features of an emboli support a diagnosis of true lymphovascular invasion (Fig. 6.19; Table 6.11):

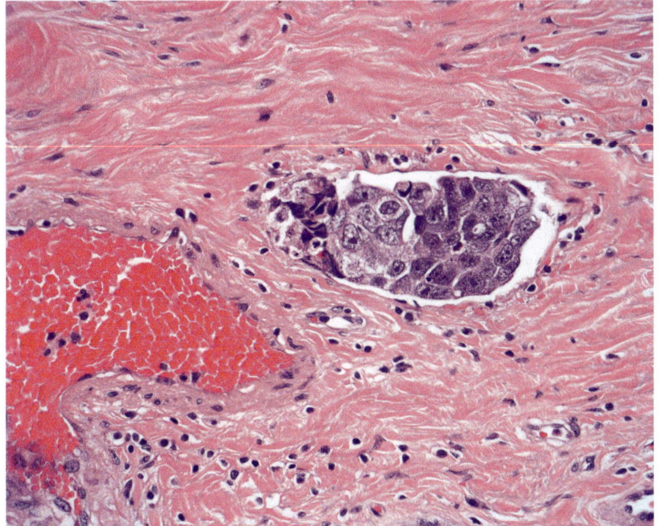

Fig. 6.19 Lymphovascular invasion by embryonal carcinoma. The embolus has characteristics including cohesion, smooth contours and adherence to the vessel wall that support true invasion

Table 6.11 Features to differentiate true lymphovascular invasion from pseudoinvasion

	True lymphovascular invasion	Pseudoinvasion
Cohesion	Yes	No
Smooth contours	Yes	No
Adherence to adjacent vessel wall	Yes	No
Tissue displacement artifact in other areas	No	Yes
Emboli predominately blood, fibrin, or inflammatory cells	No	Yes
Additional sectioning post-fixation lacks emboli	No	Yes

- Tumor cohesiveness.
- Smooth contours.
- Adherence to adjacent vessel wall.

The following are suggestive of pseudoinvasion (Fig. 6.20a, b; Table 6.11):

- Tissue displacement artifact in other areas of the tissue section.
- Discohesive tumor cells admixed with predominately blood, fibrin, and inflammatory cells.
- Additional tissue sectioning post-fixation fails to demonstrate tumor within lymphovascular spaces.

References: [10, 67]

How Can Tissue Carryover Artifact Impact the PT Category for Germ Cell Tumor and How Can This Be Pitfall Be Avoided?

Most notably, tumor displacement artifact occurs during gross prosection in which tumor is smeared on the surface and throughout the tissue sections. Tissue displacement artifact occurs in 60% of seminomas and 38% of nonseminomas. This "butter" artifact can increase discordance in the reporting of lymphovascular invasion (utilized in determining if the tumor is pT2) as it yields pseudolymphovascular tumor deposits. This is especially true for seminomas that are very friable. On secondary review, there is 6–22% discordance in interpretation of lymphovascular invasion, with overcalls more frequent. Overcalling lymphovascular invasion is the most common error identified upon review of referred testicular germ cell tumor cases.

The following are recommendations to decrease tissue displacement artifact (Table 6.12):

- Bivalve the tumor and fix the specimen overnight.

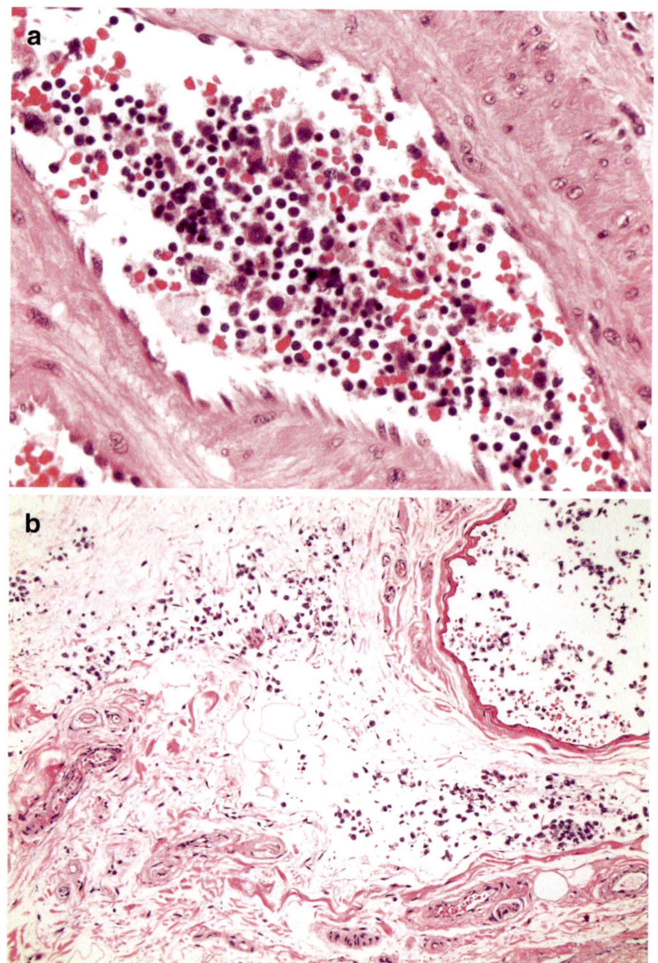

Fig. 6.20 Pseudolymphovascular invasion in seminoma. (**a**) Tumor cells are discohesive and cells within the vessel are predominately red blood cells and inflammatory cells, consistent with pseudoinvasion. (**b**) Tumor cells are scattered in a vessel but tumor displaced throughout the tissue does not support true invasion

Table 6.12 Recommendations to decrease pseudolymphovascular invasion

Gross protocol	Rationale
Bivalve the tumor and fix the specimen overnight	Fresh tumors and even tumors with a few hours of fixation are quite friable
Section the testicle from the tunica albuginea inward	Avoid central tumor displacement into peripheral lymphovascular spaces
Meticulously wipe and wash the knife blade between sectioning the tumor	Avoid tumor smeared on the surface and throughout the tissue sections

- Section the testicle from the tunica albuginea inward, so that tumor is not displaced into the peripheral lymphovascular spaces.
- Meticulously wipe and wash the knife blade between sectioning the tumor.

References: [10, 34, 65, 68]

What Is the PT Category of Lymphovascular Invasion of the Spermatic Cord? Is Lymphovascular Invasion in the Spermatic Cord Shave Margin Considered a Positive Margin?

Lymphovascular invasion of the spermatic cord is classified as pT2 as is lymphovascular invasion within the testicle (Table 6.9). However, nonseminomatous tumors with lymphovascular invasion of the spermatic cord may have a more aggressive disease course. Lymphovascular invasion in the spermatic cord shave margin is not considered a positive margin.

References: [67–71]

What Is the Significance of Tumor in the Tunica Albuginea Versus Tunica Vaginalis for Germ Cell Tumors?

Tumor in the tunica albuginea has no impact on pT classification while tumor involving the tunica vaginalis is classified as pT2 (Fig. 6.21a; Table 6.9). Tunica vaginalis invasion is extremely rare (Fig. 6.21b). Out of 148 nonseminomatous tumors, none invaded the tunica vaginalis and only 2% of seminomas had tunica vaginalis invasion.

References: [25, 27, 62]

Does Epididymal Invasion Impact PT Category for Germ Cell Tumor?

Epididymal invasion is classified as pT2 (Fig. 6.22; (Table 6.9). It is uncommon (8% of nonseminomatous tumor, 6% of seminoma). Epididymal invasion is not a predictor of higher clinical stage using multivariable analysis in either nonseminoma or seminoma.

References: [25, 27, 62]

How Is Hilar Soft Tissue Invasion Diagnosed Versus Direct Spermatic Cord Invasion and How Does It Impact the PT Category of Germ Cell Tumor?

Hilar soft tissue is defined as the stroma below the level of the epididymal head. Invasion of this stroma is classified as pT2 (Fig. 6.23; Table 6.9). Direct invasion of the soft tissue above the level of the epididymal head is considered spermatic cord invasion and is classified as pT3.

Within nonseminomatous tumors:

- Hilar soft tissue is present in 28% of cases and is significantly associated with metastasis at initial diagnosis on multivariable analysis (Table 6.10).

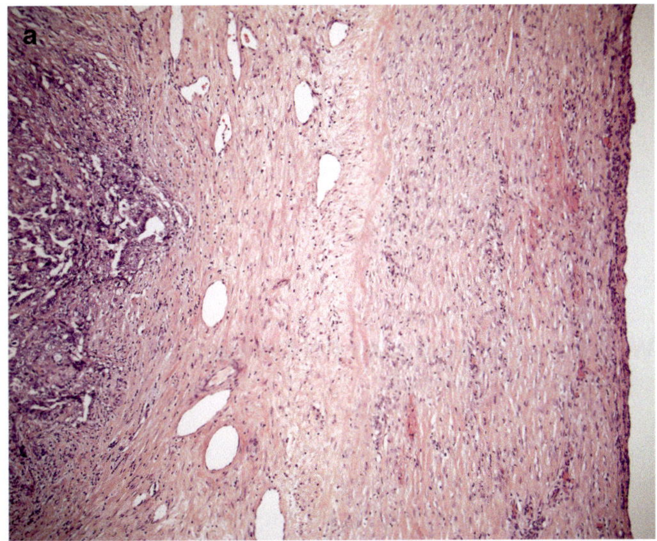

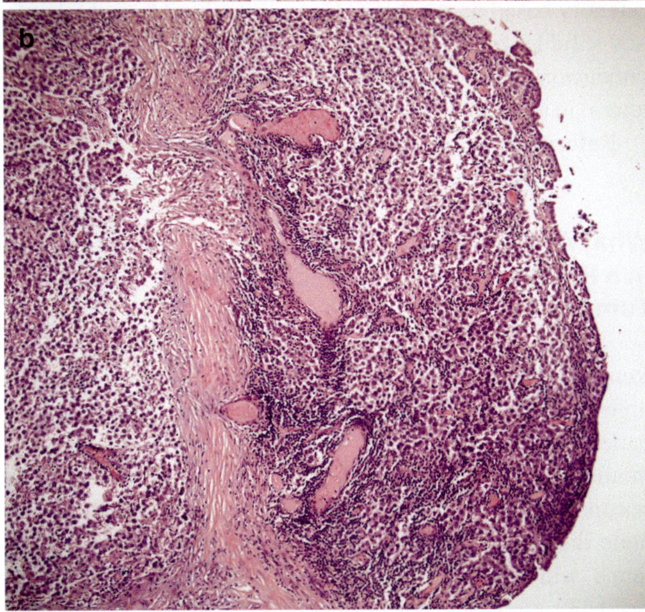

Fig. 6.21 Involvement of tunica. (**a**) The fibrous tunica albuginea is involved by embryonal carcinoma but the tunica vaginalis (flat lining far right) is not involved. This has no impact to pT category. (**b**) The tunica vaginalis (right) is eroded and ruptured by underlying seminoma. This is categorized as pT2

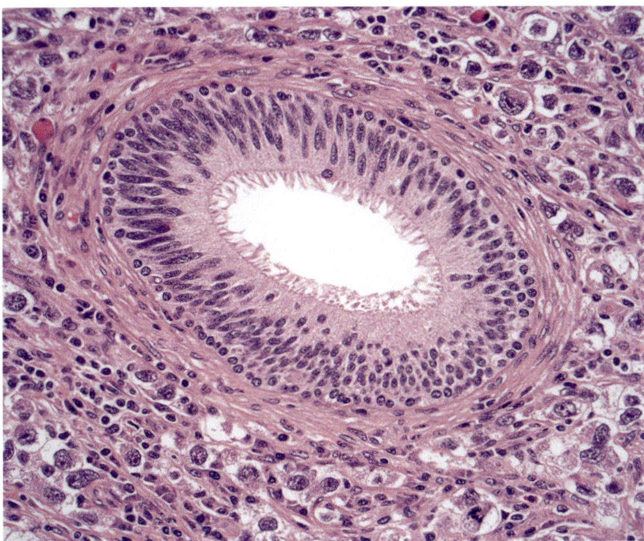

Fig. 6.22 Epididymal invasion. Seminoma surround a duct of the epididymis (center). This is categorized as pT2

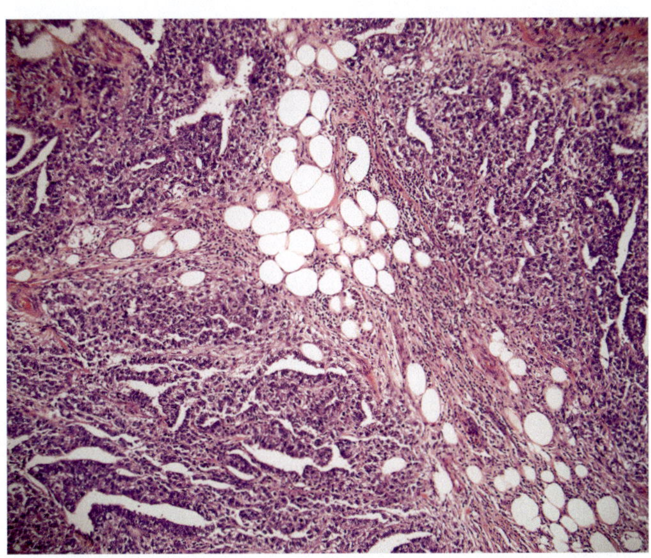

Fig. 6.23 Direct hilar soft tissue invasion by embryonal carcinoma. Below the level of the epididymal head as was present in this case is categorized as pT2 while above the epididymal head is pT3

- Direct spermatic cord invasion is present in 8% of cases and is not significantly associated with metastasis at initial diagnosis on multivariable analysis.

  Within pure seminoma tumors:

- Hilar soft tissue is present in 19–22% of cases and is not significantly associated with metastasis at initial diagnosis on multivariable analysis.
- Direct spermatic cord invasion is present in 3% of cases and is not significantly associated with metastasis at initial diagnosis on multivariable analysis.

References: [25–27, 62, 69]

How Is Discontinuous Spermatic Cord Invasion Categorized for Germ Cell Tumor?

Discontinuous invasion of the spermatic cord arises through extension from lymphovascular spaces and is classified as pM1 rather than pT3 (Fig. 6.24a, b). This method of involvement of the spermatic cord is less common than direct invasion. Of tumors with spermatic cord invasion, 81% are via direct extension, 19% are due to discontinuous invasion from lymphovascular spaces, and 4% have both patterns. A non-statistically significant trend has been demonstrated for a more aggressive course for spermatic cord involvement (pM1) compared to direct invasion (pT3).

References: [62, 67, 69]

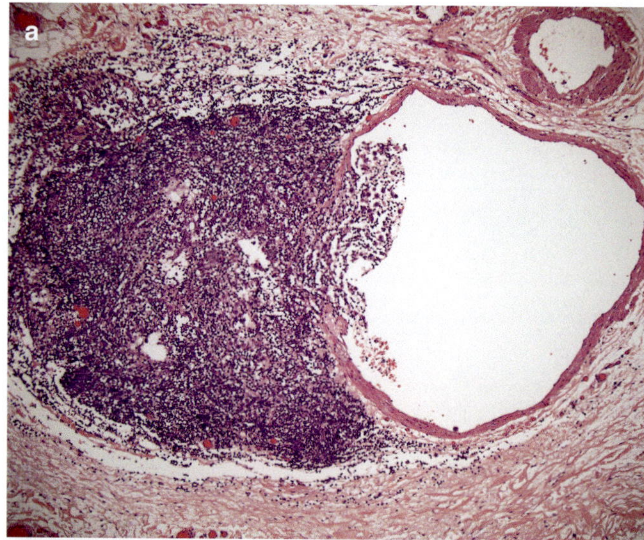

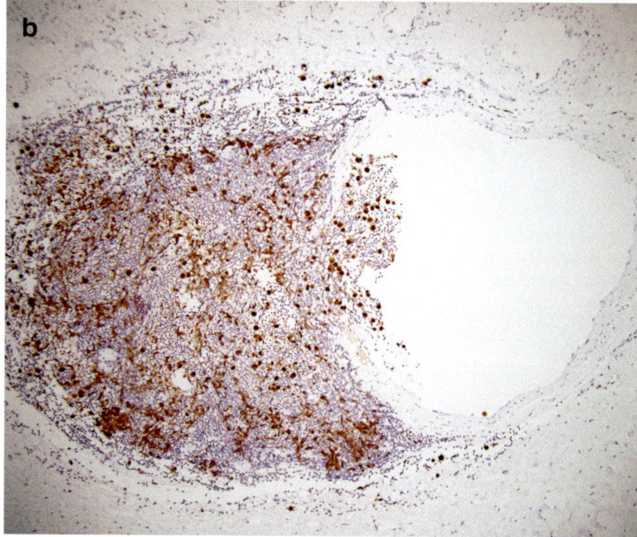

Fig. 6.24 Discontinuous invasion of the spermatic cord (pM1). (**a**) Seminoma is seen dispersed within lymphocytes in the spermatic cord soft tissue and within a ruptured vessel. (**b**) OCT3/4 highlights the tumor cells

Which Lymph Nodes Are Considered Regional for Germ Cell Tumor? How Does Prior Testicular Surgery Impact the Definition of Regional Lymph Nodes?

Regional lymph nodes that impact the pN category include interaortocaval, para/periaortic, paracaval, preaortic, precaval, retroaortic, and retrocaval nodes. Prior inguinal or scrotal surgery disrupts the lymphatic drainage after which intrapelvic and inguinal nodes are considered regional.

Reference: [62]

Table 6.13 pN category based on AJCC Cancer Staging Manual 8th edition

pNX	Cannot be assessed
pN0	No regional lymph node metastasis
pN1	1–5 involved nodes with node size ≤2 cm
pN2	>5 involved nodes OR extranodal extension OR involved nodes >2 cm and ≤5 cm
pN3	Lymph node mass >5 cm

Which Variables Impact PN Categorization of Germ Cell Tumor?

Number of involved lymph nodes, size of involved lymph node (rather than size of metastatic tumor deposit), and presence of extranodal extension are factors that impact the pN category based on the AJCC Cancer Staging Manual 8th edition (Table 6.13). As such, documenting the maximum dimension of a lymph node suspected to be involved by tumor, in addition to the size of metastatic deposit is required.

Reference: [62]

What Are the Likely Findings in a Retroperitoneal Dissection for Germ Cell Tumor?

Retroperitoneal lymph node dissection can be performed in high-risk nonseminoma in absence of imaging findings for patients that do not want or are not eligible for adjuvant chemotherapy. In nonseminoma with imaging consistent with retroperitoneal node involvement, retroperitoneal lymph node dissection is performed after chemotherapy. In seminoma with prior retroperitoneal lymph node disease and residual tumor detected postchemotherapy, a resection may be indicated. Therefore, a variety of pathologic findings should be anticipated in a retroperitoneal dissection ranging from all negative nodes to residual post-chemotherapy tumor.

The most frequent findings in a post-chemotherapy retroperitoneal lymph node dissection are necrosis and histocytic inflammation, indicative of pathologic response by the tumor to the chemotherapy. Teratoma is the most common residual germ cell tumor type. The most frequent tumor type in a retroperitoneal lymph node dissection without treatment is embryonal carcinoma, likely reflecting the higher risk nature of patients selected for this procedure.

It is critical for the pathologist to report the presence of viable germ cell tumor and their components in a retroperitoneal lymph node dissection or other sites of metastasis. In general, the presence of residual teratoma and cystic trophoblastic tumor does not warrant the use of additional chemotherapy while the presence of other tumor types does.

References: [2, 58, 72, 73]

What Are the PM Subcategories for Germ Cell Tumor?

Per the AJCC Cancer Staging Manual 8th edition, nonregional lymph node (e.g., iliac, inguinal, pelvic NOS) or lung metastasis are categorized as pM1a while pM1b consists of all distant metastatic sites other than lymph node/lungs, including discontinuous invasion of the spermatic cord (Table 6.14).

Reference: [62]

What Are the Unique Features of Spermatocytic Tumor?

- Spermatocytic tumor, previously named spermatocytic seminoma (not recommended in the current WHO classification), is a rare tumor accounting for about 1% of all testicular germ cell tumors (GCT).
- It is seen only in the testis and not associated with cryptorchism.
- Patients have a mean age of 55 years, much older than those of other GCTs.
- It is always pure and not associated with other GCT components.
- It shows the hallmark tripartite feature with 3 distinct cell groups (Fig. 6.25a):
  - Small cells with round dark nuclei and scant cytoplasm.
  - Intermediate cells with finely granular to filamentous (or spireme) chromatin and eosinophilic cytoplasm.
  - Multinuclear giant cells with similar nuclear features to the intermediate cells.
- It has frequent mitotic figures and apoptotic bodies but no necrosis.

Table 6.14 pM category based on AJCC Cancer Staging Manual 8th edition

pM1a	Non-regional lymph node (e.g., iliac, inguinal, pelvic NOS) or lung metastasis
pM1b	Distant metastasis (includes discontinuous spermatic cord, not lymph node/lungs)

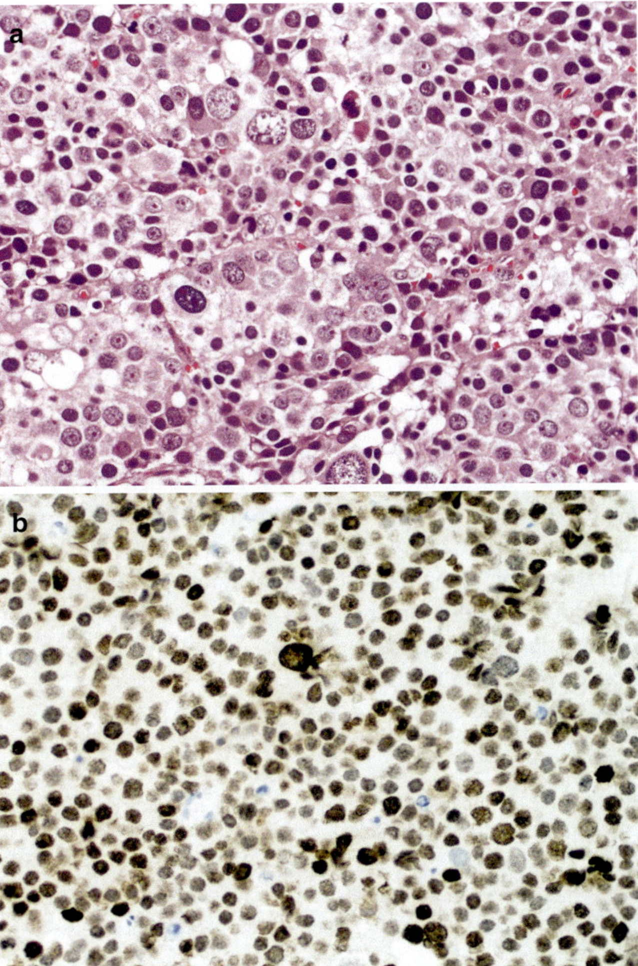

Fig. 6.25 Spermatocytic tumor. (**a**) Tumor is composed of three distinct cell types, large, intermediate, and small cells. (**b**) Tumor cells are positive for SALL4

- Lymphocytic infiltrates and granulomatous inflammation are generally absent.
- It is not associated with GCNIS.
- It shows frequent gains of chromosome 9 but lacks of isochromosome 12p.
- It is generally positive for SALL4 (Fig. 6.25b) and KIT but negative for OCT3/4, PLAP, AFP, and CD30.
- It may develop sarcomatous components sometimes, such as rhabdomyosarcoma and pleomorphic sarcoma.
- It generally has a benign clinical course, unless complicated by sarcoma.

References: [74–76]

How Is Sex Cord-Stromal Tumor Differentiated from Germ Cell Tumor?

See Table 6.15 for the differences between sex cord-stromal tumor and germ cell tumor.

References: [29, 31, 68, 77–79]

How Is a Sex Cord-Stromal Tumor Worked Up?

Sex cord-stromal tumors (SCSTs) demonstrate a number of distinct morphologies (Table 6.16). Over 90% of SCSTs are pure, but a small subset may contain more than one SCST component or even a GCT component, such as in gonadoblastoma. Among the pure SCSTs, Leydig cell tumors are the most common, followed by Sertoli cell tumors and granulosa cell tumors. In well-differentiated SCSTs, the tumor cells usually resemble the non-neoplastic Leydig cells, Sertoli cells, and stromal cells to various degrees. In poorly differentiated tumors, the resemblance is generally lost but may be present in focal areas.

Table 6.15 Comparison of clinicopathologic features between sex cord-stromal tumors and germ cell tumors

	Sex cord-stromal tumor	Germ cell tumors
Incidence	4% in adults and 25% in children	>90% in adults
Patient's age	A wide range from children to elderly	Young patients with a mean of 30 years
Common types	Leydig cell tumor	Seminoma
	Sertoli cell tumor	Embryonal carcinoma
	Granulosa cell tumor	Yolk sac tumor
		Teratoma
Growth pattern	Relatively uniform	Often heterogeneous
Cytologic atypia	Mild to moderate	Severe
Mitotic activity	Low	High
Necrosis	Uncommon	Common
Lymphovascular invasion	Uncommon	Common
Hemorrhage	Uncommon	Common
GCNIS	Absence	Often present
Iso12p	Absence	Often present
Elevated serum markers (LDH, AFP, βHCG)	Uncommon	Common
Positive IHC markers	SF1, inhibin, calretinin	Sall4, OCT3/4, and PLAP
Negative IHC markers	OCT3/4, Sall4, and PLAP	SF1, inhibin, calretinin
Metastasis	Uncommon	Common
Clinical course	5% are malignant	Most are malignant

Table 6.16 Classification of sex cord-stromal tumors of the testis

Pure tumors
Leydig cell tumor
Malignant Leydig cell tumor
Sertoli cell tumor
Malignant Sertoli cell tumor
Large cell calcifying Sertoli cell tumor
Intratubular large cell hyalinizing Sertoli cell neoplasia
Granulosa cell tumor
Juvenile-type granulosa cell tumor
Adult-type granulosa cell tumor
Tumors of fibroma/thecoma group
Thecoma
Fibroma
Mixed and unclassified tumors
Mixed sex cord-gonadal stromal tumor
Unclassified sex cord-gonadal stromal tumor
Tumor containing both germ cell and sex cord-stromal elements
Gonadoblastoma

Immunohistochemistry is an important tool in the diagnosis of SCST. Several markers, including α-inhibin, calretinin, WT-1, and Melan-A, are commonly expressed in SCSTs but not expressed in GCTs. Steroidogenic factor 1 (SF-1) is an emerging marker for SCST with a robust nuclear staining pattern. In contrast, GCT markers, such as SALL4, OCT3/4, and PLAP, are generally not expressed in SCSTs.

The main differential diagnosis of SCST is GCT in the testis (Table 6.15). Several other entities, such as metastatic carcinoma and lymphoma, also need to be distinguished from SCSTs. Metastatic carcinomas are usually seen in old patients with a clinical history of nontesticular malignancy. Metastasis typically shows intestinal growth pattern in the testis with wide-spread lymphovascular invasion. Tumor cells show greater cytologic atypia and pleomorphism than SCST. They are negative for SCST markers and positive for other tissue-specific markers. Lymphoma shows both diffuse and interstitial growth patterns. The lymphoma cells are negative for SCST markers and positive for LCA and other B-cell or T-cell markers (Table 6.16).

References: [29, 34, 77, 79]

What Are the Testicular Tumors with Both Germ Cell and Sex Cord-Stromal Elements?

- The majority of testicular tumors with mixed GCT and SCST are gonadoblastoma.
  - It is usually diagnosed in the neonates because of gonadal dysgenesis.
  - About 40% of cases are bilateral.
  - It is characterized by discrete round nests of germ cells and sex cord cells mixed with eosinophilic basement membrane material (Fig. 6.26a).

The germ cells usually resemble GCNIS and semi-noma cells.

The sex cord cells simulate the Sertoli cells of the fetal testis, with angulated nuclei and little cytoplasm.

The basement membrane materials form round deposits and often develop calcified psammomatous bodies, which may coalesce to form mulberry-like aggregates (Fig. 6.26b).

Occasionally the cellular elements regress, leaving only the calcifications, diagnostic of a regressed (so-called burnt out) gonadoblastoma.

- The germ cells are positive for SALL4, OCT3/4, C-KIT, and PLAP; the sex cord cells are positive for SF1, inhibin, calretinin, and WT1.
- At the time of diagnosis, about half of cases have developed invasive seminoma and 8% to other non-seminomatous GCTs.

- The usual treatment is bilateral orchiectomy.
- Rare cases of testicular tumors with mixed GCT and SCST are unclassified type.
  - It shows large, infiltrating nodules of germ cells and sex cord stroma cells.
  - It is a benign tumor.
  - Orchiectomy is standard therapy.

References: [80–82]

How Is Sertoli Cell Nodule Differentiated from Sertoli Cell Tumor?

See Table 6.17 for the differences between Sertoli cell nodule and Sertoli cell tumor (Figs. 6.27 and 6.28).

References: [80, 83, 84]

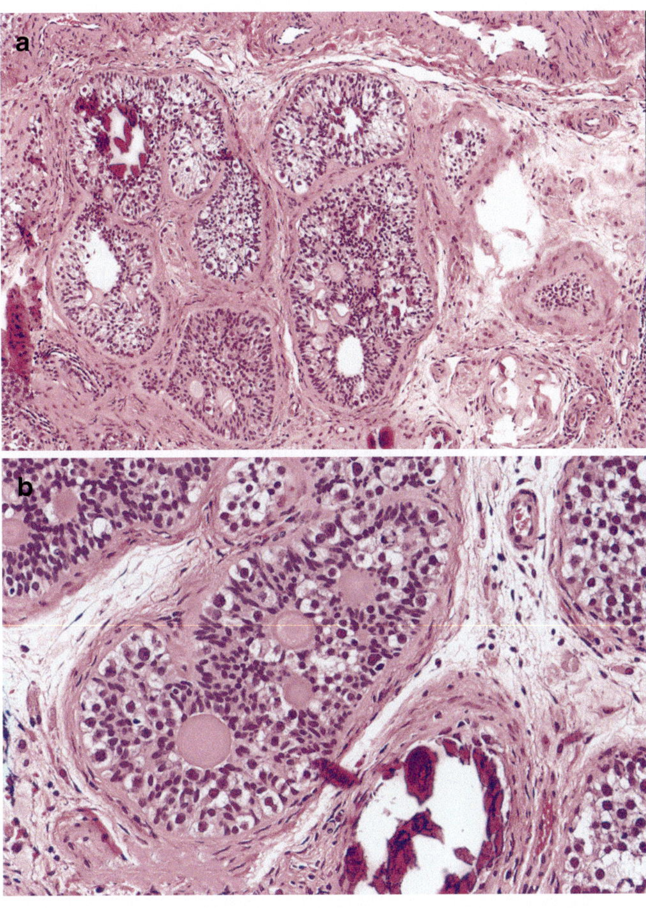

Fig. 6.26 Gonadoblastoma. (a) Tumor shows enlarged seminiferous tubules with round deposits of dense basement membrane materials and calcification. (b) The germ cells resemble GCNIS or seminoma cells, and the sex cord cells simulate the fetal Sertoli cells with angulated nuclei and scant cytoplasm, forming follicular and Call-Exner-like patterns

Table 6.17 Comparison of clinicopathologic features between Sertoli cell nodule and Sertoli cell tumor

	Sertoli cell nodule	Sertoli cell tumor
Pathology	Usually cannot be identified on gross. Sometimes may appear as small white nodules (<1 cm) Small clusters of immature tubules that often contain hyaline luminal deposits with microcalcification (Fig. 6.27a) Immature Sertoli cells lack cytologic atypia or lipid-vacuoles in cytoplasm (Fig. 6.27b). No bands of dense collagen Spermatogonia could be interspersed in some immature tubules, mimicking GCNIS and even gonadoblastoma	Usually well-circumscribed, tan-white mass (2–5 cm). Cystic changes may be present in 1/3 of cases Typically a nodular growth of tubules in scant stroma (Fig. 6.28a) Tubules may be round or elongated. Lumens may not be apparent (Fig. 6.28b) Sometimes a diffuse growth pattern with nests, cords, and clusters separated by dense collagens (Fig. 6.28c) Tumor cells have pale to eosinophilic cytoplasm that may contain lipid vacuoles (Fig. 6.28d) Cytologic atypia is usually minimal and mitotic activity is low
Clinical features	Can occur in any age Usually an incidental finding associated with testicular tumors or cryptorchidism Non-neoplastic lesion Does not need additional treatment	Usually occur in adults Asymptomatic testicular swelling with no endocrine symptoms. Most are benign, but 5% are malignant. Treated with radical orchiectomy

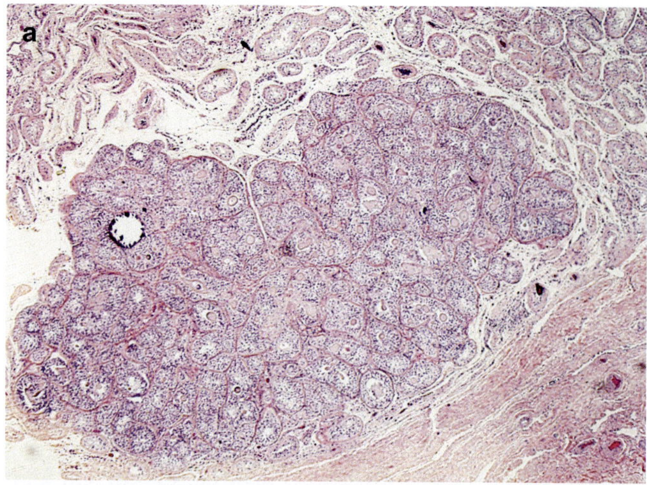

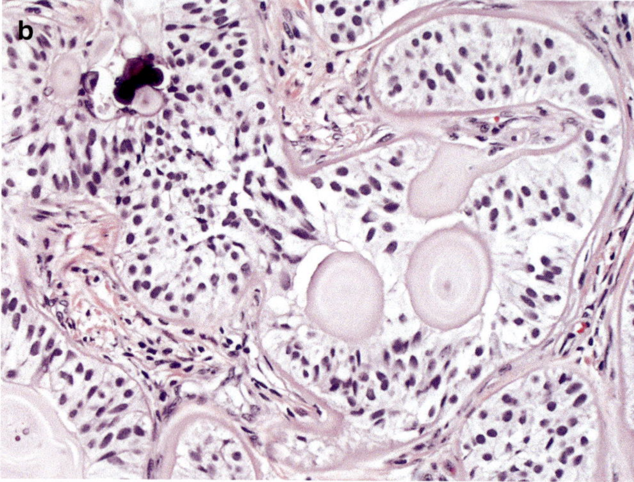

Fig. 6.27 Sertoli cell nodule. (**a**) A small nodular tumor is composed of immature tubules with focal calcification. (**b**) The tubules are lined immature Sertoli cells with minimal atypia and contain hyaline luminal deposits

What Are the Morphologic Features Are Associated with Malignancy in Sertoli Cell Tumor?

A small subset of Sertoli cell tumors (5%) are malignant and typically show two or more of the following morphologic features:

- Large size (>5 cm in largest dimension)
- Tumor necrosis
- Infiltrative border (Fig. 6.29a, b)
- Moderate-to-severe cytological atypia (Fig. 6.29c)
- Active proliferation (more than 5 mitotic figures per 10 high-power fields)
- Lymphovascular invasion (Fig. 6.29d)

If a tumor exhibits only one of the above features, it may be classified as a Sertoli cell tumor with uncertain malignant potential. Even in the absence of all these features, benign Sertoli cell tumor should not be used, as those tumors may still metastasize, although the risk is very low.

References: [85–87]

How Is Large Cell Calcifying Sertoli Cell Tumor Differentiated from Sertoli Cell Tumor, NOS?

See Table 6.18 for the differences between large cell calcifying Sertoli cell tumor and Sertoli cell tumor, NOS (Figs. 6.28 and 6.30).

References: [84, 87–90]

How Is Large Cell Calcifying Sertoli Cell Tumor Differentiated from Intratubular Large Cell Hyalinizing Sertoli Cell Neoplasia?

See Table 6.19 for the differences between large cell calcifying Sertoli cell tumor and intratubular large cell hyalinizing Sertoli cell neoplasia (Figs. 6.30 and 6.31).

References: [87, 88, 91, 92]

How Is Leydig Cell Hyperplasia Differentiated from Leydig Cell Tumor?

See Table 6.20 for the differences between Leydig cell hyperplasia and Leydig cell tumor (Figs. 6.32 and 6.33).

References: [93–95]

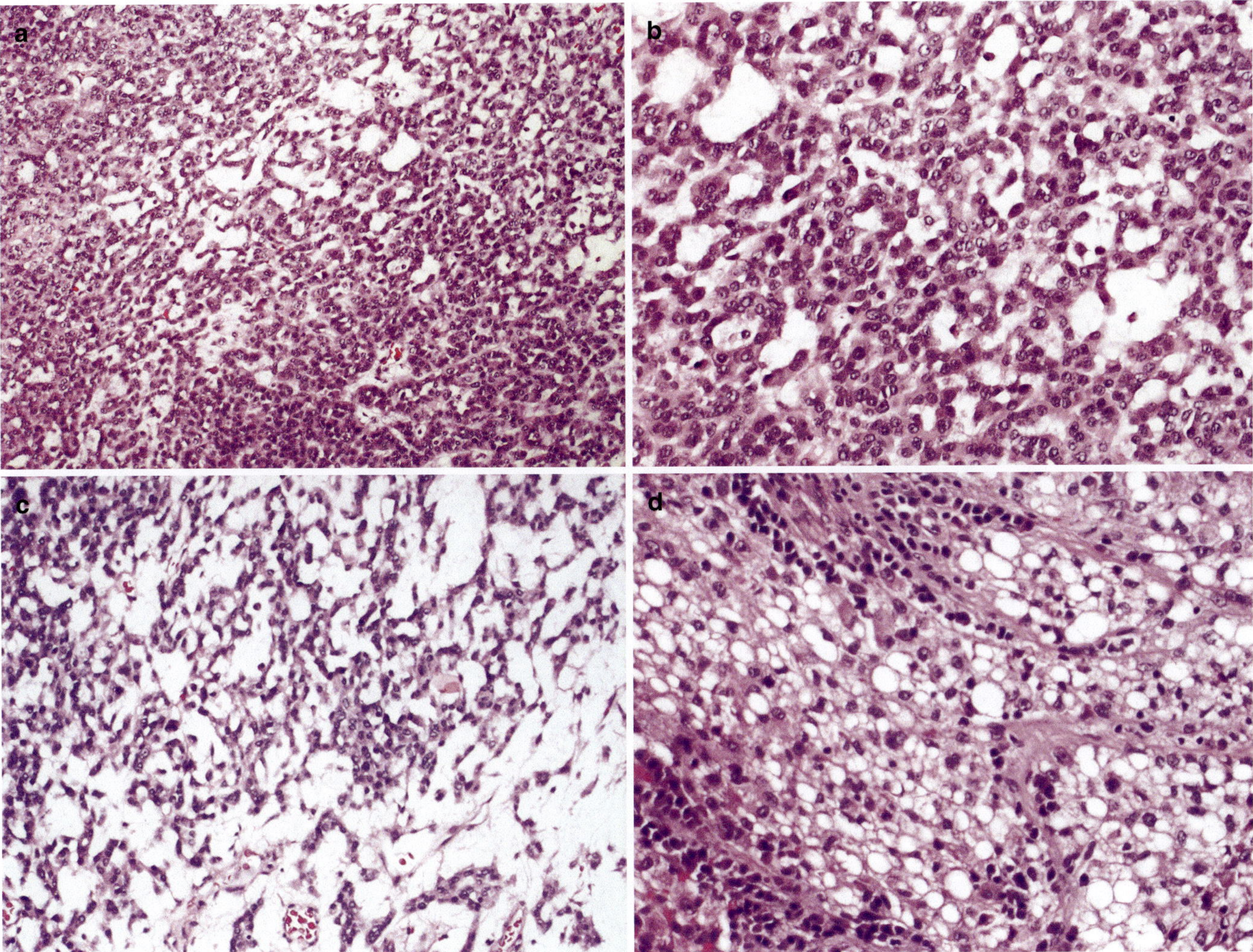

Fig. 6.28 Sertoli cell tumor. (**a**) The tumor shows a diffuse growth of tubules in scant stroma. (**b**) Some tubules have round lumens, and cytologic atypia is minimal. (**c**) Tumor cells form cords and clusters in a myxoid stroma. (**d**) Tumor cells have lipid vacuoles in the cytoplasm

What Are the Morphologic Features Are Associated with Malignancy in Leydig Cell Tumor?

Most Leydig cell tumors are benign, but approximately 5% are malignant. The average age of patients with malignant tumors is 62.5 years, in contrast to the late thirties for those with benign Leydig cell tumors. Malignant Leydig cell tumors usually demonstrate two or more of the following features: larger than 5 cm in diameter, infiltrative borders, prominent cytological atypia, >3 mitotic figures per 10 high-power fields, lymphovascular invasion, and tumor necrosis. Ancillary studies may have some value in predicting the clinical behavior of Leydig cell tumor. Aneuploidy is usually observed in metastatic Leydig cell tumors. MIB-1 staining indices show a significant increase in the malignant tumors. Staining for p53 protein may highlights

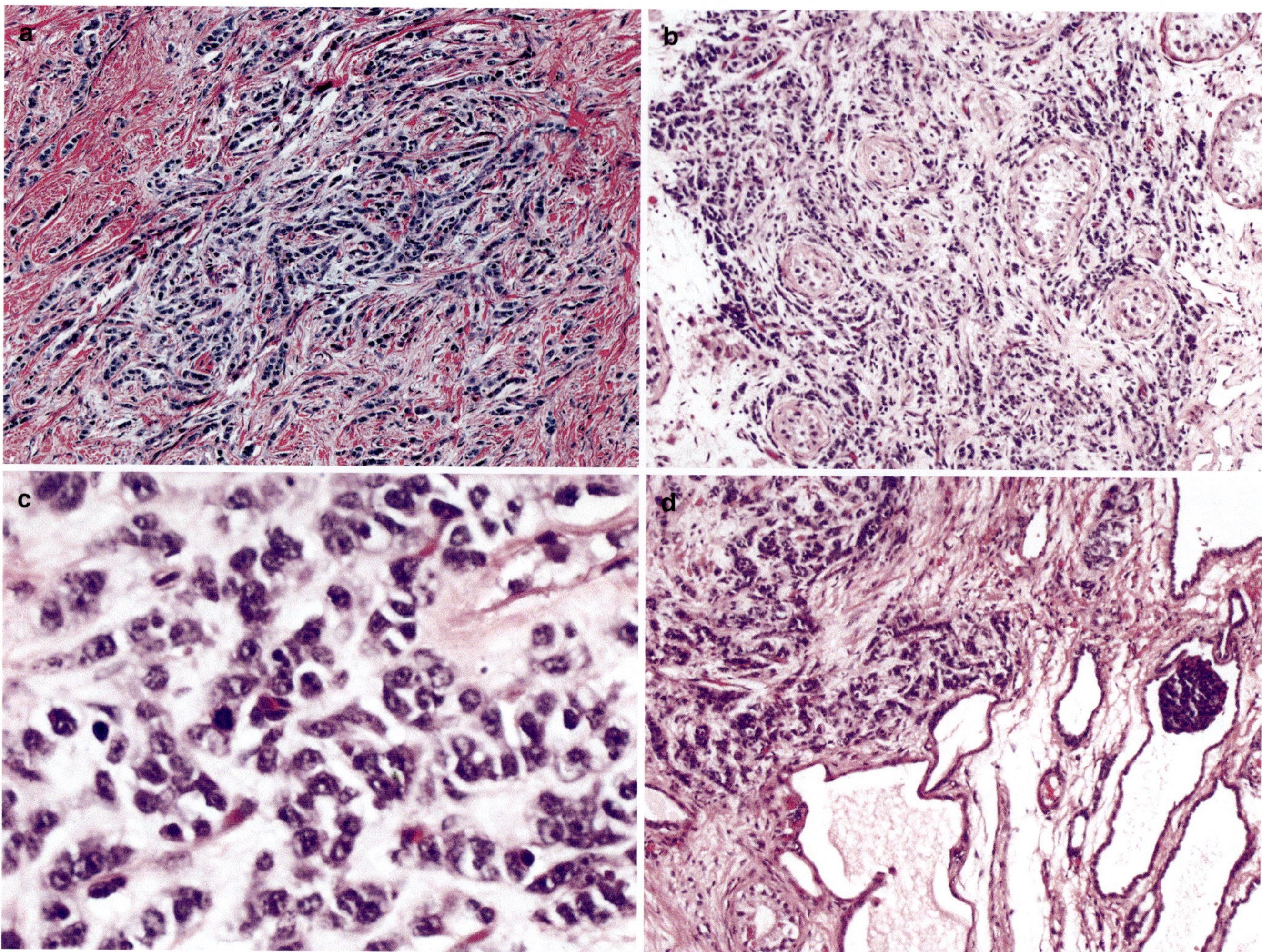

Fig. 6.29 Malignant Sertoli cell tumor. (**a**) Tumor diffusely invades the spermatic cord. (**b**) Tumor shows infiltrative growth in the testis. (**c**) Tumor cells show high-grade nuclear atypia and mitoses. (**d**) Tumor invades vascular spaces

>50% of nuclei in some malignant tumors. Malignant Leydig cell tumors usually spread to the regional lymph nodes (Fig. 6.34a, b), lungs, liver, and bones. The treatment is inguinal orchiectomy. If a tumor spread to regional lymph nodes, retroperitoneal lymph node dissection may be considered. The treatment of metastatic Leydig cell tumor has been generally unsatisfactory. Most patients die within 5 years.

References: [94, 96, 97]

How Is Adult Granulosa Cell Tumor Differentiated from Juvenile Granulosa Cell Tumor?

See Table 6.21 for the differences between adult granulosa cell tumor and juvenile granulosa cell tumor (Figs. 6.35 and 6.36).

References: [98–101]

What Are the Salient Features of Fibrothecoma?

Testicular fibrothecoma is a rare tumor that occurs in patients with a wide range of age (mean 45 years).

- It is usually a well-circumscribed, tan, and firm tumor (0.5–8 cm).
- It is characterized by spindle-shaped fibroblasts that usually shows fascicular or storiform patterns in scant stroma, resembling its ovarian counterpart (Fig. 6.37a).
- The tumor cells usually appear bland with elongated nuclei and scant cytoplasm.
- It is variably positive for inhibin (Fig. 6.37b), calretinin, cytokeratin, actin, desmin, S100, and CD34.
- All tumors follow a benign clinical course.

Table 6.18 Comparison of clinicopathologic features between large cell calcifying Sertoli cell tumor and conventional Sertoli cell tumor

	Large cell calcifying Sertoli cell tumor	Sertoli cell tumors
Pathology	Usually a well-circumscribed unilateral mass in sporadic cases Scattered small and bilateral tumors in Carney complex-related cases Tumors may show growth patterns of solid, tubules, nests, or cords in a myxoid stroma. Tumor cells are usually round to oval with abundant granular eosinophilic cytoplasm, vesicular nuclei, and prominent nucleoli (Fig. 6.30a). Calcifications vary from small psammomas to massive areas, sometimes with ossification (Fig. 6.30b) Intratubular hyalinizing Sertoli cell nodule may be seen in 40% of cases, particularly those associated with Carney complex Negative for nuclear β-catenin Malignancy is associated with the presence of two or more the following features: size >4 cm, marked nuclear atypia, >3 mitotic figures per 10 HPF, extratesticular spread, tumor necrosis, and lymphovascular invasion	Usually a well-circumscribed tan-white unilateral mass (2–5 cm). Cystic changes may be present in 1/3 of cases Typically a nodular growth of tubules in scant stroma Tubules may be round or elongated. Sometimes lumens may not be apparent Sometimes a diffuse growth pattern with nests, cords, clusters of cells separated by dense collagens Tumor cells show pale to eosinophilic cytoplasm that may become lipid vacuoles No calcifications are seen Cytologic atypia is minimal and mitotic activity is low Positive for nuclear β-catenin Malignancy is associated with the presence of two or more the following features: size >5 cm, significant nuclear atypia, >5 mitotic figures per 10 HPF, tumor necrosis, infiltrative borders, and lymphovascular invasion
Clinical features	Younger patients with a mean age of 21 years Testicular swelling in sporadic cases Patients with Carney complex may have skin myxomas, pigmented nodular adrenocortical disease, psammomatous melanotic schwannomas, etc. 60–70% of cases associated with Carney complex show germline mutations in PRKAR1A, a tumor suppressor gene Radical orchiectomy is usually performed for sporadic cases. In cases associated with Carney complex, conservative approach may be considered Most are benign, but 15% of cases are malignant	Older patients with a mean age of 46 years Asymptomatic testicular swelling with no endocrine symptoms Not asscoaited with Carney complex. Radical orchiectomy Most are benign, but 5% of cases are malignant

- It can be differentiated from fibromatous tumor of the testicular tunics because of their different cellularity and location.
- It can be differentiated from unclassified SCST, as the latter have at least focal SCST differentiation by morphology or immunohistochemistry.
- It can be differentiated from leiomyoma, as it lacks abundant eosinophilic cytoplasm and blunt-ended nuclei of the smooth muscle tumors.
- It can be differentiated from testicular fibrosarcoma, as it generally lacks nuclear atypia, mitosis and necrosis.

References: [102–104]

How Is Mesothelial Hyperplasia Is Differentiated from Malignant Mesothelioma?

See Table 6.22 for the differences between mesothelial hyperplasia and malignant mesothelioma (Figs. 6.38 and 6.39).
References: [105–108]

How Is Metastatic Adenocarcinoma Differentiated from Adenomatoid Tumor?

See Table 6.23 for the differences between adenomatoid tumor and metastatic adenocarcinoma (Figs. 6.40, 6.41, and 6.42).
References: [106–113]

What Are the Salient Features of Epididymal Adenocarcinoma?

It is a rare epithelial tumor that arises in the epididymis but commonly involves other structures, such as tunica vaginalis, testis and spermatic cord.

- The tumors may show cystic, papillary, and tubular growth pattern (Fig. 6.43a).
- Some papillary structures are lined by cuboidal and columnar cells with clear cytoplasm (Fig. 6.43b).
- Focal calcification may be present (Fig. 6.43c).
- Mitotic figures, tumor necrosis, and cytologic atypia are common.

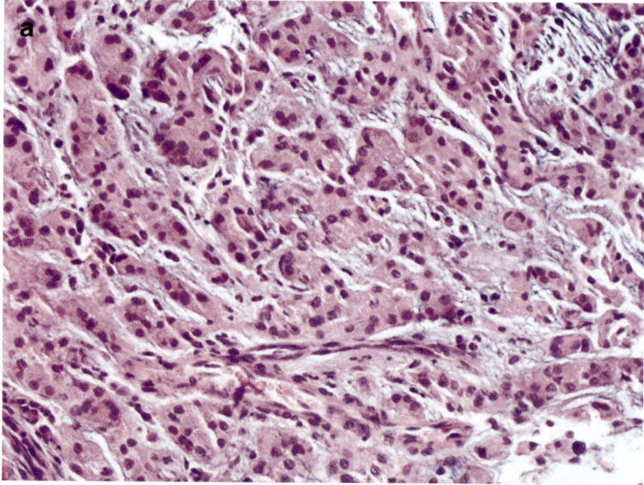

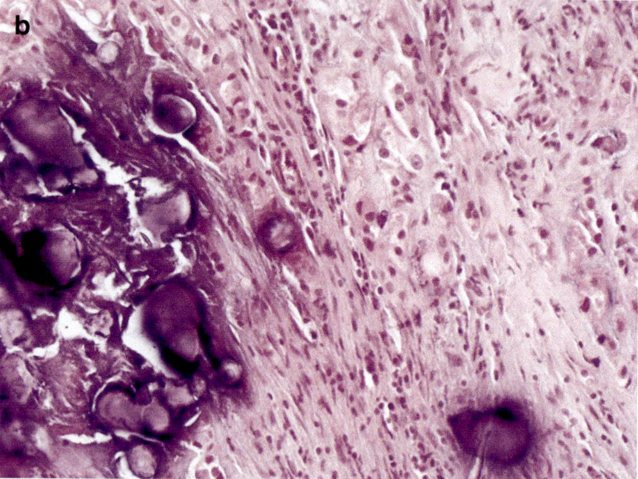

Fig. 6.30 Large cell calcifying Sertoli cell tumor. (**a**) Tumor cells have abundant granular eosinophilic cytoplasm, vesicular nuclei, and prominent nucleoli. (**b**) Tumor shows prominent microcalcification with psammoma bodies

- It is positive for CK7, carbonic anhydrase IX, and PAX8 (Fig. 6.43d), mimicking metastatic renal cell carcinoma, but it is negative for RCC antigen and AMACR.
- It is a malignant lesion that may cause death.
- It is differentiated from epididymal papillary adenoma, as the latter lacks an invasive growth pattern, tumor necrosis, and cytologic atypia.
- Other malignancies, such as metastatic carcinomas and mesothelioma, need to be differentiated, and immunohistochemistry is helpful (linage-specific markers for meta-

static carcinomas and mesothelial markers for mesothelioma).

References: [114, 115]

How Is Testicular Germ Cell Tumor Differentiated from Metastatic Adenocarcinoma to the Testis?

See Table 6.24 for the differences between germ cell tumor and metastatic adenocarcinoma (Figs. 6.41 and 6.42).
    References: [31, 68, 112, 113, 116]

How Is Paratesticular Lipoma Differentiated from Liposarcoma?

See Table 6.25 for the differences between paratesticular lipoma and well-differentiated liposarcoma (Fig. 6.44).
    References: [117–120]

How Is Leiomyoma of the Spermatic Cord Differentiated from Leiomyosarcoma?

Leiomyoma is the second most common benign mesenchymal tumor in the paratesticular region after lipoma. It often occurs in the epididymis. The tumor shows pure smooth muscle differentiation, which is characterized by fascicles of spindle cells with brightly eosinophilic cytoplasm and cigar-shaped nuclei. However, it lacks of malignant features, such as nuclear atypia, mitotic activity, and necrosis. Leiomyomas are benign and do not recur. Leiomyosarcoma is the second most common malignant mesenchymal tumor in the paratesticular region after liposarcoma. It often involves the spermatic cord or tunics. Although the tumor is often well differentiated, malignant features, including mitotic activity, necrosis, and nuclear atypia, are present at least focally (Fig. 6.45a–d). The tumors cover the entire spectrum of smooth muscle differentiation from low to high grade. Rare paratesticular leiomyosarcoma are of pleomorphic, myxoid, epithelioid, inflammatory, and dedifferentiated types. The prognosis of leiomyosarcoma is associated with histologic grade. Low grade may develop local recurrence but no

Table 6.19 Comparison of clinicopathologic features between large cell calcifying Sertoli cell and intratubular large cell hyalinizing Sertoli cell neoplasia

	Large cell calcifying Sertoli cell tumor	Intratubular large cell hyalinizing Sertoli cell neoplasia
Pathology	Unilateral in sporadic cases and bilateral in cases associated with Carney complex Usually a well-circumscribed mass (range, 1–15 cm) in sporadic cases Scattered small and bilateral tumors are characteristic of Carney complex-related cases. Tumors may show growth patterns of solid tubules, nests, clusters, or cords in a myxoid stroma Tumor cells are usually round to oval with abundant granular eosinophilic cytoplasm, vesicular nuclei, and prominent nucleoli Calcifications vary from small psammomas to massive areas, sometimes with ossification Intratubular hyalinizing Sertoli cell nodule may be seen in 40% of cases, particularly those associated with Carney complex Negative for nuclear β-catenin	Usually bilateral Multiple, small, white-light pink nodules (1–3 mm) Typically lobular clusters of expanded seminiferous tubules are scattered in the testis (Fig. 6.31a) The tubules are lined mostly by Sertoli cells, which have oval nuclei, inconspicuous nucleoli, and pale to eosinophilic cytoplasm with vacuoles The tubules are surrounded by a thickened basement membrane, which may invigilate into the tubular lumens, mimicking intraluminal globoid deposits (Fig. 6.31b) Calcification is not prominent. Cytologic atypia is minimal and mitotic activity is low Positive for aromatase
Clinical features	Young adults with a mean age of 21 years 60–70% of cases associated with Carney complex show germline mutations in PRKAR1A, a tumor suppressor gene Patients usually have testicular swelling in sporadic cases Patients with Carney complex may have skin myxomas, pigmented nodular adrenocortical disease, psammomatous melanotic schwannomas, etc. Most are benign, but 15% of cases are malignant. All malignant tumors are unilateral and unifocal and are usually not associated with Carney complex Radical orchiectomy is usually performed for sporadic cases. In cases associated with Carney complex, conservative approach may be considered	Children with a mean age of 7 years Occurs almost exclusively in patients with Peutz-Jeghers syndrome Usually shows germline mutations in the STK11 gene Patients often have gynecomastia, because of estrogen overproduction Patients with Peutz-Jeghers syndrome may have benign hamartomatous polyps in the gastrointestinal tract and hyperpigmented macules on the lips and oral mucosa (melanosis) All are benign Conservative treatment with aromatase inhibitors is recommended

metastasis, while high grade is associated with frequent metastases and mortality. The presence of mitotic activity in conjunction with nuclear atypia, infiltrative margins, or necrosis distinguishes leiomyosarcoma from leiomyoma.

References: [121–125]

How Is Paratesticular Rhabdomyosarcoma Differentiated from Leiomyosarcoma?

See Table 6.26 for the differences between leiomyosarcoma and rhabdomyosarcoma (Figs. 6.45 and 6.46).

References: [126–130]

What Types of Ovarian-Type Epithelial Tumor May Be Encountered in the Testis and Paratestis?

- A variety of ovarian surface epithelial tumors have been reported in the testis and paratestis, although they are extremely rare.
- They may arise by Müllerian metaplasia of the peritoneal lining of the tunica vaginalis or Müllerian remnants in the paratesticular connective tissue.
- Serous and mucinous tumors account for the majority, and others include endometrioid, clear cell, and Brenner tumors.
- The microscopic features are identical to their ovarian counterparts.

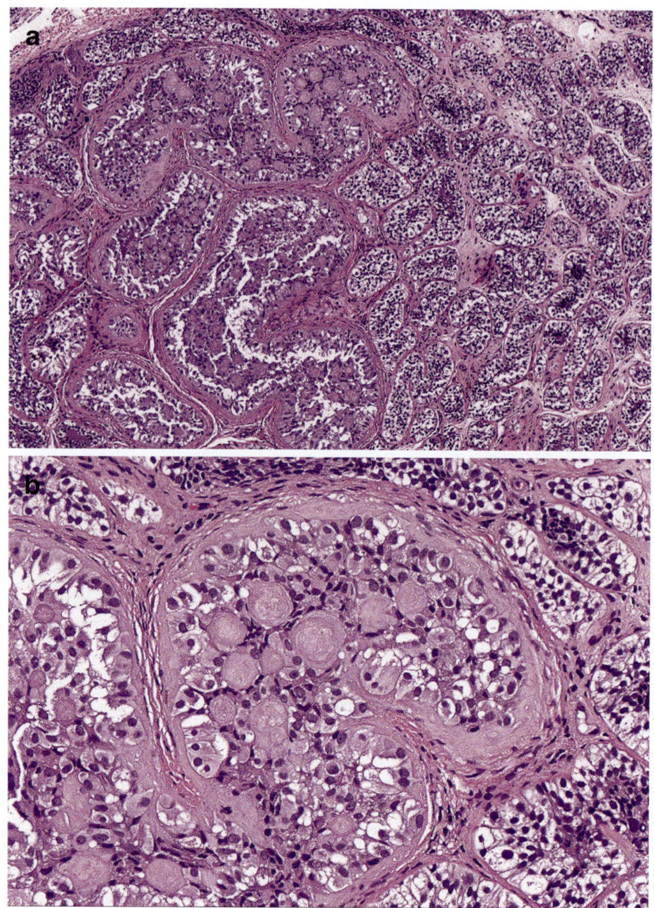

Fig. 6.31 Intratubular large cell hyalinizing Sertoli cell neoplasia. (**a**) The lesion is characterized by lobular clusters of expanded seminiferous tubules lined by mostly Sertoli cells. (**b**) The tubules are surrounded by a thickened basement membrane, which invigilates into the tubular lumens, mimicking intraluminal globoid deposits

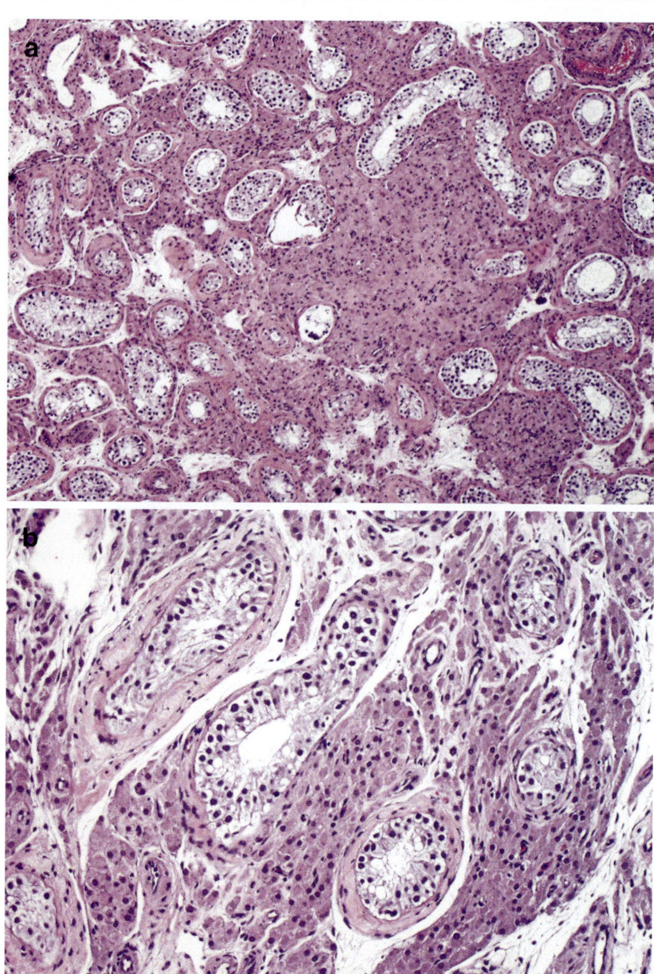

Fig. 6.32 Leydig cell hyperplasia. (**a**) It shows small clusters of Leydig cells interspersed among atrophic seminiferous tubules. (**b**) Cells show minimal cytologic atypia

Table 6.20 Comparison of clinicopathologic features between Leydig cell hyperplasia and Leydig cell tumor

	Leydig cell hyperplasia	Leydig cell tumor
Pathology	Usually bilateral	Usually unilateral
	Often grossly invisible but sometimes can produce multiple, small, yellow-brown nodules (<0.5 cm)	A well-circumscribed, homogenous, tan-yellow tumors (range, 0.5–5 cm)
	Multiple small clusters of Leydig cells interspersed among preexisting, frequently atrophic seminiferous tubules (Fig. 6.32a).	Diffuse growth pattern is the most common (Fig. 6.33a)
		Other patterns include nested (Fig. 6.33b), insular, trabecular, spindle cell, and microcystic
	Leydig cells may be present in the tunica albuginea and beyond	Tumor cells are typically uniform and round with abundant granular eosinophilic cytoplasm
	Leydig cells frequently involve nerves, which should not be misinterpreted as indicating they are neoplastic	The nuclei are round with minimal atypia and low mitotic activity
	Similar cytology to normal Leydig cells (Fig. 6.32b)	Lipofuscin pigment and Reinke crystals may be present in up to 30% of cases
Clinical features	Any age	Two incidence peaks – children (5–10 years) and adults (30–60 years)
	Usually an incident finding	Testicular swelling. Gynecomastia may be seen in one-third of patients
	Sometimes associated with infertility, precocity, undescended testis, and Klinefelter syndrome.	Most are benign but 5% are malignant
	Non-neoplastic	Ususally treated with radical orchiectomy
	No treatment is needed	

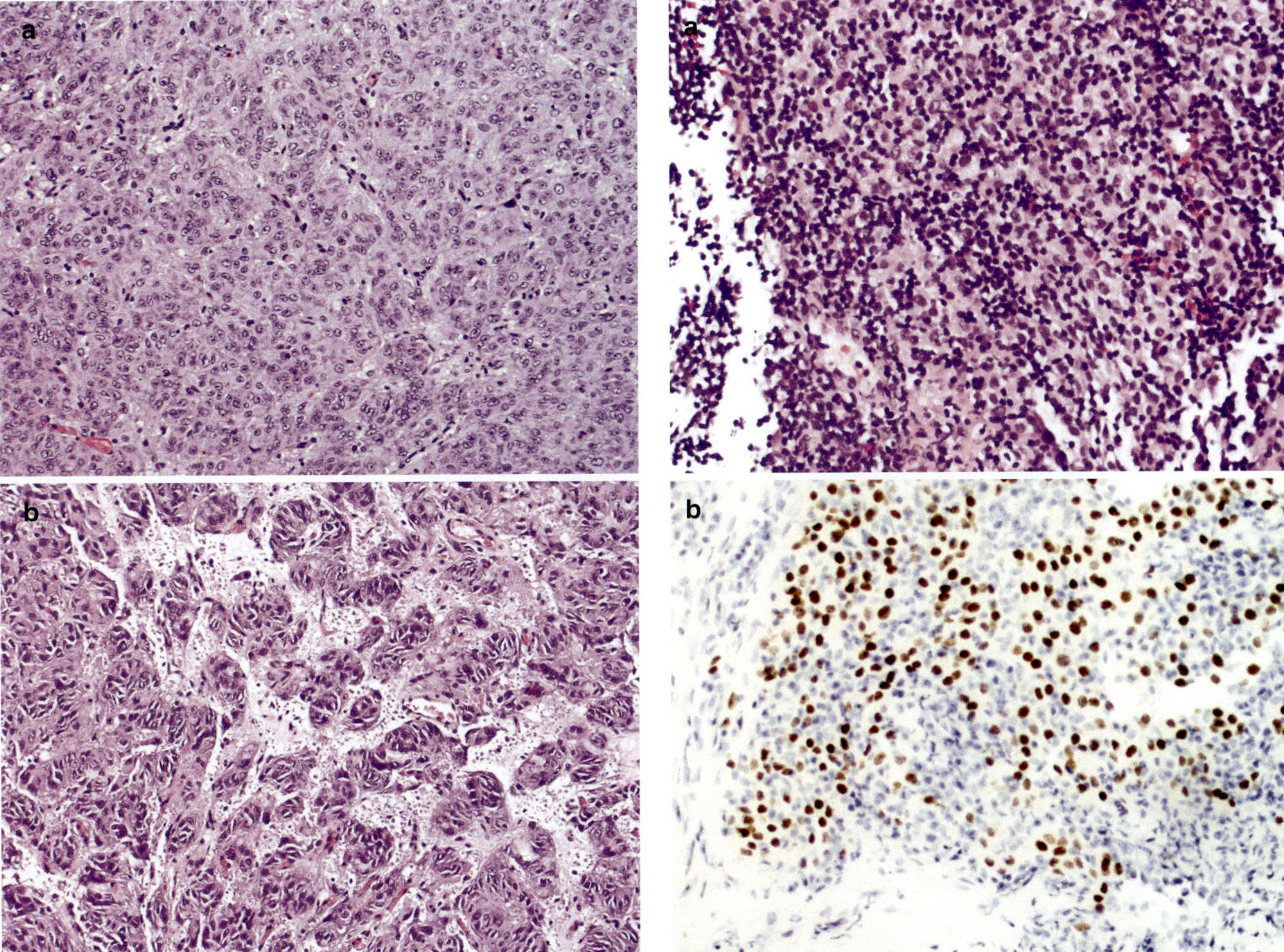

Fig. 6.33 Leydig cell tumor. (**a**) Tumor shows a diffuse growth pattern and tumor cells show minimal cytologic atypia. (**b**) Tumor shows a nested growth pattern with focal spindle cell features

Fig. 6.34 Metastatic Leydig cell tumor. (**a**) Tumor cells with high-grade nuclear atypia and abundant eosinophilic cytoplasm involve lymphoid tissue. (**b**) Tumor cells are positive for SF-1

- The criteria for benign, borderline, and malignant tumors are similar to those for their ovarian counterparts.
- Benign and borderline tumors do not recur or metastasize, whereas carcinomas have the potential for both.

References: [131–134]

What Are the Salient Features of Myoid Gonadal Stromal Tumor?

- A spindle cell neoplasm shows features of both smooth muscle and gonadal stromal differentiation.
- It occurs over a wide age range (4–59 years).
- A small, well-circumscribed tumor (1.2–3.5 cm) but not encapsulated (Fig. 6.47a).

- It is characterized by densely packed, uniform spindle cells arranged in short fascicles with variably prominent intervening collagen deposits (Fig. 6.47b).
- Tumor cells show spindle nuclei, inconspicuous nucleoli, and scant cytoplasm (Fig. 6.47c).
- Mitotic figures are uncommon.
- The tumor cells are positive for smooth muscle actin, S100 protein (Fig. 6.47d), FOXL2, and SF1, but negative for SOX9, calretinin, and inhibin.
- The tumor is differentiated from fibroma (positive for SOX9, inhibin, and calretinin; and negative for S100) and leiomyoma (negative for S100).
- All the reported tumors have exhibited benign clinical behaviors.

References: [135–138]

Table 6.21 Comparison of clinicopathologic features between adult and juvenile granuloma cell tumors

	Adult granulosa cell tumor	Juvenile granulosa cell tumor
Pathology	A well-circumscribed, predominantly solid tumor It typically shows a nodular growth pattern (Fig. 6.35a) Within nodules, diffuse, microfollicular, trabecular, nest, cord, or spindle cell (Fig. 6.35b) patterns may be present Tumor cells have elongated nuclei and scant cytoplasm Nuclear grooves are common Mitotic figures are rare Tumor cells may be luteinized	A well-circumscribed predominantly cystic tumor It typically shows cysts of various sizes with eosinophilic or basophilic fluid (Fig. 6.36a) Cysts are lined by multilayered cells. The inner cells resemble granulosa cells with round nuclei, small nucleoli, and scant cytoplasm. The outer cells resemble theca cells with elongated nuclei and scant cytoplasm (Fig. 6.36b) Tumor cells lack nuclear grooves Mitotic activity is brisk
Clinical features	Patients may be any age with a mean of 40 years Testicular swelling Gynecomastia in 25% if cases Acquired FOXL2 mutations in some cases Most are benign, but 20% are malignant Malignancy is associated with >4 cm, infiltrative borders, tumor necrosis, and lymphovascular invasion. Orchiectomy for local disease Retroperitoneal lymph node dissection may be considered for metastatic disease	Almost all patients in the first decade of life and 90% in the first 6 months Testicular swelling Cryptorchism in 30% cases Some cases show abnormal karyotypes including mosaics 45,X/47,XYY or 45,X/46,Xr(Y) All are benign Orchiectomy is curative Testis-sparing enucleation may be considered in some cases

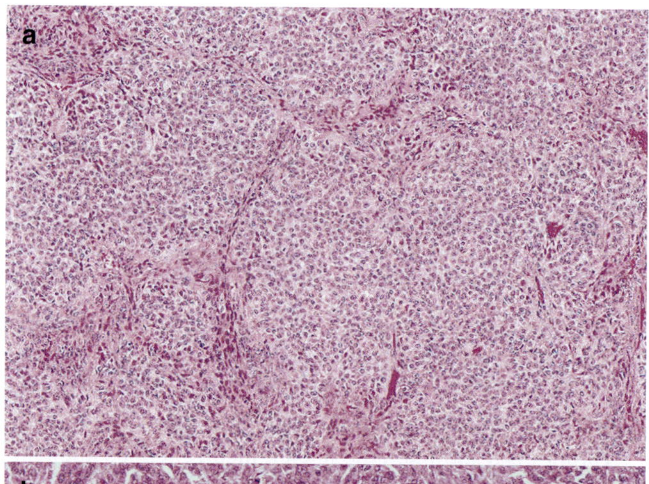

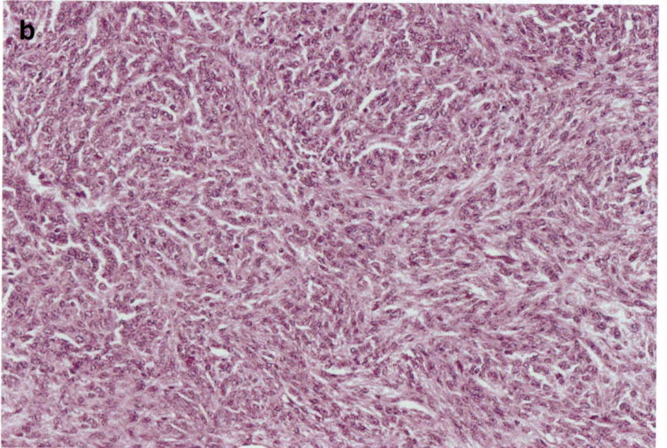

Fig. 6.35 Adult granulosa cell tumor. (**a**) Tumor usually shows nodular growth pattern. (**b**) Tumor shows focal spindle cell features

How Is Testicular Lymphoma Differentiated from Seminoma?

See Table 6.27 for the differences between seminoma and diffuse large B-cell lymphoma (Figs. 6.2 and 6.48).
References: [35, 79, 139–144]

How Is Adenomatoid Tumor Differentiated from Malignant Mesothelioma?

See Table 6.28 for the differences between malignant mesothelioma and adenomatoid tumor (Figs. 6.39 and 6.40).
References: [105–107, 109–111, 145]

How Is Rete Testis Adenocarcinoma Diagnosed?

It is a malignant glandular neoplasm arising from the rete epithelium. The tumor shows various growth patterns, such as tubuloglandular, retiform, Sertoliform, kaposiform, and spindle cell features (Fig. 6.49a). The tumor cells are cuboidal to columnar with moderate-to-eosinophilic cytoplasm and moderate-to-severe atypia (Fig. 6.49b). Necrosis, infiltrative growth, and desmoplasia are common (Fig. 6.49c). There are no specific linages associated immunohistochemical markers for rete testis. It must be differentiated from other glands-forming malignancies that occur at this site, such as malignant

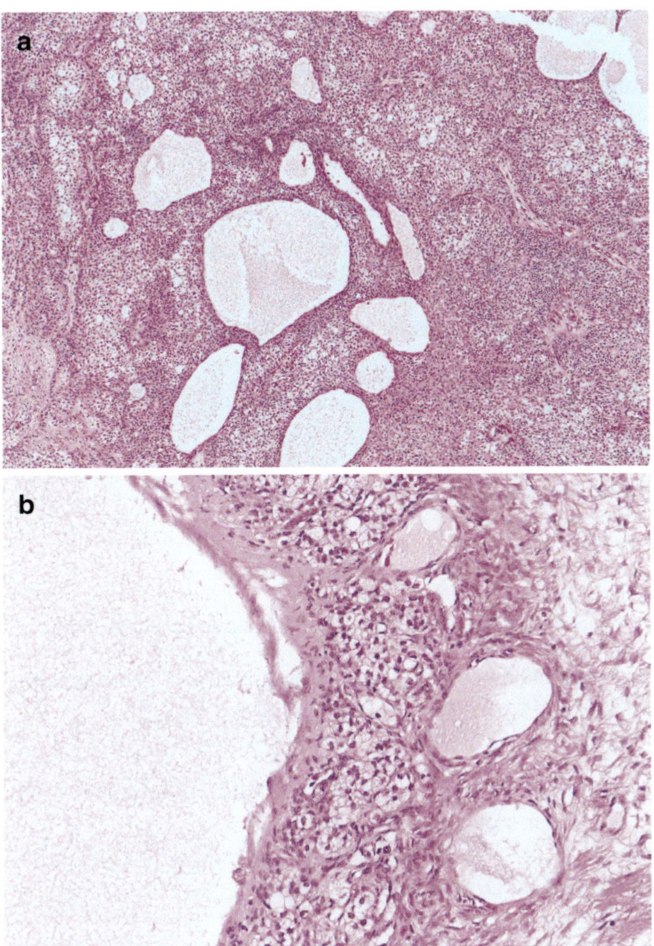

Fig. 6.36 Juvenile granulosa cell tumor. (**a**) Tumor shows cysts of various sizes with eosinophilic fluid. (**b**) Cysts are lined by multilayered cells. The inner cells resemble granulosa cells with round nuclei and scant cytoplasm. The outer cells resemble theca cells with elongated nuclei and scant cytoplasm

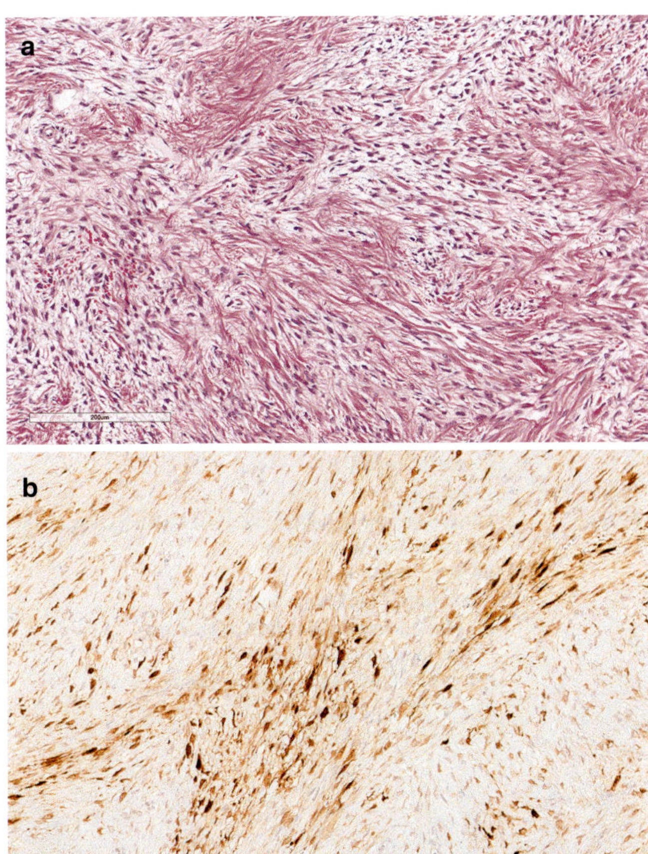

Fig. 6.37 Fibrothecoma. (**a**) Tumor is characterized by spindle-shaped fibroblasts with minimal cytologic atypia that usually shows fascicular or storiform patterns in scant stroma. (**b**) Tumor is positive for inhibin

mesothelioma, metastatic adenocarcinoma, and malignant Sertoli cell tumor. These malignancies often express lineage-associated immunohistochemical markers. The following diagnostic criteria are recommended: the tumor is grossly centered in the hilum of the testis; absence of a neoplasm elsewhere that resembles rete adenocarcinoma; morphologic and immunohistochemical features incompatible with other forms of primary testicular and paratesticular neoplasms; and at least partial tumor growth within channels of the rete testis (Fig. 6.49d). A transition from benign to malignant epithelium within the rete testis may help the diagnosis but not required, as advanced tumors may obliterate the non-neoplastic rete epithelium. Furthermore, metastatic carcinoma may grow within the rete and replace its epithelium, thereby mimicking the transition from benign to malignant.

References: [107, 146–148]

Case Presentation

Case 1

Learning Objectives
1. To become familiar with the gross and histologic features of the tumor
2. To learn the immunohistochemical features of this tumor
3. To provide the accurate pT category

Case History
A 37-year-old male with left testicular mass and elevated LDH.

Gross
Radical orchiectomy specimen with diffuse testicular involvement by a fleshy, partially nodular tumor measuring 5.8 cm with areas suspicious for epididymal invasion and hilar fat invasion (Fig. 6.50a).

Table 6.22 Comparison of clinicopathologic features between mesothelial hyperplasia and malignant mesothelioma

	Mesothelial hyperplasia	Malignant mesothelioma
Pathology	Fibrotic thickening of the walls of tunica vaginalis with no gross mass Epithelial proliferation shows simple papillary structures, tubules, and nests (Fig. 6.38). Reactive mesothelial cells have abundant cytoplasm and may contain enlarged vesicular nuclei Brisk mitotic activity may be seen in inflamed areas Lack solid and arborizing complex papillary growth patterns Lack the biphasic spindle cell pattern Often associated with inflammation An infiltrative growth pattern is absent Postive for WT-1	Usually multiple friable masses on the thickened tunica vaginalis. Sometimes tumors may invade the testicular parenchyma 75% of cases are epithelial type with broad arborizing complex papillary and tubular structures (Fig. 6.39a) 25% of cases are biphasic type with epithelial and sarcomatoid (or spindle cell) components An infiltrative component is present at least focally (Fig. 6.39b) Tumor cells may show prominent cytologic atypia with pleomorphism, mitoses, and prominent nucleoli (Fig. 6.39c) Tumor may invade the testis and paratesticular tissues Postive for WT-1 (Fig. 6.39d)
Clinical features	Any age Inflammatory irritation causes reactive hyperplasia of the mesothelial lining Scrotal swelling Sometimes inflammatory signs Hydrocele repair or needle aspiration May spontancously regress Non-neoplastic and reactive disease	Old patients (mean age 65 years) Asbestos exposure in 40% of cases Scrotal swelling Sometimes palpable ill-defined intrascrotal firm mass Radical orchiectomy for local disease Retroperitoneal lymph node dissection, radiation and chemotherapy for metastatic disease Aggressive malignant disease with a median survival of 24 months and recurrence in 60% of patients in 2 years

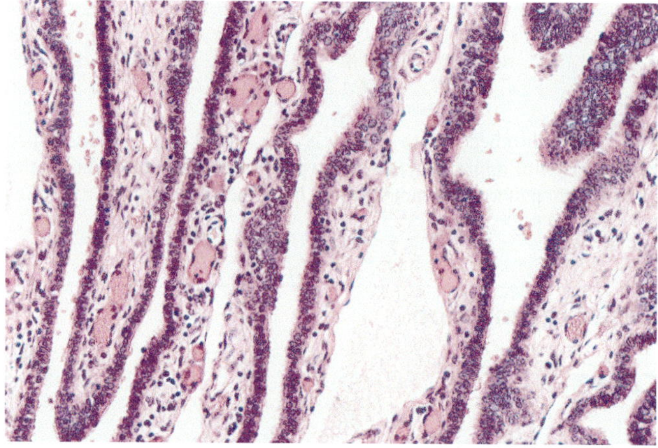

Fig. 6.38 Mesothelial hyperplasia. The epithelial proliferation is characterized by simple papillary structures lined by cells with vesicular nuclei and abundant cytoplasm

Histologic Findings
- Solid sheets with fibrous bands containing lymphocytes (Fig. 6.50b)
- Polygonal cells with distinct cell borders
- Pale eosinophilic cytoplasm
- Seminiferous tubules with atypical cells present against the basement membrane

- Invasion into the rete testis stroma, epididymal stroma and hilar soft tissue (Fig. 6.50c, d)

Differential Diagnosis
- Seminoma
- Embryonal carcinoma
- Sertoli cell tumor
- Spermatocytic tumor
- Lymphoma

IHC and Other Ancillary Studies
- Positive for PLAP, CD117/c-kit, D2-40/podoplanin, and OCT3/4
- Negative for CD30 and inhibin

Final Diagnosis
Seminoma, pT2

Take-Home Messages
1. Seminoma is a tumor with sheet-like growth and fibrous bands with lymphocytes.
2. Immunostains and the presence of GCNIS corroborate the diagnosis.
3. Hilar soft tissue invasion and epididymal invasion are a part of the pT2 category.

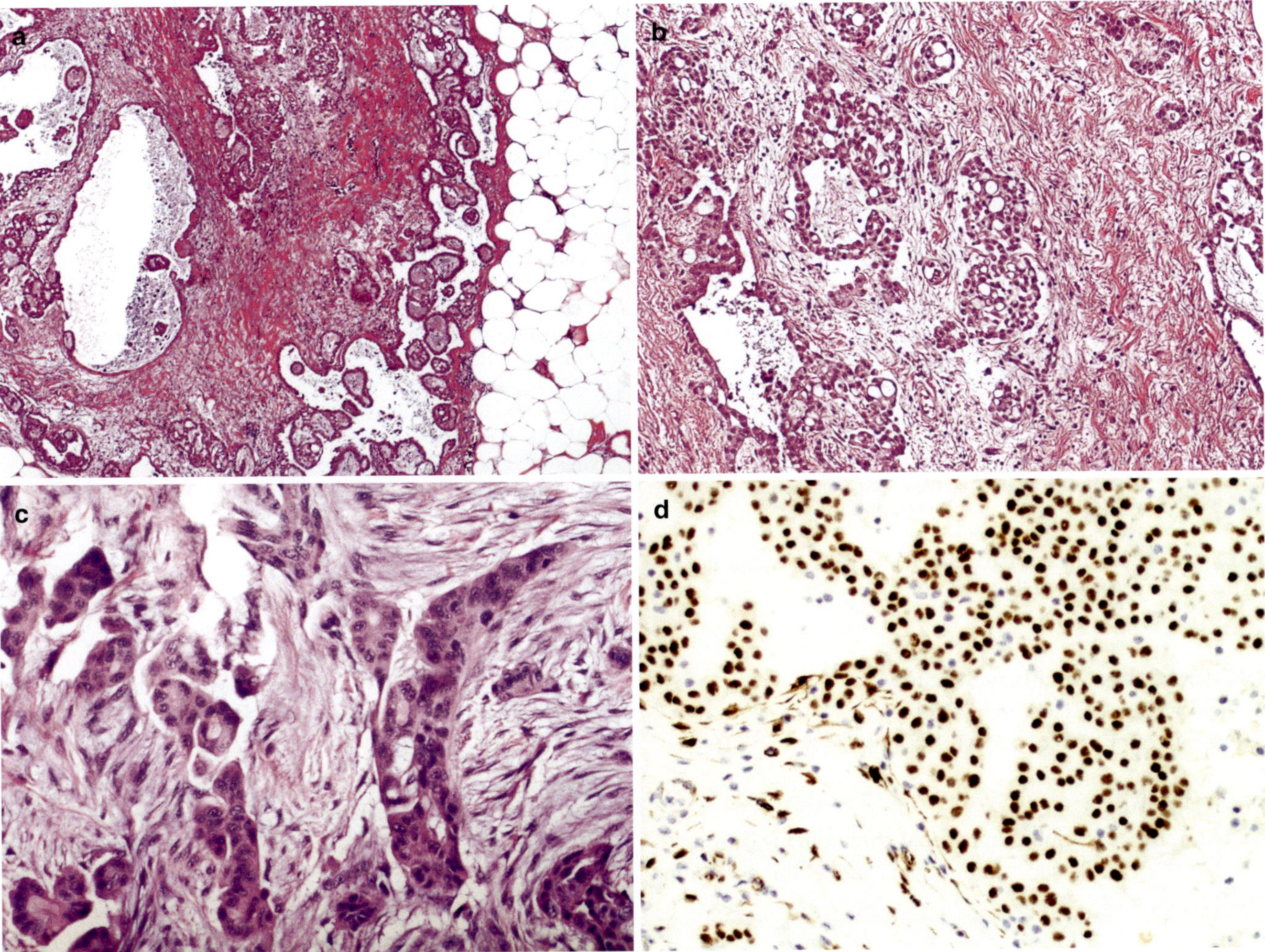

Fig. 6.39 Malignant mesothelioma. (**a**) Tumor shows complex papillary and tubular structures. (**b**) Tumor invades the fibrous stroma. (**c**) Tumor cells show prominent cytologic atypia with pleomorphism and prominent nucleoli. (**d**) Tumor is positive for WT-1

Case 2

Learning Objectives
1. To become familiar with the gross and histologic features of the tumor
2. To learn the immunohistochemical features of this tumor
3. To provide the accurate pT category

Case History
A 34-year-old male with left testicular mass with minor elevations of LDH, AFP, and HCG.

Gross
Radical orchiectomy specimen with diffuse testicular involvement by a hemorrhagic, yellow, focally cystic, and necrotic tumor measuring 7.4 cm (Fig. 6.51a)

Histologic Findings
- Predominantly tumor with sheets, papillary formation, and pseudoglandular spaces (utilized for IHC)
- Large, polygonal, pleomorphic cells with abundant mitotic figures (Fig. 6.51b)
- Amphophilic cytoplasm
- Seminiferous tubules with atypical cells present against the basement membrane
- Lymphovascular invasion (Fig. 6.51c, d)

Differential Diagnosis
- Embryonal carcinoma
- Seminoma
- Yolk sac tumor
- Choriocarcinoma
- Lymphoma
- Malignant melanoma

Table 6.23 Comparison of clinicopathologic features between adenomatoid tumor and metastatic adenocarcinoma to the testis

	Adenomatoid tumor	Metastatic adenocarcinoma
Pathology	Usually a unilateral, well-circumscribed, tan-white, small tumor (typically <2 cm) in the epididymis. Occasionally it may involve the testis It is characterized by gland-like or vascular-like spaces lined by an attenuated layer of neoplastic cells that often form thin, bridging strands across the lumen (Fig. 6.40a) Cytologic atypia is minimal (Fig. 6.40b) Prominent intracytoplasmic vacuolization component may be present (Fig. 6.40c) Necrosis, perineural invasion and lymphovascular invasion are uncommon May be positive for mesothelial markers, such as calretinin, WT1 (Fig. 6.40d), HBME1, and podoplanin	Mostly solitary nodules (62%) Sometimes multiple nodules (17%) and diffuse involvement (21%) and bilateral in 20% of cases Carcinomas of the prostate (Fig. 6.41a–d), GI tract (Fig. 6.42a–d), kidney, and lung are among the most common primary Metastases show morphologic features similar to the primary tumors Significant cytologic atypia is typical Necrosis, perineural and intravascular invasion are common Usually negative for mesothelial markers Express the lineage-specific markers of the primary tumors – NKX3.1 and Prostein, PSA for prostate cancer; TTF-1 for lung cancer; CDX-2 for colon cancer; PAX8 for kidney cancer
Clinical features	A wide age range with a mean of 36 years Usually scrotal mass, sometimes with pain May involve the scrotal skin The most common tumor in the paratesticular region Benign tumor Usually radical orchiectomy Sometimes partial orchiectomy upon confirming the diagnosis on frozen section	Usually old patients with a mean age of 60 years. Testicular or paratesticular mass Symptoms associated with the primary tumor Systemic therapy directed to primary tumor Generally poor

IHC and Other Ancillary Studies

- Positive for OCT3/4 and CD30
- Negative for glypican 3, AFP, GATA3, CK7, and HCG

Final Diagnosis

Mixed germ cell tumor, embryonal carcinoma (80%), teratoma (10%), yolk sac tumor (5%), and choriocarcinoma (5%) types, pT2

Take-Home Messages

1. Embryonal carcinoma is a pleomorphic, high-grade tumor.
2. Immunostains corroborate the diagnosis.
3. In tumors with predominant embryonal carcinoma, lymphovascular invasion is frequent yielding a pT2 categorization.

Case 3

Learning Objectives

1. To learn the gross and histologic features of this tumor
2. To learn the immunohistochemical features of this tumor
3. To distinguish this tumor from its mimics

Case History

A 68-year-old man was present with a hydrocele in the right scrotum. Image study revealed a large mass involved the testis and scrotum. His serum markers, AFP, HCG, and LDH, were within the normal ranges. He underwent an en bloc resection of the involved scrotum, testis, spermatic cord, and inguinal lymph nodes. The patient, otherwise healthy, did not have any previous cancer history.

Gross

Sections of the testis revealed a poorly defined, tan-white, solid mass (7.5 × 3.6 × 2.8 cm) with focal areas of necrosis and hemorrhage (Fig. 6.52a). The mass was centered at the rete testis and wrapped around the upper and posterior surface of the testis. The tumor also extended to the epididymis and spermatic cord.

Histologic Findings

- Tumor shows a pushing border growth with a thick fibrous capsule but does not invade the testicular parenchyma (Fig. 6.52b).
- Tumor exhibits papillary and tubulocystic structures are lined by cuboidal and flat cells and occasionally hobnail cells (Fig. 6.52c).
- The tumor cells show clear cytoplasm and high nuclear grade associated with a delicate fibrovascular vascular stroma (Fig. 6.52d).

Differential Diagnosis

- Metastatic renal cell carcinoma
- Ovarian type epithelial tumor of the paratestis
- Malignant mesothelioma
- Germ cell tumor (or yolk sac tumor)

IHC and Other Ancillary Studies (Fig. 6.52e, f)

- Positive for PAX2, PAX8, HNF-1B, and p504S
- Negative for SALL4, OCT3/4, calretinin, inhibin, and WT-1

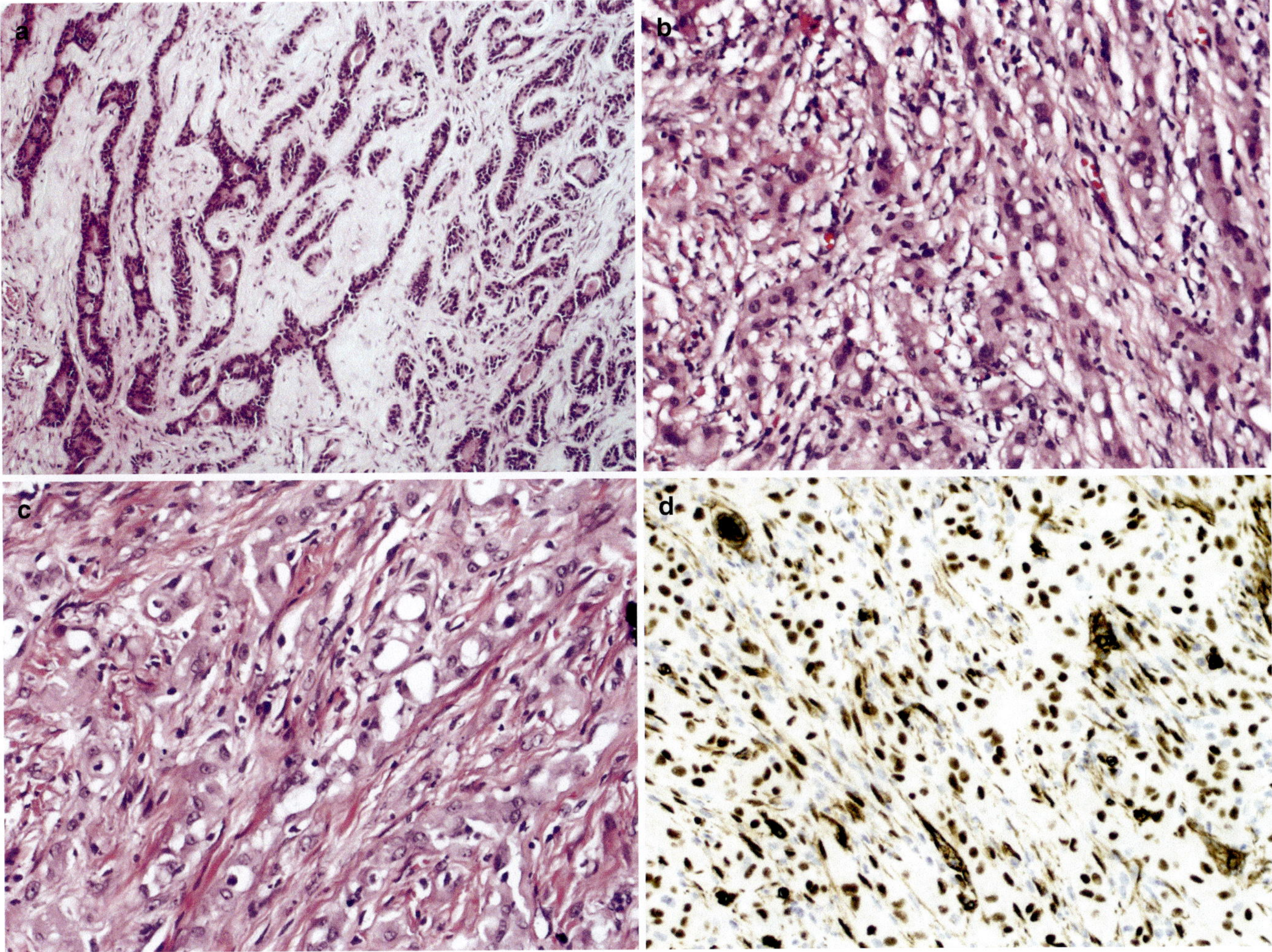

Fig. 6.40 Adenomatoid tumor. (**a**) Tumor is characterized by gland-like spaces with thin, bridging strands across the lumen. (**b**) Tumor cells have round nuclei with minimal atypia. (**c**) Intracytoplasmic vacuolization is present. (**d**) Tumor is positive for WT-1

- Ki-67 index ~30%.

Final Diagnosis
Ovarian-type epithelial tumor of the paratestis- Clear cell adenocarcinoma

Take-Home Messages
1. Clear cell adenocarcinoma may arise from the tunica vaginalis and shows microscopic and immunohistochemical features similar to its ovarian counterpart.
2. It is positive for PAX2, PAX8, HNF-1B, and p504S; and negative for germ cell tumor and mesothelial markers.
3. Clear cell adenocarcinoma cells have clear cytoplasm and form papillary structures, mimicking renal cell carcinoma, but patients do not have a previous history of RCC or renal mass.

References: [134, 149, 150]

Case 4

Learning Objectives
1. To learn the gross and histologic features of metastatic carcinoma to the testis
2. To learn how to differentiate metastatic carcinoma from other testicular malignancies
3. To learn how to use immunohistochemistry in the differential diagnosis and identifying the origin of metastatic carcinoma

Case History
A 32-year-old man presented to an emergency room with headache. He underwent evaluation that revealed a brain lesion as well as a large left lung mass. Ultrasound of the scrotum revealed bilateral testicular tumors. Interestingly, his markers were completely normal. He underwent bilateral radical inguinal orchiectomy for his presumptive diagnosis of metastatic testicular cancer.

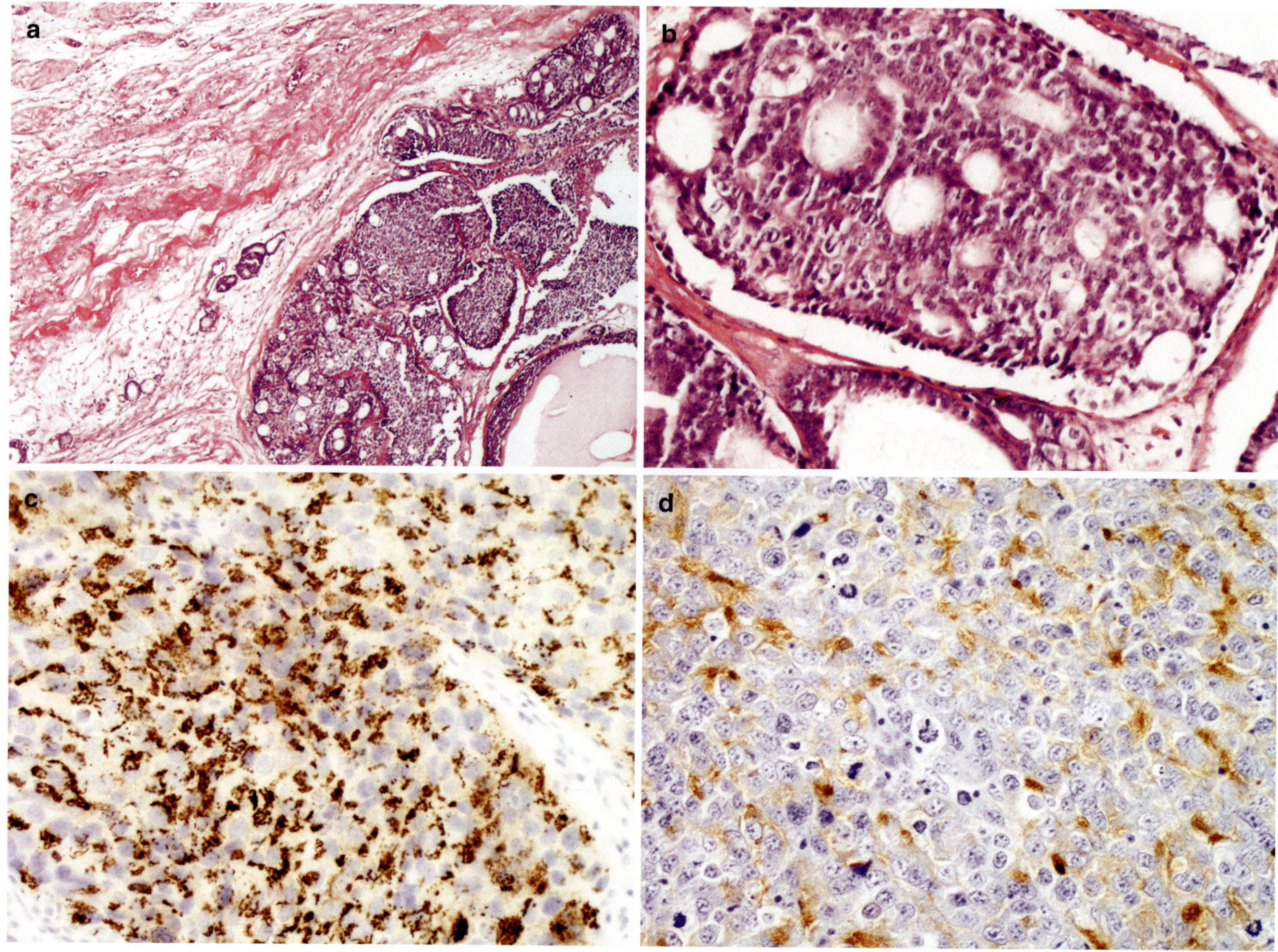

Fig. 6.41 Metastatic prostatic adenocarcinoma. (**a**) Poorly differentiated adenocarcinoma involves the testicular parenchyma. (**b**) Tumor cells form cribriform glands with prominent nucleoli. (**c**) Tumor is positive for prostein. (**d**) Tumor is positive for PSA

Gross

The right testis shows a white-tan, firm, multinodular mass (2.5 × 2.0 × 1.5 cm) with multiple miniscule satellite nodules. The left testis shows four discrete white-tan, firm nodules (0.6–2.2 cm). There was no apparent necrosis or hemorrhage on the glistening cutting surfaces. All the nodules were confined to the testis. The epididymis and spermatic cord were grossly free of tumor.

Histologic Findings

- Tumor shows large solid nodules involving the bilateral testis (Fig. 6.53a).

- Tumor cells show high-grade nuclear atypia and mitoses (Fig. 6.53b).
- The tumor involves the rete testis with lymphovascular invasion (Fig. 6.53c).
- Tumor shows an infiltrative growth pattern involving seminiferous tubules (Fig. 6.53d).

Differential Diagnosis

- Germ cell tumor (or embryonic carcinoma)
- Malignant mesothelioma
- Malignant sex cord-stromal tumor
- Diffuse large B-cell lymphoma

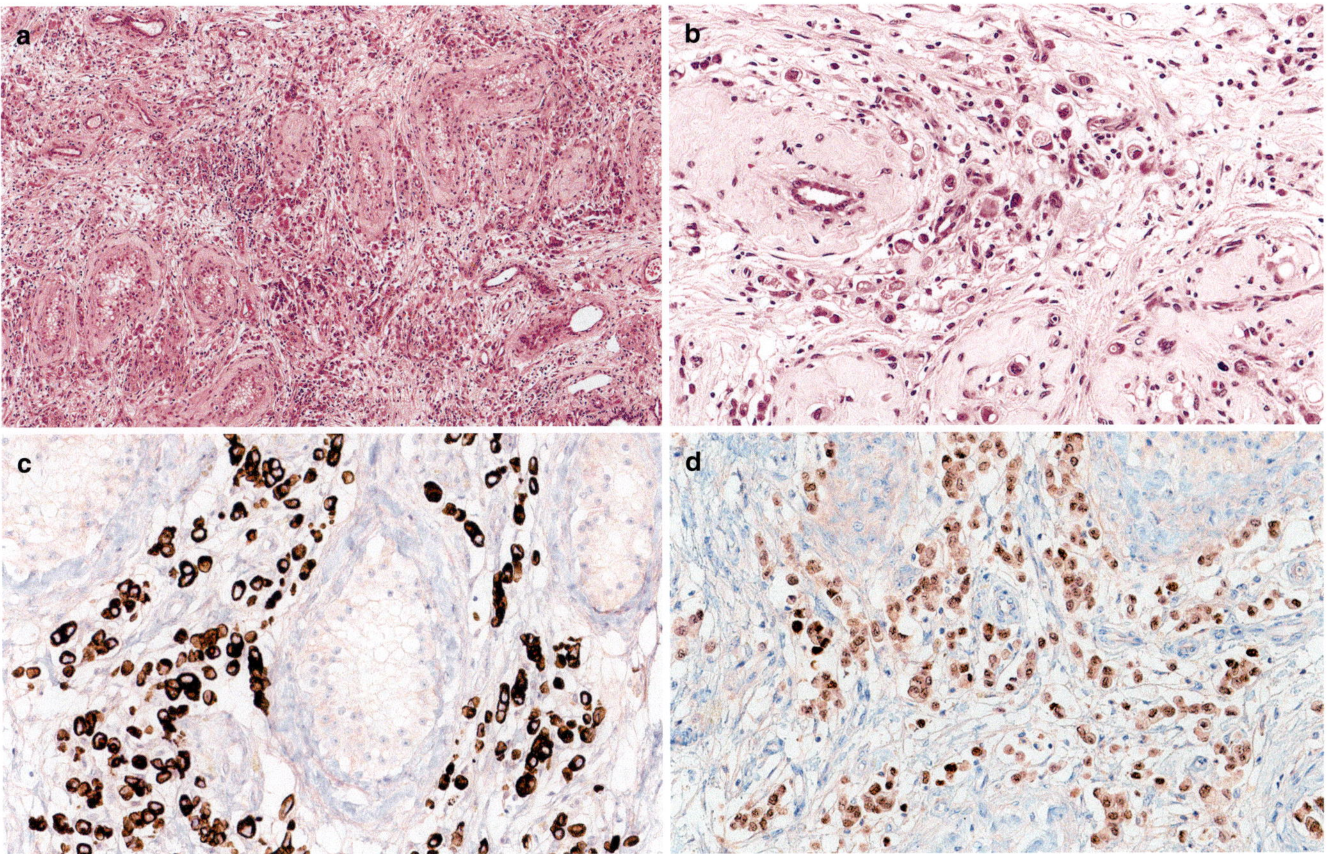

Fig. 6.42 Metastatic gastric adenocarcinoma. (**a**) Tumor diffusely invades the stroma around seminiferous tubules. (**b**) Tumor cells are poor differentiated with focal signet-ring cell features. (**c**) Tumor is positive for CK 7. (**d**) Tumor is positive for CDX2

- Metastatic lung carcinoma

IHC and Other Ancillary Studies (Fig. 6.53e–h)
- Tumor is positive for TTF-1, CK7, and Napsin
- Negative for SALL-4, OCT3/4, WT-1, SF-1, inhibin, and CD45
- DNA sequencing test shows mutations in BRAF, EGFR, and KRAS genes
- FISH test shows rearrangement of ALK gene

Final Diagnosis
Metastatic poorly differentiated lung adenocarcinoma to the testes

Take-Home Messages
1. Metastatic carcinoma often shows multiple lesions in bilateral testes.
2. Tumor may diffusely invade the testis as well as paratesticular structures with extensive lymphovascular invasion.
3. Tumor infiltrates the stroma around seminiferous tubules.
4. Immunohistochemistry is extremely valuable in the differential diagnosis and determining the origin of metastatic carcinoma.

References: [112, 151–153]

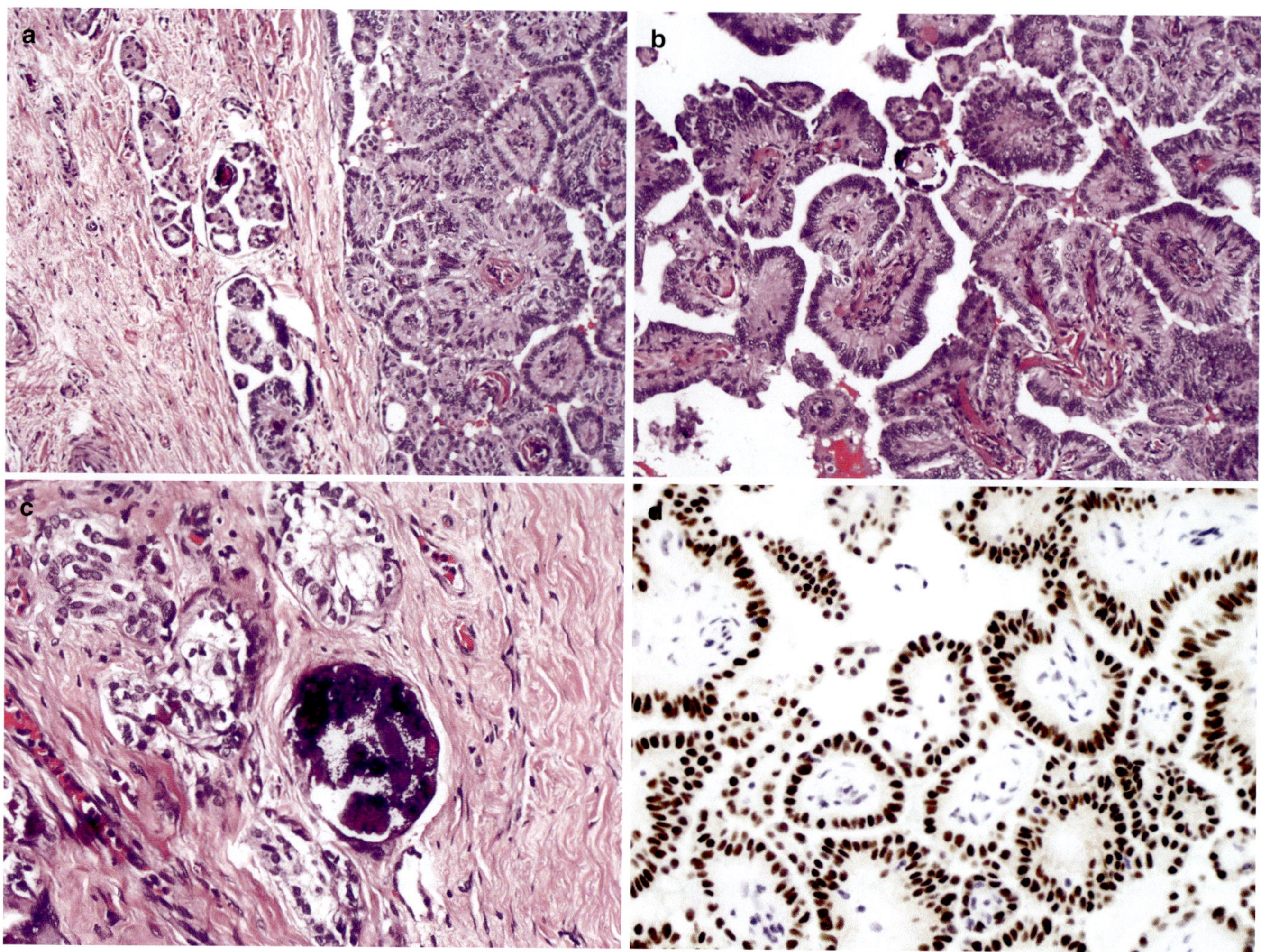

Fig. 6.43 Epididymal adenocarcinoma. (**a**) Tumor may show papillary and tubular features. (**b**) Papillary structures are lined by cuboidal cells with clear cytoplasm. (**c**) Focal calcification is present. (**d**) Tumor is positive for PAX8

Table 6.24 Comparison of clinicopathologic features between testicular germ cell tumor and metastatic adenocarcinoma to the testis

	Germ cell tumors	Metastatic adenocarcinoma
Pathology	Usually unilateral and bilateral in 5% of cases Seminoma, embryonal carcinoma, yolk sac tumor, and teratoma are among the most common types Each type shows distinct morphologic features and growth patterns GCNIS is present iso12p is present Positive for GCT markers, including OCT3/4, Sall4, and PLAP	Mostly unilateral and bilateral in 20% of cases Carcinomas of the prostate, GI tract, kidney and lung are among the most common primary Metastases show morphologic features similar to the primary tumors Lack iso12p Negative for GCTmarkers Positive for the lineage-specific markers of the primary tumors – NKX3.1 for prostate cancer; TTF-1 for lung cancer; CDX-2 for colon cancer; PAX8 for kidney cancer
Clinical features	Account for >90% of testicular tumros Young patient with a mean age of 30 years Testicular mass, sometimes with pain Elevated serum markers (LDH, AFP and βHCG) Orchiectomy, chemotherapy, or radiation therapy Most are malignant with frequent metastasis but prognosis is excellent Cure rates are close to 100% for local disease and 80% for metastasis	Account for <5% of tesituclar tumors Usually old patients with a mean age of 60 years. Testicular or paratesticular mass. Symptoms associated with the primary tumors Normal serum markers Systemic therapy directed to primary tumor Generally poor

Table 6.25 Comparison of clinicopathologic features between paratesticular lipoma and liposarcoma

	Lipoma	Liposarcoma
Pathology	A soft lobulated, well-defined mass lacking areas of hemorrhage or necrosis Mature adipocytes separated by thin fibrous septae No nuclear hyperchromasia, irregularity, or brisk mitotic activity Some lipomas may result from lipomatous hyperplasia of paratesticular soft tissue or extension of fat in an inguinal hernia rather than true neoplasms No MDM2 amplification No chromosomal abnormalities.	Well-differentiated liposarcoma appears as a soft lobulated, variably well-defined large fatty mass (3–30 cm) Dedifferentiated and pleomorphic liposarcomas may appear fleshy and often have necrosis, hemorrhage 50–60% of cases are well-differentiated type, which usually shows mature adipose tissue and a few lipoblasts characterized by nuclear indentation by intracytoplasmic lipid vacuoles (Fig. 6.44a, b). The stromal cells may have enlarged hyperchromatic nuclei Dedifferentiated type consists of an undifferentiated pleomorphic sarcoma, usually arising from a pre-existing well-differentiated liposarcoma Myxoid and pleomorphic types may also be seen and identical to those in other soft tissues locations. MDM2 amplification Giant marker/ring chromosomes in well-differentiated and dedifferentiated liposarcomas
Clinical features	A wide age range The most common paratesticular mesenchymal tumor Intrascrotal soft mass typically located in the upper portion of the spermatic cord Benign Local excision	Old patients with a mean age of 56 years Account for 20–56% of all paratesticular sarcomas Scrotal swelling near the base of the spermatic cord. Well-differentiated type often recurs but does not metastasize Dedifferentiated liposarcomas have a 5-year mortality rate of 10–30%. Conservative complete excision Radical orchiectomy, if the testis is involved

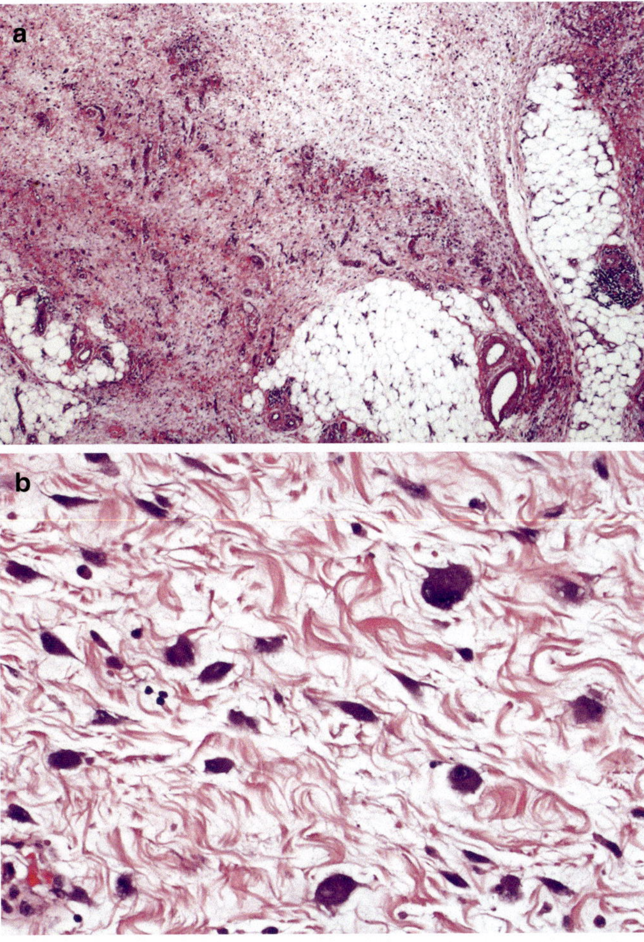

Fig. 6.44 Well-differentiated liposarcoma of the spermatic cord. (**a**) Tumor shows mature adipose tissue with bands of fibrotic stroma. (**b**) There are atypical stromal cells with enlarged hyperchromatic nuclei

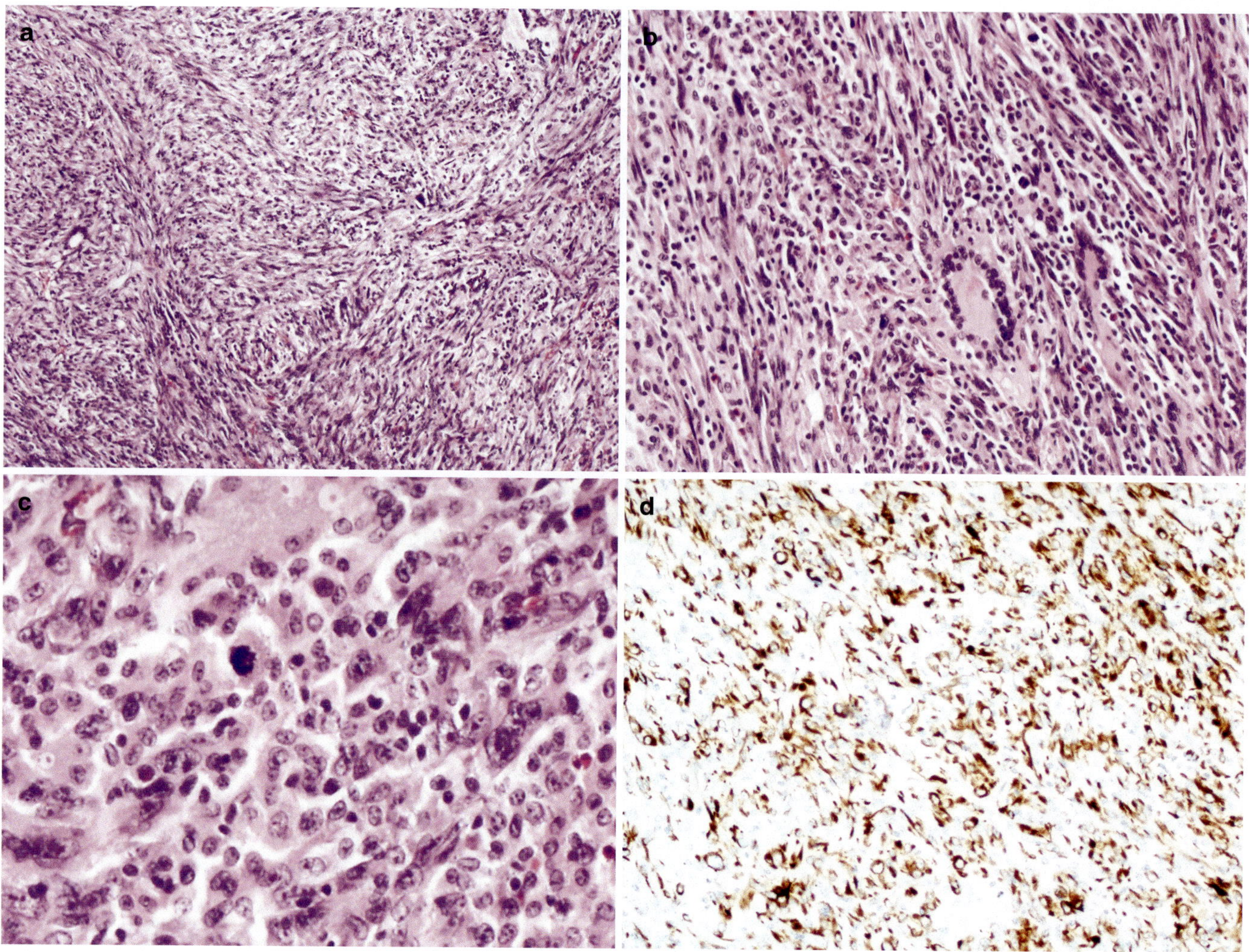

Fig. 6.45 Leiomyosarcoma of the spermatic cord. (**a**) Tumor is characterized by fascicles of atypical spindle cell proliferation. (**b**) Tumor cells show high-grade nuclear atypia. (**c**) Atypical mitosis is present. (**d**) Tumor is positive for desmin

Table 6.26 Comparison of clinicopathologic features between paratesticular rhabdomyosarcoma and leiomyosarcoma

	Rhabdomyosarcoma	Leiomyosarcoma
Pathology	Usually a lobulated, tan-white, glistening, soft tumor with focal hemorrhage and necrosis Most are embryonal type, consisting of primitive small round or spindle cells with hyperchromatic nuclei (Fig. 6.46a) Often show variable numbers of differentiated rhabdomyoblasts with distinct eosinophilic cytoplasm and discernible cross striation (Fig. 6.46b) Spindle cell type is characterized by fusiform cells arranged in a fascicle or storiform pattern. Alveolar and pleomorphic types are rare. Positive for desmin (Fig. 6.46c), muscle specific actin, myogenin (Fig. 6.46d), and MyoD1	Usually a solid, tan-white, well-circumscribed tumor with a whorled cut surface Characterized by fascicles of spindle cells with eosinophilic cytoplasm and cigar-shaped nuclei Tumor cells show variable degree (grade 1–3) of pleomorphism, tumor necrosis, and mitotic activity Tumor covers the entire spectrum of smooth muscle differentiation Other variants, such as myxoid and epithelioid, may be occasionally seen Positive for desmin and muscle specific actin Negative for myogenin and MyoD1
Clinical features	Usually occurs in children with a mean age of 6.6 years (range, 5–40 years). Painless paratesticular mass Orchiectomy for localized disease Systemic therapy for metastasis Excellent with a 5-year overall survival rate of about 90%	Usually occurs in old men with a mean age of 64 years (range, 17–92 years) Painless paratesticular mass Orchiectomy for localized disease Systemic therapy for metastasis Low grade may recur but not metastasize High grade often metastasizes and cause patient death

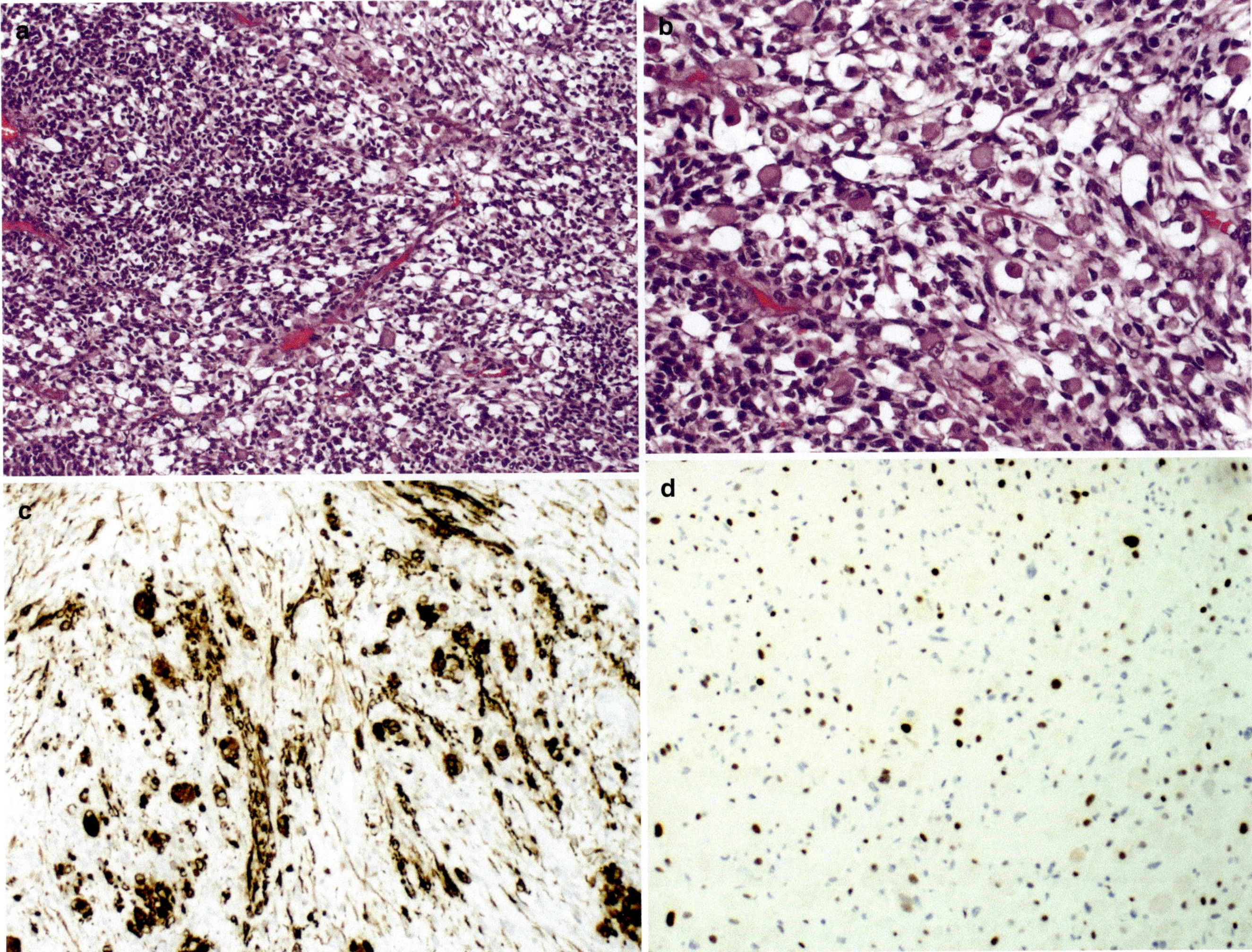

Fig. 6.46 Embryonal-type rhabdomyosarcoma. (**a**) Tumor consists of primitive small round and spindle cells with hyperchromatic nuclei. (**b**) Tumor shows a large number of differentiated rhabdomyoblasts with distinct eosinophilic cytoplasm. (**c**) Tumor is positive for desmin. (**d**) Tumor is positive for myogenin

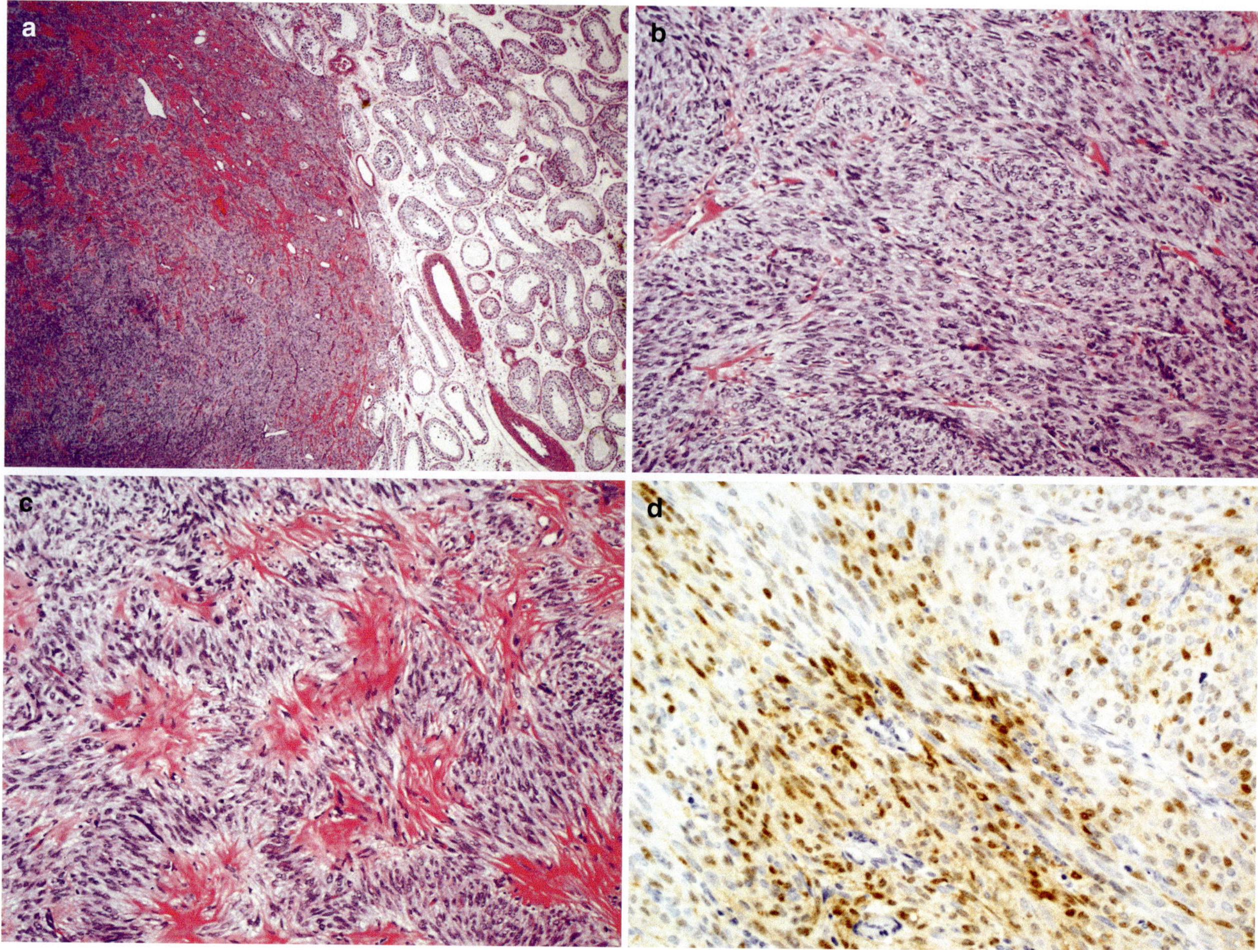

Fig. 6.47 Myoid gonadal cell tumor. (**a**) Tumor is well-circumscribed but not encapsulated. (**b**) Tumor shows densely packed, uniform spindle cells arranged in short fascicles. (**c**) Tumor cells show spindle nuclei and scant cytoplasm with prominent intervening collagen deposits. (**d**) Tumor is positive for S100

Table 6.27 Comparison of clinicopathologic features between testicular lymphoma and seminoma

	Seminoma	Testicular lymphoma
Pathology	Usually unilateral Usually a well-demarcated, tan-white multinodular mass with a mean size of 4 cm Typically shows diffuse growth pattern with solid sheets of tumor cells separated by fibrous septa. Sometimes focal cord or tubular patterns. Tumor cells show uniform and round nuclei with prominent nucleoli, distinctive cell borders, and abundant clear cytoplasm Septa usually contains abundant lymphocytes and chronic granulomatous inflammation Syncytiotrophoblasts present in 20% of cases GCNIS is present Positive for SALL4, OCT3/4, C-KIT, and PLAP Negative for CD45, CD20, and BCL2 Positive for Iso12p	Most are unilateral, but 15% of cases are bilateral A discrete fleshy, tan-white tumor with a mean of 6 cm Typically shows an interstitial growth pattern, with tumor cells surrounding but not replacing the seminiferous tubules About 80–90% of cases are diffuse large B-cell lymphomas, which are composed of atypical cells with large nuclei, prominent nucleoli, brisk mitotic activity, and scant cytoplasm (Fig. 6.48a, b). Follicular lymphoma, plasmacytoma, and other lymphomas are rare It may also involve the epididymis (60%) and spermatic cord (40%) GCNIS is absent Positive for CD45, CD20, and BCL-2 (Fig. 6.48c) Negative for SALL4, OCT3/4, C-KIT, and PLAP Negative for iso12p
Clinical features	Young patients with a mean age of 40 years The most common testicular tumor Painless scrotal swelling Orchiectomy followed by radiation and/or chemotherapy 30% of patients may have metastasis at presentation but prognosis is excellent Overall survival rate is 95%	Old patients with a mean age of 60 years The most common testicular tumor in men older than 50 years Painless testicular mass Orchiectomy followed by chemotherapy Recurrence in up to 80% of cases The 5-year survival is 60% for early stage and 20% for advanced stage

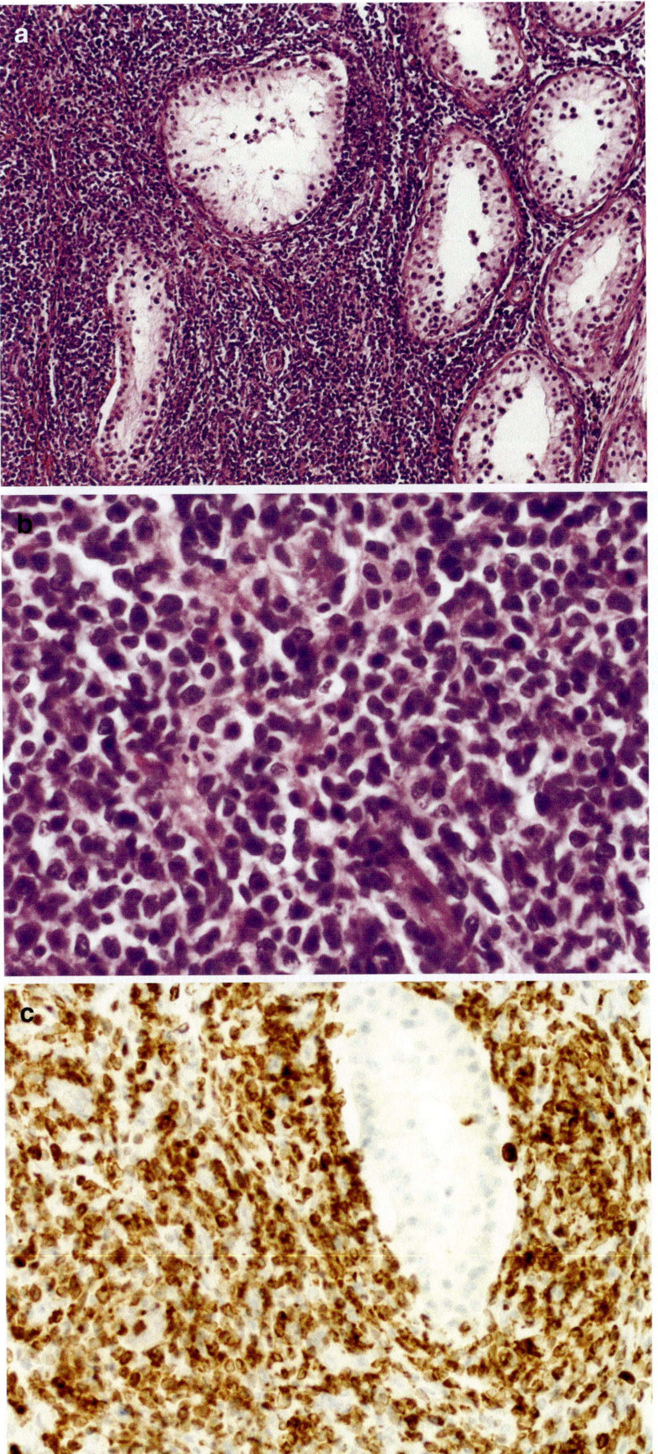

Fig. 6.48 Diffuse large B-cell lymphoma. (**a**) It shows an infiltrative growth pattern in the stroma around seminiferous tubules. (**b**) It is composed of large atypical cells with round to oval nuclei and scant cytoplasm. (**c**) It is positive for BCL-2

Table 6.28 Comparison of clinicopathologic features between adenomatoid tumor and malignant mesothelioma

	Adenomatoid tumor	Malignant mesothelioma
Pathology	Usually arise from the epididymis, sometimes from the spermatic cord and tunica Usually a unilateral, well-circumscribed, homogenous tan-white, small tumor (typically <2 cm) in the epididymis It is characterized by gland-like or vascular-like spaces lined by an attenuated layer of neoplastic cells that often form thin, bridging strands across the lumen Prominent intracytoplasmic vacuolization component may be present Cytologic atypia is minimal Necrosis, perineural invasion and lymphovascular invasion are uncommon	Usually arise from the tunica vaginalis, sometimes wrap around the testicular parenchyma The tumor coats the thickened tunica vaginalis with tan-white, solid or papillary friable nodules with focal hemorrhage and necrosis Tumor usually shows an invasive growth pattern with complex papillary or tubular architectures Tumor cells may show striking pleomorphism, with mitoses and prominent nucleoli 25% are biphasic with both epithelial and sarcomatoid components Some may have squamous, bone and cartilage differentiation
Clinical features	Younger adults with a mean age of 36 years No known risk factor The most common neoplasm in the paratesticular region. Scrotal mass Usually radical orchiectomy Sometimes partial orchiectomy upon confirming the diagnosis on frozen section Benign tumor with no metastatic potential	Old patients with a mean age of 60 years Asbestos exposure is a risking factor Scrotal mass, sometimes hydrocele Radical orchiectomy for local disease Retroperitoneal lymph node dissection, radiation and chemotherapy for metastatic disease. Aggressive malignant disease with a median survival of 24 months and recurrence in 60% of patients in 2 years

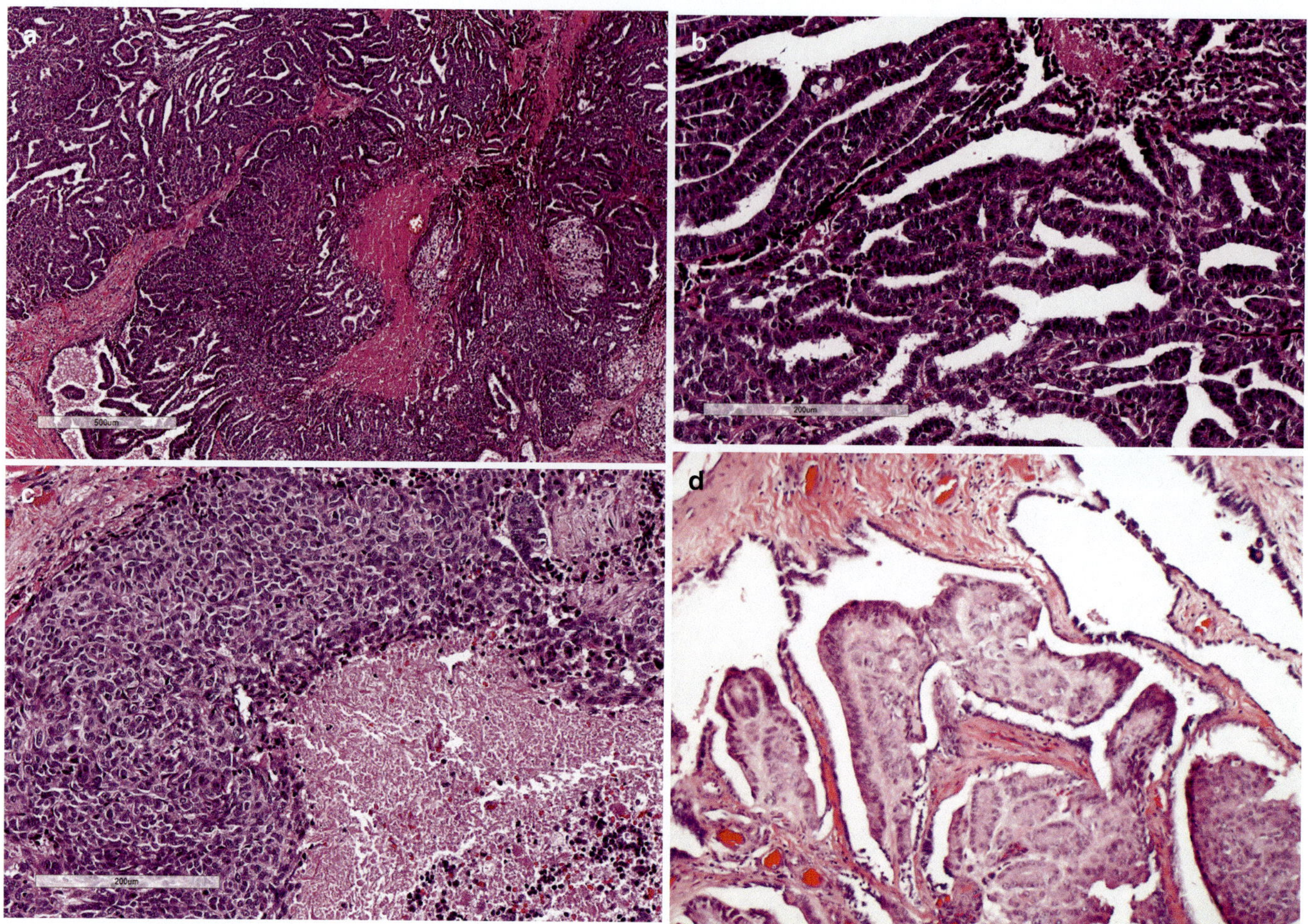

Fig. 6.49 Rete testis adenocarcinoma. (**a**) Tumor shows papillary and tubuloglandular growth patterns. (**b**) Tumor cells are cuboidal to columnar with marked nuclear atypia. (**c**) Tumor necrosis is present. (**d**) Tumor grows within channels of the rete testis

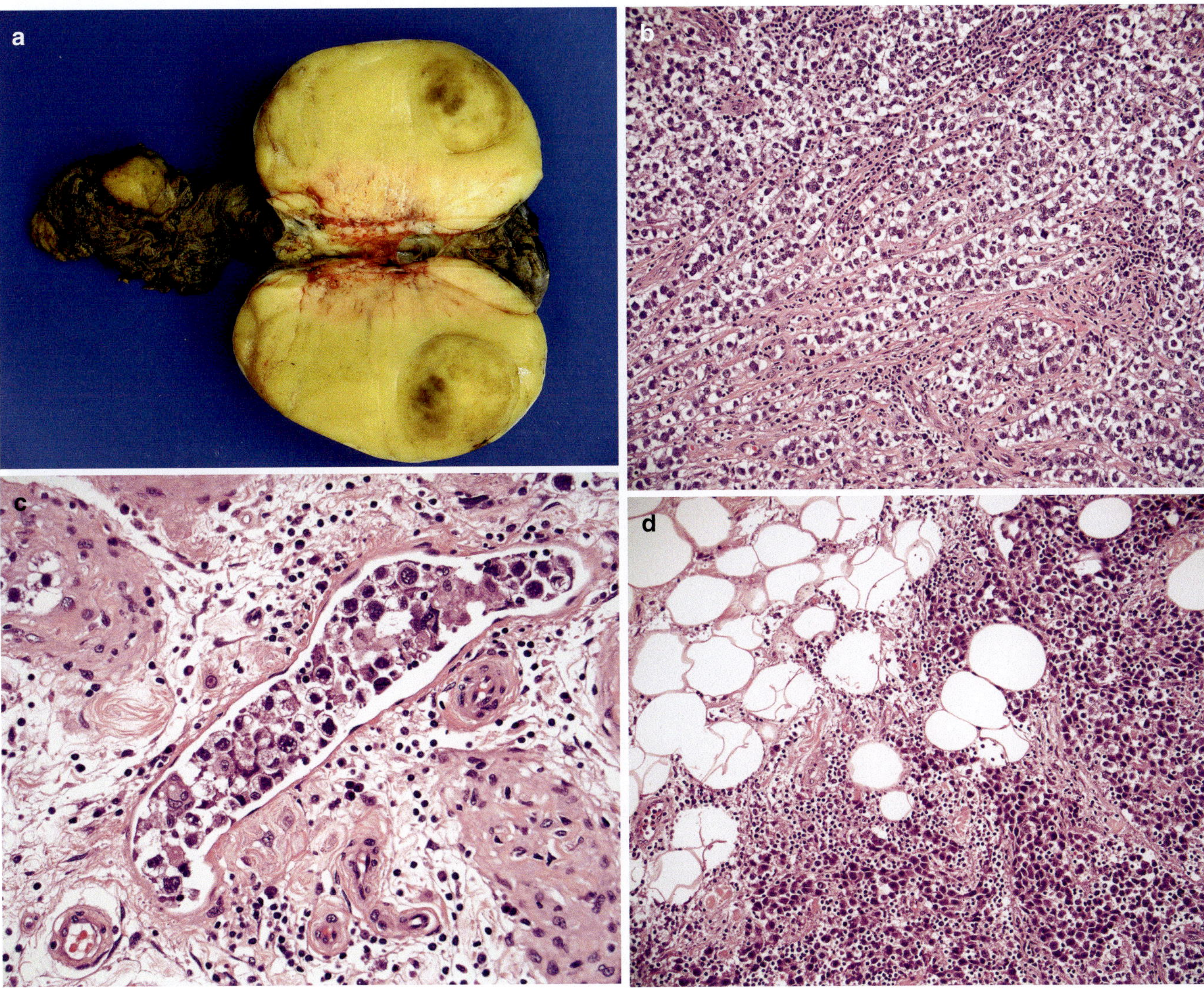

Fig. 6.50 Case 1. (**a**) Gross showing tan tumor occupying entire enlarged testis and invading surrounding hilar fat. (**b**) Tumor is separated by thin fibrous bands containing lymphocytes. Tumor cells are nonoverlapping with cleared-out cytoplasm and prominent nuclei. (**c**) Tumor is within lymphovascular spaces. This embolus is cohesive with smooth contours and is focally against the vessel wall. (**d**) Direct invasion of the hilar fat is seen

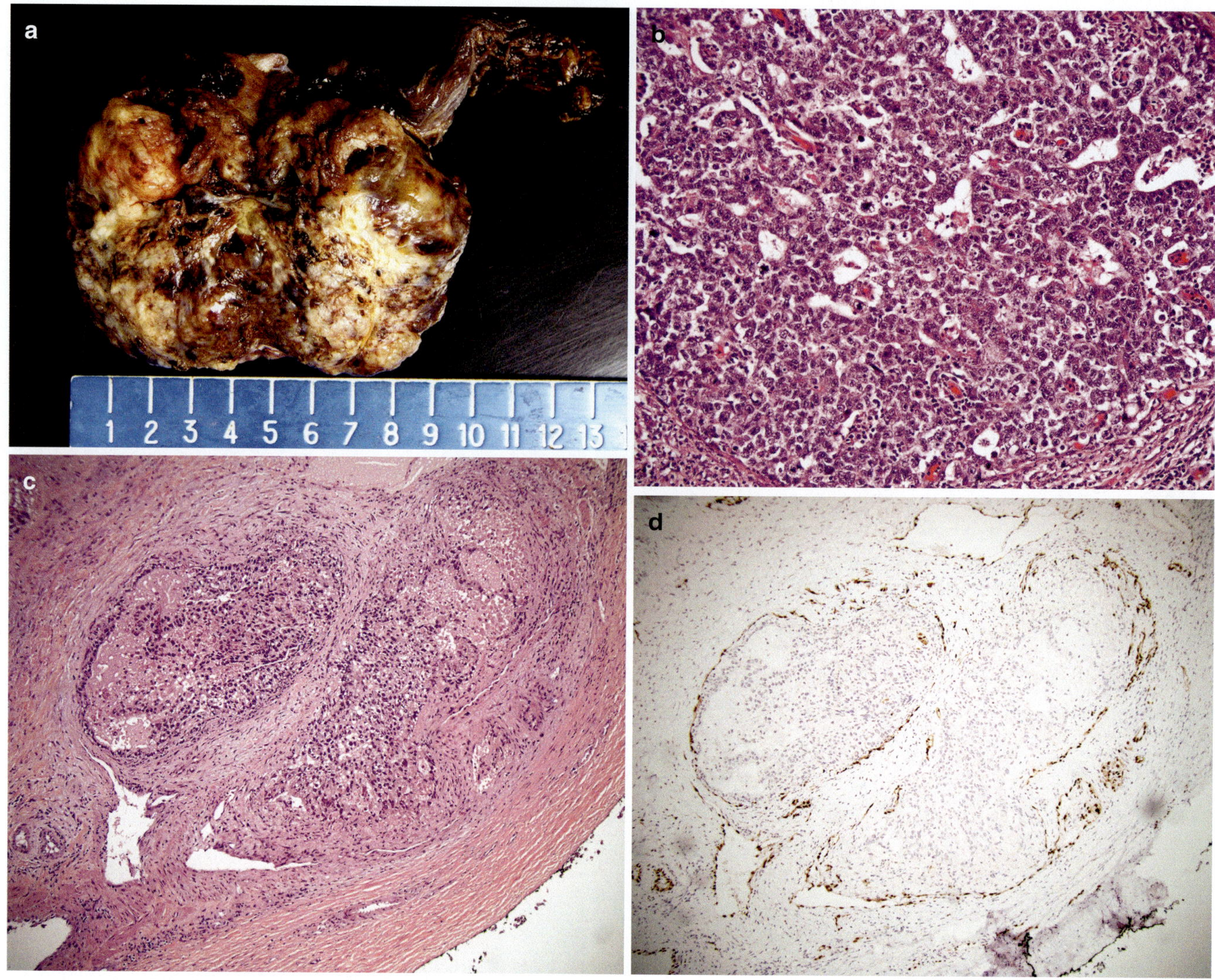

Fig. 6.51 Case 2. (**a**) Variegated, large tumor with hemorrhage and focal cyst formation. (**b**) Tumor cells are pleomorphic and overlapping and have prominent nucleoli. (**c**) Vascular emboli are difficult to appreciate as the tumor completely fills the vessels. (**d**) ERG immunostain confirms that the tumor is within vessels

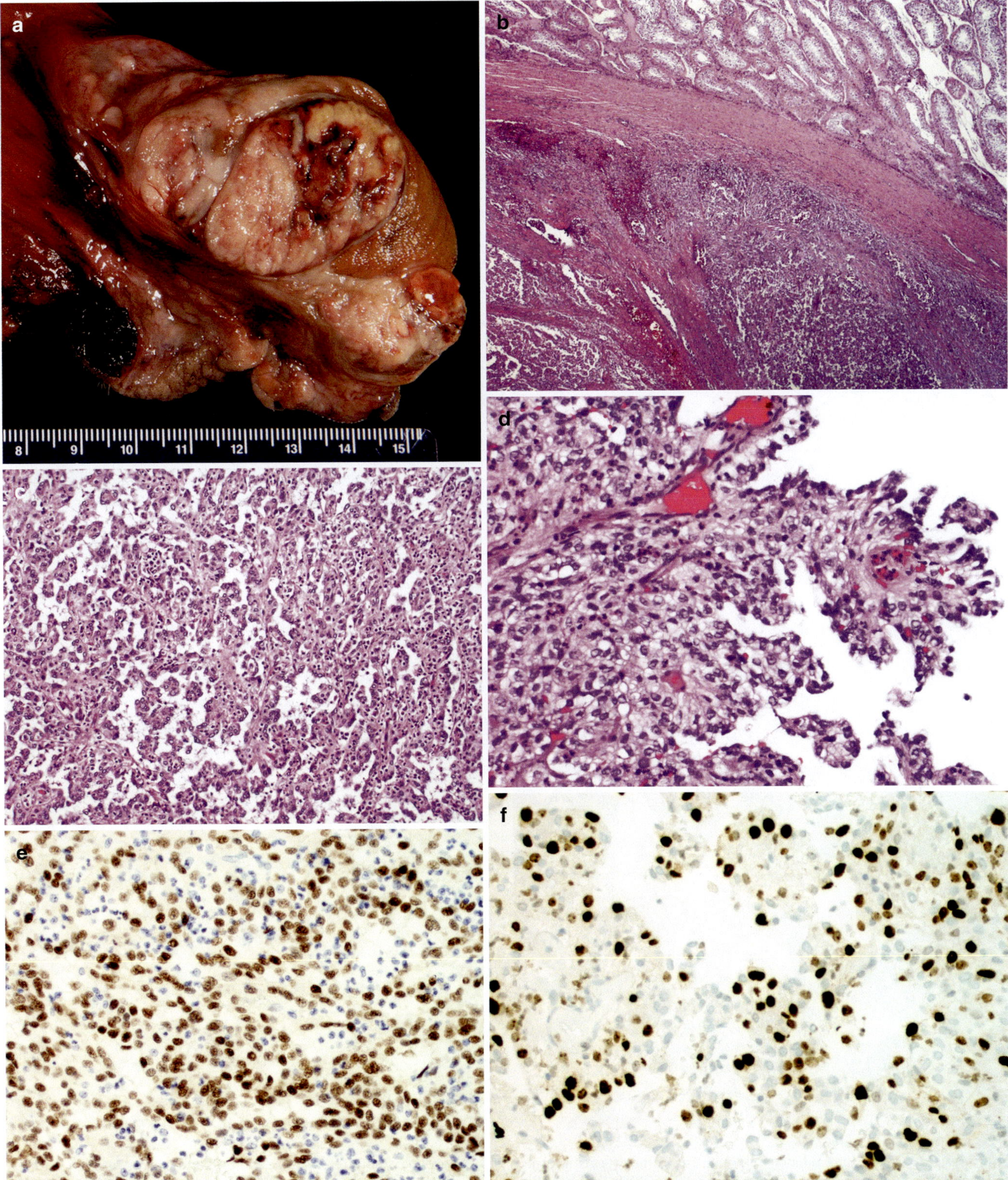

Fig. 6.52 Clear cell carcinoma of the rete testis. (**a**) Resection shows a poorly defined, tan-white mass centered at the rete testis with focal areas of necrosis and hemorrhage. (**b**) Tumor has a thick fibrous capsule and does not invade into the testicular parenchyma. (**c**) Tumor shows extensive papillary features with high nuclear grade. (**d**) Papillary structures are lined by tumor cells with clear cytoplasm. (**e**) Tumor is positive for PAX-8. (**f**) Tumor shows a Ki-67-staining index of approximately 30%

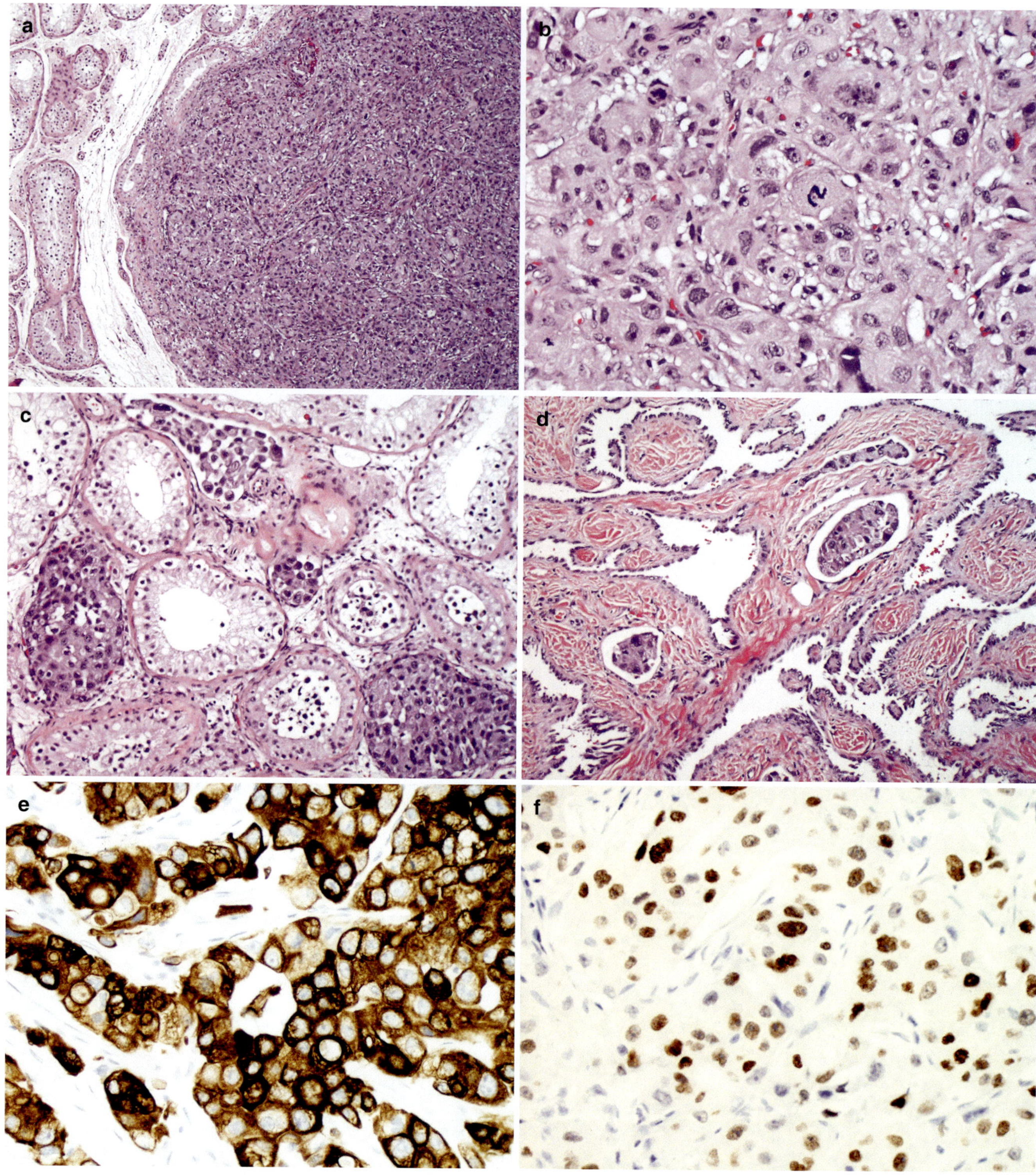

Fig. 6.53 Metastatic lung adenocarcinoma. (**a**) Tumor forms a large solid nodular involving the testicular parenchyma. (**b**) Tumor cells show high-grade nuclear atypia and mitoses. (**c**) Tumor infiltrates the stroma around seminiferous tubules. (**d**) Tumor involves the rete testis with lymphovascular invasion. (**e**) Tumor is positive for CK7 (**e**), TTF-1 (**f**), and Napsin (**g**) and negative for SALL-4 (**h**)

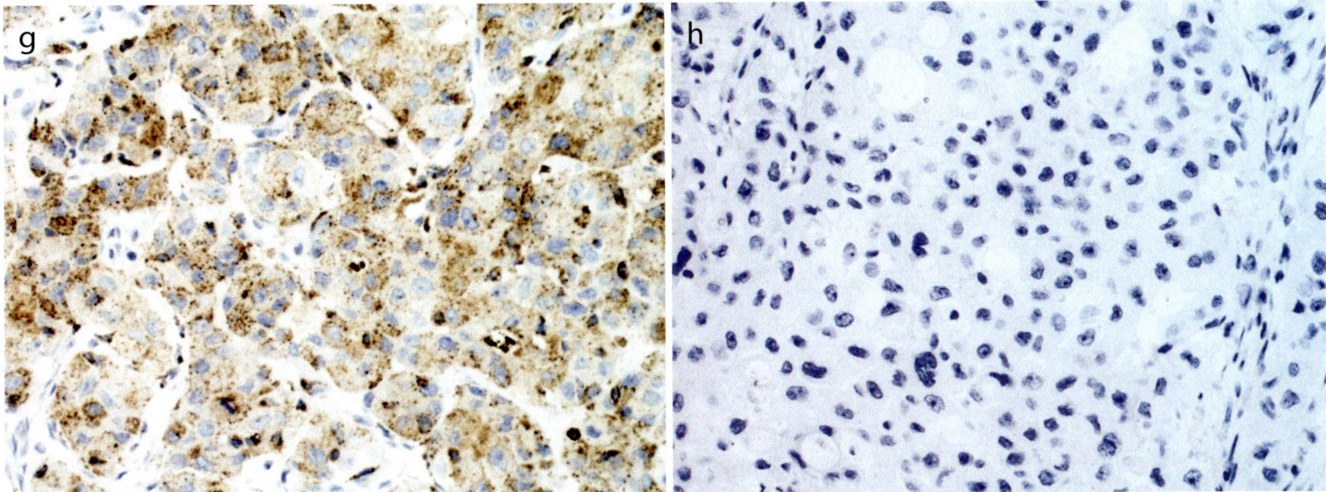

Fig. 6.53 (continued)

References

1. Spratt DE, Suresh K, Osawa T, Schipper M, Jackson WC, Abugharib A, Lebastchi A, Smith D, Montgomery JS, Palapattu GS, Priya Kunju L, Wu A, Lew M, Tomlins SA, Chinnaiyan AM, Weizer AZ, Hafez KS, Kaffenberger SD, Udager A, Mehra R. Detailed pathologic analysis on the co-occurrence of non-seminomatous germ cell tumor subtypes in matched orchiectomy and retroperitoneal lymph node dissections. Med Oncol. 2018;35(3):21.

2. Albers P, Albrecht W, Algaba F, Bokemeyer C, Cohn-Cedermark G, Fizazi K, Horwich A, Laguna MP, Nicolai N. Oldenburg J; European Association of Urology. Guidelines on testicular cancer: 2015 update. Eur Urol. 2015;68(6):1054–68.

3. Alexandre J, Fizazi K, Mahé C, et al. Stage I non-seminomatous germ-cell tumours of the testis: identification of a subgroup of patients with a very low risk of relapse. Eur J Cancer. 2001;37:576–82.

4. Alvarado-Cabrero I, Hernández-Toriz N, Paner GP. Clinicopathologic analysis of choriocarcinoma as a pure or predominant component of germ cell tumor of the testis. Am J Surg Pathol. 2014;38(1):111–8.

5. Beck SD, Foster RS, Bihrle R, Ulbright T, Koch MO, Wahle GR, Einhorn LH, Donohue JP. Teratoma in the orchiectomy specimen and volume of metastasis are predictors of retroperitoneal teratoma in post-chemotherapy nonseminomatous testis cancer. J Urol. 2002;168(4 Pt 1):1402–4.

6. Beyer J, Albers P, Altena R, et al. Maintaining success, reducing treatment burden, focusing on survivorship: highlights from the third European consensus conference on diagnosis and treatment of germ-cell cancer. Ann Oncol. 2013;24(4):878–88.

7. Boormans JL, Mayor de Castro J, Marconi L, Yuan Y, Laguna Pes MP, Bokemeyer C, Nicolai N, Algaba F, Oldenburg J, Albers P. Testicular tumour size and rete testis invasion as prognostic factors for the risk of relapse of clinical stage I seminoma testis patients under surveillance: a systematic review by the testicular cancer guidelines panel. Eur Urol. 2018;73(3):394–405.

8. Cost NG, Lubahn JD, Adibi M, et al. Risk stratification of pubertal children and postpubertal adolescents with clinical stage I testicular nonseminomatous germ cell tumors. J Urol. 2014;191:1485–90.

9. Dong P, Liu ZW, Li XD, et al. Risk factors for relapse in patients with clinical stage I testicular nonseminomatous germ cell tumors. Med Oncol. 2013;30:494–501.

10. French BL, Zynger DL. Do histopathologic variables affect the reporting of lymphovascular invasion in testicular germ cell tumors? Am J Clin Pathol. 2016;145(3):341–9.

11. Fung CY, Kalish LA, Brodsky GL, et al. Stage I nonseminomatous germ cell testicular tumor: prediction of metastatic potential by primary histopathology. J Clin Oncol. 1988;6:1467–73.

12. Hermans BP, Sweeney CJ, Foster RS, et al. Risk of systemic metastases in retroperitoneal lymph node dissection. J Urol. 2000;163:1721–4.

13. Groll RJ, Warde P, Jewett MA. A comprehensive systematic review of testicular germ cell tumor surveillance. Crit Rev Oncol Hematol. 2007;64(3):182–97.

14. Guo CC, Punar M, Contreras AL, Tu SM, Pisters L, Tamboli P, Czerniak B. Testicular germ cell tumors with sarcomatous components: an analysis of 33 cases. Am J Surg Pathol. 2009;33(8):1173–8.

15. Kollmannsberger C, Tandstad T, Bedard PL, Cohn-Cedermark G, Chung PW, Jewett MA, Powles T, Warde PR, Daneshmand S, Protheroe A, Tyldesley S, Black PC, Chi K, So AI, Moore MJ, Nichols CR. Patterns of relapse in patients with clinical stage I testicular cancer managed with active surveillance. J Clin Oncol. 2015;33(1):51–7.

16. Lorch A, Beyer J. How we treat germ cell cancers. Cancer. 2017;123(12):2190–2.

17. Magers MJ, Kao CS, Cole CD, Rice KR, Foster RS, Einhorn LH, Ulbright TM. "Somatic-type" malignancies arising from testicular germ cell tumors: a clinicopathologic study of 124 cases with emphasis on glandular tumors supporting frequent yolk sac tumor origin. Am J Surg Pathol. 2014;38(10):1396–409.

18. Mosharafa AA, Foster RS, Leibovich BC, Ulbright TM, Bihrle R, Einhorn LH, Donohue JP. Histology in mixed germ cell tumors. Is there a favorite pairing? J Urol. 2004;171(4):1471–3.

19. Moul JW, McCarthy WF, Fernandez EB, et al. Percentage of embryonal carcinoma and of vascular invasion predicts pathological stage in clinical stage I nonseminomatous testicular cancer. Cancer Res. 1994;54:362–4.

20. Oldenburg J, Fosså SD, Nuver J, Heidenreich A, Schmoll HJ, Bokemeyer C, Horwich A, Beyer J, Kataja V, ESMO Guidelines Working Group. Testicular seminoma and non-seminoma: ESMO clinical practice guidelines for diagnosis, treatment and follow-up. Ann Oncol. 2013;24(Suppl 6):vi125–32.

21. Powles T, Warde PR, Daneshmand S, Protheroe A, Tyldesley S, Black PC, Chi K, So AI, Moore MJ, Nichols CR. Patterns of relapse in patients with clinical stage I testicular cancer managed with active surveillance. J Clin Oncol. 2015;33(1):51–7.

22. Reilley MJ, Pagliaro LC. Testicular choriocarcinoma: a rare variant that requires a unique treatment approach. Curr Oncol Rep. 2015;17(2):2.

23. Stephenson AJ, Bosl GJ, Bajorin DF, et al. Retroperitoneal lymph node dissection in patients with low stage testicular cancer with embryonal carcinoma predominance and/or lymphovascular invasion. J Urol. 2005;174:557–60.

24. Vergouwe Y, Steyerberg EW, Eijkemans MJ, et al. Predictors of occult metastasis in clinical stage I nonseminoma: a systematic review. J Clin Oncol. 2003;2:4092–9.

25. Trevino KE, Esmaeili-Shandiz A, Saeed O, Xu H, Ulbright TM, Idrees MT. Pathological risk factors for higher clinical stage in testicular seminomas. Histopathology. 2018;73(5):741–7.

26. Valdevenito JP, Gallegos I, Fernández C, Acevedo C, Palma R. Correlation between primary tumor pathologic features and presence of clinical metastasis at diagnosis of testicular seminoma. Urology. 2007;70(4):777–80.

27. Yilmaz A, Cheng T, Zhang J, Trpkov K. Testicular hilum and vascular invasion predict advanced clinical stage in nonseminomatous germ cell tumors. Mod Pathol. 2013;26(4):579–86.

28. Berney DM, Warren AY, Verma M, Kudahetti S, Robson JM, Williams MW, Neal DE, Powles T, Shamash J, Oliver RT. Malignant germ cell tumours in the elderly: a histopathological review of 50 cases in men aged 60 years or over. Mod Pathol. 2008;21(1):54–9.

29. Moch H, Cubilla AL, Humphrey PA, Reuter VE, Ulbright TM. The 2016 WHO classification of tumours of the urinary system and male genital organs-part a: renal, penile, and testicular tumours. Eur Urol. 2016;70(1):93–105.

30. Ulbright TM. Recently described and clinically important entities in testis tumors. Arch Pathol Lab Med. 2019;143(6):711–21.

31. Williamson SR, Delahunt B, Magi-Galluzzi C, Algaba F, Egevad L, Ulbright TM, Tickoo SK, Srigley JR, Epstein JI, Berney DM, Members of the ISUP Testicular Tumour Panel. The World Health Organization 2016 classification of testicular germ cell tumours: a review and update from the International Society of Urological Pathology Testis Consultation Panel. Histopathology. 2017;70(3):335–46.

32. Genco IS, Ratzon F, Glickman L, Santagada E, Unger P. Intratubular teratoma: a rare form of testicular germ cell neoplasia. Int J Surg Pathol. 2019;24:1066896919836491. https://doi.org/10.1177/1066896919836491. [Epub ahead of print]. PubMed PMID: 30907201.

33. Roth LM, Lyu B, Cheng L. Perspectives on testicular sex cord-stromal tumors and those composed of both germ cells and sex cord-stromal derivatives with a comparison to corresponding ovarian neoplasms. Hum Pathol. 2017;65:1–14.

34. Ye H, Ulbright TM. Difficult differential diagnoses in testicular pathology. Arch Pathol Lab Med. 2012;136(4):435–46.

35. Ulbright TM. The most common, clinically significant misdiagnoses in testicular tumor pathology, and how to avoid them. Adv Anat Pathol. 2008;15(1):18–27.

36. Morinaga S, Ojima M, Sasano N. Human chorionic gonadotropin and alpha-fetoprotein in testicular germ cell tumors. An immunohistochemical study in comparison with tissue concentrations. Cancer. 1983;52(7):1281–9.

37. Butcher DN, Gregory WM, Gunter PA, Masters JR, Parkinson MC. The biologicaland clinical significance of HCG-containing cells in seminoma. Br J Cancer. 1985;51(4):473–8.

38. von Hochstetter AR, Sigg C, Saremaslani P, Hedinger C. The significance of giant cells in human testicular seminomas. A clinicopathological study. Virchows Arch A Pathol Anat Histopathol. 1985;407(3):309–22.

39. Hori K, Uematsu K, Yasoshima H, Sakurai K, Yamada A. Contribution of cell proliferative activity to malignancy potential in testicular seminoma. Pathol Int. 1997;47(5):282–7.

40. Zuckman MH, Williams G, Levin HS. Mitosis counting in seminoma: an exercise of questionable significance. Hum Pathol. 1988;19(3):329–35.

41. von Hochstetter AR. Mitotic count in seminomas--an unreliable criterion for distinguishing between classical and anaplastic types. Virchows Arch A Pathol Anat Histol. 1981;390(1):63–9.

42. Kao CS, Ulbright TM, Young RH, Idrees MT. Testicular embryonal carcinoma: amorphologic study of 180 cases highlighting unusual and unemphasized aspects. Am J Surg Pathol. 2014;38(5):689–97.

43. Rajab R, Berney DM. Ten testicular trapdoors. Histopathology. 2008;53(6):728–39.

44. Nogales FF, Preda O, Nicolae A. Yolk sac tumours revisited. A review of their many faces and names. Histopathology. 2012;60(7):1023–33.

45. Howitt BE, Magers MJ, Rice KR, Cole CD, Ulbright TM. Many postchemotherapy sarcomatous tumors in patients with testicular germ cell tumors are sarcomatoid yolk sac tumors: a study of 33 cases. Am J Surg Pathol. 2015;39(2):251–9.

46. Ulbright TM. Germ cell tumors of the gonads: a selective review emphasizing problems in differential diagnosis, newly appreciated, and controversial issues. Mod Pathol. 2005;18(Suppl 2):S61–79.

47. Wegman SJ, Parwani AV, Zynger DL. Cytokeratin 7, inhibin, and p63 in testicular germ cell tumor: superior markers of choriocarcinoma compared to β-human chorionic gonadotropin. Hum Pathol. 2019;84:254–61.

48. Athanasiou A, Vanel D, El Mesbahi O, Theodore C, Fizazi K. Non-germ cell tumours arising in germ cell tumours (teratoma with malignant transformation) in men: CT and MR findings. Eur J Radiol. 2009;69(2):230–5.

49. Motzer RJ, Amsterdam A, Prieto V, Sheinfeld J, Murty VV, Mazumdar M, Bosl GJ, Chaganti RS, Reuter VE. Teratoma with malignant transformation: diverse malignant histologies arising in men with germ cell tumors. J Urol. 1998;159(1):133–8.

50. Rice KR, Magers MJ, Beck SD, Cary KC, Einhorn LH, Ulbright TM, Foster RS. Management of germ cell tumors with somatic type malignancy: pathological features, prognostic factors and survival outcomes. J Urol. 2014;192(5):1403–9.

51. Malagón HD, Valdez AM, Moran CA, Suster S. Germ cell tumors with sarcomatous components: a clinicopathologic and immunohistochemical study of 46 cases. Am J Surg Pathol. 2007;31(9):1356–62.

52. Matoso A, Idrees MT, Rodriguez FJ, Ibrahim J, Perrino CM, Ulbright TM, Epstein JI. Neuroglial differentiation and neoplasms in testicular germ cell tumors lack immunohistochemical evidence of alterations characteristic of their CNS counterparts: a study of 13 cases. Am J Surg Pathol. 2019;43(3):422–31.

53. Ulbright TM, Hattab EM, Zhang S, Ehrlich Y, Foster RS, Einhorn LH, Cheng L. Primitive neuroectodermal tumors in patients with testicular germ cell tumors usually resemble pediatric-type central nervous system embryonal neoplasms and lack chromosome 22 rearrangements. Mod Pathol. 2010;23(7):972–80; Gondim DD, Ulbright TM, Cheng L, Idrees MT. Primary cystic trophoblas-

tic tumor of the testis: a study of 14 cases. Am J Surg Pathol. 2017;41(6):788–94.

54. Idrees MT, Kao CS, Epstein JI, Ulbright TM. Nonchoriocarcinomatous trophoblastic tumors of the testis: the widening spectrum of trophoblastic neoplasia. Am J Surg Pathol. 2015;39(11):1468–78.

55. Ulbright TM, Henley JD, Cummings OW, Foster RS, Cheng L. Cystic trophoblastic tumor: a nonaggressive lesion in post-chemotherapy resections of patients with testicular germ cell tumors. Am J Surg Pathol. 2004;28(9):1212–6.

56. Angulo JC, González J, Rodríguez N, Hernández E, Núñez C, Rodríguez-Barbero JM, Santana A, López JI. Clinicopathological study of regressed testicular tumors (apparent extragonadal germ cell neoplasms). J Urol. 2009;182(5):2303–10.

57. Balzer BL, Ulbright TM. Spontaneous regression of testicular germ cell tumors: an analysis of 42 cases. Am J Surg Pathol. 2006;30(7):858–65.

58. Berney DM, Lu YJ, Shamash J, Idrees M. Postchemotherapy changes in testicular germ cell tumours: biology and morphology. Histopathology. 2017;70(1):26–39.

59. Cao D, Humphrey PA, Allan RW. SALL4 is a novel sensitive and specific marker for metastatic germ cell tumors, with particular utility in detection of metastatic yolk sac tumors. Cancer. 2009;115(12):2640–51.

60. Cheng L, Zhang S, MacLennan GT, Poulos CK, Sung MT, Beck SD, Foster RS. Interphase fluorescence in situ hybridization analysis of chromosome 12p abnormalities is useful for distinguishing epidermoid cysts of the testis from pure mature teratoma. Clin Cancer Res. 2006;12(19):5668–72.

61. Kum JB, Ulbright TM, Williamson SR, Wang M, Zhang S, Foster RS, Grignon DJ, Eble JN, Beck SD, Cheng L. Molecular genetic evidence supporting the origin of somatic-type malignancy and teratoma from the same progenitor cell. Am J Surg Pathol. 2012;36(12):1849–56.

62. Amin MB. AJCC cancer staging manual. 8th ed. New York: Springer; 2017.

63. Aparicio J, Sánchez-Muñoz A, Gumà J, Domenech M, Meana JA, García-Sánchez J, Bastús R, Gironés R, González-Billalabeitia E, Sagastibelza N, Ochenduszko S, Sánchez A, Terrasa J, Germà-Lluch JR, García Del Muro X, on behalf of the Spanish Germ Cell Cancer Group. A risk-adapted approach to patients with stage I seminoma according to the status of rete testis: the fourth Spanish Germ Cell Cancer Group study. Oncology. 2018;95(1):8–12.

64. Chung P, Daugaard G, Tyldesley S, Atenafu EG, Panzarella T, Kollmannsberger C, Warde P. Evaluation of a prognostic model for risk of relapse in stage I seminoma surveillance. Cancer Med. 2015;4(1):155–60.

65. Sharma P, Dhillon J, Agarwal G, Zargar-Shoshtari K, Sexton WJ. Disparities in interpretation of primary testicular germ cell tumor pathology. Am J Clin Pathol. 2015;144(2):289–94.

66. Farooq A, Jorda M, Whittington E, Kryvenko ON, Braunhut BL, Pavan N, Procházková K, Zhang L, Rai S, Miller T, Liu J, Szabo A, Iczkowski KA. Rete testis invasion is consistent with pathologic stage T1 in germ cell tumors. Am J Clin Pathol. 2019;151(5):479–85.

67. Harari SE, Sassoon DJ, Priemer DS, Jacob JM, Eble JN, Calió A, Grignon DJ, Idrees M, Albany C, Masterson TA, Hanna NH, Foster RS, Ulbright TM, Einhorn LH, Cheng L. Testicular cancer: the usage of central review for pathology diagnosis of orchiectomy specimens. Urol Oncol. 2017;35(10):605.e9–605.e16.

68. Verrill C, Yilmaz A, Srigley JR, Amin MB, Compérat E, Egevad L, Ulbright TM, Tickoo SK, Berney DM, Epstein JI, Members of the International Society of Urological Pathology Testicular Tumor Panel. Reporting and staging of testicular germ cell tumors: the International Society of Urological Pathology (ISUP) testicular cancer consultation conference recommendations. Am J Surg Pathol. 2017;41(6):e22–32.

69. Sanfrancesco JM, Trevino KE, Xu H, Ulbright TM, Idrees MT. The significance of spermatic cord involvement by testicular germ cell tumors: should we be staging discontinuous invasion from involved lymphovascular spaces differently from direct extension? Am J Surg Pathol. 2018;42(3):306–11.

70. McCleskey BC, Epstein JI, Albany C, Hashemi-Sadraei N, Idrees MT, Jorns JM, Lu DY, Matoso A, Rais-Bahrami S, Schwartz LE, Ulbright TM, Gordetsky J. The significance of lymphovascular invasion of the spermatic cord in the absence of cord soft tissue invasion. Arch Pathol Lab Med. 2017;141(6):824–9.

71. Gordetsky J, Sanfrancesco J, Epstein JI, Trevino K, Xu H, Osunkoya A, Xiao GQ, Kao CS, Unger P, Hashemi-Sadraei N, Albany C, Jorns JM, Lu DY, Matoso A, Rais-Bahrami S, Schwartz LE, Ulbright TM, Idrees MT. Do nonseminomatous germ cell tumors of the testis with lymphovascular invasion of the spermatic cord merit staging as pT3? Am J Surg Pathol. 2017;41(10):1397–402.

72. Al-Ahmadie HA, Carver BS, Cronin AM, Olgac S, Tickoo SK, Fine SW, Gopalan A, Stasi J, Rabbani F, Bosl GJ, Sheinfeld J, Reuter VE. Primary retroperitoneal lymph node dissection in low-stage testicular germ cell tumors: a detailed pathologic study with clinical outcome analysis with special emphasis on patients who did not receive adjuvant therapy. Urology. 2013;82(6):1341–6.

73. Tarrant WP, Czerniak BA, Guo CC. Relationship between primary and metastatic testicular germ cell tumors: a clinicopathologic analysis of 100 cases. Hum Pathol. 2013;44(10):2220–6.

74. Giannoulatou E, et al. Whole-genome sequencing of spermatocytic tumors provides insights into the mutational processes operating in the male germline. PLoS One. 2017;12(5):e0178169.

75. Hu R, Ulbright TM, Young RH. Spermatocytic seminoma: a report of 85 cases emphasizing its morphologic spectrum including some aspects not widely known. Am J Surg Pathol. 2019;43(1):1–11.

76. Stueck AE, et al. Spermatocytic tumor with sarcoma: a rare testicular neoplasm. Int J Surg Pathol. 2017;25(6):559–62.

77. Idrees MT, et al. The World Health Organization 2016 classification of testicular non-germ cell tumours: a review and update from the International Society of Urological Pathology Testis Consultation Panel. Histopathology. 2017;70(4):513–21.

78. Ulbright TM. Pitfalls in the interpretation of specimens from patients with testicular tumours, with an emphasis on variant morphologies. Pathology. 2018;50(1):88–99.

79. Ulbright TM, et al. Best practices recommendations in the application of immunohistochemistry in testicular tumors: report from the International Society of Urological Pathology consensus conference. Am J Surg Pathol. 2014;38(8):e50–9.

80. Kao CS, Ulbright TM, Idrees MT. Gonadoblastoma: an immunohistochemical study and comparison to Sertoli cell nodule with intratubular germ cell neoplasia, with pathogenetic implications. Histopathology. 2014;65(6):861–7.

81. Scully RE. Gonadoblastoma. A review of 74 cases. Cancer. 1970;25(6):1340–56.

82. Kao CS, et al. "Dissecting gonadoblastoma" of Scully: a morphologic variant that often mimics germinoma. Am J Surg Pathol. 2016;40(10):1417–23.

83. Vallangeon BD, Eble JN, Ulbright TM. Macroscopic sertoli cell nodule: a study of 6 cases that presented as testicular masses. Am J Surg Pathol. 2010;34(12):1874–80.

84. Young RH, Koelliker DD, Scully RE. Sertoli cell tumors of the testis, not otherwise specified: a clinicopathologic analysis of 60 cases. Am J Surg Pathol. 1998;22(6):709–21.

85. Henley JD, Young RH, Ulbright TM. Malignant Sertoli cell tumors of the testis: a study of 13 examples of a neoplasm frequently misinterpreted as seminoma. Am J Surg Pathol. 2002;26(5):541–50.

86. Madsen EL, Hultberg BM. Metastasizing sertoli cell tumours of the human testis-a report of two cases and a review of the literature. Acta Oncol. 1990;29:946–9.

87. Kratzer SS, et al. Large cell calcifying Sertoli cell tumor of the testis: contrasting features of six malignant and six benign tumors and a review of the literature. Am J Surg Pathol. 1997;21(11):1271–80.

88. Proppe KH, Scully RE. Large-cell calcifying Sertoli cell tumor of the testis. Am J Clin Pathol. 1980;74(5):607–19.

89. Zhang C, Ulbright TM. Nuclear localization of beta-catenin in sertoli cell tumors and other sex cord-stromal tumors of the testis: an immunohistochemical study of 87 cases. Am J Surg Pathol. 2015;39(10):1390–4.

90. Veugelers M, et al. Comparative PRKAR1A genotype-phenotype analyses in humans with Carney complex and prkar1a haploinsufficient mice. Proc Natl Acad Sci U S A. 2004;101(39):14222–7.

91. Ulbright TM, Amin MB, Young RH. Intratubular large cell hyalinizing sertoli cell neoplasia of the testis: a report of 8 cases of a distinctive lesion of the Peutz-Jeghers syndrome. Am J Surg Pathol. 2007;31(6):827–35.

92. Young S, et al. Feminizing Sertoli cell tumors in boys with Peutz-Jeghers syndrome. Am J Surg Pathol. 1995;19(1):50–8.

93. Suardi N, et al. Leydig cell tumour of the testis: presentation, therapy, long-term follow-up and the role of organ-sparing surgery in a single-institution experience. BJU Int. 2009;103(2):197–200.

94. Kim I, Young RH, Scully RE. Leydig cell tumors of the testis. A clinicopathological analysis of 40 cases and review of the literature. Am J Surg Pathol. 1985;9(3):177–92.

95. Naughton CK, et al. Leydig cell hyperplasia. Br J Urol. 1998;81(2):282–9.

96. Cheville JC, et al. Leydig cell tumor of the testis: a clinicopathologic, DNA content, and MIB-1 comparison of nonmetastasizing and metastasizing tumors. Am J Surg Pathol. 1998;22(11):1361–7.

97. McCluggage WG, et al. Cellular proliferation and nuclear ploidy assessments augment established prognostic factors in predicting malignancy in testicular Leydig cell tumours. Histopathology. 1998;33(4):361–8.

98. Jimenez-Quintero LP, et al. Granulosa cell tumor of the adult testis: a clinicopathologic study of seven cases and a review of the literature. Hum Pathol. 1993;24(10):1120–5.

99. Hammerich KH, et al. Malignant advanced granulosa cell tumor of the adult testis: case report and review of the literature. Hum Pathol. 2008;39(5):701–9.

100. Lawrence WD, Young RH, Scully RE. Juvenile granulosa cell tumor of the infantile testis. A report of 14 cases. Am J Surg Pathol. 1985;9(2):87–94.

101. Young RH, Lawrence WD, Scully RE. Juvenile granulosa cell tumor--another neoplasm associated with abnormal chromosomes and ambiguous genitalia. A report of three cases. Am J Surg Pathol. 1985;9(10):737–43.

102. Zhang M, et al. Testicular fibrothecoma: a morphologic and immunohistochemical study of 16 cases. Am J Surg Pathol. 2013;37(8):1208–14.

103. Jones MA, Young RH, Scully RE. Benign fibromatous tumors of the testis and paratesticular region: a report of 9 cases with a proposed classification of fibromatous tumors and tumor-like lesions. Am J Surg Pathol. 1997;21(3):296–305.

104. Deveci MS, et al. Testicular (gonadal stromal) fibroma: case report and review of the literature. Pathol Int. 2002;52(4):326–30.

105. Chekol SS, Sun CC. Malignant mesothelioma of the tunica vaginalis testis: diagnostic studies and differential diagnosis. Arch Pathol Lab Med. 2012;136(1):113–7.

106. Perez-Ordonez B, Srigley JR. Mesothelial lesions of the paratesticular region. Semin Diagn Pathol. 2000;17(4):294–306.

107. Amin MB. Selected other problematic testicular and paratesticular lesions: rete testis neoplasms and pseudotumors, mesothelial lesions and secondary tumors. Mod Pathol. 2005;18(Suppl 2):S131–45.

108. Di Naro N, et al. Reactive pseudo-glandular mesothelial hyperplasia in testis tunica vaginalis: a case report. Pathologica. 2011;103(5):304–6.

109. Delahunt B, et al. Immunohistochemical evidence for mesothelial origin of paratesticular adenomatoid tumour. Histopathology. 2000;36(2):109–15.

110. Wachter DL, et al. Adenomatoid tumors of the female and male genital tract. A comparative clinicopathologic and immunohistochemical analysis of 47 cases emphasizing their site-specific morphologic diversity. Virchows Arch. 2011;458(5):593–602.

111. Sangoi AR, et al. Adenomatoid tumors of the female and male genital tracts: a clinicopathological and immunohistochemical study of 44 cases. Mod Pathol. 2009;22(9):1228–35.

112. Ulbright TM, Young RH. Metastatic carcinoma to the testis: a clinicopathologic analysis of 26 nonincidental cases with emphasis on deceptive features. Am J Surg Pathol. 2008;32(11):1683–93.

113. Tiltman AJ. Metastatic tumours in the testis. Histopathology. 1979;3(1):31–7.

114. Chauhan RD, et al. The natural progression of adenocarcinoma of the epididymis. J Urol. 2001;166(2):608–10.

115. Ganem JP, Jhaveri FM, Marroum MC. Primary adenocarcinoma of the epididymis: case report and review of the literature. Urology. 1998;52(5):904–8.

116. Ulbright TM, Amin MB, Balzer B, Berney DM, Epstein JI, Guo CC, Idrees MT, Looigenga LHJ, Paner G, Rajpert-De Meyts E, Skakkebark NE, Tickoo SK, Yilmaz A, Oosterhuis JW. Germ cell tumors. In: Moch H, Humphrey PA, Ulbright TM, Retuer VE, editors. WHO classification of tumours of the urinary system and male genital organs. 4th ed. Lyon: IARC Press; 2016.

117. Montgomery E, Fisher C. Paratesticular liposarcoma: a clinicopathologic study. Am J Surg Pathol. 2003;27(1):40–7.

118. Schwartz SL, et al. Liposarcoma of the spermatic cord: report of 6 cases and review of the literature. J Urol. 1995;153(1):154–7.

119. Srigley JR, Hartwick RW. Tumors and cysts of the paratesticular region. Pathol Annu. 1990;25 Pt 2:51–108.

120. Weaver J, et al. Fluorescence in situ hybridization for MDM2 gene amplification as a diagnostic tool in lipomatous neoplasms. Mod Pathol. 2008;21(8):943–9.

121. Bremmer F, et al. Leiomyoma of the tunica albuginea, a case report of a rare tumour of the testis and review of the literature. Diagn Pathol. 2012;7:140.

122. Fumo MJ, Assi OA, Liroff S. Leiomyoma of the epididymis treated with partial epididymectomy. Nat Clin Pract Urol. 2006;3(9):504–7; quiz 1 p following 507.

123. Fisher C, et al. Leiomyosarcoma of the paratesticular region: a clinicopathologic study. Am J Surg Pathol. 2001;25(9):1143–9.

124. Raspollini MR, et al. Primitive testicular leiomyosarcoma. Pathol Oncol Res. 2010;16(2):177–9.

125. Varzaneh FE, Verghese M, Shmookler BM. Paratesticular leiomyosarcoma in an elderly man. Urology. 2002;60(6):1112.

126. Jo VY, et al. Paratesticular rhabdomyoma: a morphologically distinct sclerosing variant. Am J Surg Pathol. 2013;37(11):1737–42.

127. Cooper CL, et al. Paratesticular rhabdomyoma. Pathology. 2007;39(3):367–9.

128. Keskin S, et al. Clinicopathological characteristics and treatment outcomes of adult patients with paratesticular rhabdomyosarcoma (PRMS): a 10-year single-centre experience. Can Urol Assoc J. 2012;6(1):42–5.

129. Reeves HM, MacLennan GT. Paratesticular rhabdomyosarcoma. J Urol. 2009;182(4):1578–9.

130. Ulbright TM, Young RH. Testicular and paratesticular tumors and tumor-like lesions in the first 2 decades. Semin Diagn Pathol. 2014;31(5):323–81.

131. Young RH, Scully RE. Testicular and paratesticular tumor-like lesions of ovarian common epithelial and mullerian types. A report of four cases and review of the literature. Am J Clin Pathol. 1986;86(2):146–52.

132. McClure RF, et al. Serous borderline tumor of the paratestis: a report of seven cases. Am J Surg Pathol. 2001;25(3):373–8.

133. Ulbright TM, Young RH. Primary mucinous tumors of the testis and paratestis: a report of nine cases. Am J Surg Pathol. 2003;27(9):1221–8.

134. Tulunay O, et al. Clear cell adenocarcinoma of the tunica vaginalis of the testis with an adjacent uterus-like tissue. Pathol Int. 2004;54(8):641–7.

135. Du S, et al. Myoid gonadal stromal tumor: a distinct testicular tumor with peritubular myoid cell differentiation. Hum Pathol. 2012;43(1):144–9.

136. Kao CS, Ulbright TM. Myoid gonadal stromal tumor: a clinicopathologic study of three cases of a distinctive testicular tumor. Am J Clin Pathol. 2014;142(5):675–82.

137. Nistal M, et al. Fusocellular gonadal stromal tumour of the testis with epithelial and myoid differentiation. Histopathology. 1996;29(3):259–64.

138. Weidner N. Myoid gonadal stromal tumor with epithelial differentiation (? testicular myoepithelioma). Ultrastruct Pathol. 1991;15(4–5):409–16.

139. Ferry JA, et al. Malignant lymphoma of the testis, epididymis, and spermatic cord. A clinicopathologic study of 69 cases with immunophenotypic analysis. Am J Surg Pathol. 1994;18(4):376–90.

140. Wilkins BS, Williamson JM, O'Brien CJ. Morphological and immunohistological study of testicular lymphomas. Histopathology. 1989;15(2):147–56.

141. Cheah CY, Wirth A, Seymour JF. Primary testicular lymphoma. Blood. 2014;123(4):486–93.

142. Raspollini MR. Histologic variants of seminoma mimicking lymphatic malignancies of the testis: a literature review with a report of case series focusing on problems in differential diagnosis. Appl Immunohistochem Mol Morphol. 2014;22(5):348–57.

143. Al-Abbadi MA, et al. Primary testicular and paratesticular lymphoma: a retrospective clinicopathologic study of 34 cases with emphasis on differential diagnosis. Arch Pathol Lab Med. 2007;131(7):1040–6.

144. Al-Abbadi MA, et al. Primary testicular diffuse large B-cell lymphoma belongs to the nongerminal center B-cell-like subgroup: a study of 18 cases. Mod Pathol. 2006;19(12):1521–7.

145. Jones MA, Young RH, Scully RE. Malignant mesothelioma of the tunica vaginalis. A clinicopathologic analysis of 11 cases with review of the literature. Am J Surg Pathol. 1995;19(7):815–25.

146. Ballotta MR, Borghi L, Barucchello G. Adenocarcinoma of the rete testis. Report of two cases. Adv Clin Pathol. 2000;4(4):169–73.

147. Nistal M, et al. Adenomatous hyperplasia of the rete testis. A review and report of new cases. Histol Histopathol. 2003;18(3):741–52.

148. Schwartz IS. Rete testis adenocarcinoma. Am J Surg Pathol. 1988;12(12):967.

149. Shinmura Y, Yokoi T, Tsutsui Y. A case of clear cell adenocarcinoma of the mullerian duct in persistent mullerian duct syndrome: the first reported case. Am J Surg Pathol. 2002;26(9):1231–4.

150. Thomas AZ, et al. Primary clear cell carcinoma of the rete testis: 1st report. BMJ Case Rep. 2015;2015:bcr2014209000.

151. Buck DA, et al. Testicular metastasis in a case of squamous cell carcinoma of the lung. Case Rep Oncol. 2015;8(1):133–7.

152. Ro JY, et al. Lung carcinoma with metastasis to testicular seminoma. Cancer. 1990;66(2):347–53.

153. Uchida K, et al. Testicular metastasis from squamous cell carcinoma of the lung. Int J Urol. 2003;10(6):350–2.

Liwei Jia, Qinghu Ren, Gregory T. MacLennan, and Fang-Ming Deng

Frequently Asked Questions and Answers

What Is the World Health Organization (WHO) 2016 Classification of Squamous Cell Carcinoma of Penis?

The vast majority of malignant tumors of the penis are squamous cell carcinomas (SCCs) originating in the inner mucosal lining of the glans, coronal sulcus, or foreskin. Less than 50% of the subtypes of SCCs are of the conventional type, and the majority belongs to special categories. Compared to previous exclusively morphology-based classification schemes, the 2016 WHO classification presents a new classification based on clinicopathologic properties and relation to human papillomavirus (HPV) infection (Table 7.1). The mixed category is introduced in the new classification for tumors with more than one histological pattern. The new classification also clarifies the relationships between some neoplasms. Some entities that were originally described as specific tumor types have been shown to be morphological variants. For example, carcinoma cuniculatum is a variant of verrucous carcinoma; pseudoglandular and pseudohyperplastic carcinomas are variants of usual SCC; warty-basaloid carcinoma, clear cell carcinoma, and the papillary variant of basaloid carcinoma are variants of warty carcinoma.

Table 7.1 2016 WHO classification of squamous cell carcinoma of the penis

Non-HPV-related penile SCCs	HPV-related penile SCCs	Others
SCC - Usual carcinoma - Pseudohyperplastic carcinoma - Pseudoglandular carcinoma Verrucous carcinoma - Pure verrucous carcinoma - Carcinoma cuniculatum Papillary carcinoma, NOS Adenosquamous carcinoma Sarcomatoid squamous cell carcinoma Mixed carcinoma	Basaloid carcinoma - Papillary-basaloid carcinoma Warty carcinoma - Warty-basaloid carcinoma - Clear cell carcinoma Lymphoepithelioma-like carcinoma	Unclassified carcinoma

Non-HPV-Related Squamous Cell Carcinomas

Non-HPV-related subtypes of SCC include SCC of the usual type, pseudohyperplastic carcinoma, pseudoglandular carcinoma, verrucous carcinoma and carcinoma cuniculatum and variant types of SCC (papillary, adenosquamous, and sarcomatoid SCC) (Table 7.1).

Pseudohyperplastic carcinoma occurs in older patients (typically 70–80 years old) and is associated with lichen sclerosus. Pseudoglandular carcinoma is an aggressive tumor simulating adenocarcinoma. Verrucous carcinoma is a nonmetastasizing low-grade neoplasm with carcinoma cuniculatum as a variant. Carcinoma cuniculatum is a rare low-grade tumor with a labyrinthine growth pattern with no metastatic potential. Among all penile carcinomas, sarcomatoid SCC is the most aggressive, and is associated with the worst prognosis.

L. Jia (✉)
Department of Pathology, University of Texas Southwestern Medical Center, Dallas, TX, USA
e-mail: Liwei.jia@UTSouthwestern.edu

Q. Ren · F.-M. Deng
Department of Pathology, New York University Langone Health, New York, NY, USA

G. T. MacLennan
Department of Pathology, University Hospitals Cleveland Medical Center, Cleveland, OH, USA

© Springer Nature Switzerland AG 2021
X. J. Yang, M. Zhou (eds.), *Practical Genitourinary Pathology*, Practical Anatomic Pathology,
https://doi.org/10.1007/978-3-030-57141-2_7

HPV-Related Squamous Cell Carcinomas

HPV-related carcinomas are basaloid and warty (condylomatous) SCC, and rare variants, including warty-basaloid, papillary-basaloid, and clear cell carcinoma. Very unusual HPV-related tumors are lymphoepithelioma-like and medullary SCC (Table 7.1). Basaloid SCC has a high rate of nodal metastasis, whereas warty (condylomatous) carcinoma is rarely associated with regional nodal metastasis.

Precursor Lesions

Penile intraepithelial neoplasia (PeIN) is a precursor lesion of invasive SCC. It is a penile squamous epithelial proliferation characterized by dysplastic changes and an intact basement membrane.

Differentiated PeIN is non-HPV-related. It is characterized by parakeratosis and elongation of rete ridges. Lesional cells are enlarged, with abundant eosinophilic cytoplasm, and are located predominantly in the basal layers. Differentiated PeIN is commonly associated with lichen sclerosus.

Basaloid and warty (*or mixed basaloid-warty*) *PeINs* are usually associated with HPV infection. They are typically composed of atypical small basaloid cells involving full epithelial thickness and exhibiting strong p16 immunostaining.

References: [1–4]

What Are the Microscopic Features of HPV-Related Penile Carcinomas?

HPV is frequently found in tumors with predominant basaloid cells and also in those with predominantly koilocytic cells. There is high prevalence of HPV positivity in high-grade penile carcinomas, in lesions dominated by small tumor cells, in tumors with a high number of multinucleated cells and mitoses, and in tumors with small amounts of parakeratosis.

Reference: [3]

What Is the Relationship between HPV and Histologic Subtypes of Penile Carcinoma?

HPV is frequently found in

- Basaloid and warty carcinomas and their mixtures
- Lymphoepithelioma-like
- Clear cell carcinomas
- PeIN with similar basaloid or warty morphology is frequently identified in tissues adjacent to HPV-related invasive neoplasms.

HPV is usually negative in

- Usual SCC
- Pseudoglandular carcinoma

- Sarcomatoid carcinoma
- Pseudohyperplastic carcinomas

These tumors are frequently associated with differentiated PeIN and lichen sclerosus.

What Are the Types of Non-HPV-Related Variants of Penile Carcinomas?

Squamous Cell Carcinoma, Usual Type

- Invasive SCC with a varying degree of differentiation and keratinization that cannot be classified as other histologic subtypes morphologically, also termed SCC, not otherwise specified (NOS).
- Most common histological subtype of penile SCC (60–65%).
- It is subdivided into well differentiated (Fig. 7.1a–c), moderately differentiated (Fig. 7.2a–c), and poorly differentiated (Fig. 7.3a–c) based on nuclear pleomorphism and variable amounts of keratin production.
- Tumors are usually well-differentiated or moderately differentiated SCC similar to other sites.
- Keratinization is evident in most cases.
- Squamous hyperplasia and differentiated penile intraepithelial neoplasia (PeIN) are commonly found in adjacent mucosa in the great majority of cases.
- Lichen sclerosus is present in almost 1/2 of patients.
- Tumor invasion into penile erectile tissues and multiple compartments including corpora and urethra is frequently noted.
- Assessment of depth of invasion, perineural and vascular invasion, involvement of the corpora, glans, and multifocality should be addressed in all reports.
- Usually negative for HPV by in situ hybridization and p16 by immunostain.
- Most important prognostic factors: histologic grade, anatomical level of infiltration, vascular invasion, and perineural invasion.
- Inguinal nodal metastases occur in 1/3 of patients.

Verrucous Carcinoma

- A subtype of extremely well-differentiated SCC with hyperkeratosis and acanthosis, broad papillary fronds and pushing base.
- Accounts for 3–8% of penile carcinomas.
- Usually involves the glans or foreskin, and presents as slow growing exophytic cauliflower-like gray-white mass (Fig. 7.4a).
- Extremely well differentiated, composed of acanthotic papillae with slender fibrovascular cores, with prominent keratin craters identified between papillae (Fig. 7.4b).
- Tumor is usually confined to lamina propria, with broad and pushing base (Fig. 7.4b).

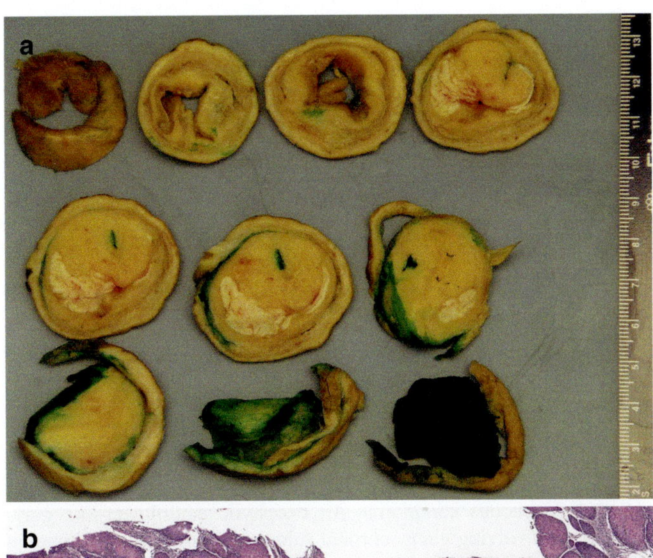

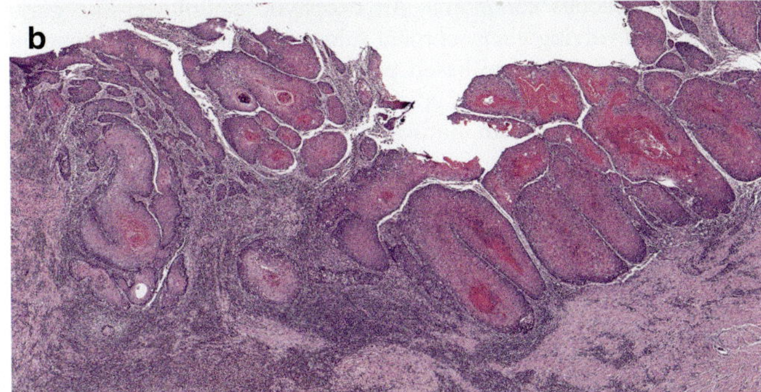

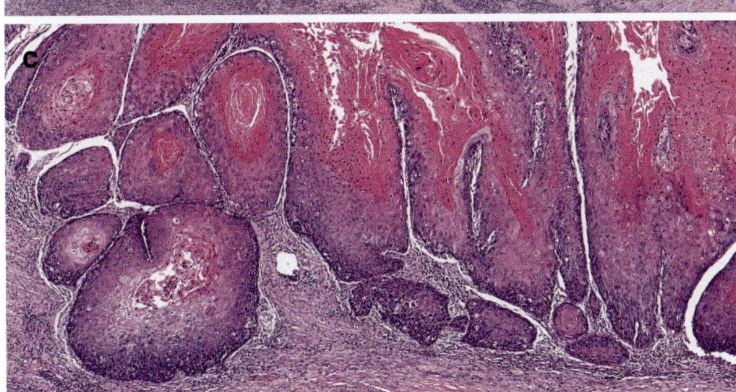

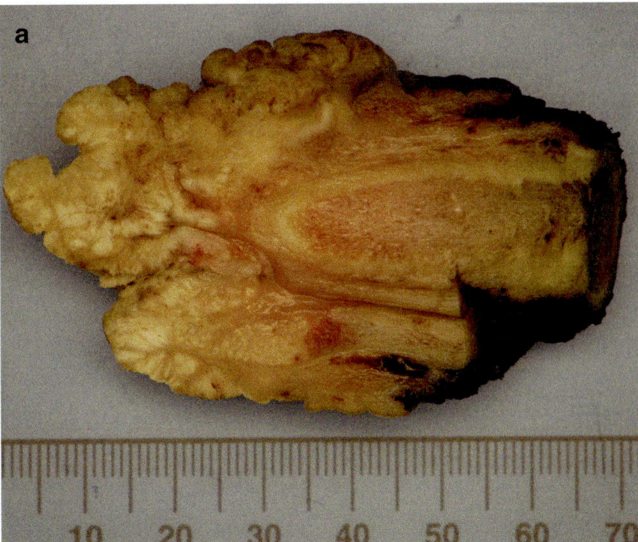

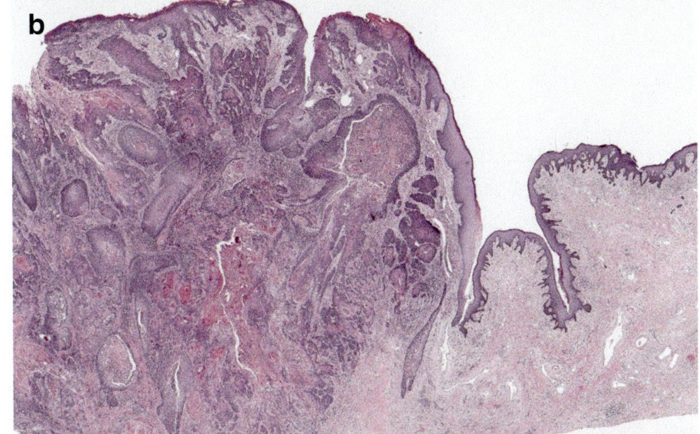

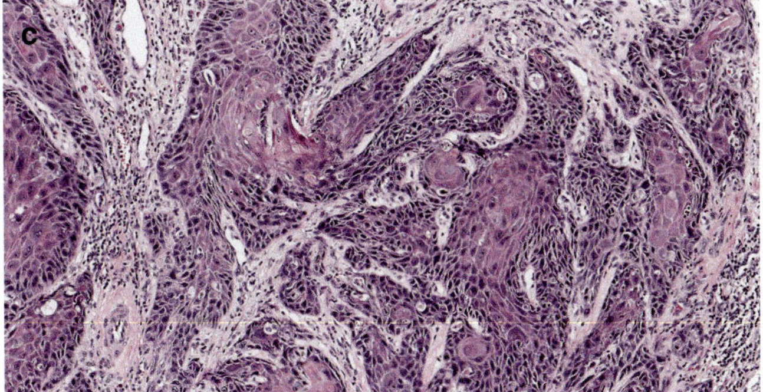

Fig. 7.1 Well-differentiated squamous cell carcinoma. (**a**) Cut surface shows a well-demarcated, pearly-white appearance. (**b**) Multiple invading tumor nests composed of well-differentiated squamous cells (**c**)

- Koilocytosis, higher-grade areas, necrosis, or infiltrative borders are absent.
- Locally aggressive but biologically indolent. No metastases reported with pure verrucous carcinoma.
- Standard recommended treatment is complete local excision with clear margins, or partial or total penectomy.
- Treatment with radiation must be avoided, as transformation to a frankly invasive squamous cell carcinoma can occur, which will have metastatic potential.

Carcinoma Cuniculatum

- Rare variant of verrucous carcinoma characterized by a deeply burrowing growth pattern mimicking rabbit burrows (cuniculi) (Fig. 7.5a).

Fig. 7.2 Moderately differentiated squamous cell carcinoma. (**a**) The tumor exhibits infiltrating whitish-gray cut surface with an irregular tumor front. (**b**) Irregular nests of tumor cells with keratinization and nuclear atypia (**c**)

- Large exoendophytic tumor with cobblestone appearance.
- Deep endophytic and interanastomosing pattern of sinus tracts mimicking rabbit burrows (Fig. 7.5b).
- Most cases show hybrid (mixed) verrucous carcinoma with peculiar deep growth pattern.
- Extremely well differentiated (verrucous carcinoma) (Fig. 7.5c).
- Acanthotic papillae separated by abundant keratin.

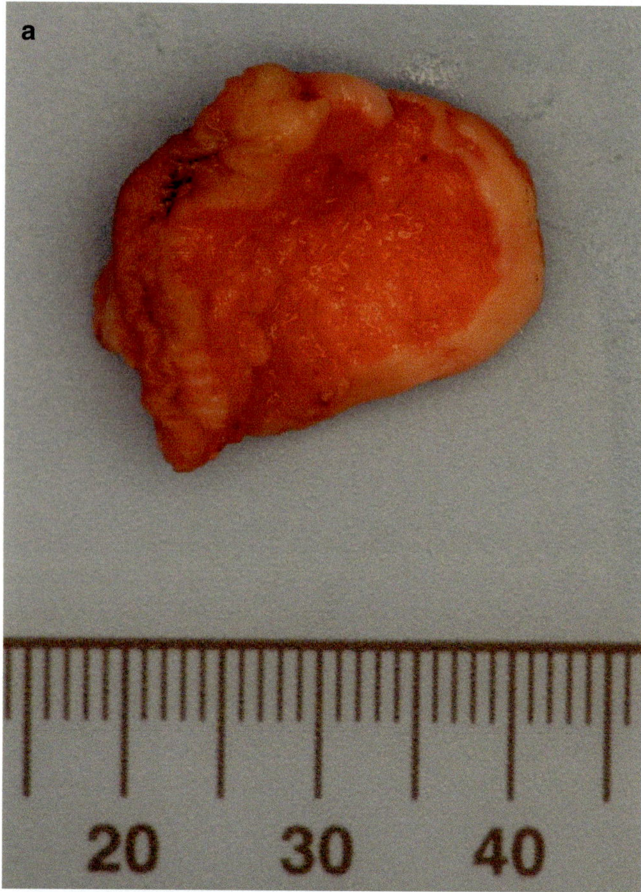

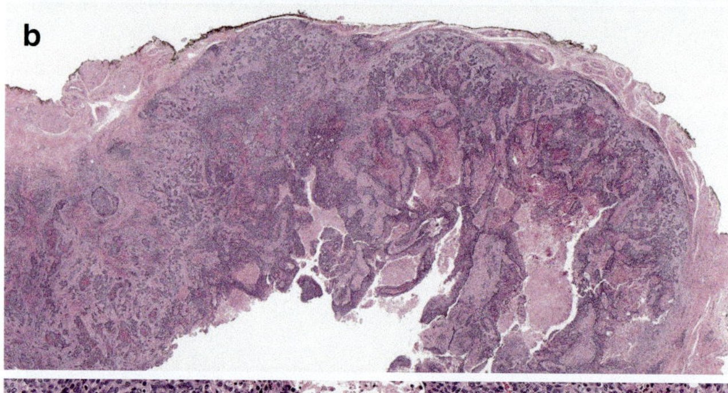

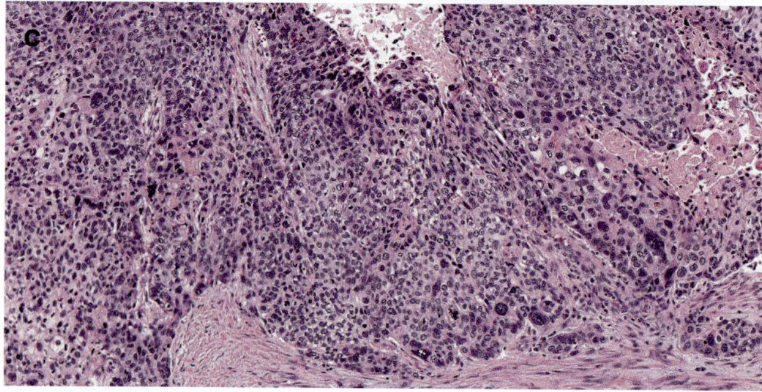

Fig. 7.3 Poorly differentiated squamous cell carcinoma. (**a**) An endophytic tumor displays tan firm cut surface with infiltrating border. (**b**) Invasive tumor composed of angulated tumor nests. (**c**) Tumor cells show poor keratinization, hyperchromatic nuclei, marked nuclear pleomorphism, and stromal reaction

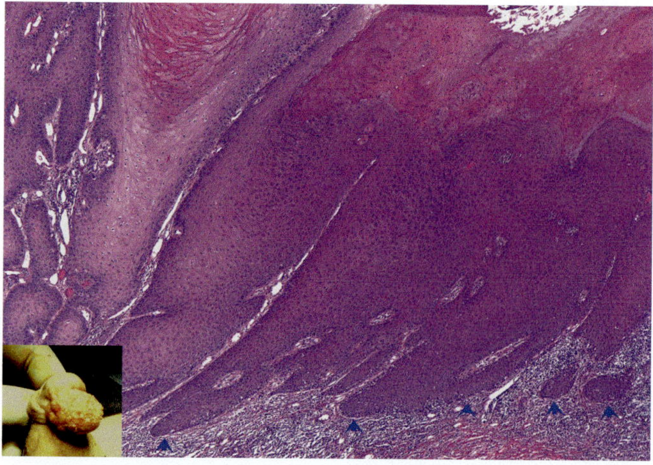

Fig. 7.4 Verrucous carcinoma. An exophytic cauliflower-like graywhite mass involving glans, coronal sulcus, and foreskin (as shown in inset). Well-defined broad-based pushing border (arrow heads) with prominent inflammatory cells present at the tumor margin. Tumor cells are well differentiated with minimal basal cell atypia

- Interanastomotic channels contain abundant keratin (Fig. 7.5b).
- Sinus tracts are commonly seen.
- Broad based pushing border.
- Focal higher-grade areas and infiltrative pattern are common.
- Lack of koilocytosis.

Papillary Carcinoma, NOS

- A variant of SCC
- A papillomatous, verruciform low-grade keratinizing neoplasm without koilocytosis
- Accounts for 5–8% of penile SCC
- Associated with lichen sclerosis, not associated with HPV infection
- Presents as a slow-growing, bulky, cauliflower-like, whitish-gray mass, most commonly involving the glans
- Irregular, complex, exophytic papillary growth (Fig. 7.6a)
- Well-to-moderately differentiated with prominent keratinization (Fig. 7.6b)
- No koilocytosis
- Less aggressive than usual penile SCC
- Standard recommended treatment is wide local excision or partial penectomy

Pseudoglandular Carcinoma

- High-grade carcinoma with prominent acantholysis and pseudoglandular features.
- Accounts for 1–2% of penile SCC.
- Unicentric large destructive, ulcerated and deeply invasive carcinoma.

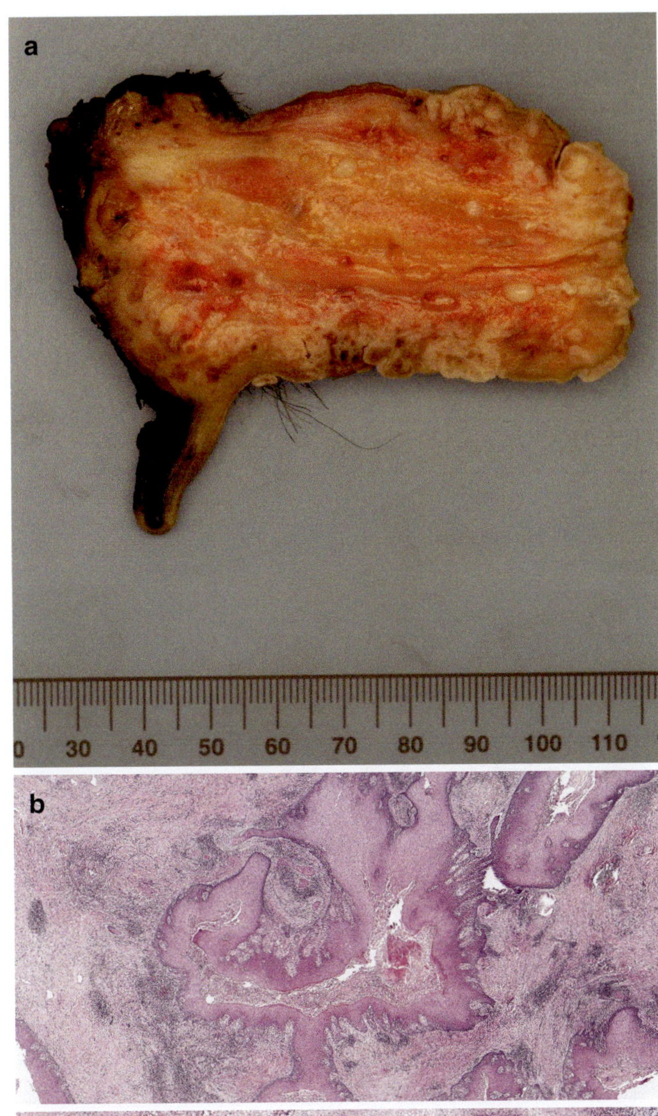

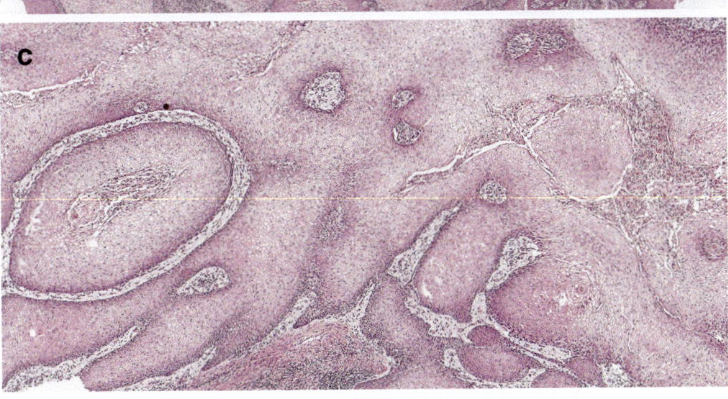

Fig. 7.5 Carcinoma cuniculatum. (**a**) A deeply burrowing growth pattern mimicking rabbit burrows. (**b**) Deep endophytic and interanastomosing pattern of sinus tracts containing abundant keratin. (**c**) Tumor cells are extremely well differentiated with minimal cytologic atypia

- Honeycomb or multicystic appearance at low magnification.
- Pseudoglandular features are noted in 30–85% of specimens.

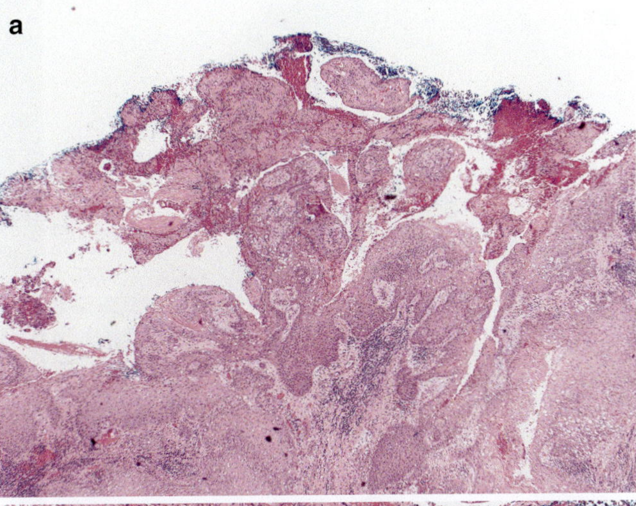

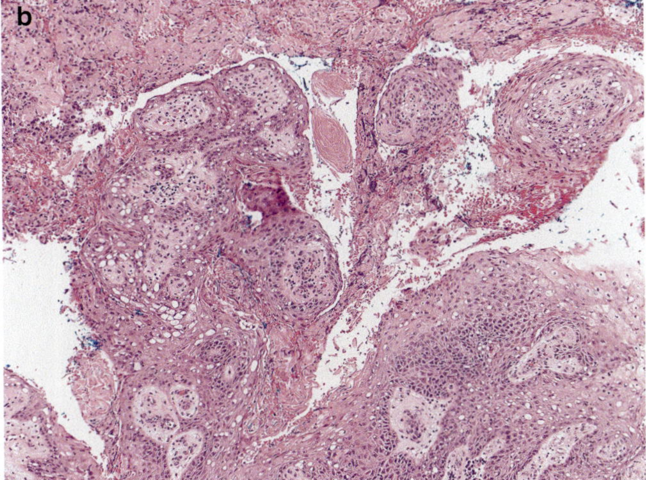

Fig. 7.6 Papillary carcinoma. (**a**) Low-power view reveals a complex papillary growth pattern with hyperkeratosis. Irregular fibrovascular cores are evident. (**b**) Papillae are lined by maturing keratinocytes with minimal to moderate nuclear atypia

- Open spaces are surrounded by high-grade cylindrical to flat squamous cells.
- Cellular debris, microabscesses, keratin, or acantholytic cells fill central pseudoglandular spaces (comedocarcinoma-like pattern).
- Deeply invasive carcinoma; most cases invade into the corpora cavernosa.
- Local recurrence and regional metastasis have been reported.
- Mortality rate is ~40%, higher than usual SCC.

Sarcomatoid Squamous Cell Carcinoma

- Squamous cell carcinoma with a malignant spindle cell or sarcomatoid component.
- ~4% of penile SCCs.
- White-gray, mixed exophytic and endophytic mass on the glans penis (Fig. 7.7a).

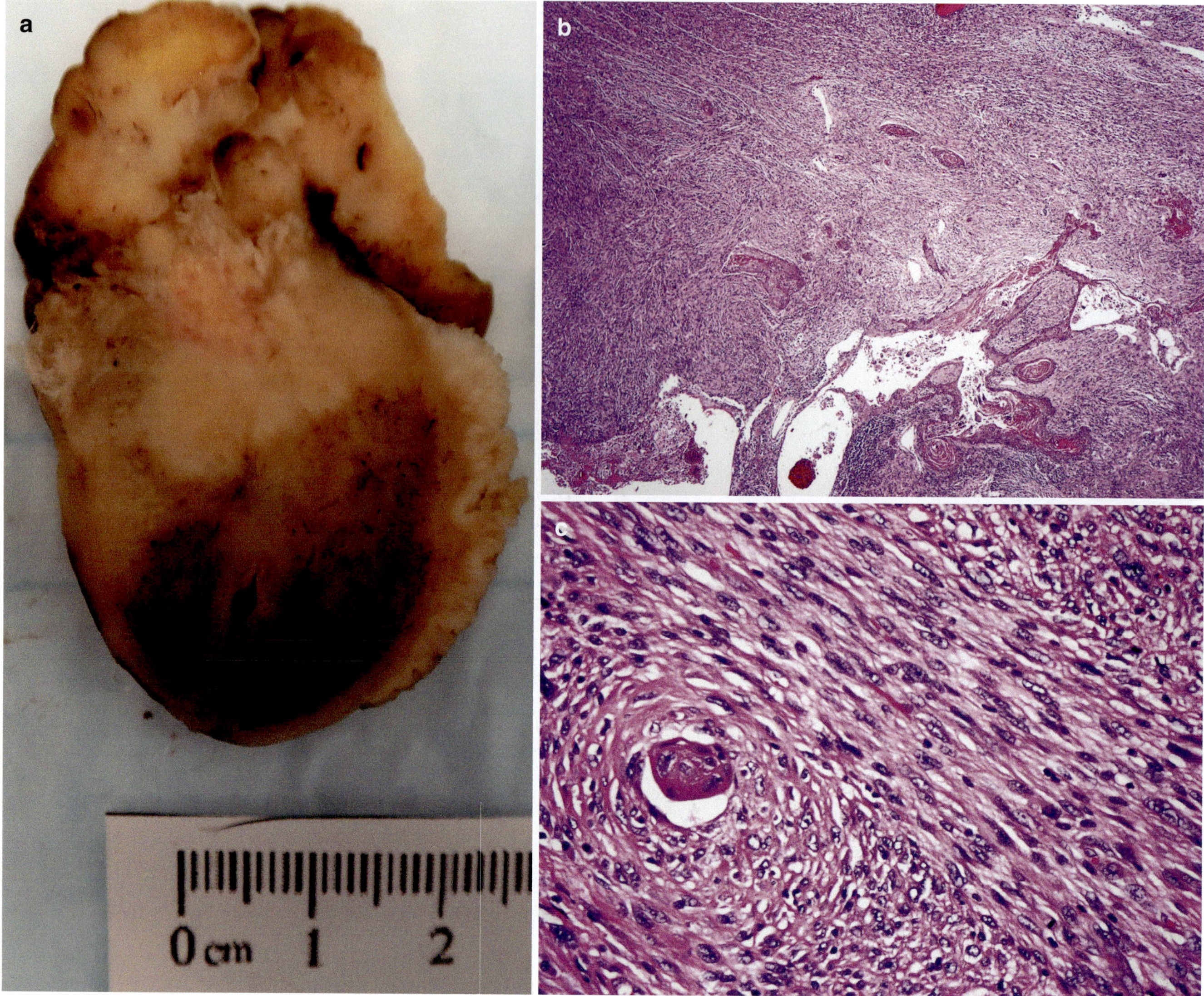

Fig. 7.7 Sarcomatoid squamous cell carcinoma. (**a**) Infiltrating tumor show tan firm cut surface, covering foreskin, coronal sulcus, and glans. (**b**) A biphasic carcinomatous and sarcomatoid spindle cell tumor. (**c**) Spindle cell component shows fibrosarcoma-like features

- The tumor is composed of high-grade SCC and a spindle cell (≥30%) component (Fig. 7.7b).
- Spindle cell component shows various histologic features, including myxoid, pseudoangiomatous, malignant fibrous histiocytoma-like, and fibrosarcoma-like (Fig. 7.7c).
- Heterologous differentiation into bone, cartilage, and muscle may be found.
- Mitotic figures are numerous, and necrosis may be prominent.
- Lymphovascular and perineural invasion are common.
- High-molecular-weight cytokeratin and p63 may be positive in sarcomatoid area.
- Clinical course usually aggressive with early lymph node metastasis and distant metastasis (e.g., lung, skin, bone, pleura).

- Most aggressive carcinoma of all penile carcinomas, with high mortality (45–75%).

Adenosquamous Carcinoma

- Biphasic malignant tumor with both squamous and adenocarcinoma components (Fig. 7.8a).
- Rare, only 11 cases reported.
- The squamous component predominates over the glandular component.
- Squamous component consists of warty or usual types of squamous carcinoma (Fig. 7.8b).
- Glandular component should have definitive gland formation (Fig. 7.8c), with or without mucin production.
- Can be deeply invasive and may show vascular invasion.

References: [5–10]

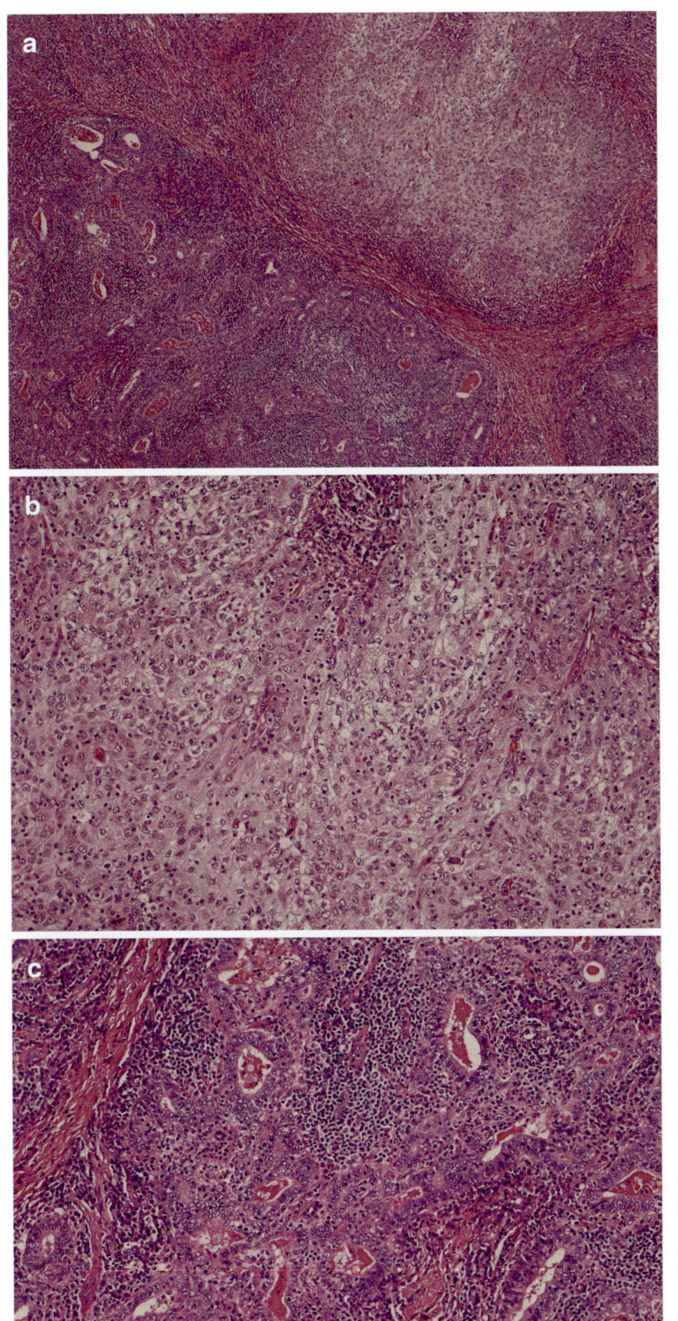

Fig. 7.8 Adenosquamous carcinoma. (**a**) Biphasic malignancy with squamous cell carcinoma and adenocarcinoma features. (**b**) Squamous component consists of usual types of squamous carcinoma. (**c**) Glandular component shows definitive gland formation

What Are the Types of HPV-Related Variants of Penile Carcinoma?

Basaloid Squamous Carcinoma
- Solid, aggressive tumor with endophytic solid growth pattern and basaloid features.

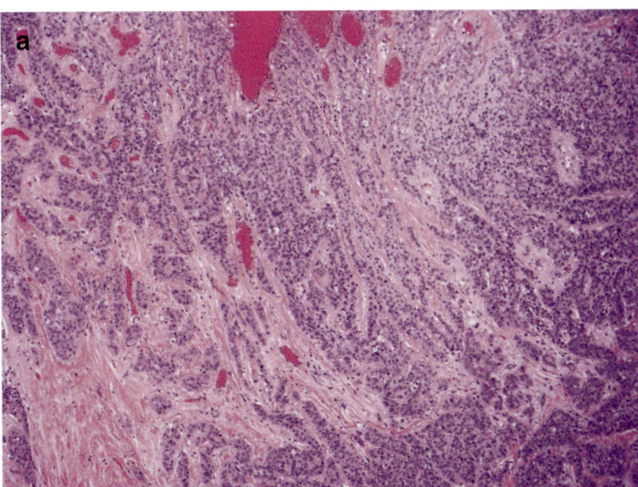

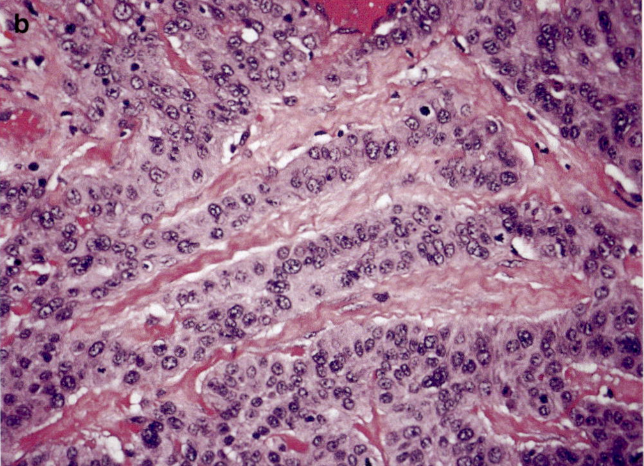

Fig. 7.9 Basaloid squamous carcinoma. (**a**) Tumor grows in a nesting pattern. (**b**) Monotonous small- to medium-sized tumor cells with high nuclear/cytoplasmic ratio and scant cytoplasm

- Most common HPV-related penile carcinoma (HPV16 most common).
- Accounts for 5–10% of penile carcinomas.
- Affects males in their 50s, ~10 years younger than patients with usual SCC.
- Grossly presents as a deeply infiltrative tumor mass with surface ulceration.
- Tumor grows in a nesting pattern with frequent comedo-necrosis (Fig. 7.9a).
- Monotonous small- to medium-sized tumor cells with high nuclear/cytoplasmic ratio and scant cytoplasm (Fig. 7.9b).
- Frequent mitotic figures and apoptotic cells may impart a "starry sky" appearance.
- Focally abrupt keratinization.
- Vascular invasion and deep invasion are frequent.
- p16 immunostain is strong and diffuse.
- Approximately half of patients may present with regional nodal metastasis.
- Mortality varies from 20% to 30%.

Papillary-Basaloid Carcinoma

- Rare variant of basaloid carcinomas, 1–2% of all penile SCCs.
- HPV-related (HPV16 most common).
- Villous exophytic tumor entirely composed of small basophilic cells indistinguishable from basaloid cells.
- Papillary configuration with a central fibrovascular core (Fig. 7.10a).
- Invasive tumor is similar to typical basaloid carcinoma (Fig. 7.10b).
- p16 immunostain is strong and diffuse.
- Prognosis depends on the stage of the carcinoma.

Warty (Condylomatous) Carcinoma

- Exophytic verruciform tumor affecting the glans, sulcus, or foreskin, accounts for 5–10% penile SCCs.
- HPV-related (HPV16 most common).
- Cauliflower or cobblestone-like gross appearance. Cut surface reveals multinodular tan to white papillomatous growth with a darker center (Fig. 7.11a).
- Condylomatous papillae with prominent central fibrovascular cores (Fig. 7.11b).
- Nuclear pleomorphism and cytoplasmic clear cells with koilocytic morphology (Fig. 7.11c).
- Commonly invasive with jagged border, moderately differentiated.
- p16 immunostain is strong and diffuse.
- Inguinal metastases are unusual, and mortality is low. Local recurrence in 17–18% cases.

Warty-Basaloid Carcinoma

- Variant of warty carcinoma of the penis and is a mixed tumor with condylomatous and basaloid features.
- HPV-related (HPV16 most common).
- Grossly large exo-/endophytic tumors. Cut surface shows a biphasic papillomatous tumor on the surface and a solid and micronodular deeply invasive tumor in erectile tissues.
- Warty and basaloid features are present and intermixed in various proportions (Fig. 7.12a, b).
- p16 immunostain is strong and diffuse.
- Inguinal metastases are present in 50% of patient and mortality is between that of basaloid and warty carcinoma, closer to that of basaloid carcinoma.

Clear Cell Carcinoma

- Aggressive, poorly differentiated variant of warty carcinoma that affects the glans or foreskin.
- HPV-related.
- Composed predominantly of clear cells, with distinctive nesting pattern.

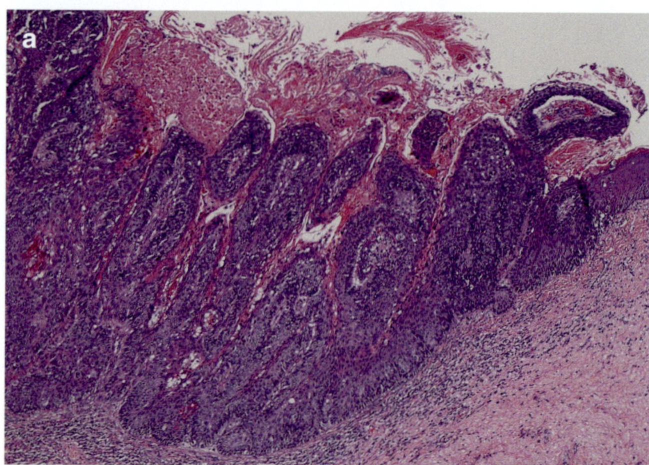

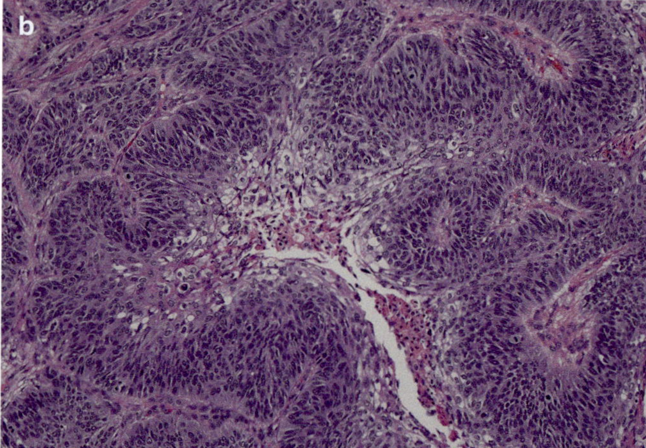

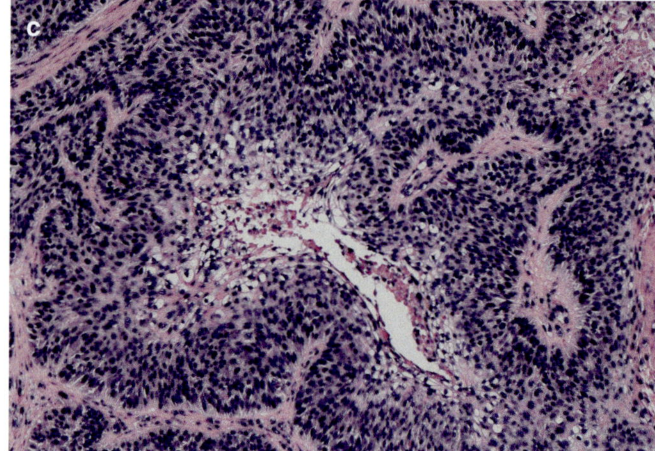

Fig. 7.10 Papillary basaloid carcinoma. (**a**) Papillary configuration with a central fibrovascular core. (**b**) Invasive tumor is similar to typical basaloid carcinoma. (**c**) Diffuse and dense staining of high-risk HPV RNA by in situ hybridization

- Comedo-like necrosis and geographic necrosis are common.
- p16 immunostain is strong and diffuse.
- Nodal metastases are present in the majority of cases.

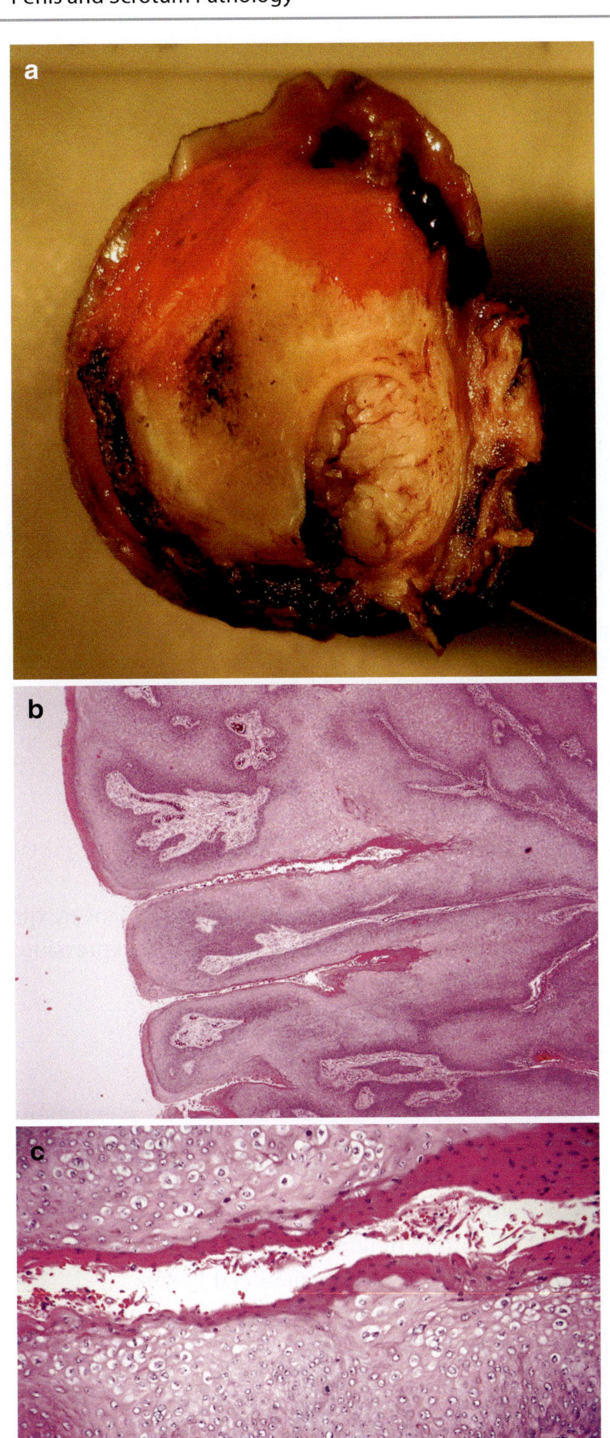

Fig. 7.11 Warty carcinoma. (**a**) Cauliflower or cobblestone-like gross appearance. Cut surface reveals multinodular tan to white papillomatous growth with a darker center. (**b**) Condylomatous papillae with prominent central fibrovascular cores. (**c**) Nuclear pleomorphism and cytoplasmic clear cells with koilocytic morphology

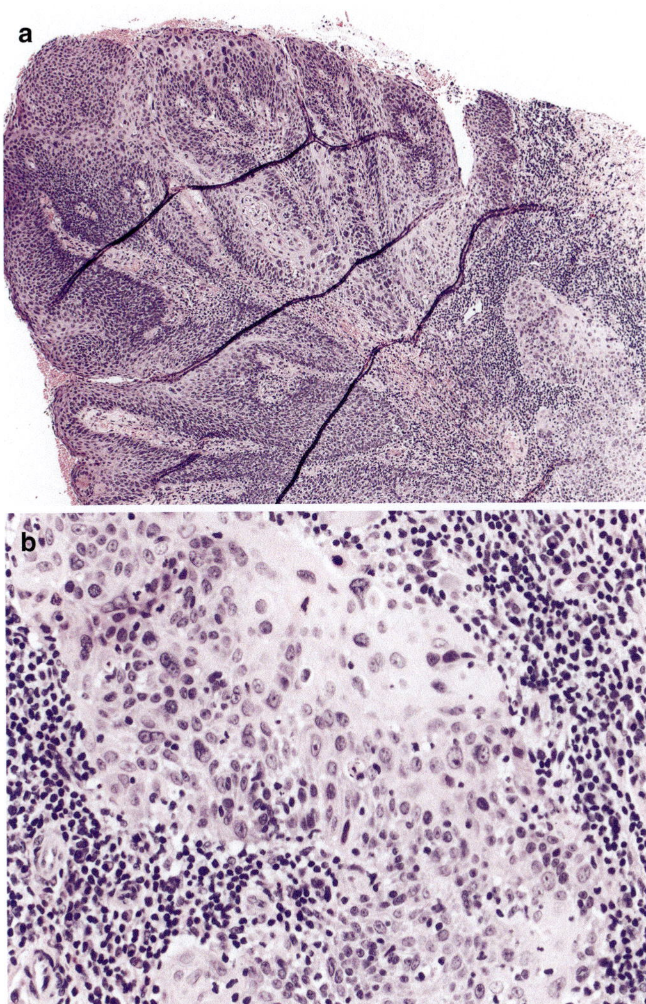

Fig. 7.12 Warty-basaloid carcinoma. (**a**) Papillomatous growth with superficial invasion of lamina propria invasion. (**b**) Dual populations of basophilic cells and clear cells. Both clear cell warty and basaloid features are present in the same invasive carcinoma nest

Lymphoepithelioma-like Carcinoma

- Poorly differentiated invasive squamous cell carcinoma resembling lymphoepithelioma or undifferentiated nasopharyngeal carcinoma.
- HPV-related.
- Large exophytic tumor located mainly in glans with extension to the foreskin.
- Invasive cords, trabeculae, nest, or sheets (Fig. 7.13a).
- Syncytial growth pattern of poorly differentiated to undifferentiated cells with indistinct cellular borders (Fig. 7.13b).
- Intermixed dense lymphoplasmacytic and eosinophilic infiltrate obscuring tumor cell boundaries.
- p16 immunostain is strong and diffuse.

References: [5, 11–16]

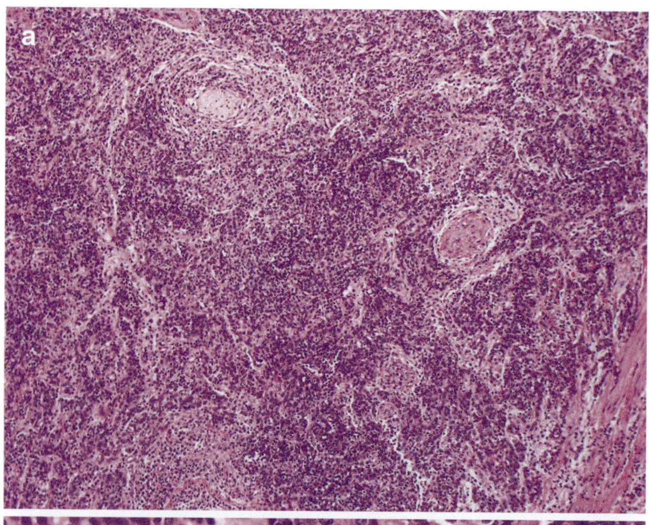

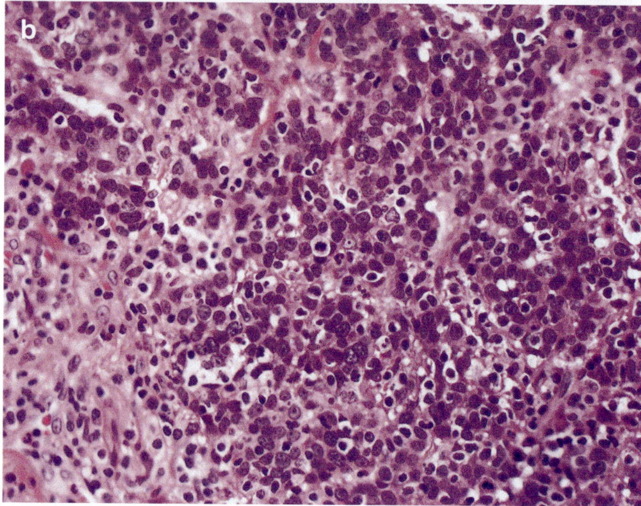

Fig. 7.13 Lymphoepithelioma-like carcinoma. (**a**) Irregular nests and trabeculae of undifferentiated tumor cells within dense lymphoplasmacytic infiltrate. (**b**) Syncytial tumor cells intermixed with inflammatory cells. (Reproduced with permission from Dr. Helen P. Cathro, University of Virginia)

What Is the Histologic Classification of Penile Intraepithelial Neoplasia (PeIN)?

PeIN is regarded as an intraepithelial (in situ) precursor lesion of invasive SCC. Synonyms include squamous cell carcinoma in situ (SCCIS), squamous intraepithelial lesion (SIL), erythroplasia of Queyrat and Bowen disease. PeIN is further subclassified into differentiated and undifferentiated types, with the latter being subdivided into basaloid, warty, and warty-basaloid subtypes.

Differentiated PeIN
- Thickened epithelium with hyperkeratosis, parakeratosis, and hypergranulosis (Fig. 7.14)
- Elongated and anastomosing rete ridges
- Subtle abnormal maturation (enlarged keratinocytes with abundant eosinophilic cytoplasm)

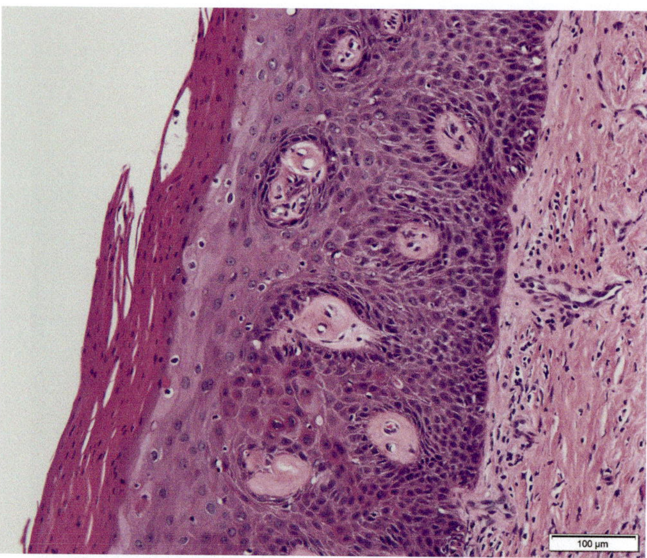

Fig. 7.14 Differentiated PeIN. Thickened epithelium with elongated rete ridges, enlarged keratinocytes with abundant eosinophilic cytoplasm, and atypical basal cells with hyperchromatic nuclei

- Keratin pearl formation
- Prominent intercellular bridges (lack of cohesion)
- Dysplastic hyperchromatic basal cells
- Unrelated to HPV infection
- p16 negative or non-block expression; p53 overexpression (suprabasal extension) or total lack of expression

Undifferentiated PeIN, Subtypes
Basaloid PeIN (Fig. 7.15)

- Epithelium replaced by a monotonous population of small- to intermediate-sized blue cells with a high nuclear/cytoplasmic ratio
- Parakeratosis with a flat surface
- Abundant mitotic figures and apoptotic bodies
- Isolated koilocytes in the superficial layers
- HPV-related, with strong/diffuse block-staining pattern of p16 positivity (Fig. 7.16a, b)

Warty PeIN (Fig. 7.17)

- Thickened epithelium with an undulating and spiking surface and striking cellular pleomorphism
- Atypical parakeratosis and dyskeratosis
- Conspicuous koilocytosis (hyperchromatic wrinkled nuclei, perinuclear halos, multinucleation)
- Abundant mitotic figures
- HPV-related, strong/diffuse block p16 positivity

Warty-basaloid PeIN (Fig. 7.18)

- Overlapping features of both warty and basaloid types

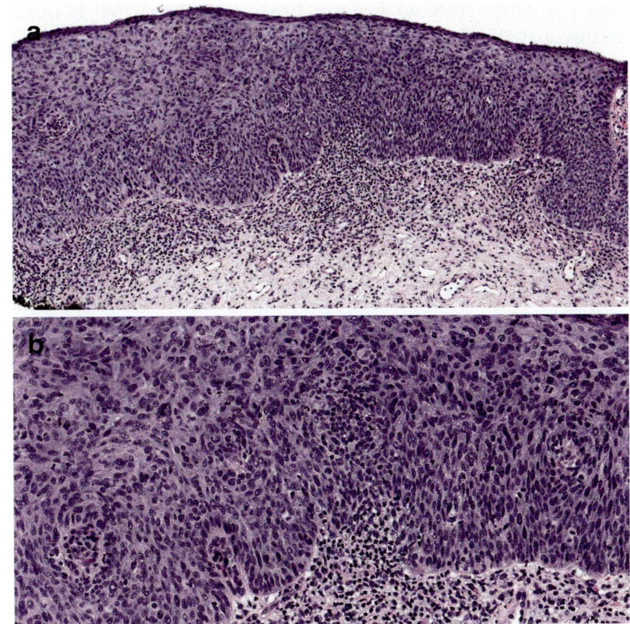

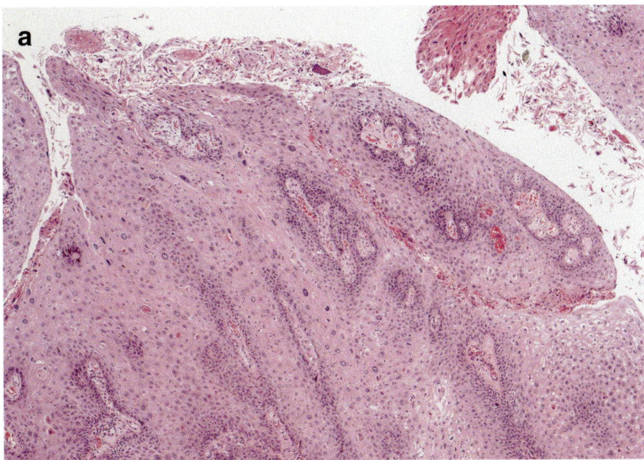

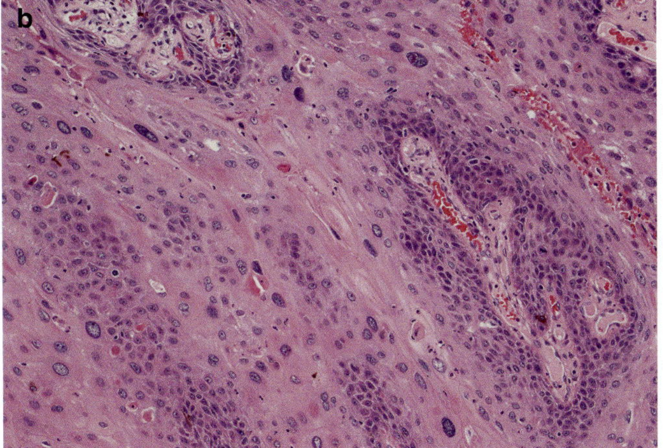

Fig. 7.15 Basaloid PeIN. (**a**) At low-power view, the lesion has flat or slightly irregular surface with parakeratosis. (**b**) At high-power view, the squamous epithelium is replaced by basophilic tumor cells with scant cytoplasm and indistinct cell borders. High mitotic rate is present

Fig. 7.17 Warty PeIN. (**a**) At low-power view, spiky or papillary parakeratotic surface is observed. (**b**) Nuclear pleomorphism is commonly found

- Spiking surface with koilocytic changes on the upper part of the epithelium
- Lower half of the epithelium is predominantly composed of small basaloid cells
- HPV-related, strong/diffuse block p16 positivity

The Lower Anogenital Squamous Terminology Standardization project (LAST) recommends a two-tiered nomenclature system for HPV-related PeIN:

- Low-grade squamous intraepithelial lesion (LGSIL): cytologic atypia limited to the lower third of the epithelium.
- High-grade squamous intraepithelial lesion (HGSIL): cytologic atypia involving more than one-third of the epithelium. When atypia involves the full thickness, it is equivalent to SCC in situ.

There is a significant association of the different types of PeIN with specific invasive SCC variants. Differentiated PeIN is seen preferentially associated with usual, papillary, pseudohyperplastic, verrucous, and sarcomatoid carcinomas.

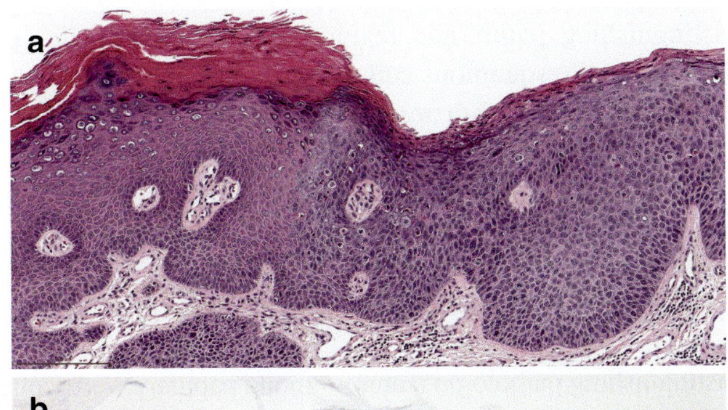

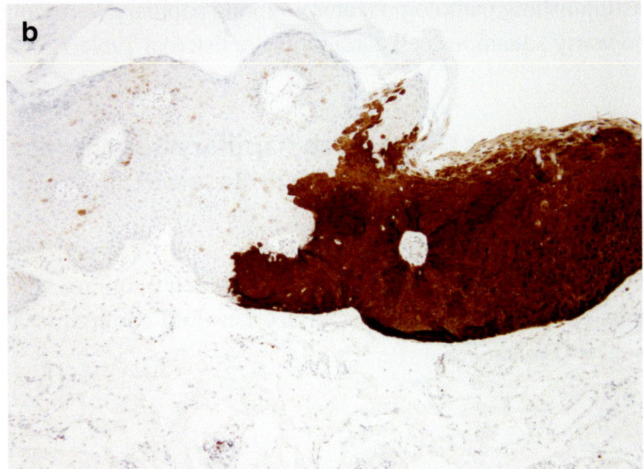

Fig. 7.16 Basloid PeIN, p16 stain. The immunopositivity for p16 is accepted as such only a dense, complete, "en block," nuclear, and cytoplasmic staining in contrast to the scattered staining pattern in normal squamous epithelium

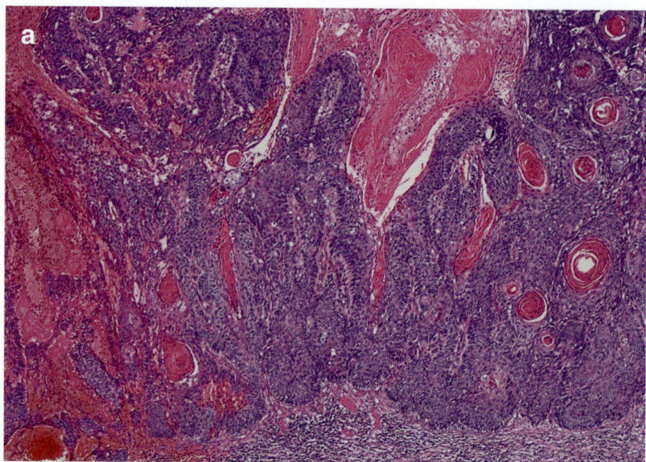

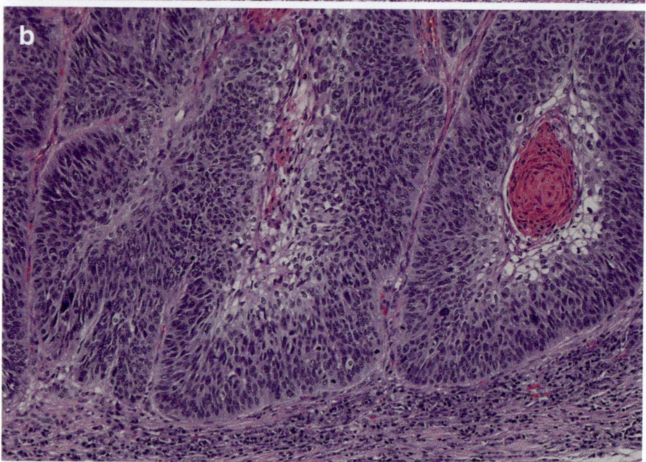

Fig. 7.18 Warty-basaloid PeIN. (**a**) Warty features in the upper third of the epithelium (spiky parakeratotic surface with koilocytosis). (**b**) Basaloid cells present in the middle and lower third of the epithelium

Undifferentiated PeIN is distinctively associated with warty, basaloid, and mixed warty-basaloid carcinomas.

References: [17, 18]

What Features Distinguish Differentiated PeIN from Undifferentiated PeIN?

Distinguishing clinicopathologic features between differentiated PeIN and undifferentiated PeIN are listed in Table 7.2.

What Features Distinguish Differentiated PeIN from Lichen Simplex Chronicus?

Distinguishing clinicopathologic features between differentiated PeIN and Lichen simplex chronicus are listed Table 7.3.

Table 7.2 Distinguishing features between differentiated PeIN and undeffirentiated PeIN

	Differentiated PeIN	Undifferentiated PeIN
Location	Foreskin	Glans
Multifocality	Sometimes	Often
HPV related	No	Yes
p16	Negative	Positive
Association with lichen sclerosus	Yes	No
Associated invasive SCC	NOS, verrucous, pseudohyperplastic, papillary, sarcomatoid SCC	Warty, basaloid, warty-basaloid SCC

What Features Distinguish Warty/Basaloid PeIN from Bowenoid Papulosis?

Distinguishing clinicopathologic features between warty/basaloid PeIN and Bowenoid papulosis are listed Table 7.4.

What Features Distinguish Penile Squamous Cell Carcinoma from Urothelial Carcinoma of Distal Urethra?

Distinguishing pathologic features and immunophenotype between penile squamous cell carcinoma and urothelial carcinoma of distal urethra are listed Table 7.5.

What Features Distinguish Papillary Squamous Cell Carcinoma, NOS, from Verrucous and Warty Carcinoma?

Distinguishing pathologic features among papillary, verrucous, and warty squamous cell carcinoma are listed in Table 7.6.

What Features Distinguish Papillary Squamous Cell Carcinoma from Papillary Basaloid Carcinoma?

Distinguishing pathologic features between papillary squamous cell carcinoma and papillary basaloid carcinoma are listed in Table 7.7.

Table 7.3 Distinguishing features between differentiated PeIN and lichen simplex chronicus

	Differentiated PeIN	Lichen simplex chronicus
Pathogenesis	Precancerous	Inflammatory/reactive
Thickened epithelium	Present	Present
Hyperkeratosis, parakeratosis and hypergranulosis	Present	Present
Basal cell atypia	Prominent	None/minimal
HPV	–	–
p16	–	–
p53	Overexpression/total loss of expression (mutated)	Basilar expression (wild type)

Table 7.4 Distinguishing features between warty/basaloid PeIN and Bowenoid papulosis

	Warty/basaloid PeIN	Bowenoid papulosis
Pathogenesis	Precancerous	<1% progress to SCC, often regresses spontaneously
Age	Older (40–60 yo)	Young, sexually active (30 yo mean)
Presentation	Solitary/multifocal	Small, multiple lesions
Regression	–	+
Basaloid cells	Present	Present
Koilocytosis	Present	Present
Spiking surface	Present	Present
HPV	+ (HPV16)	+ (HPV16)
p16	+	+
p53	Overexpression/total loss of expression (mutated)	Basilar expression (wild type)

Table 7.5 Distinguishing features between squamous cell carcinoma and urothelial carcinoma of distal urethra

	Penile squamous cell carcinoma	Urothelial carcinoma of distal urethra
Adjacent urothelial carcinoma	Absent	Present
PeIN	Present	Absent
Squamous hyperplasia	Present	Absent
p63	+	+
GATA-3	±	+
CK20	–	+
Uroplakin	–	+

Table 7.6 Distinguishing features among papillary carcinoma, verrucous carcinoma, and warty carcinoma

	Papillary carcinoma, NOS	Verrucous carcinoma	Warty carcinoma
Cauliflower-like exophytic growth	Present	Present	Present
Differentiation	Well to moderate	Well	Moderate
Papillomatosis	Present	Present	Absent
Fibrovascular core	Present	Absent	Present
Broad pushing border	Absent	Present	Absent
Koilocytosis	Absent	Present	Present
PeIN	Differentiated	Differentiated	Undifferentiated
Squamous hyperplasia	Present	Present	Present
Lichen sclerosis	Present	Present	Absent
HPV-associated	No	No	Yes
p16 immunostain	–	–	+

Table 7.7 Distinguishing features between papillary carcinoma and papillary-basaloid carcinoma

	Papillary carcinoma, NOS	Papillary-basaloid carcinoma
Cauliflower-like exophytic growth	Present	Present
Papillomatosis	Present	Present
Fibrovascular core	Present	Present
Papillae lining cells	Well-differentiated cells with eosinophilic cytoplasm (pink cells)	Poorly differentiated basophilic small cells with scanty cytoplasm (blue cells)
Broad pushing border	Absent	Absent
Koilocytosis	Absent	Absent
PeIN	Differentiated	Undifferentiated
Squamous hyperplasia	Present	Present
Lichen sclerosis	Present	Absent
HPV-associated	No	Yes
p16 immunostain	−	+

Table 7.8 Distinguishing features between sarcomatoid squamous carcinoma and primary sarcoma

	Sarcomatoid squamous cell carcinoma	Primary sarcoma
Occurrence	1–4% of penile carcinomas	Exceedingly rare
MC location	Glans	Shaft (corpora cavernosa), deeply located
History of penile carcinomas	Present	Absent
Epithelial differentiation	Present	Absent
Connection to surface epithelium	Present	Absent (deeply located)
High-grade spindle cells	Present	Present
Heterologous elements	±	±
PeIN	Present	Absent
p63/CK5/6/ HMWCK	+ (less in spindle area)	−
AE1/AE3/CAM5.2 immunostains	± (may be negative in spindle area)	−

What Features Distinguish Sarcomatoid Squamous Cell Carcinoma from Primary Sarcoma of Penis?

The distinguishing clinic–pathologic features and immunophenotype between sarcomatoid squamous cell carcinoma and primary sarcoma of the penis are listed in Table 7.8.

What Features Distinguish Verrucous Carcinoma from Giant Condylomas?

The distinguishing morphologic features between verrucous carcinoma and giant condylomas are listed in Table 7.9.

What Features Distinguish Warty-Basaloid Carcinoma from Warty Carcinoma and Basaloid Carcinoma?

The distinguishing morphologic and immunophenotypical features among warty carcinoma, basaloid squamous carcinoma, and warty-basaloid carcinoma are listed in Table 7.10.

Table 7.9 Distinguishing features between verrucous carcinoma and giant condyloma

	Verrucous carcinoma	Giant condyloma
Low-grade nuclei	Present	Present
Noninvasive, pushing border	Present	Present
Exophytic growth	Present	Present
Endophytic growth	Present	Absent
Koilocytosis	Absent	Present

Table 7.10 Distinguishing features among warty carcinoma, basaloid squamous cell carcinoma, and warty-basaloid carcinoma

	Warty carcinoma	Basaloid squamous cell carcinoma	Warty-basaloid carcinoma
Warty (condylomatous) component	Present	Absent	Present
Basaloid component	Absent	Present	Present
Koilocytosis	Present	Absent	Present
HPV-associated	Yes	Yes	Yes
p16 immunostain	+	+	+

What Features Distinguish Clear Cell Carcinoma from Warty Carcinoma with Prominent Clear Cells?

The distinguishing morphologic and immunophenotypical features between clear cell carcinoma and warty carcinoma with prominent clear cells are listed in Table 7.11.

What Features Distinguish Clear Cell Carcinoma from Metastatic Renal Cell Carcinoma?

The distinguishing pathologic and immunophenotypical features between clear cell carcinoma and metastatic renal cell carcinoma are listed in Table 7.12.

What Features Distinguish Clear Cell Carcinoma from Sweat Gland Carcinoma?

The distinguishing morphologic and immunophenotypical features between clear cell carcinoma and sweat gland carcinoma are listed in Table 7.13.

What Features Distinguish Carcinoma Cuniculatum from Verrucous Carcinoma?

The distinguishing morphologic and immunophenotypical features between carcinoma cuniculatum and verrucous carcinoma are listed in Table 7.14.

Table 7.11 Distinguishing features between clear cell carcinoma and warty carcinoma with prominent clear cells

	Clear cell carcinoma	Warty carcinoma with prominent clear cells
Papillomatosis	Absent	Present
Fibrovascular core	Absent	Present
Warty PeIN	Present	Present
HPV-associated	Yes	Yes
p16 immunostain	+	+

Table 7.12 Distinguishing features between clear cell carcinoma and metastatic renal cell carcinoma

	Clear cell carcinoma	Metastatic renal cell carcinoma
MC location	Foreskin, coronal sulcus or glans (penile mucosal compartments)	Corpus cavernosum
Lymphovascular invasion	±	Extensive
Warty/basaloid PeIN	Present	Absent
HPV-associated	Yes	No
p16 immunostain	+	−
Pax-8 immunostain	−	+

Table 7.13 Distinguishing features between clear cell carcinoma and sweat gland carcinoma

	Clear cell carcinoma	Sweat gland carcinoma
MC location	Foreskin, coronal sulcus or glans (penile mucosal compartments)	Skin shaft
Warty/basaloid PeIN	Present	Absent
HPV-associated	Yes	No
p16 immunostain	+	−

Table 7.14 Distinguishing features between carcinoma cuniculatum and verrucous carcinoma

	Carcinoma cuniculatum	Verrucous carcinoma
Cauliflower-like exophytic growth	Present	Present
Differentiation	Well to moderate	Well
Papillomatosis	Present	Present
Fibrovascular core	Absent	Absent
Burrowing pattern	Present	Absent
Focal high-grade area	Present	Absent
Focal infiltrative pattern	Present	Absent
PeIN	Differentiated	Differentiated
Squamous hyperplasia	Present	Present
Lichen sclerosis	Present	Present
HPV-associated	No	No
p16 immunostain	−	−

What Features Distinguish Pseudoglandular Carcinoma from Adenosquamous Carcinoma?

The distinguishing morphologic and immunophenotypical features between pseudoglandular carcinoma and adenosquamous carcinoma are listed in Table 7.15.

What Is the Value of P16 in the Diagnosis of HPV-Related Penile Tumors?

Although the majority of HPV-related penile tumors can be identified with routine hematoxylin and eosin (H&E) staining, p16 immunohistochemical staining can serve as a surrogate of HPV infection, which is recommended by the WHO. In a study comparing p16 with HPV detection by PCR, p16 is frequently associated with high-risk HPV, with an overall concordance of 84%. The highest rate of positivity was identified in basaloid and mixed basaloid carcinomas, while intermediate rates were present in warty and usual carcinomas.

p16 immunostaining may be helpful for accurate classification in morphologically challenging cases. For example, warty carcinoma (p16-positive) can be distinguished from papillary carcinoma, NOS and giant condylomas, both of which are p16-negative. p16 may prove to be useful as a prognostic marker as more outcome data becomes available in the future. It has been well demonstrated that patients with p16-positive carcinomas in the head and neck region have a better prognosis than those with p16-negative carcinomas. For penile carcinoma, there are fewer studies, and there is lack of consensus currently about the prognostic value of p16 immunostaining status of these tumors. In some studies, HPV presence is a good prognostic marker, whereas in other studies the findings are inconclusive.

References: [19–24]

Table 7.15 Distinguishing features between pseudoglandular carcinoma and adenosquamous carcinoma

	Pseudoglandular carcinoma	Adenosquamous carcinoma
True glandular differentiation	Absent	Present
Honeycombing (multicystic)	Present	Present/Absent
Biphasic pattern	Absent	Present
Cyst lining	High-grade cylindrical to flat squamous cells	Glandular cells
Mucin	–	+
PeIN	Differentiated	Differentiated
Squamous hyperplasia	Present	Present
Lichen sclerosis	Present	Present
HPV-associated	No	No
p16 immunostain	–	–

What Is the Prevalence Distribution of HPV Types in Penile Carcinomas?

HPV is detectable in 30–50% of penile SCCs. Most HPV infections in this setting are classified as high-risk genotypes, and the majority of these correspond to HPV-16, accounting for about 60% of HPV-attributable cases. HPV-related tumors affect younger patients, whereas tumors unrelated to HPV tend to be seen in older patients with lichen sclerosus or squamous hyperplasia (Table 7.16).

Reference: [3, 25]

What Are the Ancillary Tests for HPV Detection and Genotyping?

The detection of HPV infection in genital samples may increase the sensitivity of primary and secondary screenings of penile as well as cervical cancer. HPV testing may also improve the specificity of screening programs, resulting in the prevention of overtreatment and cost savings for confirmatory procedures.

Nucleic acid-hybridization assays

- Southern blotting
- In situ hybridization
- Dot-blot hybridization ViraPap/ViraType test (Digene Corporation, USA)

Signal-amplification assays

- Cervista HPV (Hologic, Inc., Marlborough, MA)
- Hybrid Capture II system (HC-2, Digene Corp., USA)
- *Nucleic acid-amplification methods*
- Microarray analysis
- PapilloCheck
- Polymerase chain reaction (PCR)

Table 7.16 HPV-type prevalence distribution in penile carcinomas[a]

Genotype	Frequency (%)	Relative contribution among HPV(+) cases (%)
Any type	47.0	100
HPV-16	28.3	60.23
HPV-18	6.3	13.35
HPV-6/11	3.8	8.13
HPV-31	0.5	1.16
HPV-45	0.5	1.16
HPV-33	0.4	0.87
HPV-52	0.3	0.58
Other types	1.2	2.47

[a]Data is based on a meta-analysis of 31 studies including 1466 penile carcinomas [25]

- Real-time PCR
- Abbott real time
- PCR-RFLP
- HPV genome sequencing
- INNO-LiPA (LiPA HBV GT; Innogenetics N.V., Ghent, Belgium)
- COBAS 4800 HPV test
- Linear Array HPV Genotyping (Roche Molecular Diagnostics, Pleasanton, CA)
- CLART human papillomavirus 2
- Microplate colorimetric hybridization assay (MCHA)
- PreTect Proofer (HPV-mRNA detection)
- APTIMA HPV assay (HPV-mRNA detection)

Reference: [26]

What Are the Grading Parameters for Penile Squamous Cell Carcinoma?

A three-tiered histological grading is recommended for penile SCCs: grade 1, well differentiated; grade 2, moderately differentiated; and grade 3, poorly differentiated. In penile cancers, grades 1, 2, and 3 occur with approximately equal frequency. When more than one grade is identified in the same specimen, a grade is assigned on the basis of the worst observed grade. Any proportion of grade 3 is sufficient to place the tumor in this category.

Grade 1: Well Differentiated

Tumors show extreme differentiation, keratinization, and maturation. Nuclear atypia is minimal or absent. Tumors grow in large nests. The grade of verrucous carcinoma, with minimal deviation from the histology of the normal squamous epithelium, may be used as a model for grade 1 tumors.

Grade 2: Moderately Differentiated

Tumors are intermediate in their histological features between the features of grades 1 and 3 carcinomas. They grow in irregular nests with obvious keratinization and partial cell maturation. Nuclear atypia is moderate.

Grade 3: Poorly Differentiated

Tumors are usually solid or trabecular. They show scant keratinization and are predominantly composed of undifferentiated or anaplastic cells. There is no maturation. Cells are pleomorphic and show numerous mitotic figures. Basaloid and sarcomatoid carcinomas are prototypical examples of grade 3 tumors. Any percentage of anaplastic cells (grade 3) is important in increasing the risk of inguinal metastasis.

Table 7.17 Correlation of histological grades and subtypes of penile SCCs

Grade 1	Grade 2	Grade 3
Verrucous	Warty (condylomatous)	Sarcomatoid
Papillary NOS Cuniculatum	Moderately differentiated usual	Pseudoglandular Basaloid
Pseudohyperplastic		Clear cell
Well differentiated usual		Lymphoepithelioma-like
		Poorly differentiated usual

Histological grades can be correlated with specific subtypes of penile SCCs. Many of the histological subtypes of SCC of the penis are associated with distinct grades based on the histological features of the subtypes. Usual SCC exhibits the widest range in grading (Table 7.17).

References: [27, 28]

What Are the Staging Parameters for Penile Squamous Cell Carcinoma?

The following stages are from the American Joint Committee on Cancer Staging Manual, eighth edition:

Primary Tumor (T)
- TX: primary tumor cannot be assessed.
- T0: no evidence of primary tumor.
- Tis: carcinoma in situ (preinvasive carcinoma).
- Ta: noninvasive localized carcinoma (broad pushing penetration or invasion is permitted; destructive invasion is against this diagnosis).
- T1a: tumor invades subepithelial connective tissue without lymphovascular or perineural invasion and is not high grade (ie, grade 3 orsarcomatoid).
- T1b: tumor invades subepithelial connective tissue with lymphovascular invasion and/or perineural invasion or is high grade (ie, grade 3 orsarcomatoid).
- T2: tumor invades into corpus spongiosum (either glans or ventral shaft) with or without urethral invasion.
- T3: tumor invades into corpora cavernosum (including tunica albuginea) with or without urethral invasion.
- T4: tumor invades into adjacent structures (i.e., scrotum, prostate, pubic bone).

Regional Lymph Nodes (N) (Pathological Classification)
- pNX: regional lymph nodes cannot be assessed.
- pN0: no regional lymph node metastasis.

- pN1: ≤2 unilateral inguinal metastases, no extranodal extension.
- pN2: ≥3 unilateral inguinal metastases or bilateral metastases, no extranodal extension.
- pN3: Extranodal extension of lymph node metastases or pelvic lymph node metastases.

Distant Metastasis (M)

- M0: no distant metastasis.
- M1: distant metastasis (including lymph node metastasis outside of the true pelvis).

Note: Staging of squamous cell carcinoma of the skin of the shaft or glans of the penis is different from cancer arising in the urethra.

- If the erectile tissue (corpus cavernosa, spongiosum) is involved, the tumor is pT3 or pT2.
- If the urethra is involved by cancer invading to it from the surface, through the erectile tissue, the tumor is pT3.
- If involved by surface spread via the urethral meatus, this is not pT3.
- Invasive carcinoma involving neither of these structures is pT1 [i.e., tumor only involves the lamina propria (dermis) of the penile skin].
- T1 is subdivided into T1a and T1b based on the presence or absence of lymphovascular invasion, perineural invasion or poorly differentiated cancers.
- Prostatic invasion is considered T4.
- Metastasis to lymph nodes outside of the true pelvis is M1.
  Reference: [29]

What Are the Staging Parameters for Penile Urethral Carcinoma?

Urethral carcinomas are staged using a different TNM system than carcinomas that arise on the penile shaft skin or on the glans penis. Most malignant tumors of the urethra are SCCs, followed by urothelial carcinomas and adenocarcinomas. Clear cell adenocarcinomas are rare but more common in female patients.

The following stages are from the American Joint Committee on Cancer Staging Manual, eighth edition:

Primary Tumor (T)

- pTX: primary tumor cannot be assessed.
- pTa: noninvasive carcinoma.
- pTis: carcinoma in situ.
- pT1: tumor invades subepithelial connective tissue.
- pT2: tumor invades corpus spongiosum, prostate, periurethral muscle.
- pT3: tumor invades corpus cavernosum, beyond prostatic capsule, anterior vaginal wall, bladder neck.
- pT4: tumor invades other adjacent organs.

Regional Lymph Node Metastasis (pN Stage)

- pNX: regional lymph nodes cannot be assessed.
- pN0: no regional lymph node metastasis.
- pN1: metastasis in a single lymph node 2 cm or less in greatest dimension.
- pN2: metastasis in a single node more than 2 cm in greatest dimension, or in multiple nodes.

Distant Metastasis (pM Stage)

- pM0: no distant metastasis
- pM1: distant metastasis
  Note: In the prostatic urethra, carcinoma of the urethral lining with invasion into subepithelial connective tissue is staged as pT1; invasion arising from the prostatic ducts is designated as at least pT2.
  Reference: [29]

What Are the Updates for Penile Cancer in the 8th ed. AJCC TMN Staging Manual?

Significant changes in nonurethral penile cancer have been proposed over past editions; see summary below:
- Ta Broadened to noninvasive localized squamous cell carcinoma
- T1 Tumor invasion to layers superficial to corporal tissues specified according to region's histoanatomy (glans, foreskin, or shaft)
  - Perineural invasion included to divide T1a and T1b
  - Sarcomatoid change clarified as one high-grade variable to divide T1a and T1b
- T2 Confined to tumor invasion into corpus spongiosum
  - Tumor invasion of corpus cavernosum excluded
- T3 Tumor invasion into corpus cavernosum
  - Urethral involvement no longer the determinant and can be T2 or T3
- pN1 Increased to up to two unilateral inguinal lymph node metastases without extranodal extension
- pN2 Increased to >2 unilateral or bilateral inguinal lymph node metastases without extranodal extension

Ta is now significantly expanded to all noninvasive localized squamous cell carcinoma (SCC) from the previous noninvasive verrucous carcinoma. Most verrucous carcinomas exhibit a broad pushing deep aspect, and the presence, depth and extent of invasion are often difficult to assess. The new definition does not permit any overt destructive invasion in well-sampled verrucous carcinoma. The new Ta category also includes other noninvasive SCC types such as basaloid, warty, papillary, and mixed types. Ta is analogous to noninvasive papillary urothelial carcinoma of the urinary tract, while Tis designates penile carcinoma in situ just as it designates urothelial carcinoma in situ.

The definition of T1 or noncorporal invasive cancers is revised according to penile region-specific anatomy. The corpora are covered externally by varying tissue layers in the different regions of the penis (glans, foreskin, and shaft). Having precise definitions facilitates more consistent categorization of T1 disease, as compared to previous editions which used nonspecific subepithelial tissue layers as a general definition.

T1 is subcategorized into T1a and T1b, which have different risks for lymph node (LN) metastasis (10.5–18.1% vs 33.3–50%). This subcategorization is of considerable importance in the clinical consideration of performing inguinal LN dissection.

High-grade (G3) histology is one variable used to separate T1b from T1a cancers.

Sarcomatoid carcinoma, a known aggressive histology of SCC, is now considered as a high-grade feature of T1b cancer.

Perineural invasion is recognized as a predictor for regional LN metastasis and is now added as another separation criterion between T1a and T1b tumors.

T2 is now restricted to invasion into corpus spongiosum while invasion into corpus cavernosum is upstaged to T3. In previous editions, invasion of corpus spongiosum and corpus cavernosum were grouped together as T2. Recent studies have shown that corpus spongiosum invasion is associated with a lower incidence of inguinal LN involvement than corpus cavernosum invasion (33–35.8% vs 48.6–52.5%) and better survival.

Urethral invasion, previously defined as T3 disease, can now be either T2 or T3 depending on the more important level of corporal invasion. Penile cancer near the meatus may invade directly into the distal urethra bypassing the corpora and is not associated with worse outcome.

pN1 is now increased to up to two unilateral inguinal LN metastases, while pN2 is now modified as more than three unilateral or bilateral inguinal LN metastases. The shift to the lower pN1 may avoid adjuvant chemotherapy to some patients with (two positive) LN disease since this treatment has been recommended to pN2 patients. The AJCC 7th edition pN1 (single inguinal LN) and pN2 (multiple or bilateral inguinal LNs) categories were shown in some clinical scenarios to have no significant difference in risk for death from disease. However, metastasis involving three or more unilateral or bilateral inguinal LNs have poorer outcomes compared with metastasis involving one or two unilateral inguinal LNs (60.5% vs 90.7% 3-year cancer-specific survival).

The three-tiered WHO/ISUP grading system has now replaced the four-tiered modification of the Broder's grading system for SCC (level of evidence III). Histologic grade in penile SCC is a significant predictor of regional LN metastasis and has been shown to improve the ability of the AJCC stage to predict cancer-specific mortality.

The WHO/ISUP grading for SCC considers any amount of anaplasia as grade 3 (G3). Poorly differentiated histology or anaplasia particularly when >50% is a strong predictor for LN metastasis.

The two grade extremes (G1 and G3) facilitate prognostic categorization of penile SCC.

Reference: [29]

What Are the Prognostic Markers for Penile Carcinoma?

Histologic tumor type, grade, TNM classification, and perineural invasion are the most important factors in assessing prognosis in penile cancer. A prognostic index combining tumor grade, anatomic level of tumor infiltration, and perineural invasion has been proposed. The index correlates well with incidence of nodal metastases and patient survival.

Beyond conventional pathologic parameters, no single prognostic marker has gained widespread acceptance in penile carcinoma. Expression of p16 has been shown to be associated with a better prognosis, whereas the expression of p53 indicated a dismal clinical course. At the tumor boundary, an infiltrative pattern is associated with a higher risk for lymph node metastasis as compared with a pushing pattern. Markers that indicate an epithelial-mesenchymal transition (e.g., E-cadherin) and markers that are associated with stromal degradation (e.g., metalloproteinases) are therefore also promising candidates for assessment as prognostic indicators.

Metastasis to the inguinal lymph nodes is among the most important prognostic factors in cancer of the penis. A meticulous processing of inguinal lymph node specimens is therefore mandatory. The sentinel technique with radioactive tracers can be adopted to modify the extent of inguinal dissection.

References: [30, 31]

What Is the Management of Penile Cancer?

Treatment is dependent on tumor type and staging. Traditionally, the primary management of advanced invasive carcinoma involved radical or partial penile amputation with a 2-cm margin for oncologic efficacy. When penile tumors extend into the corporeal bodies, urethra, and adjacent structures (T2–T4), a more extensive resection was typically elected. Partial penectomy has demonstrated excellent oncologic control and is the gold standard for distal invasive tumors. When a negative margin cannot be achieved or a large fungating tumor is present, total amputation with perineal urethrostomy is recommended with penile reconstruction in select cases. For patients with evidence of inguinal lymph node metastasis, lymphadenectomy is mandatory.

For small low-grade, noninvasive (PeIN, Ta, T1a) and small carefully selected high-grade or even higher stage invasive tumors, conservative excision with attempted penile preservation may be elected. Techniques include wide local excision, laser ablation, partial or total glansectomy, glans resurfacing, Mohs microsurgery, partial amputation, and radiation therapy.

Reference: [32]

What Is the Protocol for the Examination of Specimens from Patients with Carcinoma of the Penis?

Penectomy Specimen

Take measurements, describe specimen, and identify and describe tumor. Most SCCs of the penis arise from the epithelium of the distal portion of the organ (glans, coronal sulcus, and mucosal surface of the prepuce; the tumor may involve one or more of these anatomic compartments).

Take a complete cross section (shave) of the proximal shaft amputation margin, making sure to include the entire circumference of the urethra. If the urethra has been retracted, it is important to identify its resection margin and submit it entirely. The resection margin can be divided in three important areas that need to be analyzed: the skin of the shaft with underlying dartos and penile fascia; corpora cavernosa with albuginea; and urethra with periurethral cylinder that includes lamina propria, corpus spongiosum, albuginea, and penile fascia (Fig. 7.1). Since this is a large specimen, it may need to be included in several cassettes to include the entire resection margin.

Fix the rest of the specimen overnight. Then, in the fixed state and if the tumor is large and involves most of the glans, cut longitudinally and centrally by using the meatus and the proximal urethra as reference points. Separate the specimen into halves, left and right. Then bread-loaf the shaft of the penis at 3 mm intervals beginning distally and stopping 1 cm from corona. Document the size and depth of any invasive neoplasm. Indicate whether the tumor invades the landmark structures, including corpus spongiosum, corpus cavernosum, and urethra. Submit sections of tumor to demonstrate its depth of invasion and relationship to urethra, corpora cavernosa, and corpus spongiosum. A section should include the tumor and adjacent unremarkable epithelium. Sections of the foreskin and glans and shaft mucosa should also be included. For tumors involving the urethra, indicate the extent of gross involvement and submit sections to indicate this.

Sample Dictation

Specimen is received [in formalin/fresh], labeled with the patient's name and "[ ]", and consists of a [partial/total] penectomy specimen with[out] attached foreskin, measuring [ ] × [ ] × [ ] cm. There is a [ ] × [ ] × [ ] cm tumor arising in the [foreskin/glans/coronal sulcus/shaft/or a combination of these]. The lesion is [color] and [ulcerative/flat/nodular/verrucous]. Upon sectioning, the tumor invades [subepithelium/corpora cavernosa/corpus spongiosum/urethra] to a depth of [ ] cm. The tumor is [not] present at the soft tissue margin, which is inked [ ]. The remaining [foreskin/glans/shaft] appears [unremarkable/remarkable] with [describe].

Summary of Sections

- 1A Shaft shave margin (including urethra)
- 1B Foreskin shave margin (if present)
- 1C Tumor with deepest invasion
- 1D Tumor in relation to urethra, corpora cavernosa, and spongiosum
- 1E Sections of normal-appearing foreskin, glans, and shaft

What Is the Proper Way to Report the Pathologic Findings in Penile Squamous Cell Carcinoma?

The report should contain the following information: primary tumor (tumor site or sites), size in centimeters, histologic subtype, histologic grade, anatomic level of invasion, tumor thickness in millimeters, and vascular and perineural invasion.

In penectomy specimens, the margins of resection to be reported are urethral/periurethral, corporal, and skin of the shaft. In circumcision specimens, margins include coronal sulcus mucosal margin and cutaneous margin. Commonly associated lesions to be reported are penile intraepithelial neoplasia (differentiated or undifferentiated), lichen sclerosus, and other "inflammatory dermatologic" conditions. If the specimen is accompanied by inguinal nodes, the number and size of nodes should be described. All nodes should be included for microscopic examination. The number of positive nodes and total number of nodes examined should be reported as well as the presence of extracapsular extension and the number and site (e.g., inguinal vs pelvic) of metastatic nodes. The distinction between superficial and deep inguinal lymph nodes has been removed in the 8th edition TNM classification.

Case Studies

Sclerosing Lipogranuloma

Case Presentation

A 35-year-old man presented with a hard mass invading the skin and subcutaneous tissues, which had progressively

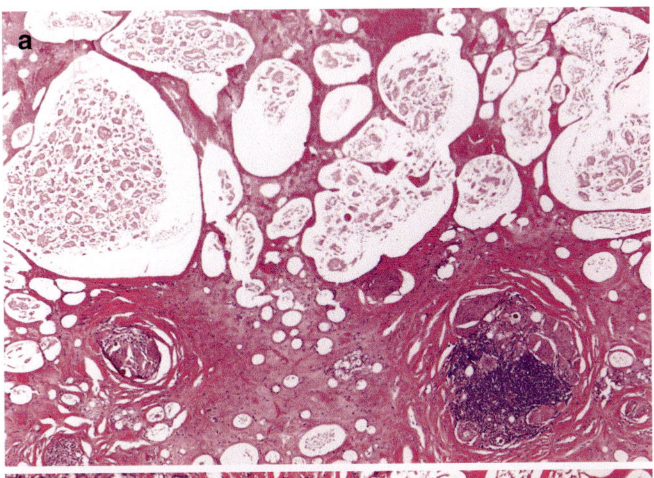

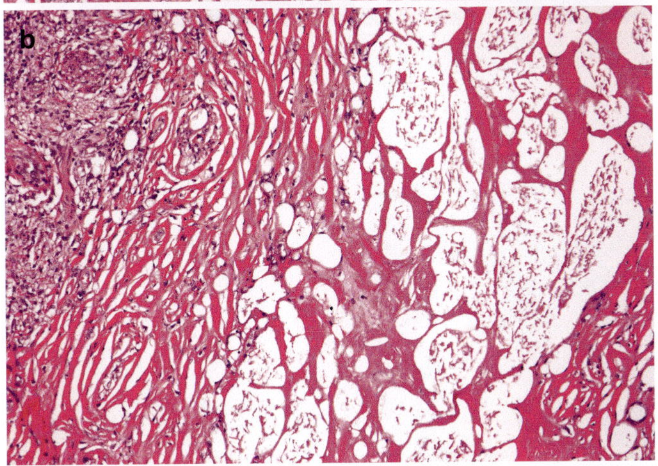

Fig. 7.19 Sclerosing lipogranuloma. (**a**) Numerous variably sized vacuolated spaces adjacent to characteristic sclerotic stroma. (**b**) Foreign body giant cells and lipid vacuoles with marked variation in size

enlarged over 3-month period. He denied the history of injecting foreign material into his external genitalia. There was no trauma to the groin. On physical examination, there were multiple non-tender, irregular masses on the penile shaft dorsally without pus discharge per meatus. The histopathology shows numerous, variably sized vacuolated spaces adjacent to characteristic sclerotic stroma (Fig. 7.19a) and foreign body giant cells and lipid vacuoles with marked variation in size (Fig. 7.19b)

Final diagnosis: sclerosing lipogranuloma

Case Report

Sclerosing lipogranuloma of the penis, also commonly referred to as penile paraffinoma, lipogranuloma, and Tancho's nodules, is a rare benign disease and presents as a peculiar granulomatous reaction that occurs after injury of the adipose tissue. It has been reported to involve many different organs. The term sclerosing lipogranuloma first appeared in Smetana and Bernhard's abstract in 1948 [33]. Subsequently, they expanded their case series to 14 cases,

9 of which involved external male genitalia [34]. They also proposed that it resulted from the reaction to endogenously broken down lipids following trauma provoking a fibrosis and foreign body reaction. Several years later, the other theory advocated by Newcomer [35] and supported by Arduino [36] was that the reaction followed the injection of foreign vegetable or mineral oils. Since then, a considerable number of cases have been reported in the English literature. Nowadays, the disease is subdivided into primary and secondary types based on precipitating factors. The primary type is caused by the reaction to endogenously broken down lipids, in which no possible etiologic factors can be identified, and is rare in Western countries. The secondary type is caused by injection of exogenous foreign bodies for variable reasons from premature ejaculation and impotence to sexual deviance. A wide variety of foreign materials, including silicone, paraffin, mineral oil, metallic mercury, petroleum jelly, vaseline, and cod liver oil, have been reported [37–40].

Clinically, patients usually present with penile deformity, painful erections and eventually, the inability to achieve sexual activities [37, 41]. Other manifestations of foreign body reaction are in the form of inflammation, induration, edema, scarring, necrosis, and ulceration. In some instance clinical presentations are alarming. Tsili et al. reported a patient presenting with painless enlargement of the penis shaft due to the presence of a hard mass invading the skin and subcutaneous tissues [42]. Reactive regional lymphadenopathy and gross deformity may lead to clinical concern for a neoplasia and often warrants biopsy.

An imaging technique accurately characterizing and assessing the extent of the disease would be valuable in the appropriate preoperative planning of these patients, although radiographical features are only described in limited number of case reports. The sonographic features include a poorly defined mass with a high level of echogenicity and an elongated appearance on a longitudinal plane [43]. Computerized tomography (CT) and multiparametric magnetic resonance imaging (MRI) findings of primary sclerosing lipogranuloma were reported in case reports. The lesion was reported to show symmetrically Y-shaped, with the arms of the Y surrounding the penile shaft. The mass showed similar and moderately high signal intensity when compared to muscles on T1- and T2-weighted images, respectively, with irregular enhancement after gadolinium administration, were often described as "Y-shaped" and were unlikely to recur. No fatty components were revealed within the mass.

Sclerosing lipogranulomas usually present indurated and sometimes tender plaque or tumor with variable sizes ranging from few centimeters to massive replacement of genital area. Correspondingly, the lesion is ill-defined with firm, yellow, granular, and gelatinous cut surfaces. Invading into adjacent skin and subcutaneous tissue and underlying muscles can be seen. Histopathological examination demonstrates lipid vacuoles embedded in a sclerotic stroma composed of epithelioid cells and a mixture of inflammatory cells infiltrates in the interstitium, including multinucleated giant cells, lymphocytes, macrophages, and monocytes. Eosinophils may be present, but usually mild. Inflammatory cells infiltrates may be multinodular or diffuse. If foreign bodies related, vacuoles of variable size corresponding to exogenous substances embedded in collagenous tissue may be obvious, which may mimic adipose tumor at lower power view. It becomes more obvious that many vacuoles are within mono- and multinucleated histiocytes at higher power examination. Immunohistochemical stain can be utilized to rule out neoplastic process, including CD68 and CD163 to confirm histiocytic nature of infiltrate. Oil Red O staining on frozen sections may be helpful to confirm the diagnosis.

Top differentials considerations include malakoplakia, liposarcoma, metastatic carcinoma with clear or signet ring cells, adenomatoid tumor and lymphangioma. Making the distinction among these differentials is critical, in view of the different therapeutic options for them. In most cases careful examination of morphologic features with H&E stain is the key to distinct sclerotic lipogranuloma from aforementioned entities. In cases that are challenging to diagnose with H&E sections, readily available immunohistochemical stains can aid in the distinction. Liposarcoma usually lacks of foreign body type giant cell reaction and foamy histiocytes, which are seen in sclerotic lipogranulomas. Metastatic carcinomas have atypical nuclei and immunoreactivity for keratin. Adenomatoid tumor is a benign mesothelial tumor and characterized by cystic or slit-like spaces lined by flattened or cuboidal cells and immunopositivity for keratin and mesothelial markers, including calretinin. Lymphangioma is another benign entity with the proliferation of dilated lymphatic vessels and positive for vascular or lymphatic markers, CD31 or D2-40, if needed, to clarify diagnosis.

Clinical management of secondary penile sclerosing lipogranuloma usually requires an aggressive treatment including partial or total excision of granulomas, with or without reconstructive skin flaps depending on the extent of excision.

Scrotal Calcinosis

Case Presentation

A 30-year-old man reports multiple itchy bumps on scrotum, which present for years. His physical examination revealed multiple and bilateral calcified cutaneous lesions of the scrotum. The lesions were completely surgically excised. Histological examination reveals basophilic granular and globular materials, which is consistent with calcium deposition (Fig. 7.20a), in various intensity and sizes in dermis and

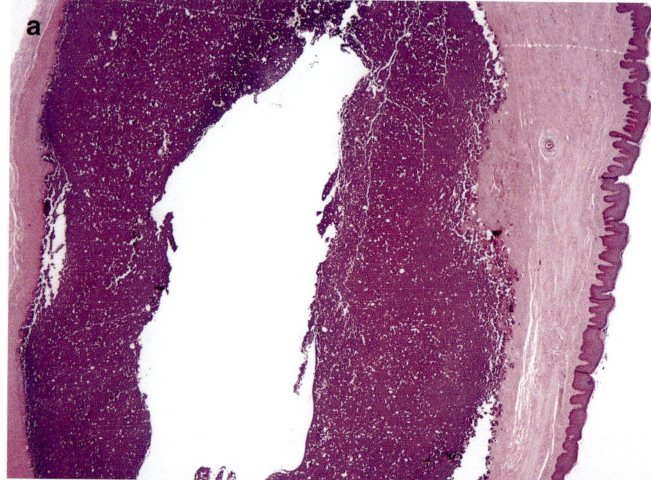

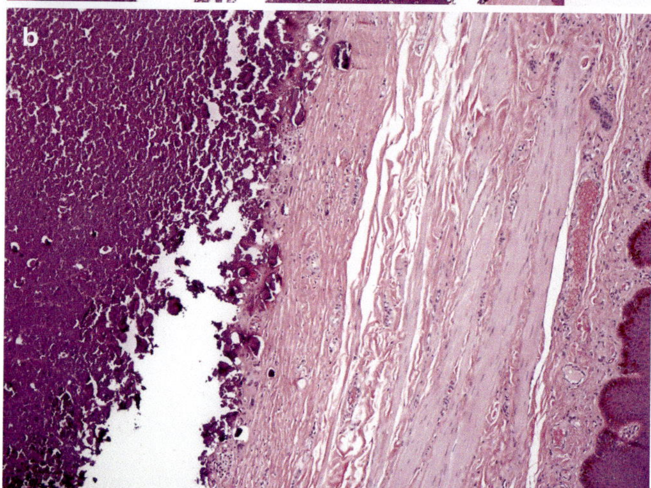

Fig. 7.20 Scrotal calcinosis. (**a**) Basophilic granular and globular materials with various intensity and size are seen in dermis, which is consistent with calcium. (**b**) Palisading histiocytes and multinucleated giant cells are present at the periphery

upper part of dartos. Palisading histiocytes and multinucleated giant cells are found at the periphery (Fig. 7.20b).

Final diagnosis: scrotal calcinosis

Case Report

Scrotal calcinosis is a rare, yet benign, disease of the scrotal skin with uncertain etiology, which was first described in 1883 by Lewinski [44]. Clinically, it usually presents as gradual growth of brown-yellow firm solitary or multiple nodules on the scrotal skin in the absence of abnormalities in calcium and phosphate metabolism [45]. Sometimes it produces a white, chalky material. Scrotal calcinosis typically begins in adolescence or early adulthood. Although it tends to increase in size and number over time [46], lesions remain discrete and do not become confluent. In addition, nodules are movable and do not attach to underlying structures. Some patients complain about pain and itching and there have also been reports of infections associated with scrotal calcinosis. Unusual presentations include pedunculated forms [47] and perineal/suprapubic pain consistent with chronic prostatitis [48]. To relieve symptoms and to preserve scrotal cosmesis are the indication for surgery [49]. Although it is controversial, surgery is still considered to be the treatment of choice and provides a good clinical outcome. The laxity of the scrotal skin, along with the decision to perform multiple elliptical excisions, allowed for good scrotal coverage and excellent cosmetic outcome. However, there are considerable controversies among clinicians as to the risk of recurrence after surgery. Some clinicians believe that all patients with scrotal calcinosis should undergo surgical intervention, in contrast, other disagree with surgical excision considering the high probability of recurrence [50].

Controversy regarding the pathogenesis of scrotal calcinosis still exists, despite its rarity and benign clinical behavior. Some investigators believe that it is truly a late presentation of epidermal inclusion cysts with dystrophic calcification [51–53]. It was previously proposed that it has been attributed to sebaceous cysts, calcified steatocystoma, fibroma, atheroma, and xanthoma [54]. More recently, it has been suggested that scrotal calcinosis is resulting dystrophic calcification from dartos muscle necrosis and degeneration [47].

Macroscopically, scrotal calcinosis shows hard white calcified deposits located in dermis and dartos. Histologically, it is characterized by basophilic granular and globular materials, which is consistent with calcium deposition, in various intensity and sizes in dermis and upper part of dartos. Palisading histiocytes and multinucleated giant cells are usually found at the periphery. Remnants of preexisting cystic lesion or adnexal neoplasm may be identified adjacent to the lesion. Calcified material can be highlighted with von Kossa stain though it is rarely necessary [55].

There almost no histologic differential diagnosis owing to very distinctive morphology of scrotal calcinosis. Nodular amyloidosis is only consideration. In contrast to scrotal calcinosis, amyloidosis exhibits homogeneous and eosinophilic material, which is positive for Congo red and crystal violet and negative for von Kossa [56].

Although the consensus on the management is still lacking, surgical intervention is the only treatment recommendation, especially for patients with multiple nodules. Nonsurgical treatment includes the use of corticosteroids and a low-calcium diet with cellulose phosphate supplementation. Surgical management corrects cosmetic deformity and enable to provide tissue sample for confirmation of the diagnosis on histologic examination.

References

1. Cubilla AL, Velazquez EF, Amin MB, Epstein J, Berney DM, Corbishley CM, et al. The World Health Organisation 2016 classification of penile carcinomas: a review and update from the International Society of Urological Pathology expert-driven recommendations. Histopathology. 2018;72(6):893–904. https://doi.org/10.1111/his.13429.
2. Moch H, Cubilla AL, Humphrey PA, Reuter VE, Ulbright TM. The 2016 WHO classification of tumours of the urinary system and male genital organs-part a: renal, penile, and testicular tumours. Eur Urol. 2016;70(1):93–105. https://doi.org/10.1016/j.eururo.2016.02.029.
3. Sanchez DF, Canete S, Fernandez-Nestosa MJ, Lezcano C, Rodriguez I, Barreto J, et al. HPV- and non-HPV-related subtypes of penile squamous cell carcinoma (SCC): morphological features and differential diagnosis according to the new WHO classification (2015). Semin Diagn Pathol. 2015;32(3):198–221. https://doi.org/10.1053/j.semdp.2014.12.018.
4. International Agency for Research on C, Moch H. WHO classification of tumours of the urinary system and male genital organs. Lyon: International Agency for Research on Cancer; 2016.
5. Guimaraes GC, Cunha IW, Soares FA, Lopes A, Torres J, Chaux A, et al. Penile squamous cell carcinoma clinicopathological features, nodal metastasis and outcome in 333 cases. J Urol. 2009;182(2):528–34; discussion 34. https://doi.org/10.1016/j.juro.2009.04.028.
6. Sanchez DF, Soares F, Alvarado-Cabrero I, Canete S, Fernandez-Nestosa MJ, Rodriguez IM, et al. Pathological factors, behavior, and histological prognostic risk groups in subtypes of penile squamous cell carcinomas (SCC). Semin Diagn Pathol. 2015;32(3):222–31. https://doi.org/10.1053/j.semdp.2014.12.017.
7. Barreto JE, Velazquez EF, Ayala E, Torres J, Cubilla AL. Carcinoma cuniculatum: a distinctive variant of penile squamous cell carcinoma: report of 7 cases. Am J Surg Pathol. 2007;31(1):71–5. https://doi.org/10.1097/01.pas.0000213401.72569.22.
8. Cunha IW, Guimaraes GC, Soares F, Velazquez E, Torres JJ, Chaux A, et al. Pseudoglandular (adenoid, acantholytic) penile squamous cell carcinoma: a clinicopathologic and outcome study of 7 patients. Am J Surg Pathol. 2009;33(4):551–5. https://doi.org/10.1097/PAS.0b013e31818a01d8.
9. Velazquez EF, Melamed J, Barreto JE, Aguero F, Cubilla AL. Sarcomatoid carcinoma of the penis: a clinicopathologic study of 15 cases. Am J Surg Pathol. 2005;29(9):1152–8. https://doi.org/10.1097/01.pas.0000160440.46394.a8.
10. Romero FR, de Castro MG, Garcia CR, Perez MD. Adenosquamous carcinoma of the penis. Clinics (Sao Paulo). 2006;61(4):363–4. https://doi.org/10.1590/s1807-59322006000400016.
11. Rubin MA, Kleter B, Zhou M, Ayala G, Cubilla AL, Quint WG, et al. Detection and typing of human papillomavirus DNA in penile carcinoma: evidence for multiple independent pathways of penile carcinogenesis. Am J Pathol. 2001;159(4):1211–8. https://doi.org/10.1016/S0002-9440(10)62506-0.
12. Cubilla AL, Lloveras B, Alemany L, Alejo M, Vidal A, Kasamatsu E, et al. Basaloid squamous cell carcinoma of the penis with papillary features: a clinicopathologic study of 12 cases. Am J Surg Pathol. 2012;36(6):869–75. https://doi.org/10.1097/PAS.0b013e318249c6f3.
13. Cubilla AL, Velazques EF, Reuter VE, Oliva E, Mihm MC Jr, Young RH. Warty (condylomatous) squamous cell carcinoma of the penis: a report of 11 cases and proposed classification of 'verruciform' penile tumors. Am J Surg Pathol. 2000;24(4):505–12. https://doi.org/10.1097/00000478-200004000-00004.

14. Chaux A, Tamboli P, Ayala A, Soares F, Rodriguez I, Barreto J, et al. Warty-basaloid carcinoma: clinicopathological features of a distinctive penile neoplasm. Report of 45 cases. Mod Pathol. 2010;23(6):896–904. https://doi.org/10.1038/modpathol.2010.69.

15. Sanchez DF, Rodriguez IM, Piris A, Canete S, Lezcano C, Velazquez EF, et al. Clear cell carcinoma of the penis: an HPV-related variant of squamous cell carcinoma: a report of 3 cases. Am J Surg Pathol. 2016;40(7):917–22. https://doi.org/10.1097/PAS.0000000000000607.

16. Mentrikoski MJ, Frierson HF Jr, Stelow EB, Cathro HP. Lymphoepithelioma-like carcinoma of the penis: association with human papilloma virus infection. Histopathology. 2014;64(2):312–5. https://doi.org/10.1111/his.12248.

17. Chaux A, Velazquez EF, Amin A, Soskin A, Pfannl R, Rodriguez IM, et al. Distribution and characterization of subtypes of penile intraepithelial neoplasia and their association with invasive carcinomas: a pathological study of 139 lesions in 121 patients. Hum Pathol. 2012;43(7):1020–7. https://doi.org/10.1016/j.humpath.2011.07.025.

18. Darragh TM, Colgan TJ, Thomas Cox J, Heller DS, Henry MR, Luff RD, et al. The lower anogenital squamous terminology standardization project for HPV-associated lesions: background and consensus recommendations from the College of American Pathologists and the American Society for Colposcopy and Cervical Pathology. Int J Gynecol Pathol. 2013;32(1):76–115. https://doi.org/10.1097/PGP.0b013e31826916c7.

19. Chaux A, Cubilla AL, Haffner MC, Lecksell KL, Sharma R, Burnett AL, et al. Combining routine morphology, p16(INK4a) immunohistochemistry, and in situ hybridization for the detection of human papillomavirus infection in penile carcinomas: a tissue microarray study using classifier performance analyses. Urol Oncol. 2014;32(2):171–7. https://doi.org/10.1016/j.urolonc.2012.04.017.

20. Cubilla AL, Lloveras B, Alejo M, Clavero O, Chaux A, Kasamatsu E, et al. Value of p16(INK)(4)(a) in the pathology of invasive penile squamous cell carcinomas: a report of 202 cases. Am J Surg Pathol. 2011;35(2):253–61. https://doi.org/10.1097/PAS.0b013e318203cdba.

21. Cubilla AL, Lloveras B, Alejo M, Clavero O, Chaux A, Kasamatsu E, et al. The basaloid cell is the best tissue marker for human papillomavirus in invasive penile squamous cell carcinoma: a study of 202 cases from Paraguay. Am J Surg Pathol. 2010;34(1):104–14. https://doi.org/10.1097/PAS.0b013e3181c76a49.

22. Djajadiningrat RS, Jordanova ES, Kroon BK, van Werkhoven E, de Jong J, Pronk DT, et al. Human papillomavirus prevalence in invasive penile cancer and association with clinical outcome. J Urol. 2015;193(2):526–31. https://doi.org/10.1016/j.juro.2014.08.087.

23. Lont AP, Kroon BK, Horenblas S, Gallee MP, Berkhof J, Meijer CJ, et al. Presence of high-risk human papillomavirus DNA in penile carcinoma predicts favorable outcome in survival. Int J Cancer. 2006;119(5):1078–81. https://doi.org/10.1002/ijc.21961.

24. Bezerra SM, Chaux A, Ball MW, Faraj SF, Munari E, Gonzalez-Roibon N, et al. Human papillomavirus infection and immunohistochemical p16(INK4a) expression as predictors of outcome in penile squamous cell carcinomas. Hum Pathol. 2015;46(4):532–40. https://doi.org/10.1016/j.humpath.2014.12.004.

25. Miralles-Guri C, Bruni L, Cubilla AL, Castellsague X, Bosch FX, de Sanjose S. Human papillomavirus prevalence and type distribution in penile carcinoma. J Clin Pathol. 2009;62(10):870–8. https://doi.org/10.1136/jcp.2008.063149.

26. Abreu AL, Souza RP, Gimenes F, Consolaro ME. A review of methods for detect human papillomavirus infection. Virol J. 2012;9:262. https://doi.org/10.1186/1743-422X-9-262.

27. Chaux A, Torres J, Pfannl R, Barreto J, Rodriguez I, Velazquez EF, et al. Histologic grade in penile squamous cell carcinoma: visual estimation versus digital measurement of proportions of grades, adverse prognosis with any proportion of grade 3 and correlation of a Gleason-like system with nodal metastasis. Am J Surg Pathol. 2009;33(7):1042–8. https://doi.org/10.1097/PAS.0b013e31819aa4c9.

28. Velazquez EF, Ayala G, Liu H, Chaux A, Zanotti M, Torres J, et al. Histologic grade and perineural invasion are more important than tumor thickness as predictor of nodal metastasis in penile squamous cell carcinoma invading 5 to 10 mm. Am J Surg Pathol. 2008;32(7):974–9. https://doi.org/10.1097/PAS.0b013e3181641365.

29. Amin MB, Edge SB, Greene FL, Byrd DR, Brookland RK, Washington MK, et al. AJCC cancer staging manual. Cham: Springer International Publishing; 2018.

30. Cubilla AL. The role of pathologic prognostic factors in squamous cell carcinoma of the penis. World J Urol. 2009;27(2):169–77. https://doi.org/10.1007/s00345-008-0315-7.

31. Chaux A, Caballero C, Soares F, Guimaraes GC, Cunha IW, Reuter V, et al. The prognostic index: a useful pathologic guide for prediction of nodal metastases and survival in penile squamous cell carcinoma. Am J Surg Pathol. 2009;33(7):1049–57. https://doi.org/10.1097/PAS.0b013e31819d17eb.

32. Wollina U, Steinbach F, Verma S, Tchernev G. Penile tumours: a review. J Eur Acad Dermatol Venereol. 2014;28(10):1267–76. https://doi.org/10.1111/jdv.12491.

33. Smetana HF, Barnhard WG. Sclerosing lipogranuloma. Am J Pathol. 1948;24(3):675–7.

34. Smetana HF, Bernhard W. Sclerosing lipogranuloma. Arch Pathol (Chic). 1950;50(3):296–325.

35. Newcomer VD, et al. Sclerosing lipogranuloma resulting from exogenous lipids. AMA Arch Derm. 1956;73(4):361–72.

36. Arduino LJ. Sclerosing lipogranuloma of male genitalia. J Urol. 1959;82(1):155–61.

37. Sasidaran R, Zain MA, Basiron NH. Low-grade liquid silicone injections as a penile enhancement procedure: is bigger better? Urol Ann. 2012;4(3):181–6.

38. Silberstein J, Downs T, Goldstein I. Penile injection with silicone: case report and review of the literature. J Sex Med. 2008;5(9):2231–7.

39. Foxton G, et al. Sclerosing lipogranuloma of the penis. Australas J Dermatol. 2011;52(3):e12–4.

40. Best EW, et al. Sclerosing lipogranuloma of the male genitalia produced by mineral oil. Proc Staff Meet Mayo Clin. 1953;28(22):623–31.

41. Bjurlin MA, et al. Mineral oil-induced sclerosing lipogranuloma of the penis. J Clin Aesthet Dermatol. 2010;3(9):41–4.

42. Tsili AC, et al. Silicone-induced penile sclerosing lipogranuloma: magnetic resonance imaging findings. J Clin Imaging Sci. 2016;6:3.

43. Jung SE, et al. Sclerosing lipogranuloma of the scrotum: sonographic findings and pathologic correlation. J Ultrasound Med. 2007;26(9):1231–3.

44. Pompeo A, et al. Idiopathic scrotal calcinosis: a rare entity and a review of the literature. Can Urol Assoc J. 2013;7(5–6):E439–41.

45. Ozgenel GY, et al. Idiopathic scrotal calcinosis. Ann Plast Surg. 2002;48(4):453–4.

46. Saad AG, Zaatari GS. Scrotal calcinosis: is it idiopathic? Urology. 2001;57(2):365.

47. Gi N, et al. Idiopathic scrotal calcinosis – a pedunculated rare variant. J Plast Reconstr Aesthet Surg. 2008;61(4):466–7.

48. Tsai YS, et al. Scrotal calcinosis presenting with prostatitis-like symptoms. Urology. 2002;59(1):138.

49. Khallouk A, et al. Idiopathic scrotal calcinosis: a non-elucidated pathogenesis and its surgical treatment. Rev Urol. 2011;13(2):95–7.
50. Ruiz-Genao DP, et al. Massive scrotal calcinosis. Dermatol Surg. 2002;28(8):745–7.
51. Swinehart JM, Golitz LE. Scrotal calcinosis. Dystrophic calcification of epidermoid cysts. Arch Dermatol. 1982;118(12):985–8.
52. Sarma DP, Weilbaecher TG. Scrotal calcinosis: calcification of epidermal cysts. J Surg Oncol. 1984;27(2):76–9.
53. Shah V, Shet T. Scrotal calcinosis results from calcification of cysts derived from hair follicles: a series of 20 cases evaluating the spectrum of changes resulting in scrotal calcinosis. Am J Dermatopathol. 2007;29(2):172–5.
54. Ito A, Sakamoto F, Ito M. Dystrophic scrotal calcinosis originating from benign eccrine epithelial cysts. Br J Dermatol. 2001;144(1):146–50.
55. Song DH, Lee KH, Kang WH. Idiopathic calcinosis of the scrotum: histopathologic observations of fifty-one nodules. J Am Acad Dermatol. 1988;19(6):1095–101.
56. Velazquez E, Cubilla A. Scrotal calcinosis. In: Amin M, Tickoo S, editors. Dignostic pathology: genitourinary: Elsevier: Philadelphia, PA 19103; 2016. p. 920–1.

Adrenal Gland Pathology

Ming Zhou and Ximing J. Yang

How to Work up Adrenal Lesions Based on Clinical, Imaging, and Laboratory Findings

Pathological diagnosis is a part of the clinical work-up of an adrenal lesion. Before reviewing the histological slides of an adrenal specimen, it is important to obtain relevant clinical, radiological, and laboratory information. Gross appearance also provides important diagnostic clues.

- Patient demographics: Both adrenal cortical tumors and pheochromocytoma tend to afflict middle-aged female. Metastatic carcinomas typically occur in older patients.
- History: In a patient with a history of malignancy, particularly, lung and kidney cancers, metastasis must be considered in the differential diagnosis.
- Functional activity of the adrenal lesion: Most patients with pheochromocytomas present with symptoms related to catecholamine synthesis such as paroxysmal or persistent hypertension, postural hypotension, palpitation, headache, or diaphoresis. Less than half of the adrenal cortical tumors are functional, and are associated with Cushing syndrome (excess of cortisol), Conn syndrome (excess aldosterone), or hyperandrogenism (excess androgen), including, hirsutism, lower voice, acne in women, and infertility.
- Laboratory tests: Pheochromocytomas produce excess catecholamine and result in elevated plasma-free metanephrine, the metabolite of epinephrine, and elevated urine catecholamine metabolites such as metanephrine, VMA, and HVA. Elevated steroid hormones can be measured in blood or urine in patients with functional adenoma or hyperplasia. Intravenous sampling for hormones may determine whether adrenal lesions are unilateral or bilateral.
- Associated genetic syndromes: The major genetic syndromes associated with pheochromocytoma are von Hippel–Lindau disease (VHLD), multiple endocrine neoplasia (MEN) types 2A and 2B, neurofibromatosis (NF) type 1, and familiar pheochromocytoma/paraganglioma syndrome due to mutations in succinate dehydrogenase (*SDH*) genes. A possibility of pheochromocytoma should be considered for patients with known aforementioned syndromes.

These criteria are summarized in Table 8.1.
References: [1, 2]

What Features in Radiographic Imaging Studies and Gross Appearance Can Be Helpful in Diagnosis of Adrenal Lesions?

- Laterality: Primary neoplastic lesions such as pheochromocytoma, cortical adenoma, and cortical carcinoma are often unilateral, while cortical hyperplasia is often bilateral. Metastatic tumors can be unilateral or bilateral.
- Focality: A cortical adenoma or pheochromocytoma is more often solitary while cortical hyperplasia is mostly multifocal, although double or even multiple adenomas have rarely been reported. Granulomatous lesions are also multifocal. Single or multifocal nodules can be seen in metastatic disease.
- Size: Cortical carcinomas are usually larger than 10 cm, while adenomas are often smaller than 5 cm.
- Color: Cortical adenomas show yellow cut surface similar to the color of normal adrenal cortex.

M. Zhou (✉)
Department of Pathology and Laboratory Medicine, Tufts Medical Center, Tufts School of Medicine, Boston, MA, USA
e-mail: mzhou3@tuftsmedicalcenter.org

X. J. Yang
Department of Pathology, Northwestern Memorial Hospital, Northwestern University Feinberg School of Medicine, Chicago, IL, USA

© Springer Nature Switzerland AG 2021
X. J. Yang, M. Zhou (eds.), *Practical Genitourinary Pathology*, Practical Anatomic Pathology,
https://doi.org/10.1007/978-3-030-57141-2_8

Table 8.1 Initial differential diagnosis of adrenal lesions based on clinical, radiological, and laboratory findings

		Radiological findings	
		Unifocal/unilateral	Multifocal/bilateral
Laboratory findings	Hyperfunctional	Adenoma, cortical carcinoma, pheochromocytoma	Cortical hyperplasia
	Nonfunctional	Adenoma, cortical carcinoma, metastasis, myelolipoma, incidentaloma	Nonhyperfunctional cortical hyperplasia metastasis

Pheochromocytomas are pink to dark on cut surface. Clear cell RCCs often show typical distinct yellow cut surface, brighter than the color of adrenal cortex or cortical adenoma, with focal hemorrhage. Myelolipomas show mixed yellow (adipose) and red (marrow elements) appearance (Fig. 8.1a–f)

- Degeneration and necrosis: Degenerative changes, including scar, and mucoid changes, can be seen in any large tumors, benign or malignant, cortical or medullary. Necrosis and hemorrhage are rare in cortical adenoma, but very commonly seen in cortical carcinoma. A pheochromocytoma is rich in blood supply, therefore, often appears hemorrhagic (Fig. 8.1a–f).
- Normal adrenal cortex ranges 0.6–1.4 (mean 1) mm. Atrophic adrenal cortex indicates the tumor secrets cortisol.

References: [3, 4]

What Are the Immunohistochemical Stains Used for the Common Differential Diagnosis?

The choice of immunohistochemical (IHC) markers depends on the purpose of differential diagnosis, which most often includes cortical tumors versus pheochromocytoma, and cortical tumors versus a metastatic clear cell renal cell carcinoma.

Cortical tumors (both adenoma and carcinoma) are positive for adrenocortical markers (Melan A, inhibin, and calretinin). Cortical carcinoma is often positive for keratins such as AE1/AE3 but cortical adenoma is not. Pheochromocytoma is positive for neuroendocrine markers such as chromogranin, synaptophysin, and neuron-specific enolase. Renal cell carcinoma is positive for PAX8 and keratins. Clear cell RCC is also positive for carbonic anhydrase (CAIX). Ki67 is generally very low in cortical adenoma and pheochromocytoma, but high in cortical carcinoma and RCC. These features are summarized in Table 8.2.

References: [5, 6]

How to Work up Adrenal Cortical Cysts?

There are four types of adrenal cysts. The most common type is vascular, which accounts for nearly 50% of the cystic lesions in adrenal gland. Other cystic adrenal lesions include pseudocysts (40%), epithelial cysts, and parasitic cysts.

Adequate tissue sampling is important to classify the cystic lesions. The cystic lining has to be carefully evaluated. Vascular cystic lesions have endothelial lining (Fig. 8.2a). An epithelial cyst has epithelial lining (Fig. 8.2b), although such a lining may be largely denuded and may be identified only after extensive sampling and search. Adrenal tumors with cystic changes are included in the "epithelial cyst" category by some authorities, although such a classification is not universally accepted. Epithelial cysts are lined by true epithelial or mesothelial lining, and by adrenal cortical (Fig. 8.2b) or medullar cells in cystic adrenal tumors. Pseudocysts do not have an epithelial or endothelial lining; rather they comprise of tissue necrosis or degenerative changes (Fig. 8.2c). Parasitic cysts are associated with parasitic organisms such as echinococcosis (hydatid cyst).

Immunohistochemistry for endothelial markers such as CD31, ERG, or D2-40 may be useful to diagnose vascular cysts. A panel of epithelial markers may be necessary to identify a neoplastic process with extensive necrosis and cystic changes such as a papillary renal cell carcinoma.

References: [7–9]

What Are the Common Adrenal Mass Lesions Encountered in Surgical Pathology?

Table 8.3 lists the types of common mass lesions resected during a 12-year period at an academic medical center in the United States (Yang X unpublished data). Based on this table, the most common adrenal mass lesion diagnosed in surgical pathology practice is cortical adenoma, which represents nearly 40% of the adrenal mass lesions. However, the percentage is much higher in an autopsy series of which 90% of the adrenal tumors are cortical adenomas. The second most common mass lesion is pheochromocytoma, probably

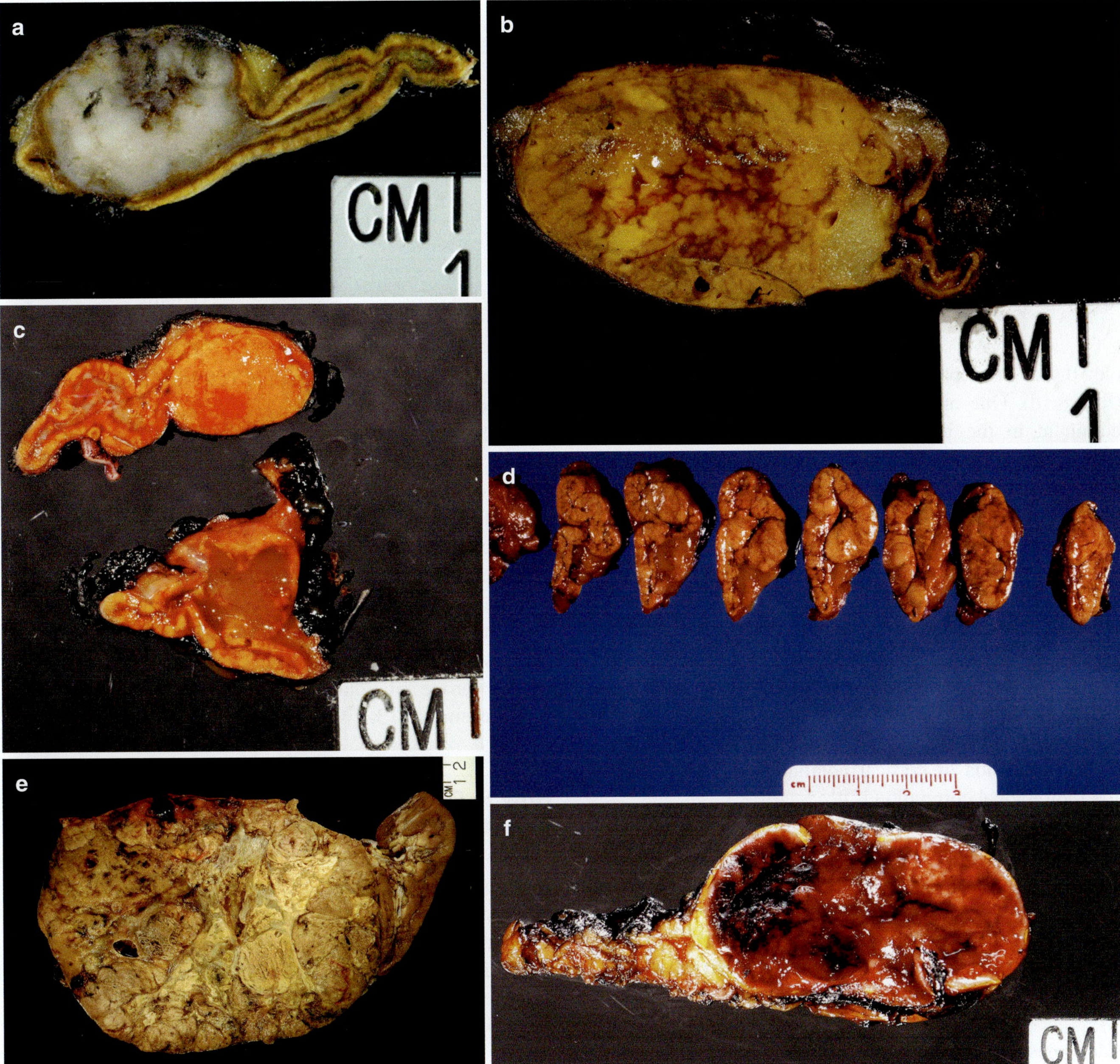

Fig. 8.1 The gross appearance of several adrenal lesions. Metastatic melanoma is white-tan with focal black pigmentation (**a**). Note the adrenal cortex is of normal thickness (1 mm). A cortisol secreting adenoma has a yellow cut surface (**b**). The adrenal cortex is atrophic. In contrast, the adrenal cortex adjacent to an aldosteronoma is of normal thickness (**c**). Adrenal cortical hyperplasia shows diffuse cortical thickening and multinodularity (**d**). An adrenalectomy specimen shows a large adrenal cortical carcinoma with multinodular appearance and necrosis (**e**). A pheochromocytoma has a friable hemorrhagic cut surface (**f**)

because most of them are symptomatic. In our series, pheochromocytomas account for nearly 20%, similar to 28.9% reported in a published study. With contemporary laboratory tests and imaging studies, these adrenal tumors can be detected earlier and resected completely. Metastatic carcinomas are seen in 10% of the adrenal surgical specimens.

References: [10, 11]

How to Distinguish Adenoma from Cortical Hyperplasia with Dominant Nodule(s)?

Adrenal cortical adenoma is usually a solitary well-defined mass without capsule (Fig. 8.3a), although double or multiple adenomas have rarely been described. Adrenal cortical hyperplasia, in contrast, is bilateral, and typically has multi-

Table 8.2 Comparison of common adrenal neoplasms

	Cortical adenoma	Cortical carcinoma	Pheochromocytoma	Renal cell carcinoma
Calretinin	Positive	Variable		
Inhibin	Positive	Positive	Negative	Negative
Melan A	Positive	Positive	Negative	Negative
AE1/AE3	Sometime positive	Variable	Negative	Positive
Vimentin	Negative	Positive	Variable	Positive
Ki67	Low (<5%)	High	Low	Low-high
S100	Negative	Negative	Positive in sustentacular cells	Negative
Synaptophysin	Often positive	Variable	Positive	Negative
Steroidogenic factor-1 (SF-1)	Positive	Positive		
PAX8	Negative	Negative	Negative	Positive

ple fused or separate large or small cortical nodules (Fig. 8.1d). One or a few nodules may become large and dominant in the background of hyperplasia (Fig. 8.3b). Adrenal cortical hyperplasia is generally treated medically, but is occasionally resected when it is no longer responsive to medical treatment or suspicious for a neoplastic lesion.

The differential diagnosis relies primarily on the clinical, imaging, and laboratory findings (Table 8.4). The nonlesional cortex provides diagnostic clues, that is, normal or atrophic in adenomas and thickened in hyperplasia. When the tissue sampling is limited as in core needle biopsy or partial resection, or severely fragmented specimen, it is prudent to sign out the case as "fragments of hyperplastic adrenal cortical tissue, the differential diagnosis includes a cortical adenoma or cortical nodular hyperplasia. Clinical and radiological correlation is necessary."

Reference: [12]

Can an Aldosteronoma (Aldosterone-Secreting Adenoma) Be Distinguished from Glucocorticoid-Secreting Adenomas Based on Morphological Features?

Adenomas secreting different classes of steroid hormones produce different symptoms and signs, upon which clinical diagnosis is based. However, some adenomas may produce more than one class of steroid hormones. Because it often causes more serious clinical symptoms, aldosteronomas are more commonly diagnosed and resected than other nonfunctional or functional cortical adenomas that secrete cortisol or androgen.

Gross appearance may provide some clues. The nonlesional cortex is usually of normal thickness in aldosteronoma (Fig. 8.1c). In contrast, it is thin and atrophic in glucocorticoid-secreting adenomas due to decreased ACTH production by the pituitary gland as the result of feedback inhibition by the elevated cortisol (Fig. 8.1b).

In aldosteronomas, tumor cells contain vacuolated eosinophilic cytoplasm and resemble zona glomerulosa (Fig. 8.4a). However, tumor cells may also resemble other layers of the adrenal cortex, ranging from large lipid rich cells (zona fasciculata) to compact oncocytic cells (zona reticularis). These different types of cells are often found in the same tumor.

Small eosinophilic intracytoplasmic inclusions (Spironolactone bodies) can sometimes be seen in the tumor cells, which are possibly related to the prior treatment with an aldosterone antagonist, such as spironolactone (Fig. 8.4b).

References: [13, 14]

How to Differentiate Cortical Adenoma from Cortical Carcinoma?

Adrenocortical carcinomas are usually large tumors, often >10 cm, and are rarely <4 cm. They often weigh >100 g, but tumors of <50 g may be malignant. Thus, neither size nor weight alone is diagnostic of malignancy. Hemorrhage and necrosis are common in cortical carcinomas (Figs. 8.1e and 8.5).

The most widely used multiparametric scoring system and algorithm to predict the biological behavior of a cortical neoplasm is the Weiss criteria, which include three categories with three parameters in each category (Fig. 8.6).

- *Nuclear atypia*: High nuclear grade (equivalent to Fuhrman III or IV); high mitotic rate (>5/50HPF); and atypical mitosis
- *Growth patterns*: <25% clear cells; >1/3 diffuse pattern; and necrosis
- *Invasiveness*: Capsular invasion; venous invasion; and sinusoidal invasion

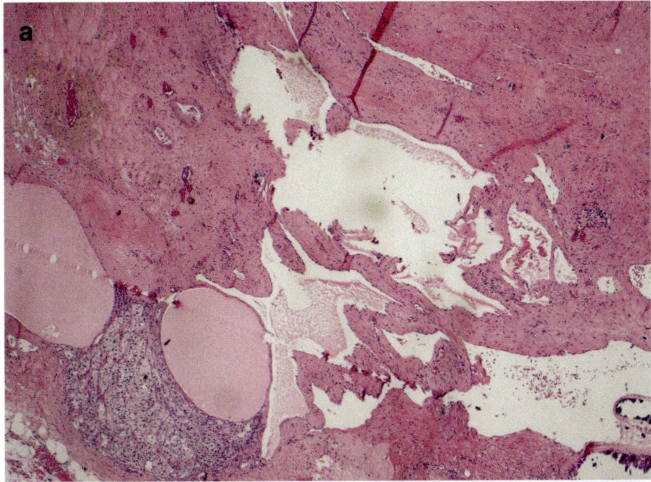

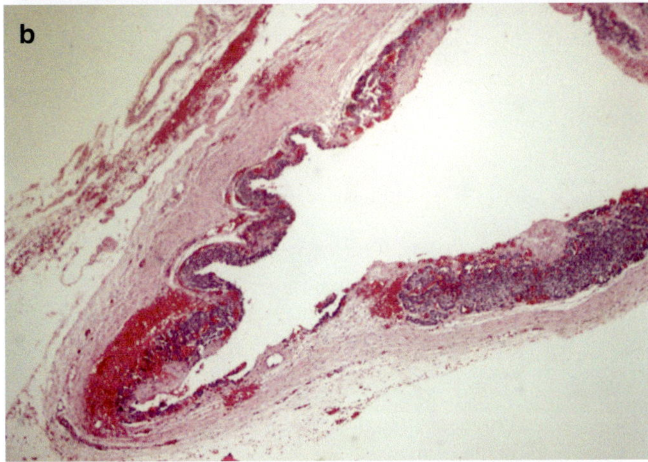

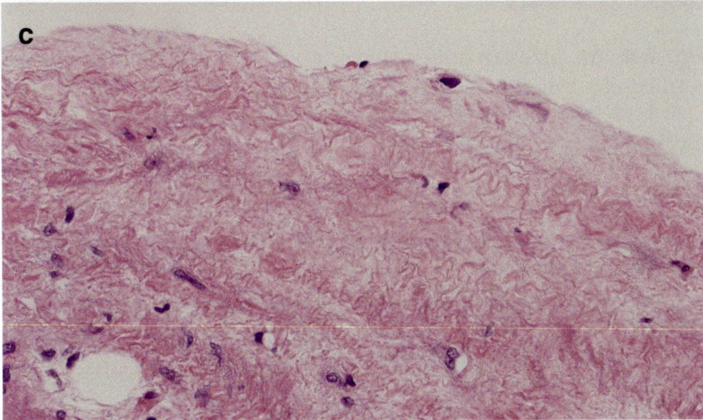

Fig. 8.2 An adrenal lymphangioma comprises of multiple cysts with fibrotic cystic walls covered with single layer of endothelial cells. Cysts contain eosinophilic material (**a**). A cystic adrenal cortical tumor is lined by cortical cells (**b**). An adrenal pseudocyst does not show any lining cells (**c**)

Table 8.3 Common adrenal mass lesions in surgical pathology[a]

Lesions	Percentage (Surgical pathology) [%]	Percentage (Autopsy) [%]
Cortical adenoma	36.9	90
Pheochromocytoma	19.8	5
Metastatic carcinoma	12.2	2
Hyperplasia	5.4	
Cortical carcinoma	3.6	2%
Myelolipoma	3.6	
Cysts	3.6	
Ganglioneuroma	2.7	
Others	12.2	

[a]Based on unpublished data from an academic institution

benign. Cortical tumors with features worrisome for but fall short of criteria for cancer should be diagnosed as "adrenal cortical tumor with uncertain malignant potential."

Reference: [15]

Do "Oncocytic" Cortical Tumors Really Have Better Prognosis?

Oncocytic cortical neoplasms are characterized by large epithelial cells with abundant eosinophilic granular cytoplasm, which can be arranged in solid, alveolar, or tubular patterns (Fig. 8.7). Most of these tumors are not functional. Oncocytic cortical neoplasms can be benign or malignant. The Weiss criteria may not be applicable in oncocytic cortical tumors, as these tumors show the loss of clear cytoplasm, prominent nuclear atypia, and diffuse growth pattern.

Bisceglia et al. proposed an algorithm to classify oncocytic adrenocortical tumors. Major criteria include high mitotic rate (>5/50 HPFs), atypical mitoses, and venous invasion, and minor criteria include large size and huge weight (>10 cm and/or >200 g), necrosis, capsular invasion, and sinusoidal invasion. One major criterion indicates malignancy, while one to four minor criteria indicate uncertain malignant potential (borderline), and the absence of all major and minor criteria indicates benign.

Reference: [16]

What Is the Current Concept on "Medullary Hyperplasia"?

Adrenal medullary proliferation with the size <1 cm is historically defined as adrenal medullary hyperplasia (AMH) while a medullary proliferative lesion >1 cm is considered a

An adrenal cortical tumor with ≥4 criteria is considered malignant, while a tumor with ≤2 criteria is considered

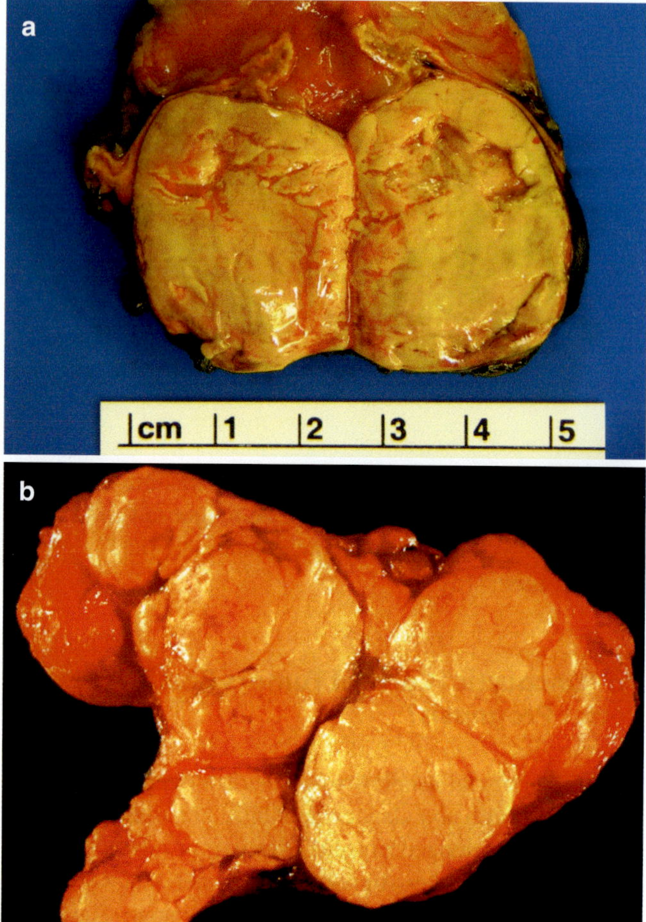

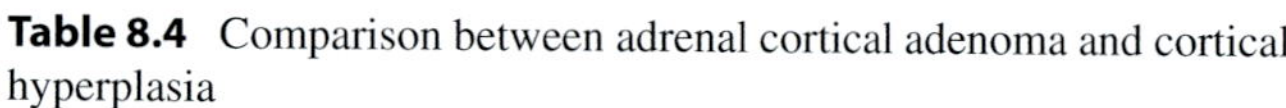

Fig. 8.3 A bisected adrenal specimen contains a 3 cm cortical adenoma which is a well-demarcated solitary mass with bright yellow cut surface (**a**). Note the nonlesional cortex is atrophic. Primary adrenal cortical hyperplasia shows several macronodules (**b**)

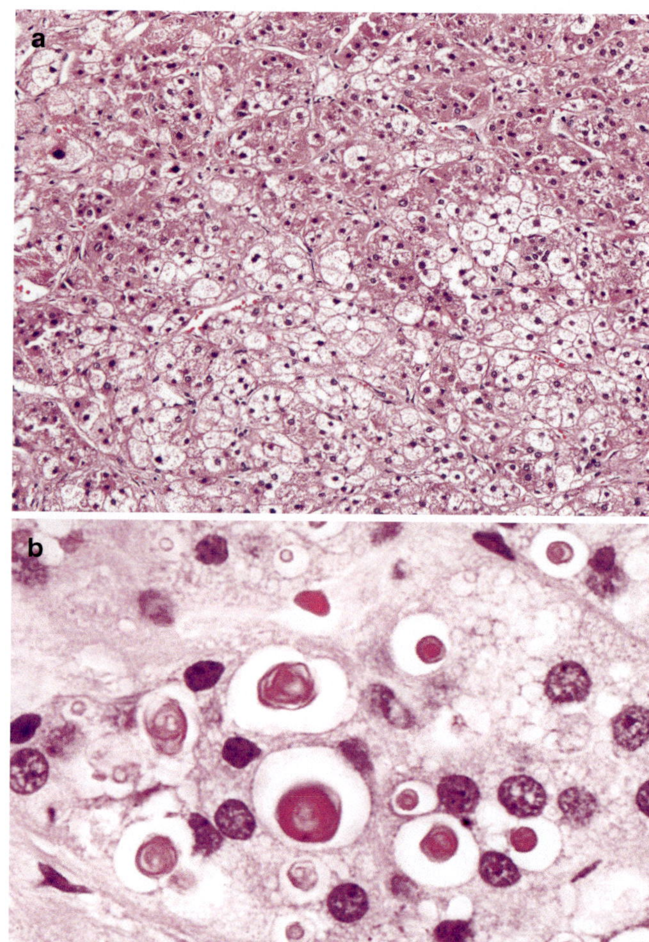

Fig. 8.4 An aldosteronoma contains mixed cells with vacuolated eosinophilic cytoplasm, large lipid-rich cells and oncocytic cells (**a**). Spironolactone bodies are small intracytoplasmic eosinophilic concentrically laminated inclusions (**b**)

Table 8.4 Comparison between adrenal cortical adenoma and cortical hyperplasia

	Adenoma	Hyperplasia with a dominant nodule
Imaging	Unilateral, unifocal	Bilateral
Intravenous sampling for hormone production	Elevated in the vein from the affected side	Elevated bilaterally
Pathology of the nonlesional cortex	Normal or atrophic	Diffuse hyperplastic

pheochromocytoma. Generally speaking, AMH produces milder symptoms, including headache, palpitation, sweating, flushing, and tremor, than pheochromocytoma. Clinically, patients with smaller adrenal lesions with mild symptoms may be followed without immediate surgery.

Macroscopically and histologically, AMH tends to present as diffuse thickening of medulla with or without forming

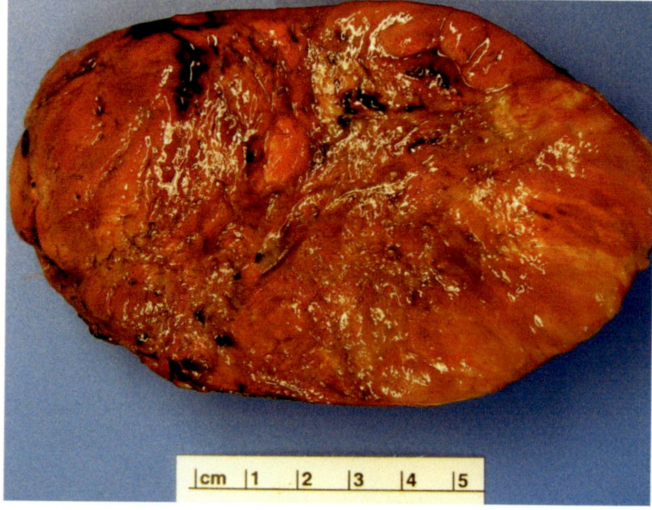

Fig. 8.5 Gross features of adrenal cortical carcinomas include large size, presence of hemorrhage, and necrosis

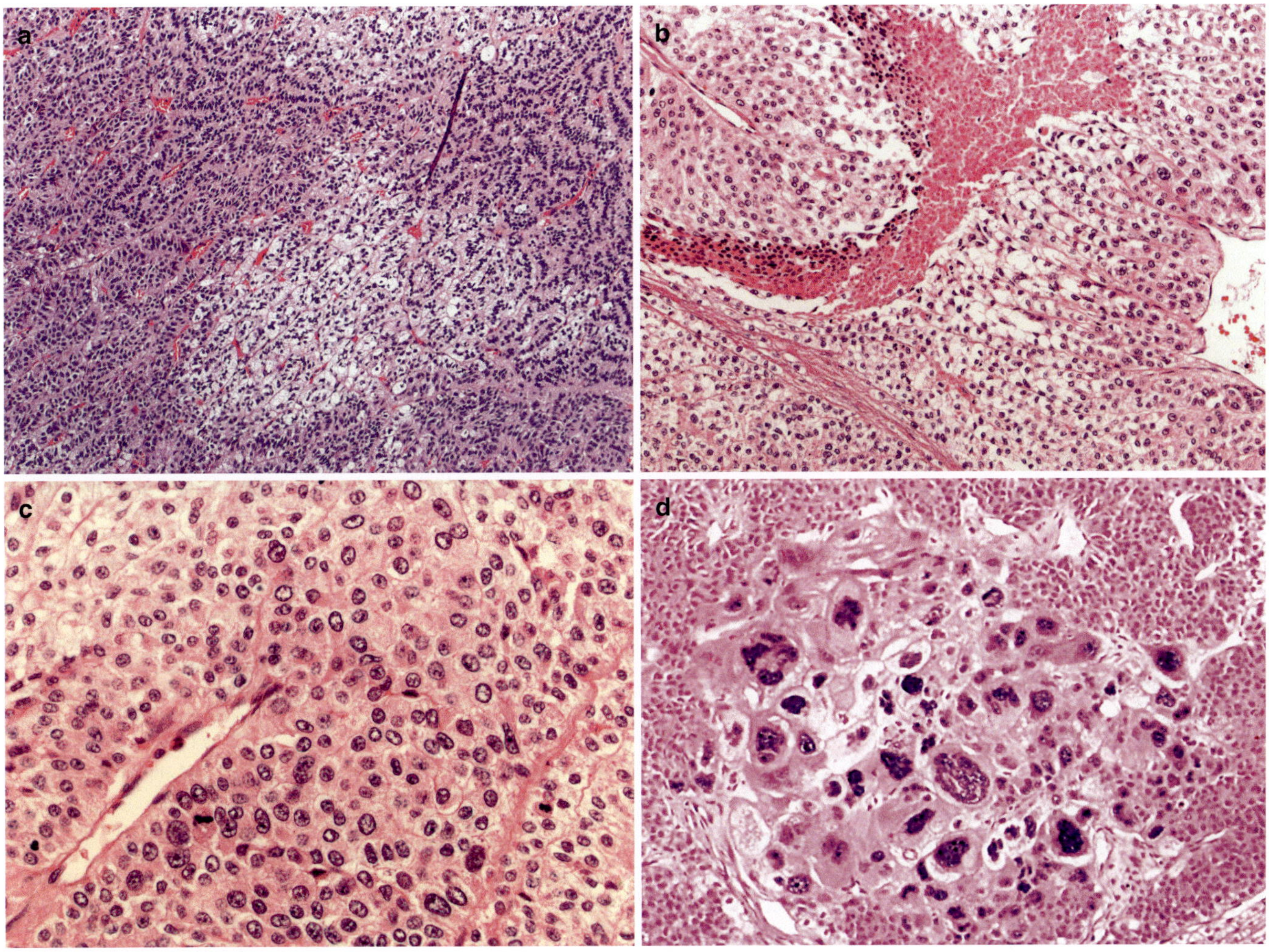

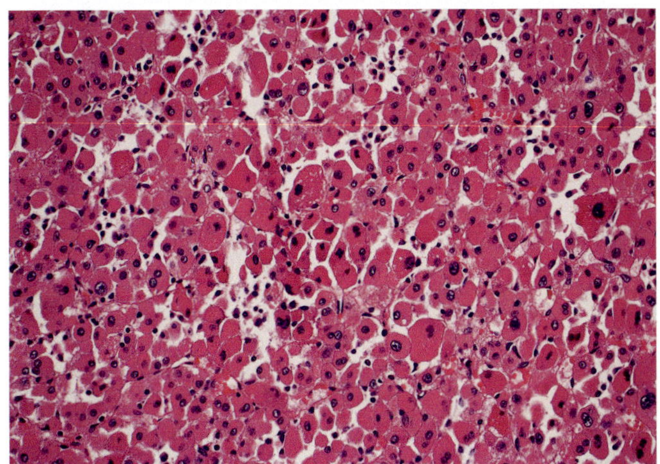

Fig. 8.6 Histological features commonly seen in adrenal cortical carcinomas include clear cells <25% of the tumor mass (**a**), necrosis (**b**), high mitotic rate (**c**), and high nuclear grade (**d**)

Fig. 8.7 An oncocytic adrenocortical tumor contains large epithelioid cells with abundant oncocytic cytoplasm and high-grade pleomorphic nuclei

a defined nodule. A pheochromocytoma is, however, a well-defined nodule without a capsule. AMH cannot be distinguished from a pheochromocytoma based on the morphology of individual cells, unless there are cytological atypia or increased mitoses or invasion.

These small lesions are usually seen in the setting of hereditary diseases, such as MEN2. They have been shown to be clonal and are therefore considered true pheochromocytomas. Some experts refer these lesions as "micropheochromocytomas."

When evaluating an adrenalectomy specimen from a symptomatic patient, the diagnosis of pheochromocytoma can be made when there is a defined nodular medullary proliferation, even when it is <1 cm. In adrenal specimens removed with radical nephrectomy for other disease without clinical features of pheochromocytoma, micropheochromocytoma can be diagnosed for a small defined medullary nodule

(<1 cm). Adrenal medullary hyperplasia can be diagnosed if there is diffuse thickening of the adrenal medulla.

References: [17, 18]

What Is the PASS Score? Can it Be Used to Predicate the Behavior of Pheochromocytoma?

All pheochromocytomas have some metastatic risk, although the only reliable feature of malignancy for pheochromocytoma is the presence of metastasis at sites such as bone, lung, liver, and lymph nodes. Risk of metastasis for a completely resected, organ-confined pheochromocytoma is very low, it is however not nil. Therefore, contemporary prognostication of pheochromocytomas is based on risk stratification models using clinical, laboratory, and pathological features. Various histological features are associated with risk of metastasis and have been factored into composite grading schemes. Phcochromocytoma of the adrenal gland scaled (PASS) score is the best-known risk stratification system. Various morphological features are assigned points, including the following:

- Vascular invasion, capsular invasion, profound nuclear pleomorphism: each 1 point.
- Invasion of periadrenal adipose tissue, large nest of diffuse growth (3–4 × Zellballen nests), presence of necrosis, high cellularity (greater amount of area accounted for by many cells with high N/C ratio), tumor cell spindling, cellular monotony, >3 mitotic figures per 10 HPF, atypical mitosis: each 2 points.
- Tumors with ≥4 points are considered malignant.

Several other systems, either completely different from, or partially based on, PASS, have also been developed. These systems require validation in large independent cohorts before they can be endorsed for routine clinical use.

The PASS criteria were created in >20 years ago. The average tumor size in the study was 7.2 cm. With contemporary imaging and lab tests, pheochromocytomas are typically 1–2 cm in size, and >95% of these patients are doing well without recurrence after complete resection.

In a large pheochromocytoma with suspicious histological features such as vascular invasion or necrosis, we recommend to provide PASS score.

References: [19, 20]

How to Distinguish Pheochromocytoma and Adrenocortical Tumors?

Such a distinction depends on clinical, radiological, laboratory, and pathological findings as listed in Table 8.5. The key histological features are presence of Zellballen (cell ball) and amphophilic cytoplasm, which are characteristics of pheochromocytoma, but not present in cortical tumors.

References: [13, 21, 22]

Table 8.5 Comparison of pheochromocytoma and adrenocortical tumors

	Pheochromocytoma	Adrenocortical tumor
Clinical	Classic triad: episodic headache, sweating, and tachycardia	Endocrine syndromes associated with over production of cortisol or aldosterone, such as hyperaldosteronism, Cushing syndrome, and virilization
Radiological	No lipid Extremely high signal intensity on MRI T2-weighted imaging	Contains lipid, although some tumors have limited amount of lipid Intermediate to high signal intensity on MRI T2-weighted imaging
Laboratory	Elevated urinary and plasma fractionated metanephrines and catecholamines	Elevated steroid hormones
Pathology: gross	Pink, fleshy, or red cut surface (Fig. 8.8)	Yellow cut surface similar to that of the adrenal cortex; cortical carcinoma usually fleshy or tan cut surface with hemorrhage and necrosis
Pathology: microscopic	Large tumor cells with amphophilic or purple cytoplasm, similar to medullary cells. Tumor cells organized in Zellballen pattern (well-defined epithelioid cell nests separated by thin fibrovascular septa) (Fig. 8.9a–c)	Diffuse and disorganized tumor cells with foamy cytoplasm due to high lipid content in cytoplasm. Cortical carcinoma may have eosinophilic cytoplasm and prominent cytological atypia
Pathology: IHC	Positive for neuroendocrine markers, negative for keratins, low in proliferative index. Presence of S100– positive sustentacular cells (Fig. 8.9d)	Positive for keratin, inhibin or melan A, negative for neuroendocrine markers, and Ki67 proliferative activities high in cortical carcinoma

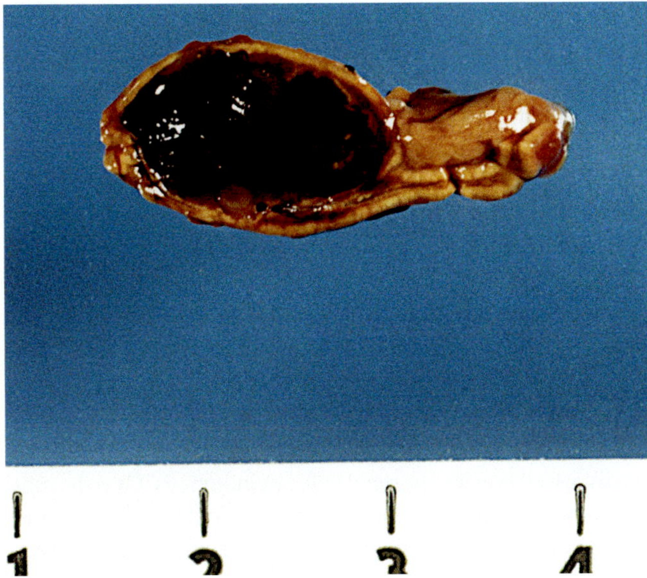

Fig. 8.8 Gross appearance of pheochromocytoma. The tumor is confined in the adrenal medulla with an intact overlying cortex

What Are the Common Metastatic Tumors to the Adrenal Gland in Surgical Pathology Practice and how to Work Them Up?

Adrenal metastases are the most common malignant lesions involving the adrenal gland and the second most common tumor of the adrenal gland after benign adenomas. In a study that comprised predominantly of autopsy cases, the most common metastatic carcinoma in the adrenal gland is the metastatic lung cancer (35%). In a cohort of the 222 adrenalectomy specimens (Yang X, unpublished data), 27 cases (12.2%) are metastatic carcinomas. The most common metastatic carcinoma was renal cell carcinoma (RCC), accounting for 44.4% of the metastatic carcinomas in the adrenal (12/27). Metastatic lung carcinoma is the second most common, accounting for 33.3% of metastatic carcinomas in the adrenal (9/27) (Fig. 8.10). The third most common one is metastatic hepatocellular carcinoma, accounting for 14.8% of metastatic carcinomas (4/27). Other malignant tumors can also metastasize to the adrenal (Fig. 8.11).

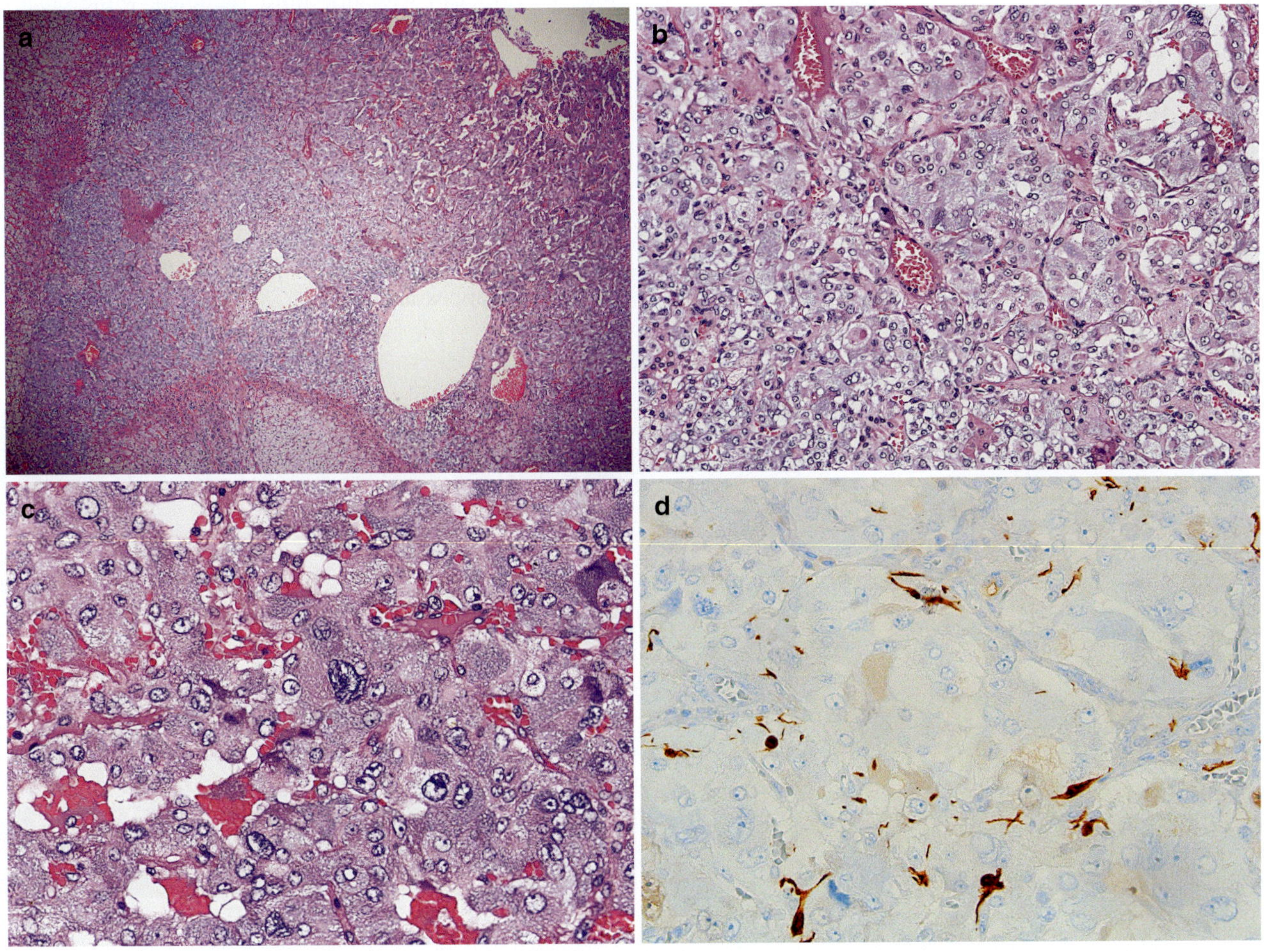

Fig. 8.9 Histological features of pheochromocytoma. The tumor (**a**, upper right) abuts the medulla and cortex (**a**, low left). At high magnification, the tumor cells are morphologically similar to but significantly larger (**b**, arrows) than medullary cells (**b**, low left). Some tumor cells show nuclear atypia (**c**) which is not an indication of malignancy. S100 immunostaining shows the presence of sustentacular cells (**d**)

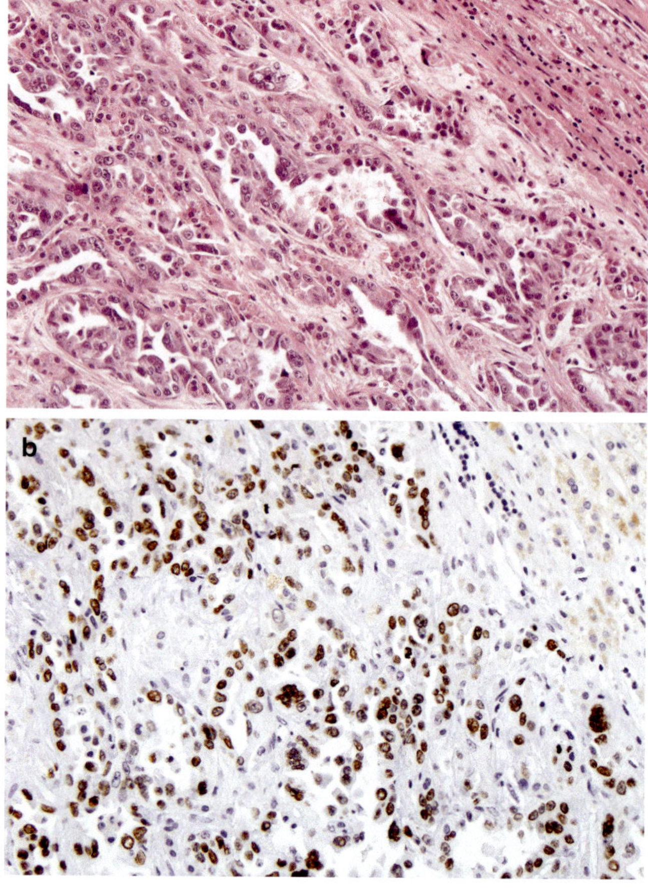

Fig. 8.10 Metastatic lung adenocarcinoma to the adrenal gland. Tumor cells with prominent cytological atypia form glandular structures (**a**) and are positive for TTF1 (**b**)

To work up a possible metastatic carcinoma to the adrenal gland, a panel of immunostains should be performed. The panel depends on patient's history, but should include adrenal cortical markers (calretinin, inhibin or melan A), pan-cytokeratins, and lineage-specific markers including lung markers such as TTF1, RCC markers such as PAX8, and HCC markers such as Hep Par 1.

Reference: [23]

How to Distinguish Metastatic Renal Cell Carcinoma from Primary Adrenal Cortical Tumors?

As discussed previously, renal cell carcinoma (RCC) is the most common metastatic carcinoma to the adrenal gland. The tumor cells of clear cell RCC contain high lipid content, and may be difficult to distinguish from cortical adenoma or carcinoma, particularly on frozen sections or small biopsy specimens.

However, careful morphological examination can yield some clues. Cytologically, adrenocortical cells contain foamy cytoplasm with fine lipid vacuoles, while clear cell RCC contain "optically clear" or "water clear" cytoplasm due to loss of cytoplasmic lipid and glycogen content during tissue processing (Fig. 8.12a).

Metastatic RCC usually displays nuclear atypia including irregular nuclear membrane and prominent nucleoli. Cortical adenomas exhibit round nuclei with smooth nuclear membrane and lack of nuclear atypia (Fig. 8.12b). Cortical carcinoma can be difficult to distinguish from RCC based on histological appearance.

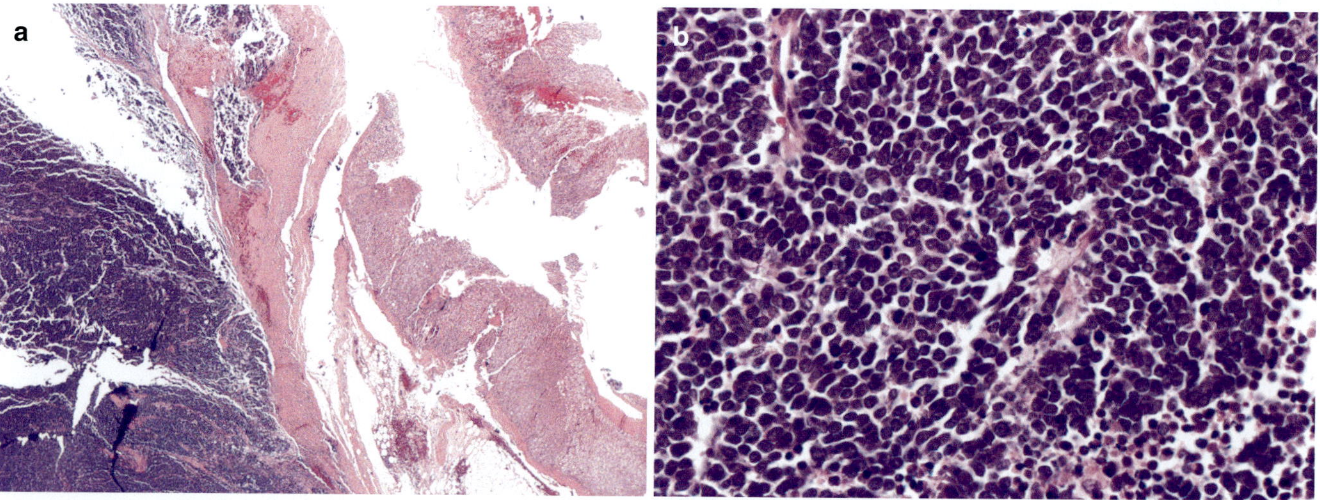

Fig. 8.11 A metastatic Merkel cell carcinoma to the adrenal gland (**a**). The tumor is a typical small round cell tumor (**b**)

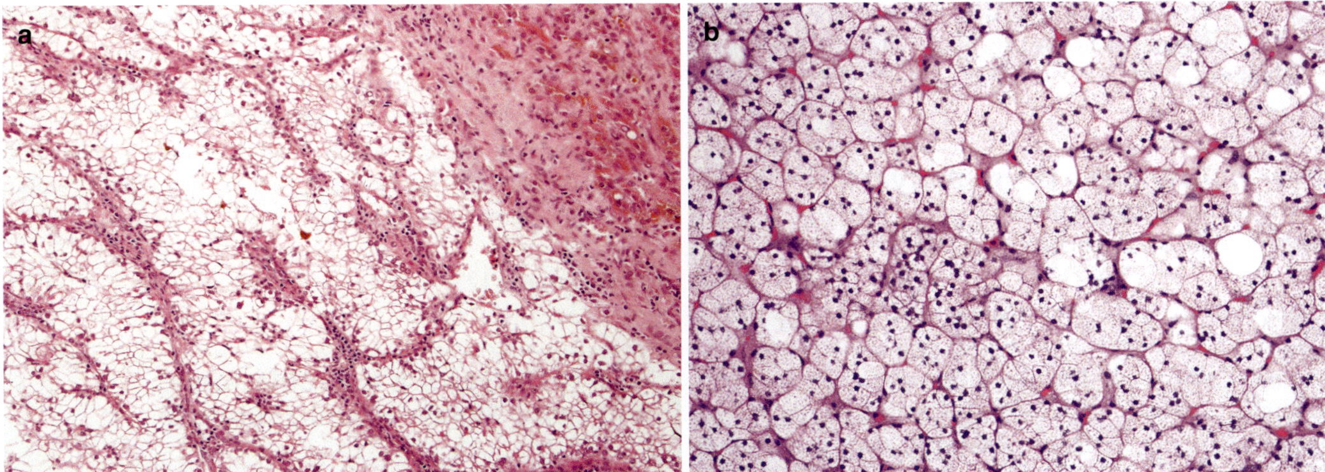

Fig. 8.12 A metastatic clear cell RCC in the adrenal gland displays "chicken-wire" vasculature, optical clear cytoplasm and irregular nuclei (**a**), while cortical adenoma cells contain foamy cytoplasm and round uniform nuclei (**b**)

In difficult cases, IHC can be very helpful. Metastatic RCC is positive for PAX8 and negative for adrenocortical markers (calretinin, inhibin, and melan A). Clear cell RCC is additionally positive for CA9 and papillary RCC is positive for AMACR. Cortical neoplasms are positive for cortical markers and negative for PAX 8 and RCC markers.

Reference: [24]

How to Distinguish Adrenocortical Tissue from Clear Cell RCC in Needle Biopsy?

Occasionally, adrenal tissue may be captured in a needle core biopsy intended for a renal mass, especially when the tumor is located in the upper pole of the kidney. Additionally, ectopic adrenal cortical tissue may be found within the renal parenchyma or in the perinephric fat that may be sampled by needle biopsy.

Architecturally, adrenal cortical tissue is arranged in three zones, namely, zona glomerulosa, zona fasciculata, and zona reticularis. However, adrenal cortical tissue sampled in needle biopsy may not have all three zones. Cortical cells are arranged in a nested pattern with delicate vascular septa (Fig. 8.13a), similar to clear cell RCC with characteristic rich "chicken-wire" vasculature. Cytologically, however, adrenal cortical cells contain foamy cytoplasm with fine lipid vacuoles, while clear cell RCC contains "optically clear" or "water clear" cytoplasm due to loss of cytoplasmic lipid and glycogen content during tissue processing (Fig. 8.13b).

Nuclei in benign adrenal cortex exhibit fine salt-and-pepper chromatin. RCC cells, even of low nuclear grades, still display cytological atypia.

Immunohistochemically, adrenal cortical tissue is positive for adrenal cortical markers (calretinin, melan A, and

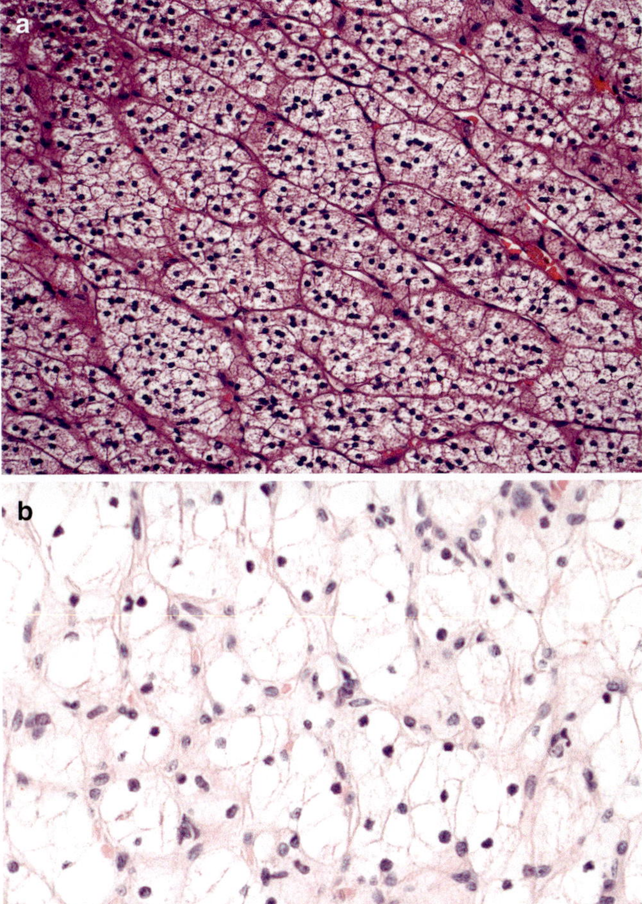

Fig. 8.13 Adrenal cortical cells are arranged in a nested pattern with delicate vascular septa and contain foamy cytoplasm with fine lipid vacuoles (**a**). Clear cell RCC has similar architectural pattern with characteristic rich "chicken-wire" vasculature. Cytologically, clear cell RCC contains "optically clear" or "water clear" cytoplasm (**b**)

inhibin) and negative for PAX8, while clear cell RCC is negative for adrenocortical markers and positive for PAX8.

Reference: [24]

How to Distinguish Neuroblastoma, Ganglioneuroblastoma, and Ganglioneuroma?

Neuroblastoma (NB) may display various degrees of ganglionic differentiation with synchronous nuclear and cytoplasmic maturation. Nuclear differentiation manifests as enlarged, eccentric nucleus with vesicular chromatin and single prominent nucleolus, while cytoplasmic differentiation manifests as abundant, eosinophilic, and amphophilic cytoplasm. However, no mature ganglion cells are present in neuroblastoma. At the end of this differentiation spectrum is ganglioneuroma, a benign tumor that represents the fully differentiated form of neural crest tumors. Ganglioneuroblastoma (GNB) shows a degree of differentiation intermediate between neuroblastoma and ganglioneuroma, composed of mixture of immature neuroblasts and mature ganglion cells. A ganglioneuroma is a benign tumor that is composed of mature ganglion cells and mature spindle neuronal cells without primitive neuroblasts or dysplastic ganglion cells. Differences between NB and GNB are summarized in Table 8.6 and Fig. 8.14.

Neuroblastoma can be divided into three subtypes:

- Undifferentiated: Tumor cells are small to medium with small amount of cytoplasm, no background neuropil.
- Poorly differentiated: <5% of tumor cells are differentiating neuroblasts with neuropil present in the background.
- Differentiating: ≥5% of tumor cells are differentiating neuroblasts with abundant background neuropil.

Ganglioneuroblastoma can be divided into two subtypes:

- Nodular: Typical ganglioneuroma with at least one well-circumscribed nodule of neuroblastoma.
- Intermixed: Predominantly mature ganglion cells with more than one microscopic foci of neuroblasts within ganglioneuromatous stroma.

Reference: [25]

How to Distinguish Neuroblastoma and Ewing Sarcoma Family Tumors?

Both neuroblastoma and Ewing sarcoma family tumors are composed of small round blue cells. Morphologically, they can be difficult to distinguish from each other as they share several pathological features such as rosettes and primitive histology. Table 8.7 summarizes the key clinical, pathological, and molecular features that distinguish between the two entities.

References: [25, 26]

What Are the Common Mistakes in Adrenal Specimen Handling?

Adrenal specimens are uncommon in daily pathology practice. The following tips ensure optimal handling and evaluation by pathologists unfamiliar with the adrenal pathology.

- Evaluation of surgical margins: Do not strip off the periadrenal fat in a specimen with mass lesions. Removal of the periadrenal adipose may allow an accurate measurement of adrenal weight, which is appropriate for adreno-

Table 8.6 Comparison of neuroblastoma, ganglioneuroblastoma, and ganglioneuroma

	Neuroblastoma	Ganglioneuroblastoma	Ganglioneuroma
Age	1st year of life	2–4 years of age	Children or adults
Histology	Primitive small neuroblasts with varying degree of differentiation Mature ganglion cells absent	Mixture of immature neuroblasts and dysplastic ganglion cells	Mature ganglion cells and spindle neuronal cells
Behavior	Malignant	Malignant Better prognosis than neuroblastoma	Benign

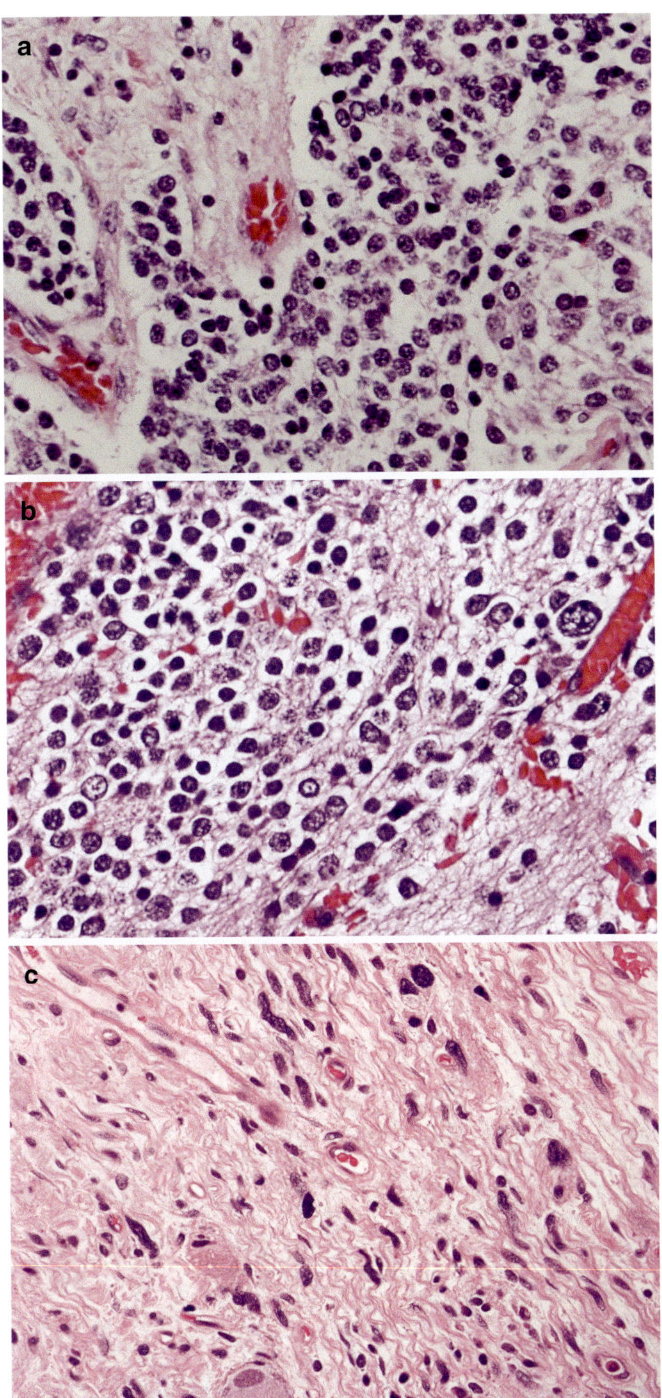

Fig. 8.14 Neuroblastic tumors. Microscopically, a neuroblastoma is characterized by primitive neuroblasts (blue cells) with scant cytoplasm in the background of neuropils (**a**). A ganglioneuroblastoma is composed of primitive neoplastic neuroblasts with scan cytoplasm and larger neoplastic cells with abundant cytoplasm resembling ganglion cells (**b**). Ganglioneuroma is composed of mature large ganglion cells and spindle neuronal cells (**c**)

cortical hyperplasia. However, it is discouraged for adrenal mass lesions as it will make evaluating surgical margins, particularly in a case of malignancy, difficult.

- Accurately measure the size of the lesion: Three-dimensional measurements are preferred, although one-dimensional measurement is acceptable for a small lesion.
- Take a close-up photo after the specimen is bisected or serially sectioned. A photo of the exterior of the specimen before it is sectioned is of limited use.
- Normally, adrenocortical tissue can be found outside the adrenal capsule in the periadrenal fat. Usually, the cortical cells form well-defined large clusters without any cytological atypia (Fig. 8.15a). Therefore, they should not be misinterpreted as extra-adrenal extension of an adrenal cortical carcinoma which displays invasive irregular nests with cytological atypia (Fig. 8.15b).

Reference: [13]

Does Morphology Correlates with the Molecular Genetics of Pheochromocytomas?

Pheochromocytomas are hereditary in at least 30–40% cases. Germline mutations in the autosomal genes, including succinate dehydrogenase (*SDH*) A-D and SDH complex assembly factor 2 (*SDHAF2*), are the most common causes of hereditary pheochromocytomas and account for up to 50% of germline mutations in these tumors.

The next most common germline mutations involve *VHL* gene in von Hippel–Lindau disease (VHLD), *RET* in multiple endocrine neoplasia type 2 (MEN2), and *NF1* in neurofibromatosis type 1. Germline mutations are rarely found in other genes *EPAS1*, *TMEM127*, *MAX*, *KIF1Bb*, *PHD2*, *FH*, *MDH2*, and *MEN1*.

Morphology may potentially suggest mutations in specific genes. Small tumor cells, presence of a myxoid stroma, and a vascularized pseudocapsule are suggestive of VHLD. Medullary hyperplasia with multiple tumor nodules is more likely seen in MEN2 (Fig. 8.16). Pheochromocytomas with *SDH* mutations often have rounded epithelioid cells sometimes with clear cytoplasm forming tightly nested balls surrounded by a well-developed capillary vasculature.

References: [18, 27, 28]

Table 8.7 Comparison of neuroblastoma and Ewing sarcoma

	Neuroblastoma	Ewing sarcoma
Age	Usually <5 years	Adolescent/young adults
Location	Adrenal most common, extra-adrenal abdomen, thorax	Skeletal system (long bones preferentially) Extraskeletal (any site)
Morphology	Small round blue cells with various degree of ganglionic differentiation Homer–Wright rosettes: cells arranged around central fibrillary cores	Uniform small round cells with round nuclei, fine chromatin and indistinct cytoplasmic membrane Homer–Wright rosettes
Immunohistochemistry	Chromogranin+ NSE+ Neurofilament protein+ GFAP+ CD99-	CD99+ Flt1+ ERG+ Focal CK+ in up to 1/3 cases Vimentin+
Molecular	MYCN amplification in ~ 1/4 cases ALK amplification, ATRK mutations	t(11;22)(q24;q12) EWS-FLI1 gene fusion in 85% cases EWSR1 fused with other ETS family members (e.g., ERG, ETV)

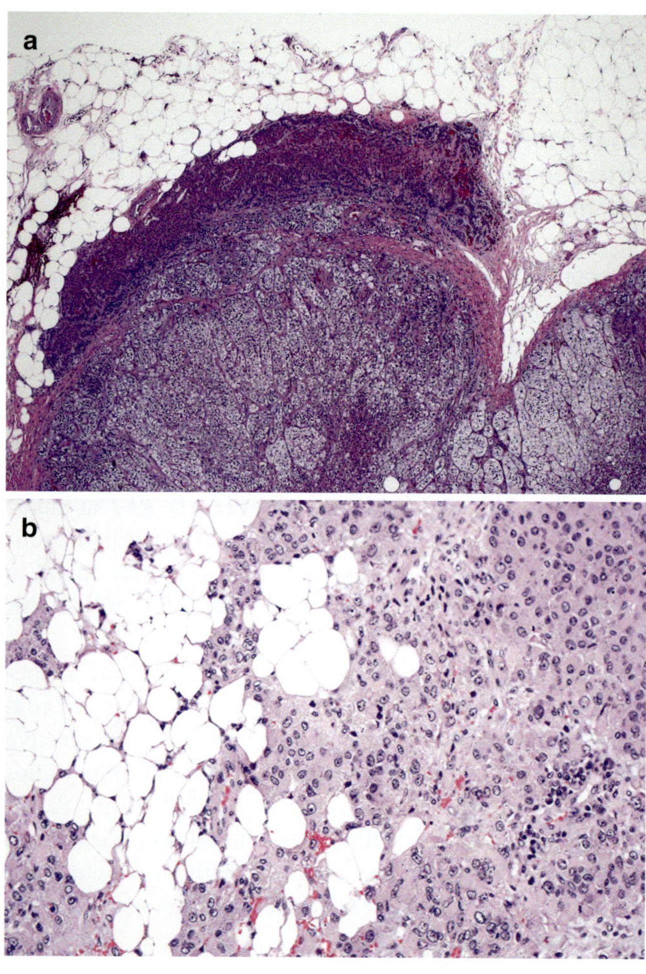

Fig. 8.15 A well-defined cluster of benign adrenocortical tissue is found in the periadrenal fat (**a**), while irregular tumor cell nests of adrenal corticocarcinoma invade the adipose tissue (**b**)

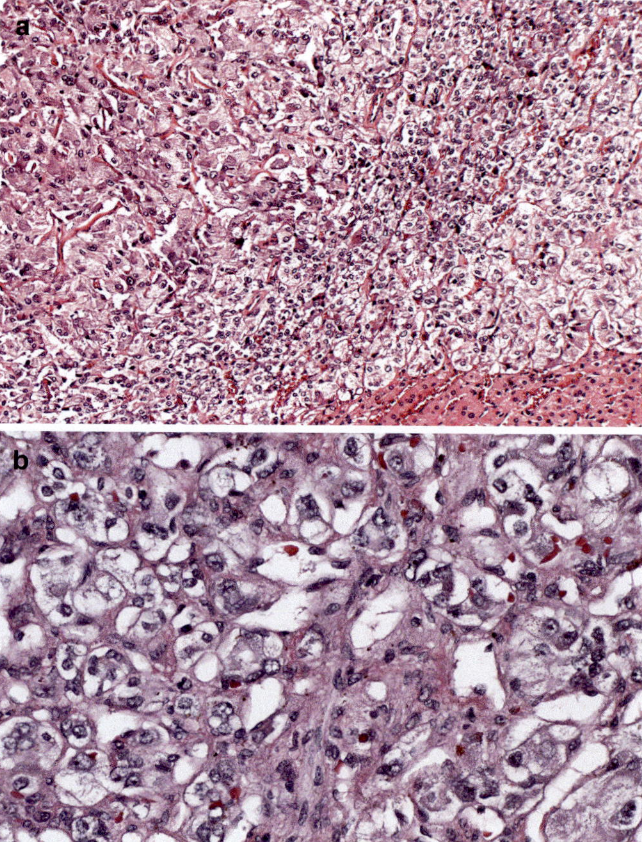

Fig. 8.16 An adrenal gland from an MEN2A patient shows multiple pheochromocytomas and confluent areas of different appearance. Adrenal cortex is at lower right (**a**). A pheochromocytoma in VHL disease is composed of small cells and small cell nests with prominent interspersed capillaries. The cytoplasm may have a myxoid or vacuolated appearance (**b**). (Photo courtesy of Dr. Art Tischler, Boston, MA)

References

1. Audenet F, Méjean A, Chartier-Kastler E, Rouprêt M. Adrenal tumours are more predominant in females regardless of their histological subtype: a review. World J Urol. 2013;31(5):1037–43. Epub 2013/01/09. https://doi.org/10.1007/s00345-012-1011-1. PubMed PMID: 23299088.

2. Bancos I, Arlt W. Diagnosis of a malignant adrenal mass: the role of urinary steroid metabolite profiling. Curr Opin Endocrinol Diabetes Obes. 2017;24(3):200–7. https://doi.org/10.1097/MED.0000000000000333. PubMed PMID: 28234802.

3. Elsayes KM, Emad-Eldin S, Morani AC, Jensen CT. Practical approach to adrenal imaging. Urol Clin North Am. 2018;45(3):365–87. https://doi.org/10.1016/j.ucl.2018.03.005. PubMed PMID: 30031460.

4. Lattin GE, Sturgill ED, Tujo CA, Marko J, Sanchez-Maldonado KW, Craig WD, et al. From the radiologic pathology archives: adrenal tumors and tumor-like conditions in the adult: radiologic-pathologic correlation. Radiographics. 2014;34(3):805–29. https://doi.org/10.1148/rg.343130127. PubMed PMID: 24819798.

5. Higgins SE, Barletta JA. Applications of immunohistochemistry to endocrine pathology. Adv Anat Pathol. 2018;25(6):413–29. https://doi.org/10.1097/PAP.0000000000000209. PubMed PMID: 30157042.

6. Mete O, Asa SL, Giordano TJ, Papotti M, Sasano H, Volante M. Immunohistochemical biomarkers of adrenal cortical neoplasms. Endocr Pathol. 2018;29(2):137–49. https://doi.org/10.1007/s12022-018-9525-8. PubMed PMID: 29542002.

7. Sebastiano C, Zhao X, Deng FM, Das K. Cystic lesions of the adrenal gland: our experience over the last 20 years. Hum Pathol. 2013;44(9):1797–803. Epub 2013/04/22. https://doi.org/10.1016/j.humpath.2013.02.002. PubMed PMID: 23618356.

8. Carsote M, Ghemigian A, Terzea D, Gheorghisan-Galateanu AA, Valea A. Cystic adrenal lesions: focus on pediatric population (a review). Clujul Med. 2017;90(1):5–12. Epub 2017/01/15. https://doi.org/10.15386/cjmed-677. PubMed PMID: 28246490; PubMed Central PMCID: PMCPMC5305088.

9. Koperski Ł, Pihowicz P, Szczepankiewicz B, Fus Ł, Cyran A, Bogdańska M, et al. Clinicopathological and immunohistochemical analysis of epithelial-lined (true) cysts of the adrenal gland with proposal of a new histogenetic categorization. Pathol Res Pract. 2017;213(9):1089–96. Epub 2017/07/21. https://doi.org/10.1016/j.prp.2017.07.022. PubMed PMID: 28781196.

10. Kanagarajah P, Ayyathurai R, Saleem U, Manoharan M. Small cell carcinoma arising from the bulbar urethra: a case report and literature review. Urol Int. 2012;88(4):477–9. Epub 2011/10/25. https://doi.org/10.1159/000332154. PubMed PMID: 22041867.

11. Chen G, Yao J, Mou L, Fang X, Huang H, Liang J, et al. Clinical analysis of 249 cases of adrenal tumors in a Chinese hospital. Urol Int. 2010;85(3):270–5. Epub 2010/07/07. https://doi.org/10.1159/000314959. PubMed PMID: 20606391.

12. Thomas AZ, Blute ML, Seitz C, Habra MA, Karam JA. Management of the Incidental Adrenal Mass. Eur Urol Focus. 2016;1(3):223–30. Epub 2016/02/03. https://doi.org/10.1016/j.euf.2015.12.006. PubMed PMID: 28723391.

13. Hodgson A, Pakbaz S, Mete O. A diagnostic approach to adrenocortical tumors. Surg Pathol Clin. 2019;12(4):967–95. Epub 2019/09/27. https://doi.org/10.1016/j.path.2019.08.005. PubMed PMID: 31672302.

14. Erickson LA. Challenges in surgical pathology of adrenocortical tumours. Histopathology. 2018;72(1):82–96. https://doi.org/10.1111/his.13255. PubMed PMID: 29239032.

15. Weiss LM, Medeiros LJ, Vickery AL. Pathologic features of prognostic significance in adrenocortical carcinoma. Am J Surg Pathol. 1989;13(3):202–6. https://doi.org/10.1097/00000478-198903000-00004. PubMed PMID: 2919718.

16. Bisceglia M, Ludovico O, Di Mattia A, Ben-Dor D, Sandbank J, Pasquinelli G, et al. Adrenocortical oncocytic tumors: report of 10 cases and review of the literature. Int J Surg Pathol. 2004;12(3):231–43. https://doi.org/10.1177/106689690401200304. PubMed PMID: 15306935.

17. Turchini J, Cheung VKY, Tischler AS, De Krijger RR, Gill AJ. Pathology and genetics of phaeochromocytoma and paraganglioma. Histopathology. 2018;72(1):97–105. https://doi.org/10.1111/his.13402. PubMed PMID: 29239044.

18. Kloeppel GLR, Osamura R, Rosai J, editors. Pathology and genetics of endocrine organs. 4th ed. Lyon: IACR Press; 2017.

19. Thompson LD. Pheochromocytoma of the Adrenal gland Scaled Score (PASS) to separate benign from malignant neoplasms: a clinicopathologic and immunophenotypic study of 100 cases. Am J Surg Pathol. 2002;26(5):551–66. https://doi.org/10.1097/00000478-200205000-00002. PubMed PMID: 11979086.

20. Kimura N, Takayanagi R, Takizawa N, Itagaki E, Katabami T, Kakoi N, et al. Pathological grading for predicting metastasis in phaeochromocytoma and paraganglioma. Endocr Relat Cancer. 2014;21(3):405–14. Epub 2014/05/06. https://doi.org/10.1530/ERC-13-0494. PubMed PMID: 24521857.

21. Sbardella E, Grossman AB. Pheochromocytoma: an approach to diagnosis. Best Pract Res Clin Endocrinol Metab. 2019:101346. Epub 2019/10/22. https://doi.org/10.1016/j.beem.2019.101346. PubMed PMID: 31708376.

22. Mihai R. Diagnosis, treatment and outcome of adrenocortical cancer. Br J Surg. 2015;102(4):291–306. https://doi.org/10.1002/bjs.9743. PubMed PMID: 25689291.

23. Lam KY, Lo CY. Metastatic tumours of the adrenal glands: a 30-year experience in a teaching hospital. Clin Endocrinol. 2002;56(1):95–101. https://doi.org/10.1046/j.0300-0664.2001.01435.x. PubMed PMID: 11849252.

24. Lapinski JE, Chen L, Zhou M. Distinguishing clear cell renal cell carcinoma, retroperitoneal paraganglioma, and adrenal cortical lesions on limited biopsy material: utility of immunohistochemical markers. Appl Immunohistochem Mol Morphol. 2010;18(5):414–21. https://doi.org/10.1097/PAI.0b013e3181ddf7b9. PubMed PMID: 20861762.

25. Shimada H, Umehara S, Monobe Y, Hachitanda Y, Nakagawa A, Goto S, et al. International neuroblastoma pathology classification for prognostic evaluation of patients with peripheral neuroblastic tumors: a report from the Children's Cancer Group. Cancer. 2001;92(9):2451–61. https://doi.org/10.1002/1097-0142(20011101)92:9<2451::aid-cncr1595>3.0.co;2-s. PubMed PMID: 11745303.

26. Sbaraglia M, Righi A, Gambarotti M, Dei Tos AP. Ewing sarcoma and Ewing-like tumors. Virchows Arch. 2020;476(1):109–19. Epub 2019/12/04. https://doi.org/10.1007/s00428-019-02720-8. PubMed PMID: 31802230.

27. Toledo SP, Lourenço DM, Sekiya T, Lucon AM, Baena ME, Castro CC, et al. Penetrance and clinical features of pheochromocytoma in a six-generation family carrying a germline TMEM127 mutation. J Clin Endocrinol Metab. 2015;100(2):E308–18. Epub 2014/11/12. https://doi.org/10.1210/jc.2014-2473. PubMed PMID: 25389632.

28. Gill AJ. Succinate dehydrogenase (SDH)-deficient neoplasia. Histopathology. 2018;72(1):106–16. https://doi.org/10.1111/his.13277. PubMed PMID: 29239034.

Index

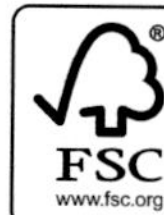